OCULAR PATHOLOGY

A TEXT AND ATLAS

MYRON YANOFF, M.D., F.A.C.S.

**Clinical Professor of Ophthalmology and Pathology,
School of Medicine, University of Pennsylvania;
Chief, Section of Ophthalmic Pathology,
Department of Ophthalmology,
Hospital of the University of Pennsylvania and Scheie Eye Institute,
Philadelphia, Pennsylvania**

BEN S. FINE, M.D.

**Research Associate, Ophthalmic Pathology Division,
Armed Forces Institute of Pathology;
Associate Research Professor of Ophthalmology,
The George Washington University;
Senior Attending Ophthalmologist,
The Washington Hospital Center,
Washington, D.C.**

OCULAR PATHOLOGY

A TEXT AND ATLAS

WITH 25 FULL COLOR ILLUSTRATIONS

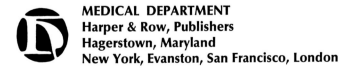

MEDICAL DEPARTMENT
Harper & Row, Publishers
Hagerstown, Maryland
New York, Evanston, San Francisco, London

Library of Congress Cataloging in Publication Data

Yanoff, Myron.
  Ocular pathology.

  Bibliography.
  Includes index.
  1. Eye—Diseases and defects—Outlines, syllabi, etc.
2. Eye—Wounds and injuries—Outlines, syllabi, etc.
I. Fine, Ben S., joint author. II. Title.
RE50.Y36   617.7′1′0202   75–5568
ISBN 0–06–142779–9

to our wives and children

contents

forewords

During this year of the observance of the 100th anniversary (1874–1974) of the University of Pennsylvania's Department of Ophthalmology, it is exciting to have the publication of a volume whose coauthors have contributed significantly to the strides in ocular pathology taken by the Department in the past several years.

Myron Yanoff, a highly regarded member of our staff, began a residency in ophthalmology in 1962, upon graduating from the University's School of Medicine. The residency continued for the next five years, during the first two of which he also held a residency in the Department of Pathology. His keen interest and ability in ocular pathology were readily apparent, and I encouraged him to apply for a fellowship at the Armed Forces Institute of Pathology (AFIP), Washington, D.C. From July 1964 through June, 1965, he carried out exceptional research at the AFIP in both ophthalmology and pathology. He returned to our Department in July, 1965, where the caliber both of his clinical and research work was of the highest. When he completed his residency in June, 1967, I invited him to join the staff, and he has recently attained the rank of full professor. During the ensuing years he has contributed substantially to the literature, particularly in the fields of ophthalmic and experimental pathology. He is Board certified in ophthalmology and in pathology.

Ben Fine, noted for his work in electron microscopy at AFIP and at George Washington University, has shared his expertise in the field through lectures presented as part of the curriculum of the annual 16-week Basic Science Course in the Department's graduate program.

It can be said that 100 years ago ophthalmology was a specialty that had been gradually evolving during the preceding 100 years, dating from the time of the invention of bifocals by Benjamin Franklin in 1785. Few American physicians of that era, however, knew how to treat diseases of the eye, but as medical education became more specialized it was inevitable that ophthalmology would also become a specialty.

With the invention of the ophthalmoscope in 1851, great advances were made in the teaching and practice of ophthalmology. This contributed greatly, of course, to setting the scene for the establishment of the University's Department of Ophthalmology. It was on February 3, 1874, that Dr. William F. Norris was elected First Clinical Professor of Diseases of the Eye. Similar chairs had been established earlier in only three other institutions. The chair at the University of Pennsylvania later became known as the William F. Norris and George E. de Schweinitz Chair of Ophthalmology.

Both Dr. Norris and Dr. de Schweinitz actively engaged in the study of ocular pathology. Dr. Norris stressed the importance of the examination of the eye by microscopy and of the correlation of findings from pathology specimens with the clinical signs. Dr. de Schweinitz was instrumental in having a member of his staff accepted as ophthalmic pathologist with the Department of Pathology.

In the years that followed under succeeding chairmen of the Department, other aspects of ophthalmology were stressed. Then, in 1947, during the chairmanship of Dr. Francis Heed Adler, Dr. Larry L. Calkins was appointed to a residency. Dr. Calkins, like Dr. Yanoff, displayed a keen interest in ocular pathology. Accordingly, he was instrumental in its study being revitalized during the three years of his residency. Another resident, Dr. William C. Frayer, who came to the Department in 1949, joined Dr. Calkins in his interest in ocular pathology. Dr. Frayer received additional training in the Department of Pathology and then became the ophthalmic pathologist of the department.

The importance of ocular pathology was increasingly evident, but facilities for carrying out the work in the Department of Ophthalmology were unfortunately limited. Until 1964, the pathology laboratory had been confined to a small room in the outpatient area of the Department. Then we were able to acquire larger quarters in the Pathology Building of the Philadelphia General Hospital located next door to the Hospital of the University of Pennsylvania. Although the building was earmarked for eventual demolition, the space was fairly adequate for research and also for conducting weekly ophthalmic pathology teaching conferences. Despite the physical aspects, we saw to it that Dr. Yanoff and his team of workers had a well equipped laboratory.

During the next several years as I saw that my dream for an eye institute with facilities for patient care, teaching and research under one roof was to become a reality, I was delighted to be able to include prime space on the research floor for the ever enlarging scope of ocular pathology. In addition to all that Dr. Yanoff has had to build upon from the past tradition of our Department of Ophthalmology, I would like to think that the new facilities at the Institute have in some measure contributed to the contents of this excellent volume. With grateful appreciation, therefore, I look upon this book as the authors' birthday present to the Department. From these same facilities, as Dr. Yanoff and Dr. Fine continue to collaborate, I can hope will come insights and answers for which all of us are ever searching in the battle against eye disease.

HAROLD G. SCHEIE, M.D.
Chairman, Department of Ophthalmology,
University of Pennsylvania;
Director, Scheie Eye Institute

October, 1974
Philadelphia, Pennsylvania

From their earliest days in ophthalmology Myron Yanoff and Ben Fine impressed me as exceptional students. As they have matured and progressed up the academic ladder, they have become equally dedicated and effective teachers. Their anatomical studies of normal and diseased tissues have always been oriented toward providing meaningful answers to practical as well as esoteric clinical questions. Their ability to draw upon their large personal experience in clinical ophthalmology, ocular pathology, and laboratory investigation for their lectures at the Armed Forces Institute of Pathology and at the University of Pennsylvania have contributed immeasurably to the success of those courses. Now they have used the same time-tested approach in assembling their material for this book. Beginning with their basic lecture outlines, then expanding these with just enough text to substitute for what would have been said verbally in lecture, adding a remarkable amount of illustrative material for the amount of spaced consumed, and then providing pertinent references to get the more ambitious student started in his pursuit of a subject, Drs. Yanoff and Fine have provided us with a sorely needed teaching aid for both the student and the teacher of ocular pathology. It should prove to be especially popular among medical students and residents in both ophthalmology and ocular pathology. With it one gets good orientation from the well-conceived outlines and fine clinicopathologic correlations from the selection of appropriate illustrations.

It is with considerable pride and admiration that I've watched the evolution of the authors' work and its fruition in the form of this latest book. I am proud that both authors launched their respective careers with periods of intensive study at the Armed Forces Institute of Pathology and that ever since, they have remained loyal, dedicated, and highly ethical colleagues. I admire their youthful energy, their patient, careful attitude, their friendly cooperative nature, and their ability to get important things accomplished. I'm appreciative of this opportunity to express my gratitude for the work they have been doing. If it is true that "by his pupils, a teacher will be judged," I could only wish to have had several dozen more like Drs. Yanoff and Fine.

LORENZ E. ZIMMERMAN, M.D.
Chief, Ophthalmic Pathology Division,
Armed Forces Institute of Pathology,
Washington, D.C.

April, 1975

preface

OCULAR PATHOLOGY is an outgrowth of a series of lectures presented at the annual postgraduate courses in ophthalmology at the Scheie Eye Institute in Philadelphia and at the Lancaster Course in Colby College, Maine, and at the biannual course in ophthalmic pathology at the Armed Forces Institute of Pathology, Washington, D.C.

The aim of the book is to present ocular pathology in a simplified, systematic manner useful both to the student and to the practitioner. To achieve this goal the text is presented in expanded outline form. In order to minimize repetition, the text is extensively cross referenced by page number, thus keeping the book as short as possible. A bibliography covering each section in the outline is included at the end of each chapter; although extensive and quite up to date, the bibliography is not intended to be exhaustive, but rather to guide the reader to further literature in particular areas.

The topics included in each chapter have been determined by two main considerations. First, some topics have been grouped into a traditional type of discussion of individual ocular tissues, e.g., cornea and sclera, retina, lens. Second, other topics have been grouped together according to disease entities, e.g., congenital anomalies, granulomatous inflammation, ocular melanotic tumors. Additionally, Chapter 1, Basic Principles of Pathology, reviews many of the underlying concepts in general pathology and immunopathology.

The topics are illustrated generously. To achieve meaningful clinicopathologic correlations, a clinical or macroscopic picture, or both, have been inserted into the photomicrograph whenever possible. Often, the clinical (and macroscopic) illustration is from the same case as the photomicrograph; however, good clinical examples illustrative of the problem but not from the same case also are used. In addition, where appropriate, electronmicrographs, both transmission and scanning, have been provided. In order to shorten the legends and to make them more readable, all credits have been placed in a separate appendix at the end of the book. By the use of multiple photographic insets and by deleting credits from the legends, considerably more illustrative material has been included than otherwise could have been shown. The color plates have been kept to a minimum and have been used mainly to illustrate techniques, such as positive iron staining with the Prussian blue reaction, which are difficult, if not impossible, to demonstrate adequately in black and white.

We wish to thank all who have helped in the preparation of this text. In particular, we wish to dedicate this book in part to the 100th Anniversary of the Department of Ophthalmology of the University of Pennsylvania and to its Chairman, Dr. Harold G. Scheie, and to Dr. Lorenz E. Zimmerman, our inspirational teacher and mentor, whose prodding and example have encouraged us continuously over the years and who directly and indirectly is responsible for most of what is in this book.

Our special thanks to Drs. Ralph C. Eagle, Jr., and David M. Kozart for their review of the entire manuscript and their encouragement and editorial comments; to Dr. B. Allen Flaxman for his review and thoughtful comments on the chapters on skin and ocular melanotic tumors; to Dr. William C. Frayer for his review and thoughtful comments on the chapters on nongranulomatous inflammation and on nonsurgical and surgical trauma and for his continuing encouragement; to Shelly D. Yanoff, Fruma I. Fine, and Drs. James A. Katowitz, Mark O. M. Tso, Ramon L. Font, and Jay L. Helfgott for their advice and encouragement; and to the many people listed in the Appendix who so kindly allowed us to use their material or illustrations. In addition, we are grateful to Mr. Martin Cohn and Mr. William C. Nyberg for their help in preparing the clinical, macroscopic, and microscopic pictures, and to Elisabeth W. McDonnell of the Armed Forces Institute of Pathology for her help with many of the line drawings.

We are especially grateful to Carol A. Brown for her expert typing of the manuscript. We are deeply saddened by the fact that this delightful, quixotic young woman's life and magic were snuffed out much too soon, making life a little less meaningful for all who knew her.

Finally, we extend our sincere appreciation to Nestor G. Menocal and Efrain Perez-Rosario whose loyalty and dedication in the histologic preparation and sectioning techniques have provided us with the material for our various publications and for this book.

M.Y.
B.S.F.

OCULAR PATHOLOGY

A TEXT AND ATLAS

chapter 1

Basic Principles of Pathology

INFLAMMATION

DEFINITION*

In its broadest sense the process of inflammation may be considered as the response of a tissue or tissues to a noxious stimulus. The tissue may be predominantly cellular (the retina), composed mainly of extracellular materials (the cornea), or a mixture of both (the uvea). The response may be localized or generalized, the noxious stimulus infectious or noninfectious. In a general way inflammation is an immune (nonspecific or specific) response to a foreign stimulus or agent.

CAUSES

I. Noninfectious
   A. Exogenous causes of noninfectious inflammation include physical injury (surgical or nonsurgical trauma; thermal and other forms of radiant energies), chemical injury (acid and alkali), and allergic reactions to external antigens (conjunctivitis secondary to ragweed pollen).
   B. Endogenous causes include necrosis of intraocular tumor (either on an ischemic or immune basis), a corneal ulcer causing a sterile hypopyon, allergic reactions to internal antigens (e.g., phacoanaphylactic endophthalmitis, i.e., cellular immunity to one's own

lens antigen), and such conditions of unknown cause as sarcoidosis and most cases of uveitis.
II. Infectious causes include viral, rickettsial, bacterial, fungal and parasitic agents.

PHASES OF INFLAMMATION

I. Acute (immediate or shock) phase
   A. The five cardinal signs of the acute phase (Fig. 1–1): 1) rubor or redness and 2) color or heat, both due to increased rate and volume of blood flow; 3) tumor or mass, due to exudation of fluid (edema) and cellular migration; and 4) dolor or pain and 5) functio laesa or loss of function, both due to outpouring of fluid and irritating chemicals such as histamine and serotonin. These signs are due to the local tissue and cellular phenomena that occur at the site of the noxious agent.
   B. The acute phase seems to be related to or initiated by histamine release from mast cells and maintained by kinins and other chemicals. Unless a continuous stimulus is present the phase is transient, lasting from 3 to 5 hours. Chemical mediators* cause smooth muscle contraction (arteriolar constriction) and local increase in vascular permeability.

   The chemical mediators seem to increase vascular permeability by causing the usually "tight" junctions between adjacent vessel endothelial cells (especially endothelia of venules) to open, allowing luminal fluid to leak into the surrounding

---

* Inflammation is *not* synonymous with infection. Inflammation may be caused by an infection, e.g., postoperative staphylococcal endophthalmitis, but it may also be caused by noninfectious agents, such as thermal burns (cautery to produce chorioretinal adhesions in retinal detachment surgery). Conversely, infection is not always accompanied by significant inflammation. For example, in certain diseases of the immune mechanism widespread infection may be present, but the individuals are incapable of mounting an inflammatory response.

* The chemical mediators include histamine, serotonin, kinins, plasmin, complement, prostaglandins and slow-reacting substance of anaphylaxis. All directly or indirectly can cause smooth muscle contraction and localized increased vascular permeability.

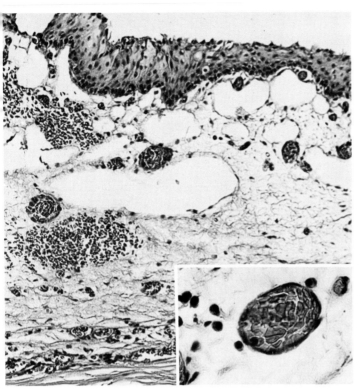

FIG. 1–1. Acute inflammation. Conjunctival blood vessels and lymphatics (clear spaces) are dilated. Subepithelial tissue is spread out by edema fluid and inflammatory cells. **Inset** shows dilated, engorged blood vessel surrounded by edematous tissue, which contains plasma cells and lymphocytes. **Main figure,** H&E, ×110; **inset,** H&E, ×300.

tissue spaces. Leukocytes can force themselves between the endothelial cells (active emigration of leukocytes). Erythrocytes, on the other hand, pass between endothelial cells passively by the process called diapedesis.

1. *Histamine* is found in the granules of mast cells where it is stored by electrostatic binding to a heparin–protein complex; it is also present in the polymorphonuclear leukocyte.
2. *Serotonin* (5-hydroxytryptamine) is found in the granules of mast cells and platelets. Although it is a vaso-active amine like histamine, its true role in inflammation is not known.
3. The *kinins* are peptides formed by the enzymatic action of kallikrein on the α-globulin plasma substrate kininogen. Kallikrein can be activated by the coagulation factor XII, the *Hageman factor,* or by plasmin.
4. *Plasmin,* the proteolytic enzyme responsible for fibrinolysis, has the capacity to liberate kinins from their precursors and probably to activate kallikrein. The formation of plasmin from plasminogen is

brought about by factor XII, the Hageman factor.

The Hageman factor then is quite important in the early stages of inflammation because of its relationship to kinins and plasmin. In addition, the Hageman factor activates plasmin, which in turn initiates the complement sequence, one of the functions of which is histamine release.

5. The complement system consists of at least nine discrete protein substances, eight of which are either α- or β-globulins and one of which is a γ-globulin. Complement achieves its effect via a cascade of at least the nine separate components working in a special sequence; the Hageman factor by activating plasmin can initiate the complement sequence.

The biologic functions of the complement components include histamine release, facilitation of phagocytosis of foreign protein, generation of anaphy-latoxin, which leads to vasodilatation, immune adherence or fixation of an organism to a cell surface, poly-morphonuclear leukocytic chemotaxis

3

and, finally, lysis of bacteria, red cells, etc. Complement, therefore, plays a key role in the inflammatory process.

6. Prostaglandins are 20-carbon cyclical unsaturated fatty acids with a 5-carbon ring and 2 aliphatic side chains. Although they can cause contraction of smooth muscle and vasodilatation, their exact role in inflammation is unknown.*

7. Slow-reacting substance of anaphylaxis (SRS-A), an acidic lipid substance, seems to be involved in inflammation related to immediate hypersensitivity. Its exact function is as yet unknown but seems to be related to IgE (see section Humoral Immunoglobulin below).

C. Immediately following an injury there is a brief (about 5 minutes) contraction of arterioles followed by a gradual relaxation and dilatation of the arterioles coincident with a general vasodilatation of all vessels due to the chemical mediators discussed above as well as to antidromic axon reflexes.

After the transient arteriolar constriction terminates, blood flow increases above the normal rate for a variable period of time up to a few hours, but then the flow diminishes to below normal (or even to cessation) even though the vessels are still dilated. Part of the decrease in flow is due to increased viscosity as a result of fluid loss through the capillary and venular wall. The release of heparin by mast cells during this period probably helps to prevent widespread coagulation in the hyperviscous intravascular blood.

During the early period following an injury the leukocytes (predominantly the polymorphonuclear leukocytes) start to stick to the vessel walls, at

first momentarily but then prolonged, an active process called *margination* (Fig. 1–2). The polymorphonuclear leukocytes (PMN) then actively move by an ameboid activity through the vessel wall via the endothelial cell junctions (generally takes 2 to 12 minutes), a process called *emigration.* Erythrocytes also escape into the surrounding tissue, pushed out of the blood vessels through similar but larger openings between the endothelial cells, a passive process called *diapedesis.*

D. *Chemotaxis* or a positive unidirectional response to a chemical stimulus by inflammatory cells may be initiated by lysosomal enzymes released by dead cells, peptide extracts from bacteria, the complement system and the kinins.

E. The *PMN* (Fig. 1–3) is the main inflammatory cell in the acute phase of inflammation.

1. The PMN is born in the bone marrow and is considered "the first line of cellular defense."

2. It is the most numerous of the circulating leukocytes, making up 50 to 70 percent of the total.

3. The PMN functions at an alkaline pH, is drawn to a particular area by chemotaxis, and removes noxious material as well as bacteria by phagocytosis and lysosomal digestion.

Lysosomes are saclike cytoplasmic structures that contain digestive enzymes and other active polypeptides. The term lysosome currently is used to include a group of disparate organelles divisible roughly into four principal varieties: *storage granules* or primary lysosomes, e.g., specific granules of PMNs (Figs. 1–3 and 1–5) and eosinophils are lysosomes that as yet have not participated in digestion but can be shown to contain two or more lytic enzymes within the granules; *digestive vacuoles* (secondary lysosomes or phagolysosomes) result when the membranes of storage granules merge with ingested, intravacuole particles (proteins, microorganisms or inert particles), i.e., the vacuoles or phagosomes merge with storage granules, receive

---

* Prostaglandins have a marked platelet aggregation inhibitory action; they inhibit catecholamine-induced lipolysis and have an insulinlike lipogenic effect, possibly affecting a nonspecific inhibition of the formation of cyclic AMP. They affect the iris musculature in response to mechanical stimulation and, perhaps, intraocular pressure. The action of aspirin and aspirinlike drugs may be due in part to an inhibition of prostaglandin synthesis.

FIG. 1–2. Margination. **A.** Polymorphonuclear leukocytes "stick" to walls of dilated blood vessels in acutely inflamed conjunctiva. **B.** Leukocytes are adherent to blood vessel wall. Leukocytes also have emigrated through endothelial cell junctions into edematous surrounding tissue. **A,** H&E, ×40; **B,** H&E, ×101.

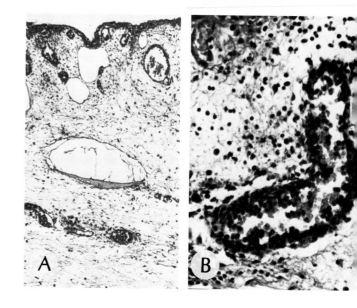

FIG. 1–3. Polymorphonuclear leukocyte (PMN). **Upper left** shows collection of PMNs in hypopyon (purulent exudate) secondary to corneal ulcer. *D*, Descemet's membrane. **Lower left** compares size of PMN (*arrows*) to plasma cell (*P*) and monocyte (*M*). **Right** electron micrograph shows segmented nucleus of typical PMN and its cytoplasmic spherical and oval granules (storage granules or primary lysosomes). **Upper left,** Brown & Brenn, ×250; **lower left,** H&E, ×1,000; **right,** ×15,600.

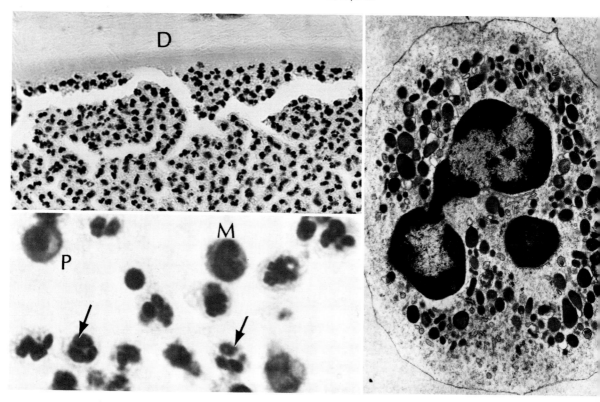

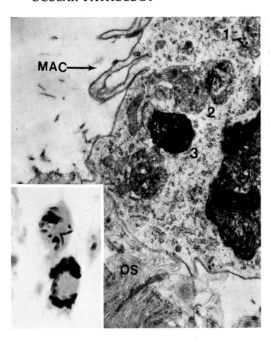

FIG. 1–4. Digestive vacuoles. Electron micrograph shows ingestion of necrotic photoreceptor outer segments (*OS*) within digestive vacuoles (sequence *1, 2, 3*) of adjacent macrophage (*MAC*). **Inset** shows 1.5 μ section of pigment-filled macrophages in subretinal space. **Main figure,** ×16,000; **inset,** PD, ×970.

lysosomal hydrolases and become digestive vacuoles (Fig. 1–4); *autophagic vacuoles* result from a cell sacrificing a portion of its own cytoplasm as a result of fasting, anoxia, focal necrosis or active catabolism; and *residual bodies* are the end result when lysosomes have carried out their digestive functions and appear filled with debris, generally lipid. Lysosomal dysfunction or lack of function has been associated with numerous heritable storage diseases: Pompe's disease (glycogen storage disease type II) has been traced to a lack of the enzyme α-1,4-glucosidase in liver lysosomes (see p. 443 in Chap 11); Gaucher's disease is due to a deficiency of the lysosomal enzyme β-D-galactosidase (see p. 445 [Table 2] in Chap. 11); metachromatic leukodystrophy is due to a deficiency of the lysosomal enzyme arylsulfatase A (see p. 445 [Table 2] in Chap. 11); most of the common lipid or polysaccharide storage diseases are due to a deficiency of a lysosomal enzyme specific for the disease (see under appropriate diseases in Chap. 11); and Chediak-Higashi syndrome may be considered a general disorder of organelle formation (see section Congenital Anomalies in Chap. 11) with abnormally large and fragile leukocyte lysosomes.

FIG. 1–5. Eosinophils are characterized by their bilobed nucleus and granular cytoplasm. **Inset** electron micrograph shows segmentation of nucleus and dense cytoplasmic "crystalloids" within many cytoplasmic storage granules. There appears to be degradation of some granules. **Main figure,** H&E, ×1,000; **inset,** ×6,000.

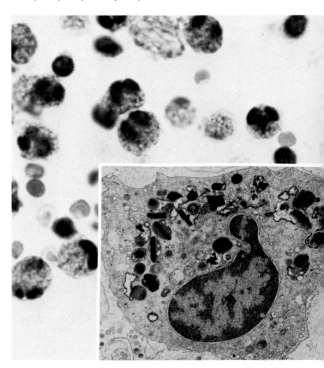

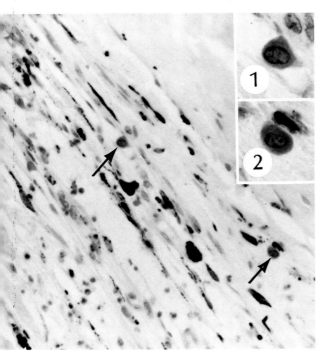

FIG. 1–6. Mast cells (*arrows*) are seen as the only cells in which cytoplasm stains with alcian blue stain for acid mucopolysaccharides. **Insets 1** and **2** show higher magnification of two mast cells. **Main figure,** alcian blue, ×252; **inset 1,** alcian blue, ×630; **inset 2,** alcian blue, ×630.

FIG. 1–7. Serous exudate present in choroid between long ciliary nerve (*double arrows*) and sclera (*S*). *Single arrow* shows retinal pigment epithelium. H&E, ×52.

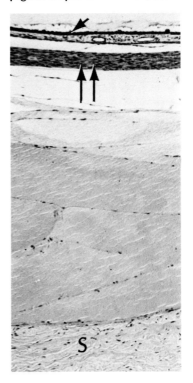

4. The PMN is an end cell; it lives for a few days and then dies. It liberates proteolytic enzymes on death, producing tissue necrosis.
F. Eosinophils and mast cells (basophils) may be involved in the acute phase of inflammation.
   1. Eosinophils (Fig. 1–5) originate in bone marrow, constitute 1 to 2 percent of circulating leukocytes, increase in number in parasitic infestations and allergic reactions and decrease in number following steroid administration or stress.
   2. Mast cells (basophils) (Fig. 1–6) elaborate heparin and histamine and are imperative for the initiation of the acute inflammatory reaction.

   Mast cells seem to be identical to basophils except for location; mast cells are fixed tissue cells, whereas basophils are circulating leukocytes constituting about 1 percent of circulating leukocytes. Basophils generally are recognized by the presence of a segmented nucleus, whereas the nucleus of a mast cell is large and nonsegmented.

G. The acute phase is an exudative* phase, i.e., an outpouring of cells and fluid from the circulation. The nature of the exudate often determines and characterizes an acute inflammatory reaction.
   1. Serous exudate (Fig. 1–7) is composed primarily of protein, e.g., as

* Exudation implies the passage of protein-containing fluid (and cells) through opened endothelial vascular junctions into the surrounding tissue (inflammatory exudate). Transudation implies the passage of fluid through an intact vessel wall into the surrounding tissue so that its protein content is low or nil (aqueous fluid).

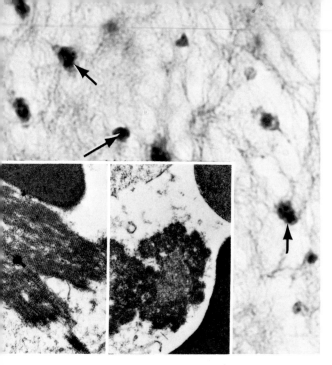

FIG. 1–8. Fibrinous exudate has a cobweb appearance in light micrograph. Cells (*arrows*) use fibrin as scaffold for moving and on which to lay down reparative materials. **Inset** shows electron micrograph of fibrin as cut in longitudinal section showing periodicity (left) and in cross-section (right). **Main figure,** PAS, ×680; **insets,** both ×25,600.

seen clinically in the aqueous "flare" within the anterior chamber.

2. Fibrinous exudate (Fig. 1–8) has a high content of fibrin, e.g., as seen clinically in a "plastic" aqueous.
3. Purulent exudate (Figs. 1–3 and 1–9) is composed primarily of PMNs and necrotic products, e.g., as seen in a hypopyon.

The term pus as commonly used is synonymous with a purulent exudate.

4. Sanguinous exudate (Fig. 1–10) is composed primarily of erythrocytes, e.g., as in a hyphema.

II. Subacute (intermediate or reactive counter-shock and adaptive) phase*
   A. The subacute phase is a phase of great variability concerned with healing and restoration of normal homeostasis (formation of granulation tissue and healing) or the exhaustion of local defenses resulting in necrosis, recurrence or chronicity.
   B. The PMNs at the site of injury release lysosomal enzymes (generally when they die) into the area. The enzymes

---

* Although the immune reaction is described separately in this chapter, it is intimately related to inflammation, especially to this phase. Many of the processes described herein are a direct result of the immune process.

FIG. 1–9. Purulent exudate composed of polymorphonuclear leukocytes is present in anterior chamber (hypopyon). **Inset 1** shows the edge of corneal ulcer from the main figure stained to demonstrate a colony of gram-positive cocci (*arrow*). **Inset 2** shows clinical picture of corneal ulcer with hypopyon. **Main figure,** Brown & Brenn, ×75; **inset 1,** Brown & Brenn, ×75; **inset 2,** clinical.

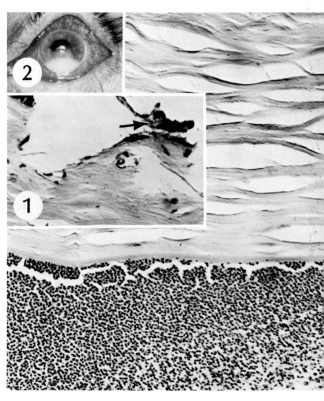

directly increase capillary permeability and cause tissue destruction and indirectly increase inflammation by stimulating mast cells to release histamine by activating the kinin-generating system and by inducing the chemotaxis of mononuclear (MN) phagocytes.

C. MN cells (Fig. 1–11) are derived from circulating monocytes (3 to 7 percent of circulating leukocytes), fixed tissue histiocytes (reticuloendothelial system) and possibly lymphocytes.

1. The MN cells or macrophages are the "second line of cellular defense," arrive after the PMN and are dependent on PMN release of a chemotactic factor for their arrival.

2. MN cells can live for weeks, have the ability to proliferate, are phagocytic and utilize proteolytic digestion. They cause much less tissue necrosis than is produced by PMNs and are more efficient phagocytes than are PMNs.

Mononuclear cells have an enormous phagocytic capacity and generally are named for the phagocytosed material, e.g., blood-filled macrophages (erythrophagocytosis), pigment-filled macrophages (pigment usually melanin or hemosiderin) (Fig. 1–12), lipid-laden macrophages (Fig. 1–13), lens-filled macrophages (as in phacolytic glaucoma) (Fig. 1–14), gitter cells filled with lipid material in the central nervous system, etc.

3. MN cells seem to have to fix antigen on their surface for the antigen to behave as an immunogenic substance.

4. The MN cells can change into epithelioid cells and inflammatory giant cells.

D. Lysosomal enzymes, including collagenase, are released by PMN, MN cells and other cells (e.g., epithelial cells and keratocytes in corneal ulcers) and result in considerable tissue destruction.

E. If the area of injury is tiny, the PMNs and MN cells alone can handle and "clean up" the area with resultant healing.

F. In larger injuries *granulation tissue* is produced. Granulation tissue (Fig. 1–15) is composed of leukocytes, proliferating blood vessels and fibroblasts.

1. MN cells arrive first after the PMNs, followed by an ingrowth of capillaries, which proliferate from the endothelium of preexisting blood vessels. The new blood vessels tend to leak fluid and leukocytes, especially PMNs.

2. Fibroblasts (Fig. 1–16) arise from fibrocytes and possibly from other cells (monocytes). Fibroblasts proliferate, lay down collagen and elaborate ground substance.

3. With time the blood vessels involute and disappear, the leukocytes disappear, and the fibroblasts re-

FIG. 1–10. Sanguinous exudate is shown by hyphema filling anterior chamber. H&E, ×50.

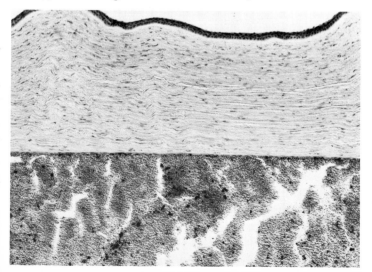

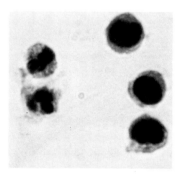

FIG. 1–11. Monocytes on the right have folded, large vesicular nuclei and moderate amount of cytoplasm. Compare in size to two polymorphonuclear leukocytes on the left. H&E, ×1,000.

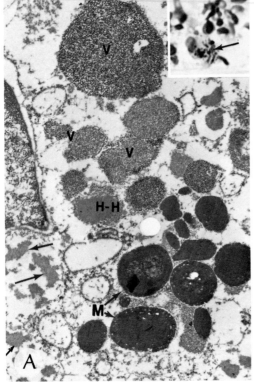

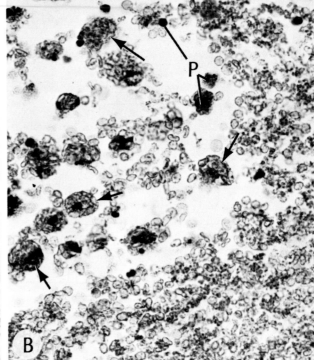

FIG. 1–12. Erythrophagocytosis. **A.** Electron micrograph of pigment (hemosiderin)-filled macrophage, similar to that in **inset** (*arrow*), showing hemoglobin-hemosiderin (*H-H*) and hemosiderin (*V*)-filled vesicles. Clumps of hemoglobin (*arrows*) are outside the cell. *M,* neuroepithelial melanin granules. **B.** Erythrocytes are seen free in the vitreous and in macrophages (*arrows*). Some hemoglobin has been oxidized to hemosiderin and appears as pigment (*P*). **A,** ×15,000; **inset,** H&E, ×530; **B,** H&E, ×275.

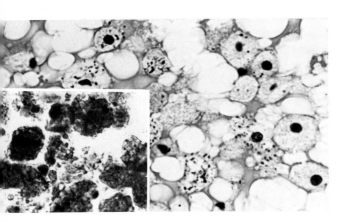

◄ **FIG. 1–13.** Foamy and clear lipid-laden macrophages in subretinal space. **Inset** shows staining with oil red-O technique to demonstrate fat. **Main figure,** H&E, ×275; **inset,** oil red-O, ×275.

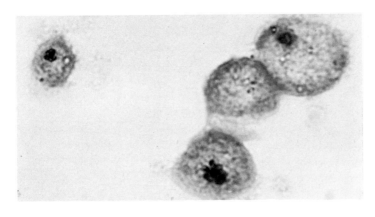

FIG. 1–14. Lens-filled macrophages in anterior chamber in eye with phacolytic glaucoma. PAS, ×800.

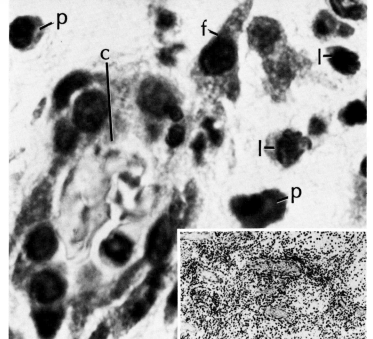

FIG. 1–15. Granulation tissue. **Main figure** is higher magnification of **inset** to show three components of granulation tissue: capillaries (c), fibroblasts (f) and leukocytes (l, lymphocyte; p, plasma cell). **Main figure,** H&E, ×1,000; **inset,** H&E, ×40.

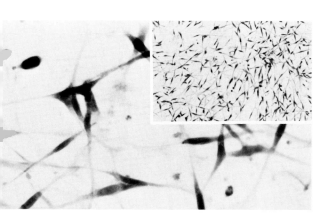

FIG. 1–16. Fibroblasts in tissue culture showing typical spindly, stellate form. **Inset** shows low magnification of **main figure. Main figure,** H&E, ×252; **inset,** H&E, ×40.

FIG. 1–17. Lymphocyte. **A.** Electron micrograph of B-cell (bone marrow derived) lymphocyte. Nucleus is surrounded by small ring of cytoplasm containing several mitochondria (m), diffusely arrayed ribonucleoprotein particles and many surface protrusions or microvilli. *rbc,* red blood cell; *pl,* platelet. **Inset** shows group of lymphocytes in inflamed iris. In tissue sections lymphocytes have almost no cytoplasm around small dark nuclei. **B.** Platelet with vacuoles (v), glycogen particles (g), chromomeric granules (ch) and mitochondria. **A,** ×8,000; **inset,** H&E, ×400; **B,** ×20,000.

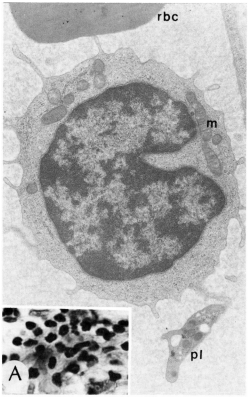

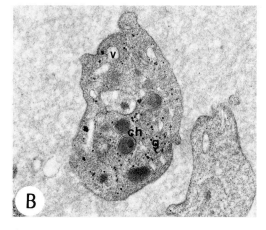

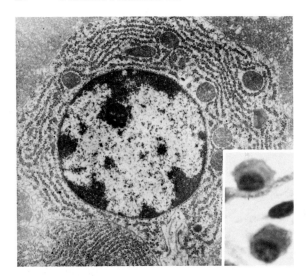

FIG. 1–18. Plasma cell. Electron micrograph shows nucleus surrounded by exceedingly prominent granular endoplasmic reticulum, which accounts for cytoplasmic basophilia in light microscopy. Mitochondria also are present in cytoplasm. **Inset** shows two plasma cells, each with clumping of chromatin in eccentrically located nucleus, halo around nucleus and tapering of cytoplasm. **Main figure,** ×10,500; **inset,** H&E, ×1,000.

turn to their resting state (fibrocytes). This involutionary process results in contracture of the collagenous scar and a reorientation of the remaining cells into a parallel arrangement along the long axis of the scar.

4. If the noxious agent persists, the condition may not heal as above but rather may become chronic. If the noxious agent that caused the inflammation is immunogenic, introduction of a similar agent at a future date can start the cycle anew (recurrence).

III. Chronic phase. The chronic phase is the result of a breakdown in the preceding two phases, or it may start initially as a chronic inflammation, e.g., with irritating material such as silica or asbestos, when there is a near balance between the resistance of the body and the inroads of an infecting agent such as the organisms of tuberculosis

or syphilis, in conditions of unknown cause such as sarcoidosis, following long-continued mechanical irritation such as might be caused by a jagged tooth, or as a result of impaired nutritional conditions such as in anterior segment ischemia (which occurs following removal of rectus muscles and loss of anterior ciliary blood supply).

A. *Chronic nongranulomatous inflammation* is a proliferative inflammation characterized by a cellular infiltrate of lymphocytes and plasma cells (and sometimes PMNs and/or eosinophils).
   1. The *lymphocyte* (Fig. 1–17) comprises 15 to 30 percent of circulating leukocytes, is produced in thymus, spleen and lymph node, is capable of proliferation, and is the competent immunocyte.
   2. The *plasma cell* (Fig. 1–18), produced by the bone marrow-derived lymphocyte, produces immunoglobulins (antibodies). Certain modified forms of the plasma cell may be recognized in tissue sections:
      a. *Plasmacytoid cell* (Fig. 1–19) has a single eccentric nucleus and slightly eosinophilic granular cytoplasm (instead of the normal basophilic cytoplasm of the plasma cell).
      b. *Russell bodies* (Fig. 1–19) are plasma cells changed so that their cytoplasm is filled and enlarged with eosinophilic grape-like clusters in a morular form, with single eosinophilic globular structures or with eosinophilic crystalline structures; generally the nucleus appears as an eccentric rim or has disappeared.

      The eosinophilic material in plasmacytoid cells and in Russell bodies appears to be immunoglobulin which has become inspissated as if the plasma cells can no longer release the material ("constipated" plasma cells).

B. *Chronic granulomatous inflammation* is a proliferative inflammation characterized by a cellular infiltrate of epithe-

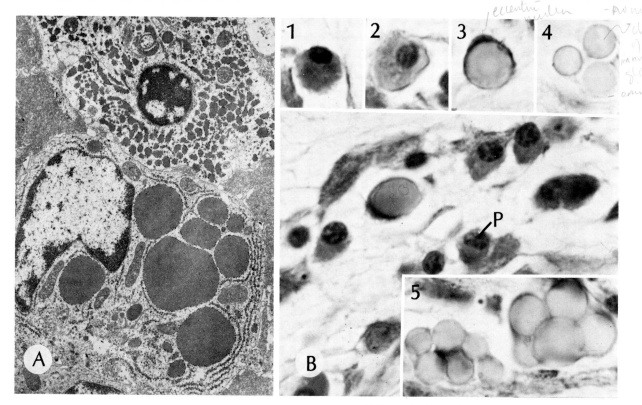

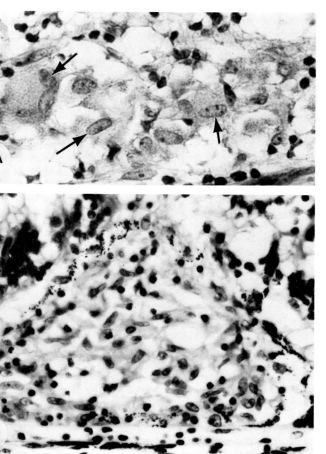

FIG. 1–19. Altered plasma cells. **A.** Electron micrograph of plasmacytoid cells with upper cell showing many small pockets of inspissated material (γ-globulin?) in segments of rough endoplasmic reticulum and lower cell containing large globules (γ-globulin?) of inspissated material, which appear as eosinophilic globules in light microscopy. **B. Main figure** shows numerous plasma cells, plasmacytoid cell (*P*) and Russell body with narrow rim of nucleus. **Insets 1** through **4** show transition from plasmacytoid cells (**insets 1** and **2**) to Russell bodies (**inset 4**). **Inset 5** shows clusters of Russell bodies. **A,** ×6,000; **B,** H&E, ×1,000; **inset 1,** H&E, ×1,000; **inset 2,** H&E, ×1,000; **inset 3,** H&E, ×720; **inset 4,** H&E, ×1,000; **inset 5,** H&E, ×1,000.

FIG. 1–20. A. Epithelioid cells in early formation in sympathetic uveitis. Macrophages come together, lose their cell borders and form syncytium. Vesicular macrophagic nuclei (*arrows*) can still be recognized. **B.** Same phenomenon of epithelioid formation has occurred in this Dalen-Fuchs's nodule (epithelioid cells between Bruch's membrane and retinal pigment epithelium) in sarcoidosis. **A,** H&E, ×400; **B,** H&E, ×252.

lioid cells (and sometimes inflammatory giant cells, lymphocytes, plasma
cells, PMNs and eosinophils).

1. Epithelioid cells (Fig. 1–20) are a
syncytium of cells formed by macrophages coming together and losing
their distinct cell boundaries—large
vesicular nuclei of macrophages
with their tiny nucleoli are identified easily within the syncytium of
abundant eosinophilic cytoplasm.

It is this special syncytial arrangement
of macrophages that superficially resembles an epithelium. The cells of
this syncytium therefore are called
epithelioid *cells.*

2. Inflammatory giant cells are formed
by fusion of macrophages and/or
by amitotic division of macrophages. Three forms predominate:
a. Langhans' giant cell (Fig. 1–21),
when sectioned through its
center, shows a perfectly homogeneous eosinophilic central
cytoplasm with a peripheral rim
of nuclei.

It is important to note that the central cytoplasm is perfectly homogeneous. If not, material such as
fungi or foreign bodies may be
present, and then the cell is not a
Langhans' giant cell but rather a
foreign body giant cell. When sectioned through the peripheral portion of the cell, the Langhans' giant
cell appears as a foreign body giant
cell. Langhans' giant cells are seen
in tuberculosis but also may be
seen in many other granulomatous
processes.

b. Foreign body giant cell (Fig.
1–22) has its nuclei randomly
distributed through its eosinophilic cytoplasm.

c. Touton giant cell (Fig. 1–23),
frequently associated with lipid
disorders such as juvenile
xanthogranuloma, appears much
like a Langhans' giant cell with
the addition of a rim of foamy
(fat positive) cytoplasm peripheral to the rim of nuclei.

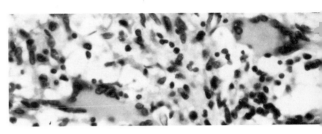

FIG. 1–21. Langhans' giant cells in ocular
tuberculosis. Homogeneous central cytoplasm is surrounded by rim of nuclei. H&E,
×252.

3. Three patterns of inflammatory
reaction may be found in granulomatous inflammations:
a. *Diffuse type* (Fig. 1–24*A*) with
the epithelioid cells (sometimes
with macrophages and/or inflammatory giant cells) distributed randomly against a
background of lymphocytes and
plasma cells occurs typically in
sympathetic uveitis, disseminated histoplasmosis and other
fungal infections, lepromatous
leprosy, juvenile xanthogranuloma, Vogt-Koyanagi-Harada
disease, cytomegalic inclusion
disease, toxoplasmosis, etc.
b. *Discrete (sarcoidal or tuberculoidal)* type (Fig. 1–24*B*) with
accumulation of epithelioid cells
(sometimes with inflammatory
giant cells) into nodules (tubercles) surrounded by a narrow
rim of lymphocytes (and perhaps plasma cells) occurs typically in sarcoidosis, tuberculoid
leprosy, miliary tuberculosis, etc.
c. *Zonal type* (Fig. 1–24*C*) with a
central nidus (necrosis, lens, foreign body, etc.) surrounded by
palisaded epithelioid cells (sometimes with PMNs, inflammatory
giant cells, and macrophages), in
turn surrounded by lymphocytes
and plasma cells, in turn frequently surrounded by granulation tissue, occurs in caseation
tuberculosis, some fungal infections, rheumatoid scleritis, cha-

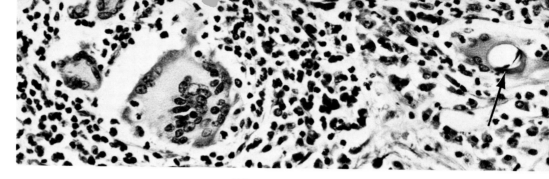

FIG. 1–22. Foreign body giant cells resemble Langhans' giant cells except for presence of foreign material (*arrow*) in cytoplasm of former. H&E, ×500.

FIG. 1–23. Touton giant cell resembles closely Langhans' giant cell except for addition of peripheral rim of foamy (fat positive) cytoplasm in former. H&E, ×495.

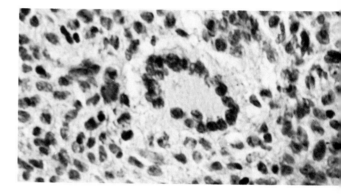

FIG. 1–24. Patterns of granulomatous inflammation. **A.** Diffuse type in case of sympathetic uveitis. **B.** Discrete (sarcoidal or tuberculoidal) type in case of sarcoidosis. **C.** Zonal type in case of phacoanaphylactic endophthalmitis. **A,** H&E, ×110; **B,** H&E, ×170; **C,** H&E, ×100.

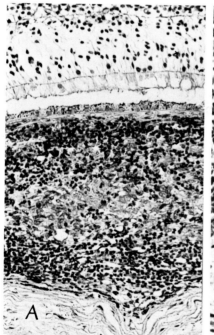

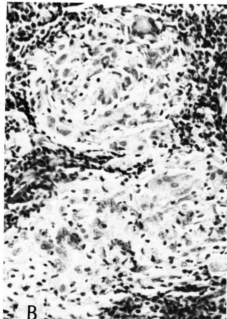

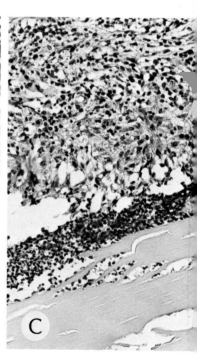

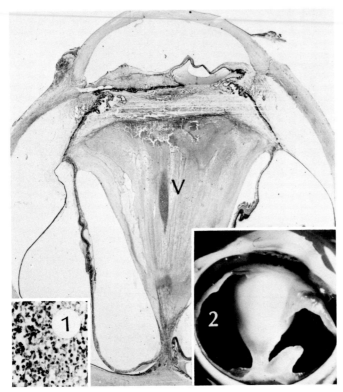

FIG. 1–25. Staining patterns of inflammation. Diffuse abscess, here filling vitreous (*V*), is characteristic of bacterial infection. **Inset 1** shows higher magnification of purulent vitreous abscess. **Inset 2** shows macroscopic appearance of vitreous abscess. **Main figure,** H&E, ×3; **inset 1,** H&E, ×101; **inset 2,** macroscopic.

FIG. 1–26. Staining patterns of inflammation. Multiple microabscesses, here in anterior vitreous, are characteristic of fungal infections. **Inset** shows fungi from same case stained with special stain to demonstrate fungi. **Main figure,** H&E, ×5; **inset,** Gomori's methenamine silver, ×300.

lazion, phacoanaphylactic endophthalmitis, nematode endophthalmitis, cysticerosis, etc.

STAINING PATTERNS OF INFLAMMATION

I. Patterns of inflammation are best observed microscopically under the lowest (scanning) power.

II. With the hematoxylin and eosin (H&E) stain a deep blue (basophilic) infiltrate generally is caused by a chronic nongranulomatous inflammation. The deep basophilia is produced by lymphocytes that have blue nuclei with practically no cytoplasm and by plasma cells that have blue nuclei and blue cytoplasm.

III. A deep blue infiltrate with scattered gray (pale pink) areas ("pepper and salt") generally is caused by a chronic granulomatous inflammation with the blue areas lymphocytes and plasma cells and the gray areas islands of epithelioid cells.

IV. A "dirty" gray infiltrate generally is caused by a purulent reaction with PMNs and necrotic material.

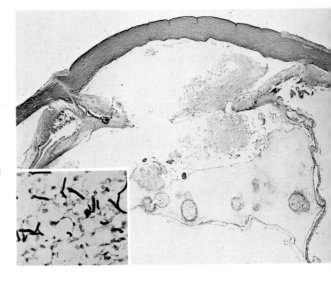

A. If the infiltrate is diffuse (Fig. 1–25), e.g., filling the vitreous (vitreous abscess), the cause is probably bacterial.

B. If the infiltrate is localized into two or more small areas (Fig. 1–26) (i.e., multiple abscesses or microabscesses), the cause is probably fungal.

IMMUNOBIOLOGY

BACKGROUND

I. All lymphocytes in mammalian lymph nodes and spleen have a remote origin in the bone marrow: those that have undergone an intermediate cycle of proliferation in the thymus (thymus-derived lymphocytes) probably mediate cellular immunity, whereas those that seed directly into lymphoid tissue (bone marrow-derived lymphocytes) probably provide the precursors of cells that produce circulating antibody.

II. The long-lived, recirculating lymphocytes derived from the thymus initiate cellular immunity (delayed hypersensitivity), are responsible for graft-versus-host reactions and initiate the reactions of the body against foreign grafts such as skin and kidneys (host-versus-graft reactions). When sensitized, they interact with antigen to liberate a substance that immobilizes macrophages (*migration inhibitory factor* or *MIF*), a factor that will kill some varieties of mammalian cells in vitro (lymphotoxin), a chemotactic factor, a factor inducing mitosis in other lymphocytes and another that increases the permeability of skin blood vessels.

III. The long-lived, recirculating lymphocytes derived from bone marrow (without an intermediate cycle in the thymus) can be stimulated by antigen to enlarge, divide and differentiate to form antibody-secreting plasma cells.

Under most circumstances the thymus-derived lymphocytes collaborate with the bone marrow-derived lymphocytes during the induction of antibody-forming cells by the latter (see section Humoral Immunoglobin).

CELLULAR IMMUNITY
(DELAYED HYPERSENSITIVITY)*

I. Two distinct cell types participate in cellular immunity: the thymus-derived lymphocyte and the bone marrow-derived monocyte (macrophage).

* The terms cellular immunity and delayed hypersensitivity will be used as synonyms in the following discussion.

A. Phagocytic cells of the monocytic line (monocytes, reticuloendothelial cells, histiocytes, macrophages, epithelioid cells and inflammatory giant cells are all different forms of the same cell) are devoid of antibody and immunologic specificity. The phagocytic cells, however, seem to have to attach the antigen to itself, probably to an RNA template, before the thymus-derived lymphocytes can react with the antigen.

At this time, i.e., attachment of antigen, the phagocytes most likely are incapable of further phagocytic activity. Very likely the RNA template of the phagocyte with its attached antigen is passed into the lymphocyte where it triggers proliferation and differentiation to a protein-synthesizing end cell.

B. All thymic-derived lymphocytes seem to be precommitted to make only one type of antibody, which is cell bound. When an antigen is attached to a phagocytic cell, each small lymphocyte precommitted to that antigen responds by becoming a large, rapidly dividing cell and gives rise to many committed, or sensitized, lymphocytes (Fig. 1–27). The individual is now sensitized and with subsequent exposure to the same antigen will provoke a hypersensitivity reaction (cellular immunity).

II. When the sensitized lymphocytes interact with antigen, they release MIF, which inhibits macrophages within 24 hours and kills fibroblasts in two to three days. Also MIF may act as a macrophage-activating factor. Other factors released include a macrophage and PMN chemotactic factor; cytotoxic factors; growth, cloning and DNA-synthesis inhibiting factors; mitogenic factors; and interferon.

III. The nature of the cell-bound antibody produced by the sensitized lymphocyte is poorly understood.

IV. The delayed hypersensitivity reaction begins with perivenous accumulation of sensitized lymphocytes and other mononuclear cells (i.e., monocytes, which constitute 80 to 90 percent of the cells mobilized to the lesion). The infiltrative

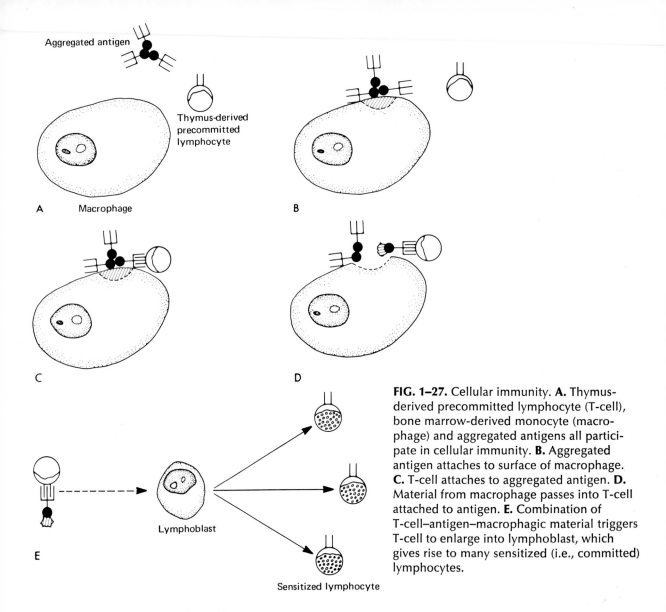

FIG. 1–27. Cellular immunity. **A.** Thymus-derived precommitted lymphocyte (T-cell), bone marrow-derived monocyte (macrophage) and aggregated antigens all participate in cellular immunity. **B.** Aggregated antigen attaches to surface of macrophage. **C.** T-cell attaches to aggregated antigen. **D.** Material from macrophage passes into T-cell attached to antigen. **E.** Combination of T-cell–antigen–macrophagic material triggers T-cell to enlarge into lymphoblast, which gives rise to many sensitized (i.e., committed) lymphocytes.

lesions enlarge and multiply (e.g., in tuberculosis where the lesions take a granulomatous form), and there is cellular invasion and destruction of tissue.

Sensitized lymphocytes arrive at the antigenic site (e.g., at the site of tubercle bacilli within an infected phagocyte) along with monocytes sensitized by transfer of cytophilic antibody* (Fig. 1–28). Release of chemotactic

* Migration inhibitory factor (MIF) is released by a sensitized lymphocyte when it encounters its specific soluble antigen. MIF stops the migration of monocytic leukocytes by making them "sticky," and it may also affect the venular endothelium. As a result, monocytes adhere to the endothelium. The monocytes then gradually are transformed into macrophages.

factor by the sensitized (committed) lymphocyte draws nonsensitized monocytes and PMNs to the area. Release of cytotoxin (lymphotoxin) causes tissue necrosis. Release of mitogenic factor causes proliferation of cells. The result is the formation of a consolidated tubercle.

V. Delayed hypersensitivity is involved in transplantation immunity, in the pathogenesis of various autoimmune diseases (e.g., phacoanaphylactic endophthalmitis, sympathetic uveitis and the "garden variety" uveitis) and in defense against most viral, fungal, protozoal and many bacterial (e.g., tuberculosis and leprosy) diseases. Perhaps the most important role

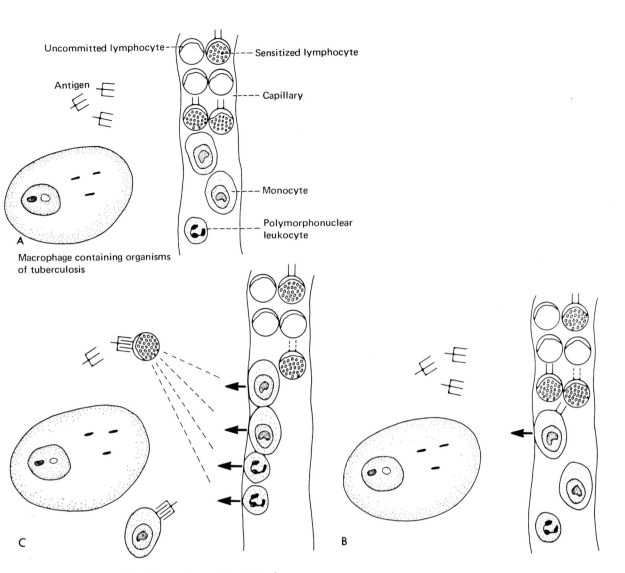

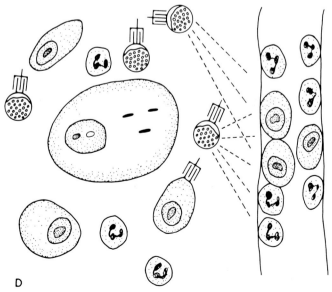

FIG. 1–28. Cellular immunity. **A.** Sensitized lymphocytes (SL) in capillary arrive with other leukocytes, including monocytes, at antigenic site where macrophage contains tubercle bacilli and antigens are present in surrounding tissue. **B.** Monocytes become sensitized by transfer of cytophilic antibody from SL and leave circulation to migrate toward antigenic stimulus. **C.** SL encounter specific antigen and release biologically active molecules that draw monocytes and other leukocytes to area. **D.** When monocytes arrive at site, they become immobilized by migration inhibitory factor (MIF) released by SL. SL also release cytotoxin, which causes tissue necrosis (caseation), and mitogenic factor, which causes proliferation of cells, some of which undergo transformation into epithelioid cells; hence, tuberculoma is formed.

is to act as a natural defense against cancer, i.e., the immunologic rejection of vascularized tumors and immunologic surveillance of neoplastic cells.

HUMORAL IMMUNOGLOBULIN (ANTIBODY)

I. Four distinct cell types participate in humoral immunoglobulin (antibody) formation: the thymus-derived lymphocyte, the bone marrow-derived lymphocyte, the bone marrow-derived monocyte and the plasma cell (Fig. 1–29).
   A. Cells of the monocytic line attach the antigen to themselves as in the early stage of the formation of cellular immunity.
   B. Specifically precommitted cells of both thymus-derived and bone marrow-derived lymphocytes attach to different determinants of the antigen.

   Recent evidence has shown that only aggregated antigen can be fixed by macrophages and, therefore, capable of illiciting an antibody response. Monomeric or deaggregated forms of antigen have been shown to be *tolerogenic*, i.e., causing immunologic unresponsiveness.

   C. As a result of some type of synergistic action whereby passage of information goes from the thymic to the bone marrow lymphocyte, the bone marrow lymphocyte differentiates and proliferates into plasma cells that elaborate specific immunoglobulins.
II. Humoral immunoglobulins (antibodies) are all made up of multiple polypeptide chains and are the predominant mediator of immunity in certain types of infection such as acute bacterial infection (those caused by streptococci and pneumococci) and viral diseases (hepatitis).
III. Five major classes of human immunoglobulin have been identified. All are γ-globulins and have been named γA-globulin (IgA), γD-globulin (IgD), γE-globulin (IgE), γG-globulin (IgG) and γM-globulin (IgM).
   A. IgA (β_2A or γ_1A) is the "first line of defense" and is dominant in all fluids bathing the organs and systems that are in continuity with the external environment, e.g., tears, saliva, gastrointestinal secretions, breast milk and colostrum. IgA probably regulates the normal flora found in tears and in the respiratory and gastrointestinal tracts, i.e., gives localized protection in external secretions.
   B. IgD is found in the serum in concentrations of only 0.03 mg/cc. Its function is not known.
   C. IgE includes the skin sensitizing or reagin antibodies found in increased amounts in allergic individuals. IgE is attached to basophilic leukocytes, and the combination of allergen and basophil-bound IgE results in the release of histamine. A second chemical mediator of IgE activity is the slow-reacting substance of anaphylaxis or SRS-A.
   D. IgG (γ, 7Sγ or γ_2) is the most common immunoglobulin, is formed after IgM and seems to have a regulatory effect on IgM. It functions in complement fixation and placental transfer.
   E. IgM (γ_1A or γ-macroglobulin) is the first immunoglobulin to appear after a primary antigenic stimulus. It decreases as IgG increases. IgM functions in early immune response and in complement fixation.
IV. Once a lymphocyte has become committed (sensitized) to the production of immunoglobulin to a specific antigen, it makes that immunoglobulin and none other, as does its progeny. It, or its progeny, may produce immunoglobulin or become resting memory cells to be reactivated at an accelerated rate (*amnestic response*) if confronted again by the same antigen.

TRANSPLANTATION TERMINOLOGY

I. *Autograft* is a transplantation of tissue excised from one place and grafted to another in the same individual.
II. *Syngraft (isograft)* is a transplantation of tissue excised from one individual and grafted to another who is identical genetically.
III. *Allograft (homograft)* is a transplantation of tissue excised from one individual and grafted to another of the same species.

1–33), ciliary body atrophy in high myopia and retinal vascular atrophy in retinopathia (retinitis) pigmentosa.

DYSPLASIA

I. Dysplasia is an abnormal growth of tissue during embryonic life.

II. Examples of ocular dysplasia include retinal dysplasia, dysplasia of the optic nerve (coloboma of the optic nerve) and mesodermal dysgenesis of the cornea and iris.

NEOPLASIA

I. Neoplasia is a continuous increase above the normal number of cells in a tissue. It differs from hyperplasia in that its growth never attains an equilibrium. The neoplasm* may be benign or malignant.

II. A malignant neoplasm differs from a benign one in being *invasive* (infiltrate *and* actively destroys surrounding tissue), in having the ability to *metastasize* (develop secondary centers of neoplastic growth at a distance from the primary focus) and in showing *anaplasia* [histologic attempt to depict malignancy (Fig. 1–34) by showing a variation from the normal structure and/or behavior in the sense of a loss of specialized or "adult" characteristics of the cell or tissue, e.g., loss of cellular or tissue polarity, loss of special secretory abilities or inability to form photoreceptors].

DEGENERATION AND DYSTROPHY

I. A dystrophy is a primary (bilateral), inherited disorder with distinct clinicopathologic findings. The dystrophies are discussed under the individual tissues.

II. A degeneration (monocular or binocular) is a secondary phenomena resulting from previous disease. It occurs in a tissue that had reached its full growth.

A clear differentiation between a degeneration and a dystrophy is seen in combined corneal dystrophy (Fuchs). The bilateral,

* Neoplasm is a tumor, but not all tumors are neoplasms. Tumor simply means mass and may be secondary to neoplasm, inflammation, edema, etc.

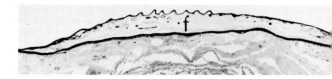

FIG. 1–32. Fibrous metaplasia, or transformation of lens epithelium into fibrous tissue (*f*), in anterior subcapsular cataract. PAS, ×40.

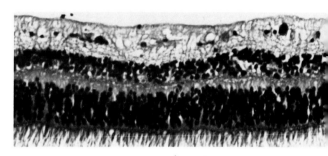

FIG. 1–33. Atrophy, or loss of tissue, is present in inner retinal layers in case of long-standing glaucoma. H&E, ×101.

central endothelial abnormality, corneal gutatta, is the dystrophy that is primary and causes secondarily chronic corneal edema. The chronic corneal edema can lead to secondary epithelial changes such as epithelial edema and pannus degenerativus. The secondary epithelial changes are degenerative.

A. *Cloudy swelling* is a reversible change in cells secondary to relatively mild infections, intoxications, anemia or circulatory disturbances. The cells are enlarged and filled with granules or fluid and probably represent an intracellular edema.

B. *Hydropic degeneration* is a reversible change in cells also secondary to relatively mild infections, intoxications, anemia or circulatory disturbances. The cells are enlarged and contain cytoplasmic vacuoles and probably represent an early stage of swelling of the endoplasmic reticulum.

C. *Fatty change* results when fat accumulates within cells following damage by a variety of agents, e.g., chloroform and carbon tetrachloride.

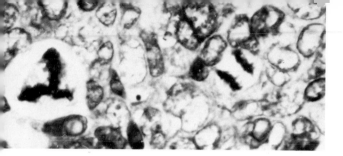

FIG. 1–34. Neoplasia is depicted by normal mitotic figure on right and abnormal tripolar mitotic figure on left in case of sebaceous carcinoma of lid. H&E, ×630.

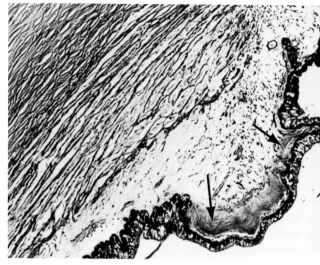

FIG. 1–35. Hyaline degeneration (*arrows*) is present in ciliary processes. PAS, ×40.

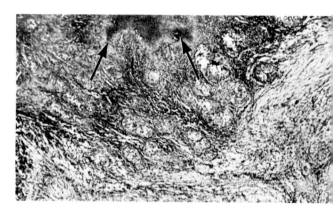

FIG. 1–36. Caseation necrosis (*arrows*) is seen in center of intraocular tuberculous granuloma. H&E, ×16.

D. *Glycogen infiltration* results from diseases such as diabetes mellitus, e.g., lacy vacuolation of iris pigment epithelium (see p. 566 in Chap. 15) and from a lack of nutrition, e.g., in many pathologic retinal conditions such as long-standing retinal detachment, central retinal vein occlusion and proliferating retinal pigment epithelial cells.

E. *Amyloid* may be found in ocular tissues in primary amyloidosis (see p. 248 in Chap. 7 and p. 480 in Chap. 12) e.g., in primary familial amyloidosis and lattice corneal dystrophy, in which case it is a dystrophic change, or in secondary amyloidosis (see p. 248 in Chap. 7), in which case it is a degenerative change.

F. *Hyaline* degeneration is quite common, consists of an acellular, amorphous, eosinophilic material and may be found in such places as the walls of arteriolarsclerotic vessels or in the ciliary processes in elderly individuals (Fig. 1–35).

NECROSIS

I. Coagulative necrosis. This is a "firm, dry" necrosis generally formed in tissue that has been shut off from its blood supply.

A. The gray, opaque retina seen clinically following a central retinal artery occlusion has undergone coagulative necrosis ("ischemic necrosis").

B. Caseation (Fig. 1–36), characteristic of tuberculosis, is a form of coagulative necrosis.

II. Hemorrhagic necrosis. This type is caused by occlusion of venous blood flow but with retention of arterial blood flow, as seen classically in central retinal vein thrombosis.

III. Liquefaction necrosis. Necrosis of this type results from autolytic (see section Autolysis and Putrefaction below) decomposition, generally in tissue that is rich in proteolytic enzymes, e.g., suppuration is a form of liquefaction necrosis in which rapid digestion is brought about by the proteolytic enzymes from the leukocytes present in the area.

IV. Fat necrosis. This results in a lipogranulomatous reaction to the liberated free fatty acids and glycerol.

CALCIFICATION

I. Dystrophic calcification. Dystrophic calcification occurs when calcium is deposited in dead or dying tissue, e.g., in long-standing cataracts, especially in traumatic cataracts found in adults whose trauma dates back to childhood; in the necrotic areas of retinoblastoma (Fig. 1–37); and in pannus in band keratopathy in chronically edematous corneas.

II. Metastatic calcification. This type of calcification occurs when calcium is deposited in previously undamaged tissue, e.g., in the cornea in the form of a horizontal band in individuals with high serum calcium levels (hyperparathyroidism, vitamin D intoxication).

AUTOLYSIS AND PUTREFACTION

I. Autolysis is, in part, the self-digestion of cells utilizing their own cellular digestive enzymes contained within lysosomes (so-called "suicide bags") and, in part, other unknown factors.

II. When necrotic (autolytic) tissue is invaded by certain bacteria (especially *Clostridia*), the changes catalyzed by destructive bacterial enzymes are called *putrefaction*.

PIGMENTATION

I. In ocular histologic sections stained with H&E, four main pigments commonly found may resemble each other closely: 1) melanin and lipofuscin; 2) hemosiderin; 3) exogenous iron; and 4) acid hematin.

II. Melanin is found in uveal melanocytes as fine, powdery, brown granules barely resolvable with the light microscope and in pigment epithelial cells of the retina, ciliary body and iris as rather large, black granules. Lipofuscin occurs in aged cells and in the RPE and may look similar to melanin with conventional light microscopy but differs considerably in morphology and density with electron microscopy.

III. Hemosiderin results from intraocular hemorrhage when hemoglobin is oxidized to hemosiderin. It occurs as an orange-brown pigment within macrophages and when plentiful in the eye is called *hemosiderosis bulbi*.

A. Systemic *hemochromatosis* consists of portal cirrhosis and elevated iron con-

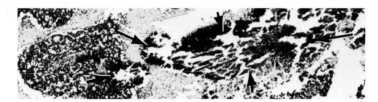

FIG. 1–37. Dystrophic calcification (*arrows*) is present within retinoblastoma. H&E, ×40.

FIG. 1–38. A. Acid hematin, a formaldehyde artifact, appears in routine sections as dark pigment. **B.** Pigmented area is birefringent to polarized light. **A,** H&E, ×101; **B,** H&E, polarized, ×101.

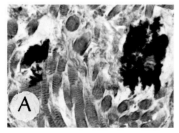
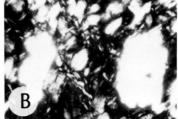

TABLE 1–1
Deposition of Iron in the Eye in Local* and Systemic (Hemo) Siderosis†

Tissue	Local siderosis and hemo-siderosis	Systemic hemo-chromatosis
Corneal epithelium	Yes	No
Trabecular meshwork	Yes	No
Iris epithelium	Yes	No
Iris dilator and sphincter muscles	Yes	No
Ciliary epithelium	Yes	Yes
Lens epithelium	Yes	No
Vitreous body	Yes	No
Sclera	No	Yes
Blood vessels	Yes	No
Sensory retina	Yes	No
Retinal pigment epithelium	Yes	Yes

* With local iron foreign body, iron usually will be deposited in all adjacent (contiguous) tissues.

† Modified from Roth AM, Foos RY: Ocular pathologic changes in primary hemochromatosis. Arch Ophthalmol 87:507, 1972.

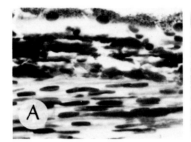
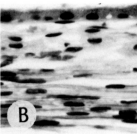

FIG. 1–39. A. In routine sections retinal pigment epithelium and choroid are pigmented. B. Bleaching adjacent section removes the melanin pigment. A, H&E, ×252; B, H&E, bleached, ×252.

tent in parenchymal cells of multiple organs; when increased amounts of iron are deposited in tissues of multiple organs but cirrhosis and its complications are lacking, systemic *hemosiderosis* is present.

B. The distribution of iron in the eye differs in local ocular disease causing deposition of iron (hemosiderosis bulbi and siderosis bulbi) and systemic disease (see Table 1–1).

IV. Exogenous iron results from an intraocular iron foreign body. The resultant ocular iron deposition is called siderosis bulbi (see Table 1–1).

V. Acid hematin is an artifact produced by the action of acid fixatives, particularly formaldehyde, on hemoglobin.

VI. Differentiation of the pigments:

A. Only acid hematin is birefringent to polarized light (Fig. 1–38).

B. Only melanin bleaches with oxidizing agents such as hydrogen peroxide (Fig. 1–39).

C. Only iron stains positively with the common stains for iron (see Color

Color Plate I. A. Hudson-Stahli line. Iron is present within epithelial cells. B. Fleischer ring of keratoconus. Iron is present within epithelial cells. C. Kayser-Fleischer ring of Wilson's disease (hepatolenticular degeneration). Copper is deposited within Descemet's membrane. D. Copper is present within capsule of lens in cataract of Wilson's disease. E. Blood staining of the cornea. Loose hemoglobin (or red blood cell fragments) is widely distributed throughout collagenous lamellas. Conversion of hemoglobin to hemosiderin by keratocytes causes cytoplasm of cells to stain blue with iron stain. F. Iron is taken up by lens epithelium in siderosis bulbi. G. Siderosis bulbi with dense staining of necrotic lens epithelium. A cortical cataract also is present. H. Siderosis bulbi. Heavy accumulation of iron within nonpigmented epithelial cells of ciliary body (posterior pars plana). I. Edge of band keratopathy. Myriad granules of calcium are deposited within Bowman's membrane. A, Perl's stain, ×500; B, Perl's stain, ×500; C, rhodanine, ×500; D, H&E, ×500; E, Perl's stain, ×500; F, Perl's stain, ×500; G, Perl's stain, ×500; H, Perl's stain, ×500; I, alizarin red, ×300.

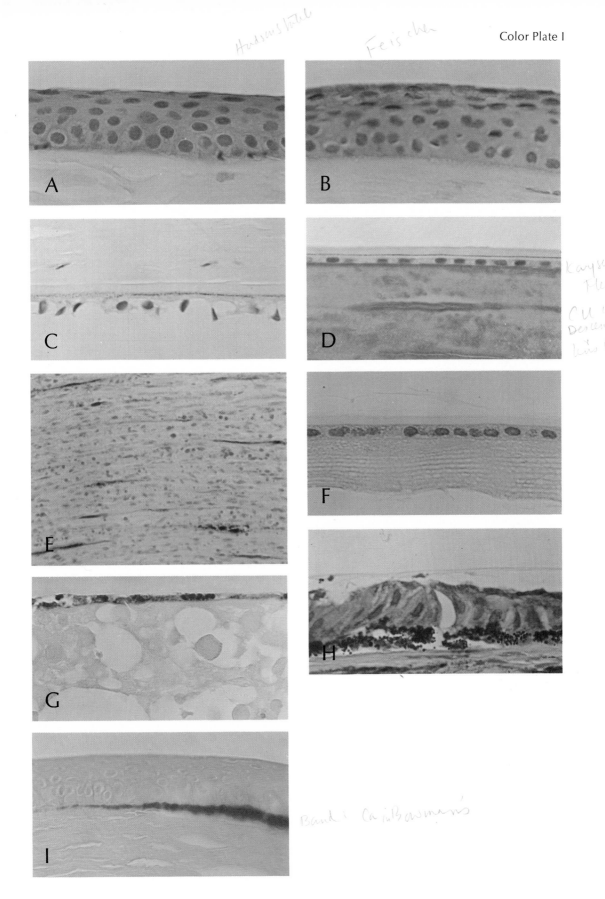

Hudsenstahl

Feischer

Kayser-Fleischer

CH in Descemet bis Bupula

Band: Ca in Bowmans

chapter 2

Congenital Anomalies

PHAKOMATOSES (DISSEMINATED HEREDITARY HAMARTOMAS)

GENERAL INFORMATION

I. The phakomatoses are a heredofamilial group of congenital tumors having in common the presence of disseminated, usually benign, hamartomas.

A hamartoma is a congenital tumor composed of tissues that are normally found in the involved area, in contrast to a choristoma, which is a congenital tumor composed of tissues not normally present in the involved area.

II. In each of the types of phakomatosis the hamartomas tend to affect predominantly one type of tissue, e.g., blood vessels in angiomatosis retinae and neural tissue in neurofibromatosis.

ANGIOMATOSIS RETINAE
(von Hippel's Disease) (Fig. 2–1)

I. General information
   A. The onset of ocular symptoms generally is in young adulthood.
   B. Retinal hemangioblastomas are bilateral in 50 percent of cases, and cerebellar hemangioblastomas occur in 20 percent of cases.

   The combination of retinal plus cerebellar hemangioblastomas (and hemangioblastomas of medulla and spinal cord) is called *von Hippel-Lindau disease*. Historically the retinal component, von Hippel's disease, was the first to be described.

   C. An autosomal dominant inheritance pattern with incomplete penetrance is found.
II. Ocular findings
   A. A retinal hemangioblastoma (see p. 528 in Chap. 14) may occur in any part of the retina and generally is supplied by large feeder vessels.
   B. Retinal hemorrhages and exudates result from leakage of blood and serum from the abnormal blood ves-

sels in the hemangioblastic tumor.
   C. Ultimately formation of organized fibroglial bands and retinal detachment may develop. Secondary angle closure glaucoma also may be found.
III. Systemic findings
   A. A hemangioblastoma may occur in the cerebellum, medulla and spinal cord (Lindau's component).
   B. Cysts of pancreas and kidney commonly are found.
   C. Hypernephroma and pheochromocytoma may occur infrequently.
IV. Histology
   A. The basic lesion is a hemangioblastoma (see p. 528 in Chap. 14) that is practically the same histologically whether found in the retina or in the cerebellum.
   B. Secondary complications such as retinal exudates and hemorrhages, fixed retinal folds and organized fibroglial membranes, retinal detachment, rubeosis iridis, peripheral anterior synechias and secondary chronic retinal detachment may be found.

MENINGOCUTANEOUS ANGIOMATOSIS
(Encephalotrigeminal Angiomatosis; Sturge-Weber Syndrome) (Fig. 2–2)

I. General information
   A. The syndrome generally consists of unilateral (rarely bilateral) meningeal calcification, facial nevus flammeus (port wine stain) frequently along the distribution of trigeminal nerve and congenital glaucoma.
   B. The condition is congenital.
      1. Heredity does not seem to be an important factor.
      2. There is a suggestion that the syndrome may be transmitted as an irregular autosomal dominant, but proof is lacking.
II. Ocular findings
   A. A cavernous hemangioma (see p. 528 in Chap. 14) of the choroid on the side of the facial nevus flammeus is the most common intraocular finding.
   B. A cavernous hemangioma or telangi-

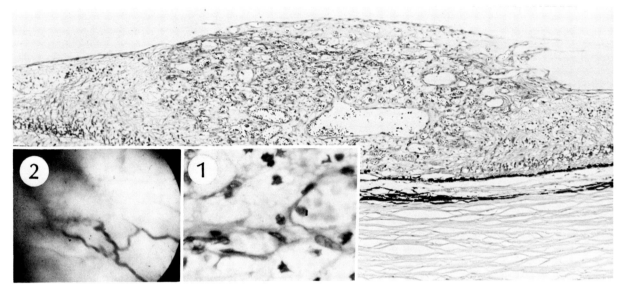

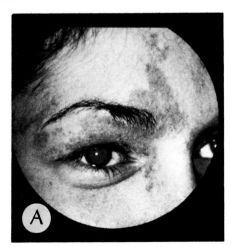

FIG. 2–1. Angiomatosis retinae. Vascular tumor (hemangioblastoma) replaces full thickness of retina. **Inset 1** is higher magnification to show capillary blood spaces intimately associated with characteristic pale, foamy, polygonal, stromal cells. **Inset 2** shows fundus picture of retinal angioma. **Main figure,** H&E, ×40; **inset 1,** H&E, ×252; **inset 2,** fundus picture.

FIG. 2–2. Meningocutaneous angiomatosis. **A.** Facial nevus flammeus (port wine stain) is seen along distribution of first division of trigeminal nerve. **B.** Choroid is thickened posteriorly by cavernous hemangioma. **Inset 1** is higher magnification to show large blood-filled spaces separated by thin, endothelial-lined, fibrous septa. **Middle insets** show fundus appearance of choroidal hemangioma before (**2**) and after (**3**) fluorescein (late phase). **A,** clinical; **B,** H&E, ×5; **inset 1,** H&E, ×40; **insets 2** and **3,** fundus pictures.

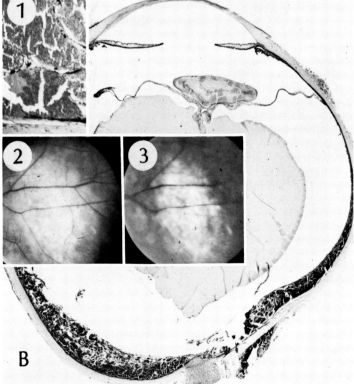

ectasis (see pp. 528, 532 in Chap. 14) of the lids on the side of the facial nevus flammeus is common and associated frequently with congenital glaucoma.
   C. Congenital glaucoma may be present. In about 30 percent of cases the glaucoma is associated with hemangioma of the facial skin.
      1. When glaucoma is present, the lids usually are involved with a facial hemangioma, especially the upper.
      2. A hemangioma of the choroid on the side of the facial hemangioma is common when glaucoma is present.
      3. The cause of the glaucoma is unknown, but it is not related to the choroidal hemangioma in most cases.
III. Systemic findings
   A. Cavernous hemangioma or telangiectasis of the skin of the face ("birthmark" or port wine stain) is the most common visible sign.
   B. Hemangioma of the meninges and brain on the side of the facial hemangioma generally is present.

   Meningeal or intracranial calcification frequently is present and allows the area of the hemangioma to be located radiographically.

   C. Seizures and mental retardation are common.

IV. Histology
   A. The basic lesion in the skin of the face (including lids), the meninges and the choroid is a cavernous hemangioma (see p. 528 in Chap. 14). In addition, telangiectasis (see p. 528 in Chap. 14) of the skin of the face may occur.
   B. The histology of glaucomatous eyes seems identical to that seen in genetic congenital glaucoma (see section on congenital glaucoma in Chap. 16) and in most instances is not related to a hemangioma.
   C. Secondary complications such as microcystoid degeneration of the overlying retina (see p. 418 in Chap. 11) and leakage of serous fluid into the subretinal space (see p. 423 in Chap. 11) are common.

NEUROFIBROMATOSIS
(von Recklinghausen's Disease)
(Figs. 2–3 through 2–6)

I. General information
   A. The onset of symptoms generally occurs in late childhood.
   B. Multiple tumors derived from Schwann cells of peripheral and sensory nerves and glial cells of the central nervous system are found.
   C. A superimposed malignant change (fibrosarcoma, neurofibrosarcoma, malignant schwannoma) may occur.
   D. The disease is transmitted as an irregular autosomal dominant with variable penetrance.
II. Ocular findings
   A. Eyelids
      1. "Cafe au lait" spot
      2. Neurofibromas
         a. Fibroma molluscum, i.e., the common neurofibroma, which results from a proliferation of the distal end of a nerve, producing a small localized skin tumor
         b. Plexiform neurofibroma ("bag of worms"), i.e., a diffuse proliferation within the nerve sheath, producing a grossly thickened and tortuous nerve
         c. Elephantiasis neuromatosa, i.e., a diffuse proliferation outside the nerve sheath, producing a marked thickening and folding of the skin
   B. Eyeball
      1. Thickening of corneal and conjunctival nerves
      2. Hamartomas in trabecular meshwork, uvea, retina and optic nerve head
         a. Mainly melanocytic nevi in trabecular meshwork and uvea

         The multiple, small, spider-like, melanocytic iris nevi clinically appear characteristic.

         b. Mainly glial hamartomas in retina and optic nerve head
      3. Congenital glaucoma

         If a plexiform neurofibroma of the eyelid is present (especially in the upper

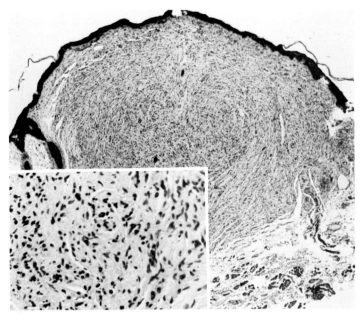

FIG. 2–3. Neurofibromatosis. Skin fibroma molluscum results from proliferation (mainly of Schwann cells) of the distal end of nerve. **Inset** is higher magnification to show neural elements. **Main figure,** H&E, ×21; **inset,** H&E, ×101.

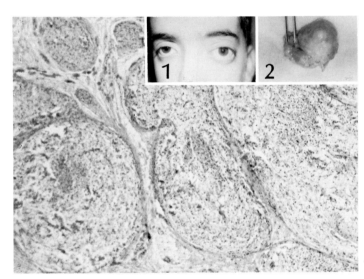

FIG. 2–4. Neurofibromatosis. Plexiform neurofibroma, diffuse proliferation of Schwann cells within nerve sheath, produces grossly thickened and tortuous nerves. **Main figure** shows section from gross specimen (**inset 2**) removed from left orbit and causing proptosis (**inset 1**). **Main figure,** H&E, ×16; **inset 1,** clinical; **inset 2,** macroscopic.

FIG. 2–5. Neurofibromatosis. **Inset** shows typical iris neurofibromas, which consist of collections of nevus cells (**main figure**) on surface of iris. **Main figure,** H&E, ×40; **inset,** clinical.

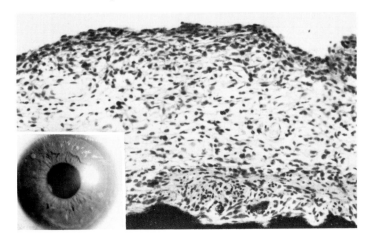

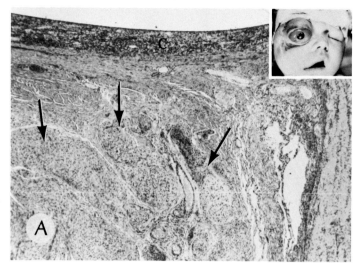

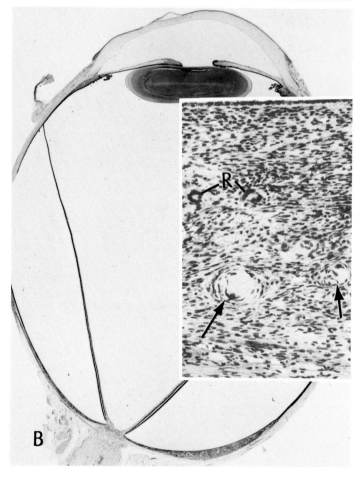

FIG. 2–6. Neurofibromatosis. **A. Inset** shows child born with neurofibromatosis. Plexiform neurofibroma (*arrows*) behind globe caused proptosis. Choroid (*c*) is thickened by hamartoma. **B.** Whole eye removed at autopsy from child shown in **A. Inset** shows high magnification of diffuse choroidal hamartoma. The hamartoma is composed of structures resembling tactile nerve endings (*arrows*), rosette formations (**R**) and cells resembling nevus cells. **A,** H&E, ×21; **inset,** clinical. **B,** H&E, ×3; **inset,** H&E, ×101.

eyelid), 50 percent of the eyes will have glaucoma.

C. Optic nerve
Optic nerve glioma

About ten percent of patients with gliomas of the optic nerve have neurofibromatosis.

D. Orbit
1. Plexiform neurofibroma
2. Neurilemmoma (schwannoma)
3. Absence of greater wing of sphenoid
4. Pulsating exophthalmos

The pulsating exophthalmos may be associated with an orbital encephalocele.

5. Enlarged optic foramen
III. Systemic findings
A. Hamartomas of the brain, spinal cord, meninges, cranial nerves, peripheral nerves and sympathetic nervous system may occur.
B. Pheochromocytoma has been reported infrequently.
C. Hamartomas of gastrointestinal tract and other viscera may be found.
IV. Histology
A. In the skin and orbit a diffuse, irregular proliferation of peripheral nerve elements (predominantly Schwann cells) results in an unencapsulated neurofibroma. The tumor is composed of numerous cells with elongated, basophilic nuclei and faintly granular cytoplasm associated with fine, wavy, "maidenhair," immature collagen fibers.
1. Nerve fibers can be seen frequently with special stains.
2. Vascularity is quite variable from tumor to tumor and within the same tumor.

Histologically neurofibromas are often confused with dermatofibromas, neurilemmomas or schwannomas (see p. 541 in Chap. 14) and leiomyomas (see p. 347 in Chap. 9).

B. In the eye the lesion may be a melanocytic nevus (see p. 656 in Chap. 17), slight or massive involvement of the uvea (usually choroid) by a mixture of hamartomatous neural and nevus elements or a glial hamartoma (see p. 36 in Chap. 2).

TUBEROUS* SCLEROSIS
(Bourneville's Disease; Pringle's Disease)
(Figs. 2–7 and 2–8)

I. General information
A. Onset of symptoms generally occurs during the first three years of life.
B. The triad of mental deficiency, seizures and adenoma sebaceum (angiofibroma) is the characteristic finding.

* The name originates from the shape of the tumors, i.e., like a potato or tuber in shape.

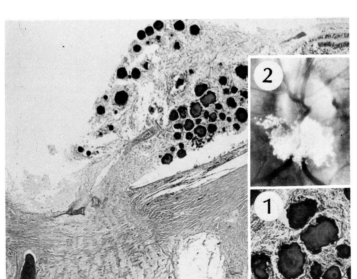

FIG. 2–7. Tuberous sclerosis. Glial hamartoma containing calcospherites replaces full thickness of retina next to optic disc. **Inset 1** is higher magnification of calcospherites presumably formed by glial cells. **Inset 2** shows clinical, "mulberry" appearance of retinal glial hamartoma. **Main figure,** H&E, ×40; **inset 1,** H&E, ×60; **inset 2,** clinical.

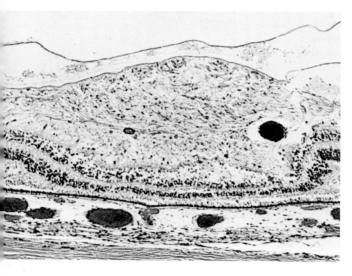

FIG. 2–8. Tuberous sclerosis. "Young" glial hamartoma in same eye shown in Figure 2–7 is composed of glial cells, without calcospherites, occupying the inner part of the retina. H&E, ×40.

C. The prognosis is poor with 75 percent dead by 20 years of age.

D. The disease is transmitted as in irregular autosomal dominant with low penetrance.

II. Ocular findings

   A. Lids

      Adenoma sebaceum (angiofibroma)

   B. Eyeball

     1. Glial hamartoma of retina in 53 percent of cases

      "Young" glial hamartomas of the retina have a smooth, spongy appearance with fuzzy borders, are gray white and may be mistaken for retinoblastoma. Older lesions appear condensed with an irregular surface, are white and appear as a *mulberry*. The whitened, wrinkled clinical appearance is due mainly to avascularity rather than to calcium deposition. The lesions frequently are multiple and vary in size from one-fifth to two disc diameters.

     2. Glial hamartoma of optic disc anterior to lamina cribrosa (*giant drusen*)

      The giant drusen of the optic nerve head may be mistaken for a swollen disc, i.e., pseudopapilledema. Most patients seen clinically with drusen of the optic nerve do not have tuberous sclerosis.

III. Systemic findings

   A. Glial hamartomas of the cerebrum occur quite commonly and result in epilepsy in 93 percent of cases, in mental deficiency in 62 percent of cases and in intracranial calcification in 51 percent of cases.

   B. Adenoma sebaceum (angiofibroma) of the skin of the face occurs in 83 percent of cases.

   C. Hamartomas of lung, heart and kidney may also be found.

IV. Histology

   A. Giant drusen of the optic disc occur anterior to the lamina cribosa and are glial hamartomas (see p. 510 in Chap. 13).

   B. Adenoma sebaceum are not tumors of the sebaceous gland apparatus but are angiofibromas (see p. 217 in Chap. 6).

   C. The glial hamartoma in the cerebrum (generally in the walls of the lateral ventricles over the basal ganglia) and retina are composed of large, fusiform astrocytes separated by a coarse and nonfibrillated, or finer and fibrillated, matrix formed from the astrocytic cell processes. Whereas the cerebral tumors usually are well vascularized, the retinal tumors generally are sparsely or nonvascularized. Calcospherites may be prominent, especially in older lesions.

ATAXIA–TELANGIECTASIA
(Louis-Bar Syndrome)

I. General information
   A. Ataxia–telangiectasia has its onset in infancy.
   B. The condition consists of progressive cerebellar ataxia, oculocutaneous telangiectasia and frequent pulmonary infection.
   C. The disease is transmitted as an autosomal recessive.

II. Ocular findings
   A. Telangiectasis (see p. 528 in Chap. 14) of conjunctiva occurs in 100 percent of cases.
   B. Peculiarity of eye movements (mainly nystagmus) also occurs in 100 percent of cases.
   C. Fixation nystagmus is found in 87 percent of cases.

III. Systemic findings
   A. Frequent findings are dysarthria and drooling, and dry coarse hair and skin.
   B. Infrequent findings are mental retardation and statural growth retardation.
   C. A number of immunologic defects may be found:
      1. Deficiency of immunoglobulin A (IgA).
      2. Structural abnormalities of thymus and lymph nodes.
      3. Prolonged survival of skin homografts.
      4. Impaired lymphocyte transformation.
      5. Lymphopenia.
      6. Lymphoreticular malignancies.
   D. Recurrent sinopulmonary infections are probably related to the immunologic defects.
   E. Diabetes mellitus may be found in these patients.

IV. Histology
   The basic lesion is one of telangiectasis (see p. 528 in Chap. 14).

ARTERIOVENOUS COMMUNICATION OF RETINA AND BRAIN
(Wyburn-Mason Syndrome) (Fig. 2–9)

I. General information
   A. The onset occurs in adolescence or early adulthood.
   B. Arteriovenous communication (arteriovenous aneurysm; cirsoid, racemose, serpentine, plexiform and cavernous angiomas) of the midbrain and retina associated with facial nevi and mental changes are found.
   C. The retinal lesion usually is unilateral and differs from that of angiomatosis retinae and ataxia–telangiectasia in that:

FIG. 2–9. Arteriovenous communication is present within retina.

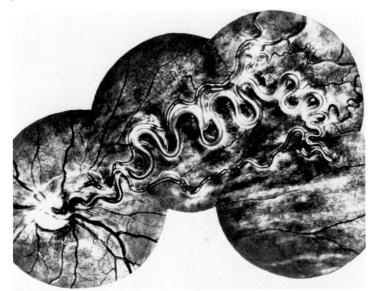

1. Angiomatosis retinae's retinal lesion is a tumor of blood vessels and stromal cells, i.e., a hemangioblastoma (see p. 528 in Chap. 14).
2. Ataxia–telangiectasia's retinal lesion is an excess of normal capillaries, i.e., a vascular malformation or telangiectasis (see p. 528 in Chap. 14) or capillary formations consisting of abnormally dilated and tortuous capillaries.
3. Wyburn-Mason's retinal lesion is a lack of normal capillaries, i.e., a vascular malformation, or arteriovenous communication (see p. 528 in Chap. 14) or arteriovenous connection, lacking a capillary bed between artery and vein.

D. The syndrome has a familial occurrence.

II. Ocular findings
  A. Nonprogressive arteriovenous aneurysms.
  B. Strabismus, gaze palsies and diplopia.
  C. Pulsating exophthalmos.
  D. Visual loss.
  E. Ptosis.

III. Systemic findings
  A. Arteriovenous aneurysm of midbrain.
  B. Weber's syndrome.
  C. Intracranial calcification.

IV. Histology
The basic lesion is an arteriovenous connection, bypassing a capillary bed (see p. 528 in Chap. 14).

CHROMOSOMAL ABERRATIONS

Normally the human cell is *diploid* and contains 46 chromosomes: 44 autosomal chromosomes and 2 sex chromosomes (XX in a female and XY in a male). The individual chromosomes may be arranged in an array according to morphologic characteristics. The resultant array of chromosomes is called a *karyotype*. A karyotype is made by photographing a cell in metaphase, cutting out the individual chromosomes and arranging them in pairs in chart form according to predetermined morphologic criteria i.e., karyotype (Fig. 2–10). The paired chromosomes are designated in numbers in one system and in letters in another system. In genetic shorthand 46 (XX) means that there are 46 chromo-

somes with a female pattern and 46 (XY) means that there are 46 chromosomes with a male pattern. Paired chromosomes 13, 14 and 15 appear morphologically identical (unless special techniques such as autoradiography or chromosomal band patterns as shown with fluorescent quinacrine are used) and therefore are called the 13–15 group in one system and the D group in another system. In trisomy 13–15 there is an extra chromosome in the 13–15 group. Trisomy 13–15 may be written 47, 13–15+ or 47, D+, meaning 47 chromosomes with an extra chromosome (+) in the 13–15 or D group. Similarly, the paired chromosomes 18 are part of the E group and the paired chromosomes 21 are part of the G group. Therefore, 47, 18+ (E+) means trisomy 18, and 47, 21+ (G+) means trisomy 21 or mongolism. Chromosomes may be normal in total number, i.e., 46, but may have structural alterations of individual chromosomes. The genetic shorthand for structural alterations of individual chromosomes is as follows: p = short arm; q = long arm; + = increase in length; − = decrease in length; r = ring form; and t = translocation. Therefore 46, 18 p− means a normal number of chromosomes, but one of the two number 18 chromosomes has a deletion (decrease in length) of its short arms. Similarly, 46, 18q− and 46, 18r means a normal number of chromosomes but a deletion of the long arms or a ring form, respectively, of one of the two 18 chromosomes. There may be too few chromosomes, e.g., in 45(X) (Turner's syndrome),

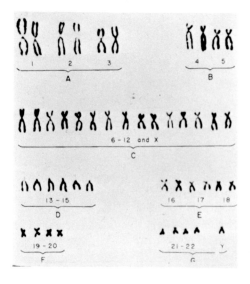

FIG. 2–10. Normal male karyotype with 44 autosomal chromosomes and 2 sex chromosomes (XY).

where there are only 45 chromosomes with one of the sex chromosomes missing. The type of chromosomal abnormality, however, has little to do with specific ocular malformations. In fact, except for the presence of cartilage in a ciliary body coloboma in trisomy 13–15, no ocular malformations or combinations thereof appear specific for any chromosomal abnormality.

TRISOMY 13–15
(47, 13–15+ [D+]; Patau's Syndrome)
(Figs. 2–11 through 2–16)

I. General information
   A. Trisomy 13–15 results from an extra chromosome in the 13–15 (D) group of autosomal chromosomes, i.e., one set of chromosomes exists in triplicate rather than as a pair. An accidental failure of disjunction of one pair of chromosomes during meiosis (meiotic nondisjunction) causes the abnormality.

   Autoradiographic studies have shown that the extra chromosome belongs in the number 13 chromosome group.

   B. The condition, which is present in 1 in 14,000 live births, usually is lethal by 6 months of age. There is no sex predilection.
   C. Because the condition was described in the prekaryotype era, many names refer to the same entity: arhinencephaly, oculocerebral syndrome, encephaloophthalmic dysplasia, bilateral retinal dysplasia (Reese-Blodi-Straatsma syndrome), anophthalmia and mesodermal dysplasia (cleft palate).
   D. Ocular anomalies, generally quite severe, occur in all cases.
II. Systemic findings. These include mental retardation; low set and malformed ears; hairlip or cleft palate or both; sloping forehead; facial angiomas; cryptorchidism; narrow, hyperconvex fingernails; fingers flexed or overlapping or both; polydactyly of hands or feet or both; posterior prominence of the heels ("rocker bottom feet"); characteristic features of the dermal ridge pattern, including transverse palmar creases; cardiac and renal abnor-

malities; absence or hypoplasia of the olfactory lobes (arhinencephaly); bicornuate uterus; apneic spells; apparent deafness; minor motor seizures; and hypotonia.
III. Ocular findings
   A. Bilateral microphthalmos is common and may be extreme so as to mimic anophthalmos, i.e., clinical anophthalmos. In rare instances synophthalmos (cyclops) can occur.

   Anophthalmos is a difficult diagnosis to make clinically. Only through serial histologic sections of the orbital contents can the diagnosis of anophthalmos be substantiated.

   B. Coloboma of the iris and ciliary body, cataract and persistent hyperplastic primary vitreous (PHPV) are present in most (about 80 percent) of the eyes.
   C. Retinal dysplasia is found in at least 75 percent of eyes. Retinal folds and microcystoid degeneration of the retina also are common findings.

   When retinal dysplasia is unilateral and the other eye is normal, the condition generally is unassociated with trisomy 13–15 or other systemic anomalies.

   D. Mesodermal dysgenesis of the cornea and iris is present in at least 60 percent of eyes.
IV. Histology
   A. The coloboma of the iris and ciliary body frequently contains a mesodermal

FIG. 2–11. Trisomy 13–15. Karyotype shows extra chromosome (7 instead of 6) in 13–15 or D group. (#13)

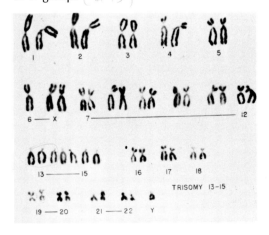

TRISOMY 13-15

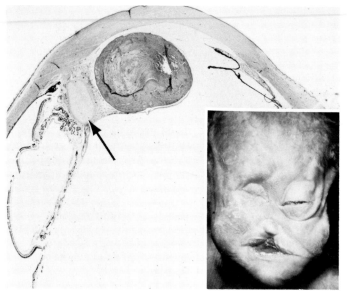

FIG. 2–12. Trisomy 13–15. Coloboma of iris and anterior ciliary body is filled with mesodermal tissue containing cartilage (*arrow*). Retina just behind cartilage is dysplastic. **Inset** shows apparent anophthalmos of right eye, microphthalmos of left eye, abnormal nose and cleft upper lip. **Main figure,** H&E, ×6; **inset,** clinical.

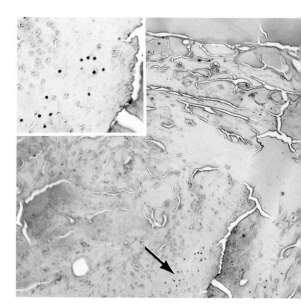

FIG. 2–13. Trisomy 13–15. Cataractous lens shows retention of lens cell nuclei in the embryonic lens nucleus (*arrow*), which is under higher magnification in **inset. Main figure,** H&E, ×100; **inset,** H&E, ×200.

FIG. 2–14. Trisomy 13–15. Persistent posterior hyaloid system (*arrow*) present. Falciform retinal fold (*R*) is also seen. Macroscopic.

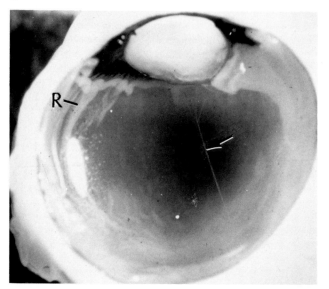

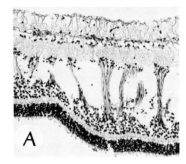 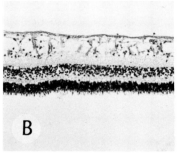

FIG. 2–15. Trisomy 13–15. Both typical (**A**) and reticular (**B**) microcystoid degeneration of the retina are seen. **A,** H&E, ×100; **B,** H&E, ×37.

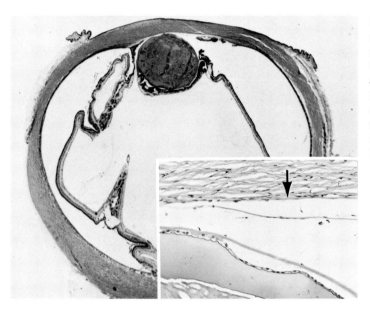

FIG. 2–16. Trisomy 13–15. Mesodermal dysgenesis of iris and cornea (Rieger's syndrome) is present. **Inset** is higher magnification of central cornea to show localized absence of central corneal endothelium and Descemet's membrane (Peters' anomaly or ectodermal–mesodermal dysgenesis of cornea). *Arrow* shows ending of Descemet's membrane. **Main figure,** H&E, ×3; **inset,** H&E, ×100.

connection between sclera and the retrolental area. Cartilage is present within the mesodermal tissue in about 65 percent of cases, most commonly when the eyes are small, i.e., 10 mm or under.

Although ocular cartilage has been reported in embryonal medulloepithelioma, in chromosome 18 deletion defect, in angiomatosis retinae and in an otherwise healthy individual, it is not present in these conditions within a coloboma of the ciliary body. Intraocular cartilage within a coloboma of the ciliary body, therefore, seems diagnostic of trisomy 13–15.

B. The cataract may be quite similar to that seen in rubella with retention of lens cell nuclei in the embryonic lens nucleus. Anterior subcapsular, anterior and posterior cortical, nuclear, and posterior subcapsular cataractous changes also may be seen.

C. The pathology of PHPV (see p. 698 in Chap. 18), retinal dysplasia (see p. 390 in Chap. 11) and typical and reticular microcystoid degeneration of the retina (see section Microcystoid Degeneration in Chap. 11) is discussed elsewhere.

D. Mesodermal dysgenesis in the form of Peters' anomaly (p. 265 in Chap. 8), Rieger's syndrome (p. 268 in Chap. 8) and an immature anterior chamber angle is noted frequently.

TRISOMY 18
(47, 18+ [E+]; Edwards' Syndrome) (Fig. 2–17)

I. General information
    A. Trisomy 18 results from an extra chromosome in the 17–18 (E) group of autosomal chromosomes.
    B. The condition has about the same incidence as trisomy 13–15, i.e., 1 in 14,000 live births, and similarly proves fatal at an early age. Females are predominantly affected.
    C. Ocular malformations, generally of a minor nature, occur in about 50 percent of cases.
II. Systemic findings. Included are mental retardation; low set, malformed and rotated ears; micrognathia; narrow palatal arch; head with prominent occiput, relatively flattened laterally; short sternum; narrow pelvis, often with luxation of hips; fingers flexed, with the index overlapping third and/or fifth overlapping fourth; hallux short, dorsiflexed; characteristic features of the dermal ridge pattern including an exceptionally high number of arches; cardiac and renal malformations; Meckel's diverticulum; heterotopic pancreatic tissue; severe debility; and moderate hypertonicity.
III. Ocular findings. These tend to be minor and mainly involve the lids and bony orbit. They include narrow palpebral fissures, ptosis, epicanthus, hypoplastic supraorbital ridges, exophthalmos, hypertelorism or hypotelorism and nystagmus. Rare ocular anomalies include corneal opacities, anisocoria, uveal and optic disc colobomas, cataract, microphthalmos, severe myopia, megalocornea, keratitis, scleral icterus, bluish sclera, persistent hyaloid artery, absent retinal pigmentation, and irregular retinal vascular pattern.
IV. Histology—mainly related to hyperplasia, hypertrophy and cellular abnormalities.
    A. Corneal epithelium, mainly in the basal layer, may show cellular hypertrophy, swelling, disintegration, bizarre chromatin patterns, and atypical mitoses. Hyperplasia of the corneal endothelium may be present and may be focal or diffuse.
    B. Posterior subcapsular cataracts, minor

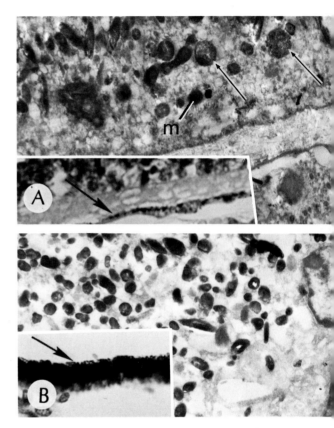

FIG. 2–17. Trisomy 18. **A.** Electron micrograph of hypopigmented posterior retinal pigment epithelium showing many immature melanosomes (*arrows*) but only a few mature melanosomes (*m*). **Inset** shows light microscopic appearance of hypopigmented posterior retinal pigment epithelium (*arrow*). **B.** Electron micrograph of anterior retinal pigment epithelium, which contains mainly mature melanosomes. **Inset** shows light microscopic appearance of relatively normal anterior retinal pigment epithelium (*arrow*). **A,** ×6,000; **inset,** H&E, ×256. **B,** ×6,000; **inset,** H&E, ×256.

retinal changes (gliosis, hemorrhage) and optic atrophy may be seen. The retinal pigment epithelium may show hypopigmented and hyperpigmented areas. In addition, severe optic disc colobomas have been reported.

TRISOMY 21
(47, 21+ [G+]; Down's Syndrome; Mongolism)
(Figs. 2–18 and 2–19)

I. General information
   A. Trisomy 21 results from an extra chromosome in the 21 (G) group of autosomal chromosomes.
   B. The condition is the most common autosomal trisomy with an incidence of 1 in 700 live births (in white populations). Major ocular malformations are rare.
II. Systemic findings. These include severe mental retardation; flat nasal bridge; an open mouth with a furrowed, protruding tongue and small, malformed teeth; prominent malformed ears with absent lobes; a flat occiput with a short broad neck; loose skin at the back of the neck and over the shoulders (in early infancy); short, broad hands; short, curved little fingers with dysplastic middle phalanx; specific features of the dermal ridge, including a transverse palmar crease; cardiovascular defects; Apert's syndrome; and anomalous hematological and biochemical traits.
III. Ocular findings. Included are hypertelorism, oblique or arched palpebral fissures, epicanthus, ectropion, speckled iris (*Brushfield spots*), esotropia, high myopia, excessive retinal vessels crossing the margin of the optic disc, chronic conjunctivitis, keratoconus (sometimes acute), and lens opacities.
IV. Histology
   A. Brushfield spots consist of areas of relatively normal iris stroma that are surrounded by a ring of mild iris hypoplasia.
   B. The cataract may have abnormal anterior lens capsular excrescences similar to that seen in Lowe's syndrome and Miller's syndrome.
   C. Keratoconus is discussed elsewhere (see p. 306 in Chap. 8).

The above three trisomies are all autosomal chromosomal trisomies. An example of a sex chromosomal trisomy is *Klinefelter's syndrome* (47, XXY); the ocular pathology in this condition is not

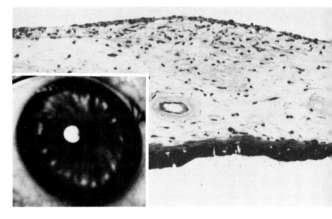

FIG. 2–18. Trisomy 21. **Inset** shows Brushfield spots in iris of person with Down's syndrome. **Main figure** shows light microscopy of same iris. Brushfield spot seen as area of relatively normal iris stroma surrounded by hypoplastic iris. **Main figure,** PAS, ×101; **inset,** clinical.

FIG. 2–19. Trisomy 21. Posterior subcapsular cataract seen in lens showing many artifactitious disruptions. **Inset** shows higher magnification of posterior subcapsular cortical degeneration. **Main figure,** H&E, ×16; **inset,** PAS, ×252.

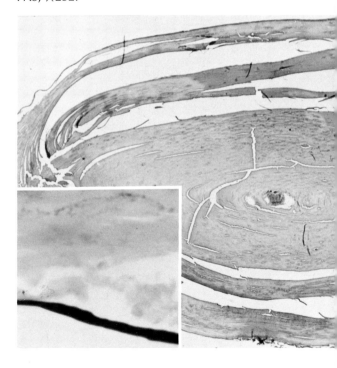

striking. In *XYY* syndrome (47, XYY) the patients have normal height, psychic and social problems, gonadal atrophy, luxated lenses and iris and choroid colobomas.

46 5p—

CHROMOSOME 5 DELETION DEFECT
(46, 5p—; Cri du Chat Syndrome)

I. General information
  A. Chromosome 5 deletion defect results from a deletion of part of the short arm of chromosome 5 (46, 5p—). Only one of the two chromosomes of the chromosome 5 pair is affected.
  B. Many newborn infants with the defect have an abnormal cry that sounds like a cat, hence the name "cri du chat" syndrome. The abnormal cry generally disappears as the child grows older.
  C. The defect is compatible with longevity.
II. Systemic findings. Included are severe mental retardation, low set ears, microcephaly, micrognathia, "moon-shaped" face, short neck, transverse palmar creases, scoliosis and kyphosis, curved fifth fingers, limitation of flexion or extension of fingers and abnormalities of the cardiovascular system and kidneys.
III. Ocular findings. These include hypertelorism, epicanthus, mongoloid or antimongoloid eyelid fissures, exotropia, optic atrophy, tortuous retinal artery and veins and pupils supersensitive to 2.5 percent methacholine.
IV. Histologic ocular findings have not been reported.

CHROMOSOME 13 DELETION DEFECT

See p. 686 in Chap. 18. *(Retinoblastoma)*

CHROMOSOME 18 DELETION DEFECT   *46, 18p— or*
(46, 18p—; 46, 18q—; or 46, 18r; Partial 18 Monosomy)
(Figs. 2–20 through 2–22)

I. General information
  A. Chromosome 18 deletion defect results from a straight deletion of part of the short arm of chromosome 18 (46, 18p—), part of the long arm (46, 18q—) or parts or all of the long and short arms resulting in a ring form (46, 18r). Only one of the two chromo-

somes of the chromosome 18 pair is affected.
  B. No specific ocular abnormalities relate to the different forms of deletion.
  C. The defect is compatible with longevity.
II. Systemic findings. These include low set ears, nasal abnormalities, external genital abnormalities, hepatosplenomegaly, cardiovascular abnormalities and holoprosencephaly.
III. Ocular findings. Included are hypertelorism; epicanthus; ptosis; strabismus; nystagmus; myopia; glaucoma; microphthalmos; microcornea; corneal opacities; posterior keratoconus; Brushfield spots; cataract; uveal colobomas, including microphthalmos with cyst; retinal abnormalities; optic atrophy; and cyclops.
IV. Histology
  A. Microphthalmos with cyst (see p. 516 in Chap. 14) and uveal colobomas are discussed elsewhere (see p. 329 in Chap. 9).
  B. Intrascleral cartilage and intrachoroidal smooth muscle may be present anterior to and associated with a coloboma of the choroid.
  C. Other findings include hypoplasia of the iris, immature anterior chamber angle, persistent tunica vasculosa lentis, cataract, retinal dysplasia and retinal nonattachment.

45 X

Turner's syndrome (Figs. 2–23 and 2–24) (gonadal dysgenesis; Bonnevie-Ullrich syndrome; ovarian agenesis; and ovarian dysgenesis) generally is due to only one sex chromosome being present, the X chromosome (45, X). Some cases, however, are due to X long arm isochromosome (46, X [Xqi]), X deletion defect of the short arm (46, X [Xp—]) or X deletion (partial or complete) of all arms resulting in a ring chromosome (46, X [Xr]). Ocular findings include epicanthus, blepharoptosis, myopia, strabismus and nystagmus. In *Noonan's syndrome* ocular anomalies are even more frequent than in Turner's syndrome and include antimongoloid slant of the palpebral fissures, hypertelorism, epicanthus, blepharoptosis, exophthalmos, keratoconus, high myopia and posterior embryotoxon. Noonan's syndrome (Bonnevie-Ullrich or Ullrich syndrome; XX Turner phenotype or "female Turner"; and XY Turner phenotype or "male Turner") is an inherited (inherited pattern is controversial) condition in which the individuals (either men or women) phenotypically resemble Turner's syndrome but have a normal karyotype (46, XY or XX).

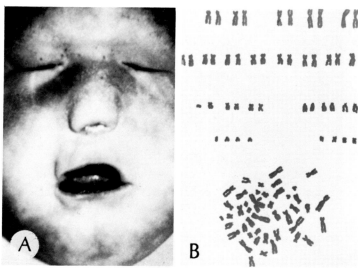

FIG. 2–20. Chromosome 18 deletion defect. **A.** Abnormal facies showing nose with single opening. **B.** Karyotype of child shown in **A** (46, XX, 18r). **A,** clinical; **B,** karyotype.

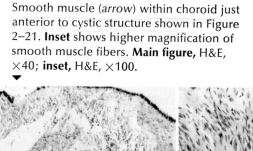

FIG. 2–22. Chromosome 18 deletion defect. Smooth muscle (*arrow*) within choroid just anterior to cystic structure shown in Figure 2–21. **Inset** shows higher magnification of smooth muscle fibers. **Main figure,** H&E, ×40; **inset,** H&E, ×100.

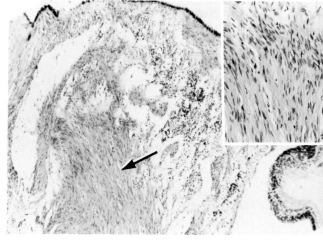

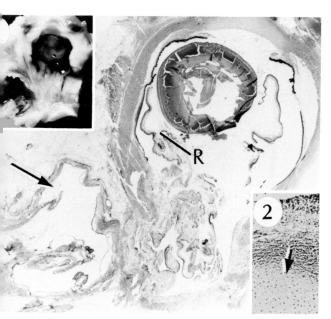

FIG. 2–21. Chromosome 18 deletion defect. Microphthalmic eye from child shown in Figure 2–20A. Retina (*R*) nonattached and dysplastic. Large cyst (*arrow*) connected to eye. **Inset 1** shows macroscopic appearance of eye. **Inset 2** shows cartilage (*arrow*) within sclera. **Main figure,** H&E, ×4; **inset 1,** macroscopic; **inset 2,** H&E, ×50.

FIG. 2–23. Turner's syndrome. Leukokoria with telangiectatic vessels on surface of an exudatively detached retina in a child with Turner's syndrome (45 ×). **Inset** shows opened enucleated eye from same child. **Main figure,** clinical; **inset,** macroscopic.

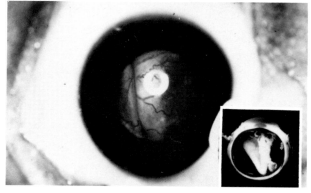

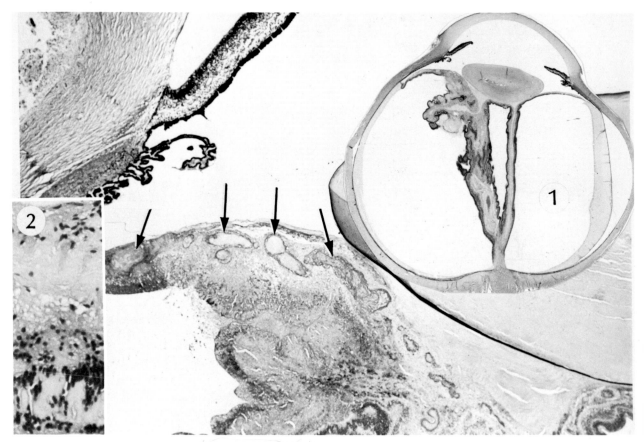

FIG. 2–24. Turner's syndrome and Coats's disease. Microscopic appearance of eye seen in Figure 2–23 shows abnormal telangiectatic retinal vessels characteristic of Coats's disease (*arrows*), rubeosis iridis and peripheral anterior synechia. **Inset 1** shows whole eye with exudatively detached retina. **Inset 2** shows area of retina near abnormal retinal vessels, demonstrating exudate spreading out, and causing necrosis of, outer retinal layers. **Main figure,** PAS, ×32; **inset 1,** H&E, ×3; **inset 2,** H&E, ×136.

MOSAICISM

I. General information
   A. When two or more populations of karyotypically distinct chromosomes are found in cells from a single individual, chromosomal mosaicism is present.

   It is now usual to refer to individuals containing mixtures of cells derived from different zygotes as *chimeras* (e.g., in a true hermaphrodite 46 XX, 46 XY) and to reserve the term mosaic for individuals with cell mixtures arising from a single zygote.

   B. Mosaicism may occur in most of the previously described chromosomal abnormalities.

II. Tetraploid–diploid mosaicism (92/46) (Fig. 2–25)

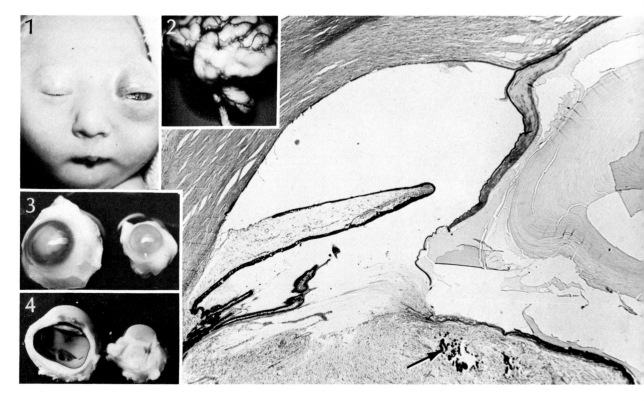

FIG. 2–25. Tetraploid–diploid mosaicism.
Inset 1 shows child with peculiar facies.
Proptosis of left eye due to orbital cellulitis
and endophthalmitis. **Inset 2** shows abnormal
brain. **Insets 3** and **4** show unopened (**3**) and
opened (**4**) mildly microphthalmic right eye
(left) and markedly microphthalmic and
phthisical left eye (right). **Main figure** of right
eye demonstrates peripheral anterior
synechia, ectropion uveae, cataract adherent
to posterior cornea and detached, gliotic
retina containing calcium (*arrow*). **Main
figure,** H&E, ×25; **inset 1,** clinical; **inset 2,**
macroscopic of brain; **inset 3,** macroscopic
unopened eyes; **inset 4,** macroscopic opened
eyes.

A. In tetraploid–diploid mosaicism two karyotypically distinct populations of cells exist: a large size cell with increased DNA content containing 92 chromosomes (tetraploid) and a normal size cell with a normal complement of 46 chromosomes (diploid). The condition is incompatible with longevity.

B. Systemic findings include micrognathia, horizontal palmar creases, deformities of the fingers and toes, cardiovascular abnormalities, microcephalus and maturation arrest of the forebrain.

C. Ocular anomalies include microphthalmos, corneal opacities and leukokoria.

D. Histologically the eyes may show rubeosis iridis, anterior peripheral synechias, luxated and cataractous lens, nonattachment of the retina and massive hyperplasia of the pigment epithelium.

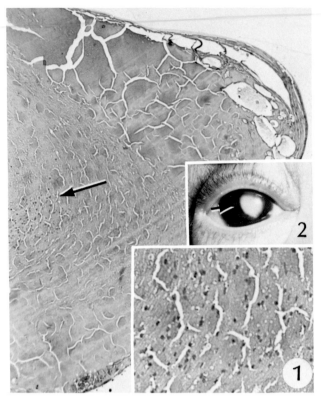

FIG. 2–26. Rubella. Anterior and equatorial cortical and nuclear (*arrow*) cataract present. **Inset 1** is higher magnification of area near arrow in main figure showing retention of lens cell nuclei in the embryonic nucleus. **Inset 2** shows dense nuclear cataract surrounded by less dense cortical cataract (*arrow* shows edge of pupil). **Main figure,** H&E, ×38; **inset 1,** H&E, ×120; **inset 2,** clinical.

INFECTIOUS EMBRYOPATHY

TOXOPLASMOSIS

See p. 94 in Chapter 4.

CYTOMEGALIC INCLUSION DISEASE

See p. 98 in Chapter 4.

CONGENITAL RUBELLA SYNDROME
(Gregg's Syndrome) (Figs. 2–26 through 2–30)

   I. Congenital rubella syndrome consists of cataracts, cardiovascular defects, mental retardation and deafness. The syndrome results from maternal rubella infection during pregnancy (50 percent of fetuses affected if mother contracts rubella during first four weeks of pregnancy; 20 percent affected if contracted during first trimester).

  II. Systemic findings. These include low birth weight; deafness; congenital heart defects (especially patent ductus arteriosus); central nervous system abnormalities; thrombocytopenic purpura; diabetes mellitus; osteomyelitis; dental abnormalities; pneumonitis; hepatomegaly; and genitourinary anomalies.

 III. Ocular findings include cataract, congenital glaucoma, iris abnormalities and a secondary pigmentary retinopathy.

     In one study of 328 cases of congenital rubella the rubella retinopathy was the most characteristic finding and was shown to be progressive in at least nine cases. In the same study 30 percent had cataracts and 9 percent had glaucoma. When rubella cataract was present, congenital glaucoma was present in 9 percent of cases, and when congenital glaucoma was present, cataract was present in 33 percent of cases. Congenital rubella cataract and glaucoma, therefore, occur together at the frequency expected of coincidental events occurring independently.

 IV. The rubella virus can pass through the placenta, infect the fetus and thereby cause abnormal embryogenesis.

     The rubella virus can survive within the lens for at least three years after birth. Surgery on rubella cataracts may release the virus into the interior of the eye and cause an endophthalmitis. To prevent this it has been suggested that needling and aspiration of congenital rubella cataracts should be done as a one-step procedure.

  V. Histology
    A. Retention of lens cell nuclei in the embryonic lens nucleus is characteristic (but not pathognomonic—see trisomy 13–15 above and Leigh's disease below). Anterior and posterior cortical lens degenerative and dysplastic lens changes also may be seen.
    B. The iris shows poor development of its dilator muscle and necrosis of its epithelium along with a chronic, nongranulomatous inflammatory reaction.

     The combination of the dilator muscle abnormality and chronic inflammation

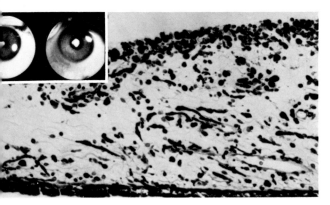

FIG. 2–27. Rubella. Iris is atrophic, infiltrated with plasma cells and lymphocytes (chronic nongranulomatous iritis) and shows loss of its dilator muscle. **Inset** shows same eye before (left) and after (right) maximal dilatation with mydriatics. Dense nuclear cataract is seen in the minimally dilated pupil. **Main figure,** H&E, ×130; **inset,** clinical.

FIG. 2–28. Rubella. Chronic nongranulomatous inflammatory infiltrate present in ciliary body. Some necrosis of pigment epithelium is seen. H&E, ×130.

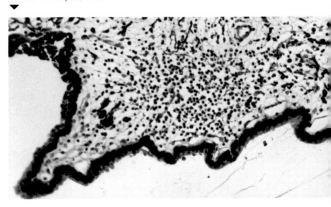

FIG. 2–29. Rubella. The mottled, "salt and pepper" appearance in the peripheral fundus (**main figure**) and the coarse pigmentation seen near the macula (**inset 1**) is due to alternating areas of retinal pigment epithelial atrophy (*arrow* in **inset 2**) and hypertrophy (**inset 3**). **Main figure,** fundus; **inset 1,** fundus; **inset 2,** H&E, ×630; **inset 3,** H&E, ×630.

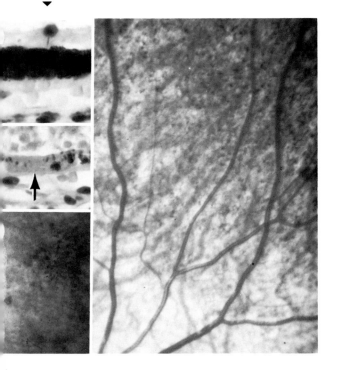

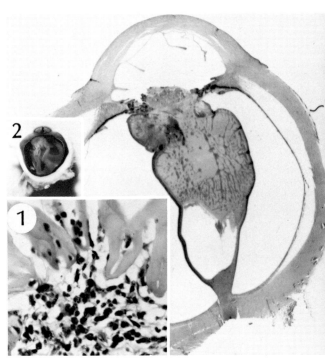

FIG. 2–30. Rubella. Total retinal detachment due to cyclitic membrane, seemingly centered around lens remnants. **Inset 1** demonstrates lens remnants in pupillary region surrounded by chronic nongranulomatous inflammation. **Inset 2** shows macroscopic appearance of same eye in which needling and aspiration for rubella cataract was done some months prior to enucleation. **Main figure,** H&E, ×5; **inset 1,** H&E, ×200; **inset 2,** macroscopic.

frequently causes the iris to dilate poorly and to appear "leathery."

C. The ciliary body shows necrosis of its pigment epithelium with pigment phagocytosis by macrophages and a chronic nongranulomatous inflammatory reaction.

D. With congenital glaucoma the anterior chamber angle appears as it does in the genetic congenital glaucoma (see section Congenital Glaucoma in Chap. 16).

E. Atrophy and hypertrophy, frequently in alternating areas of retinal pigment epithelium (RPE), is seen in most, if not all, cases.

It is this RPE abnormality that results in the clinically observed "salt and pepper" fundus of rubella retinopathy.

F. Following cataract or iris surgery, complications due to virus infection may cause a chronic nongranulomatous inflammatory reaction around lens remnants and secondary disruption of intraocular tissues with fibroblastic overgrowth, resulting in cyclitic membrane and retinal detachment.

CONGENITAL SYPHILIS

See p. 272 in Chapter 8.

DRUG EMBRYOPATHY

THALIDOMIDE (Fig. 2–31)

I. Thalidomide ingestion during the first trimester of pregnancy may result in a condition known as phocomelia, i.e., the condition of having the limbs extremely shortened so that the feet or hands arise close to the trunk.

II. Ocular findings include paresis of ocular muscles, uveal colobomas, microphthalmos or anophthalmos.

III. Histologically hypoplasia of the iris and colobomas of the uvea (see pp. 329–332 in Chap. 9) and optic nerve (see p. 486 in Chap. 13) may be seen.

LYSERGIC ACID DIETHYLAMIDE (LSD) (Fig. 2–32)

I. LSD ingestion during the first trimester of pregnancy may result in multiple central nervous system and ocular abnormalities.

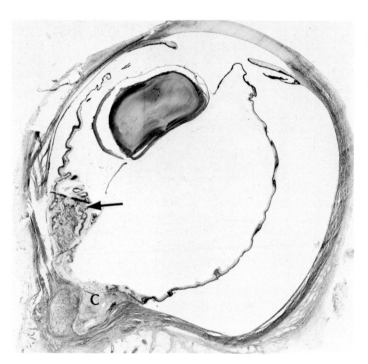

FIG. 2–31. Thalidomide embryopathy. Coloboma of optic disc (c), focal areas of retinal dysplasia over choroidal coloboma (arrow) and hypoplasia of iris (especially on left side). H&E, ×4.

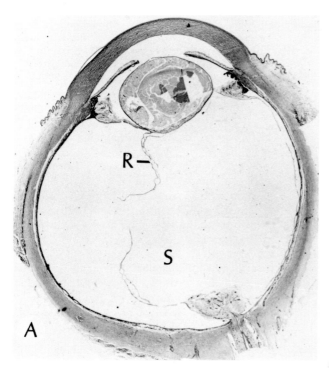

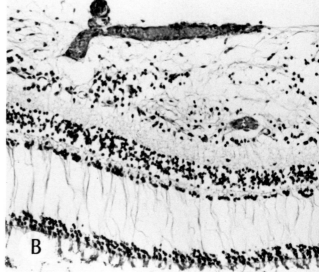

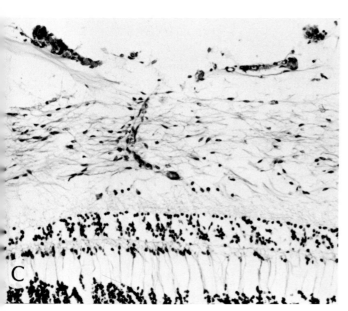

FIG. 2–32. LSD embryopathy. Mother took LSD (and other drugs) during entire pregnancy. **A.** Microphthalmic right eye shows cataract, nonattachment of retina and retinoschisis. *R*, retina with narrow part of schisis; *S*, large schisis cavity. **B** and **C.** Posterior retina of left eye demonstrates areas of neovascularization with new vessels growing out of the retina onto the internal surface of the retina simulating retrolental fibroplasia (baby weighed 7 lb, 8 oz at birth and had no oxygen administration). **A,** PAS, ×6; **B,** H&E, ×101; **C,** H&E, ×101.

II. CNS abnormalities include arhinencephaly; fusion of the frontal lobes; Arnold-Chiari malformation with hydrocephalus; and absence of the normal convolutional pattern in cerebral hemispheres and of foliar markings in the cerebellum.

III. Ocular findings include cataract and microphthalmia.

IV. Histologically the lens may show anterior and posterior cortical degeneration and posterior migration of lens epithelial nuclei, and the retina may contain a posterior retinitis proliferans and juvenile retinoschisis.

OTHER CONGENITAL ANOMALIES

CYCLOPIA AND SYNOPHTHALMOS (Fig. 2–33)

I. Cyclopia (or synophthalmos) is a condition in which anterior brain and midline mesodermal structures develop anomalously. The condition is incompatible with life.

II. In the brain there is a failure in division of the telencephalon (future cerebral hemispheres), a development of a large dorsal cyst and a lack of midline structures such as the corpus callosum, septum pel-

lucidum, olfactory lobes and neurohypophysis.

III. The orbital region is grossly deformed due to a failure of the frontonasal bony processes to develop so that the maxillary processes fuse, resulting in an absent nasal cavity and a single central cavity or "pseudoorbit." The nose generally is present as a rudimentary proboscis above the pseudoorbit.

IV. If only one eye is present (i.e., complete and total fusion of the two eyes) in the pseudoorbit, the condition is called cyclopia. A much more common situation is synophthalmos wherein two eyes are present in differing degrees of fusion, but never complete fusion.

V. Histologically in cyclopia the one eye may be relatively normal, completely anomalous, or all degrees in between. In synophthalmos the partially fused two eyes may

FIG. 2–33. Synophthalmos. Incomplete fusion of two eyes, each of which is relatively normal. *Arrow* points to intrascleral cartilage shown with higher magnification in **inset 1. Inset 2** is picture of child from whom eye was obtained; note proboscis above pseudorbit. **Main figure,** H&E, ×5; **Inset 1,** H&E, ×16; **inset 2,** clinical.

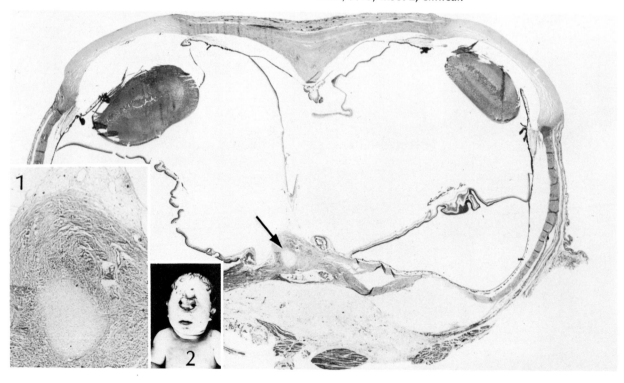

be relatively normal, totally anomalous, or all degrees in between.

ANENCEPHALY

I. Anencephaly is the most serious congenital malformation that occurs spontaneously in man and is compatible with completion of pregnancy. The condition is characterized by absence of the cranial vault, and the cerebral hemispheres are missing completely or reduced to small masses attached to the base of the skull.

II. Macroscopically the eyes are normal. Histologically the main finding is hypoplasia (or atrophy) of the retinal ganglion cell and nerve fiber layers and of the optic nerve. Uncommonly, uveal colobomas, retinal dysplasia, corneal dermoids, anterior chamber angle anomalies and vascular proliferative retinal changes may be seen.

ANOPHTHALMOS

I. The differentiation between anophthalmos or complete absence of the eye and extreme microphthalmos or a rudimentary small eye can only be made by the examination of serial, histologic sections of the orbit. The differentiation cannot be made clinically.

The term *clinical anophthalmos* is applied to the condition where no eye can be found clinically.

II. Three types of anophthalmos are recognized:

A. *Primary anophthalmos* due to a suppression of the optic anlage during the mosaic differentiation of the optic plate after formation of the rudiment of the forebrain—occurs before the 2-mm stage of embryonic development.

B. *Secondary anophthalmos* due to the complete suppression or grossly anomalous development of the entire anterior portion of the neural tube.

C. *Consecutive or degenerative anophthalmos* due to atrophy or degeneration of the optic vesicle after it has been initially formed.

III. Histologically serial sections of the orbit fail to show any ocular tissue.

MICROPHTHALMOS

I. The differentiation between microphthalmos and anophthalmos is discussed above.

II. Three types of microphthalmos are recognized:

A. Pure microphthalmos (*nanophthalmos*) wherein the eye is smaller than normal in size but has no other gross abnormalities. These eyes generally are hypermetropic, may have retinal macular hypoplasia and are susceptible to acute angle closure glaucoma.

B. Microphthalmos with cyst—see p. 332 in Chapter 9 and p. 516 in Chapter 14.

C. Microphthalmos associated with other systemic anomalies, e.g., in trisomy 13–15 and congenital rubella. This type of microphthalmos is discussed in the appropriate sections.

III. Histologically the eye ranges from essentially normal in nanophthalmos to rudimentary in clinical anophthalmos, and all degrees in between (see under appropriate sections).

OCULOCEREBRORENAL SYNDROME OF MILLER (Fig. 2–34)

I. Miller's syndrome consists of Wilms's tumor, congenital nonfamilial aniridia* and genitourinary anomalies. Mental and growth retardation, microcephaly and deformities of the pinna also may be present.

II. In individuals without Wilms's tumor the incidence of aniridia* is 1 in 50,000; with Wilms's tumor the incidence is 1 in 73. The cause of this association is not known.

III. Histologically the iris is hypoplastic and rudimentary.* The cataract shows cortical degenerative changes and capsular excrescences similar to that seen in trisomy 21 and Lowe's syndrome (see p. 360 in Chap. 10).

SUBACUTE NECROTIZING ENCEPHALOMYELOPATHY (Leigh's Disease)

I. Leigh's disease is a central nervous system disorder characterized by onset between two months and six years of age; feeding difficul-

---

* Aniridia is a misnomer. The iris is not absent but is hypoplastic and rudimentary.

ties; failure to thrive; generalized weakness; hypotonia; and death in several weeks to 15 years. The disease has an autosomal recessive inheritance pattern. The symptoms are non-specific and a familial history helps make the diagnosis.

II. Ocular findings include blepharoptosis, nystagmus, strabismus, Parinaud's syndrome, pupillary abnormalities, field defects, absent foveal retinal reflexes and optic atrophy.

III. Histologically the eyes show glycogen-containing, lacy vacuolation of the iris pigment epithelium; no cataracts but persistence of lens cell nuclei in the deep cortex similar to that seen in congenital rubella and trisomy 13–15 lenses; atrophy of retinal ganglion cell and nerve fiber layers; and optic atrophy.

DELANGE SYNDROME

I. The deLange syndrome consists of mental and growth retardation; characteristic facial appearance; multiple skeletal abnormalities; and a feeble, low-pitched cry. No cause is known definitely, but an autosomal recessive inheritance pattern has been suggested.

II. Constant ocular findings include bushy eyebrows with synophrys, long arcuate eyelashes, telecanthus, blue sclera and antimongoloid palpebral fissures. Inconstant findings include nystagmus, strabismus, blepharoptosis, myopia and abnormal fundi.

III. Ocular pathology is not available.

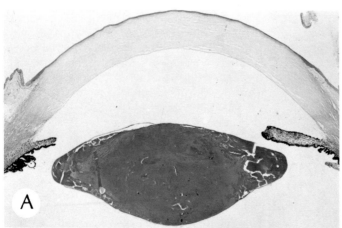

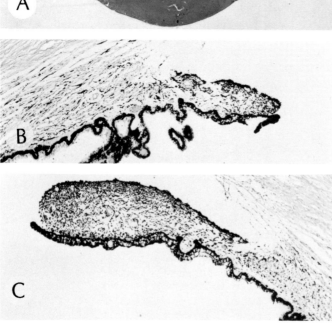

FIG. 2–34. Oculocerebrorenal syndrome of Miller. **A.** Rudimentary hypoplastic iris leaves are present along with congenital cortical and nuclear cataract in eye from 6½-month-old, mentally retarded, microcephalic baby, who had bilateral Wilms's tumor. **B** and **C** show different planes of section to demonstrate very rudimentary iris with both uveal and neuroepithelial layers present but with sphincter and dilator muscles absent. **A,** H&E, ×10; **B,** H&E, ×50; **C,** H&E, ×50.

MECKEL SYNDROME
(Dysencephalia Splanchnocystic; Gruber Syndrome)

I. The Meckel syndrome consists of posterior encephalocele, polydactyly and polycystic kidneys as the most important diagnostic features, but also includes sloping forehead, microcephaly, cleft lip and palate and ambiguous genitalia. The condition has an autosomal recessive inheritance pattern.

II. Ocular findings include cryptophthalmos, cysts on lower lids, small fissures, mongoloid or antimongoloid lid fissures, hypertelorism or hypotelorism, clinical anophthalmos, microphthalmos and cataract.

III. Histologically microphthalmos, mesodermal dysgenesis of cornea and iris, cataract, uveal colobomas, retinal dysplasia and optic atrophy may be found.

DWARFISM

I. Ocular anomalies occur frequently in many different types of dwarfism.
  A. Dwarfism secondary to mucopolysaccharidoses—see p. 302 in Chapter 8.
  B. Dwarfism secondary to osteogenesis imperfecta—see p. 314 in Chapter 8.
  C. Dwarfism secondary to stippled epiphyses (Conradi's syndrome) with cataracts.
  D. Dwarfism secondary to Cockayne's syndrome with retinal degeneration and optic atrophy (see p. 438 in Chap. 11).
  E. Dwarfism secondary to Lowe's syndrome (see p. 360 in Chap. 10).
  F. The syndrome of dwarfism, myotonia, diffuse bone disease, myopia and blepharophimosis.
  G. The syndrome of dwarfism with disproportionately short legs, reduced joint mobility, hyperopia, glaucoma, cataract and retinal detachment.
  H. The syndrome of dwarfism, congenital trichomegaly, mental retardation and retinal pigmentary degeneration.
  I. Achondroplastic dwarfism with mesodermal dysgenesis of cornea and iris.
  J. Ateleiotic dwarfism with soft, wrinkled skin of lids.
  K. Diastrophic dwarfism with mild retinal pigment epithelial disturbance in macular and perimacular areas.
  L. Spondyloepiphyseal dysplastic dwarfism with retinal degeneration (including lattice degeneration), retinal detachment, myopia and cataracts.
  M. Cartilage-hair hypoplastic dwarfism with fine sparse hair of eyebrows and cilia and trichiasis.

II. The histology is described in the appropriate sections under the individual tissues.

BIBLIOGRAPHY

PHAKOMATOSES

Angiomatosis Retinae

Apple DJ, Goldberg MG, Wyhinny GJ: Argon laser treatment of von Hippel-Lindau retinal angiomas. II. Histopathology of treated lesions. Arch Ophthalmol 92:126, 1974

Font RL, Ferry AP: The phakomatoses. Int Ophthalmol Clin 12:1, 1972

Hagler WS, Hyman BN, Waters WC III: Von Hippel's angiomatosis retinae and pheochromocytoma. Trans Am Acad Ophthalmol Otolaryngol 75:1022, 1971

Jesberg DO, Spencer WH, Hoyt WF: Incipient lesions of von Hippel-Lindau disease. Arch Ophthalmol 80:632, 1968

Manschot WA: Juxtapapillary retinal angiomatosis. Arch Ophthalmol 80:775, 1968

Melmon KL, Rosen SW: Lindau's disease: review of the literature and study of a large kindred. Am J Med 36:595, 1964

Meningocutaneous Angiomatosis

Alexander GL, Norman RM: The Sturge-Weber Syndrome. Bristol, England, Wright, 1960

Berkow JW: Retinitis pigmentosa associated with Sturge-Weber syndrome. Arch Ophthalmol 75:72, 1966

Font RL, Ferry AP: The phakomatoses. Int Ophthalmol Clin 12:1, 1972

Tasman W: The Phakomatoses, in Tasman W (ed): Retinal Diseases in Children. New York, Harper & Row, 1971, 71.

Neurofibromatosis

Font RL, Ferry AP: The phakomatoses. Int Ophthalmol Clin 12:1, 1972

Graham JH, Johnson WC, Helwig EG (eds): Dermal Pathology. Hagerstown, Harper & Row, 1972, pp 647–648

Grant WM, Walton DS: Distinctive gonioscopic findings in glaucoma due to neurofibromatosis. Arch Ophthalmol 79:127, 1968

Nordmann J, Brini A: Von Recklinghausen's disease and melanoma of the uvea. Br J Ophthalmol 54:641, 1970

Yanoff M, Zimmerman LE: Histogenesis of malignant melanomas of the uvea. III. The relationship of congenital ocular melanocytosis and neurofibromatosis to uvea melanomas. Arch Ophthalmol 77:331, 1967

Tuberous Sclerosis

Bjonberg A: Adenoma sebaceum. Review, case reports and discussion of eugenic aspects. Acta Derm Venerol (Stockh) 41:213, 1961

Font RL, Ferry AP: The phakomatoses. Int Ophthalmol Clin 12:1, 1972

Golden GS: Tuberous sclerosis. Minn Med 47:881, 1964

Harley RD, Grover WD: Tuberous sclerosis. Description and report of 12 cases. Ann Ophthalmol 1:477, 1970

Kinder RSL: The ocular pathology of tuberous sclerosis. J Pediatr Ophthalmol 9:106, 1972

Lagos JC, Gomez MR: Tuberous sclerosis: reappraisal of a clinical entity. Mayo Clin Proc 42:26, 1967

Ataxia–Telangiectasia

Boder E, Sedgwick RP: Ataxia–telangiectasia. A familial syndrome of progressive cerebellar ataxia, oculo-cutaneous telangiectasia and frequent pulmonary infections. Pediatrics 21:526, 1958

Font RL, Ferry AP: The phakomatoses. Int Ophthalmol Clin 12:1, 1972

Schalch DS, McFarlin DE, Barlow MH: An unusual form of diabetes mellitus in ataxia telangiectasia. N Engl J Med 282:136, 1970

Arteriovenous Communication of Retina and Brain

Archer DB, Deutman A, Ernest JT, Krill AE: Arteriovenous communications of the retina. Am J Ophthalmol 75:224, 1973

Baurmann H von, Meyer F, Oberhoff P: Komplikationen bei der arteriovenösen Anastomose der Netzhaut. Klin Monatsbl Augenheilkd 153:562, 1968

Brown DG, Hilal SH, Tenner HS: Wyburn-Mason syndrome. Arch Neurol 28:67, 1973

Font RL, Ferry AP: The phakomatoses. Int Ophthalmol Clin 12:1, 1972

Wyburn-Mason R: Arteriovenous aneurysm of the midbrain and retina with facial naevus and mental changes. Brain 66:12, 1943

CHROMOSOMAL ABERRATIONS

Trisomy 13–15

Boué J, Deluchat C, Albert DM, Lahav M: The eyes of embryos with chromosomal abnormalities. Am J Ophthalmol 78:167, 1974

Ginsberg J, Bove KE: Ocular pathology of trisomy 13. Ann Ophthalmol 6:113, 1974

Hoepner J, Yanoff M: Ocular anomalies in trisomy 13–15: an analysis of 13 eyes with two new findings. Am J Ophthalmol 74:729, 1972

Mottet NK, Jensen H: The anomalous embryonic development associated with trisomy 13–15. Am J Clin Pathol 43:334, 1965

Rodrigues MM, Valdes-Dapena M, Kistenmacher M: Ocular pathology in a case of 13 trisomy. J Pediatr Ophthalmol 10:54, 1973.

Taylor AI: Autosomal trisomy syndromes: a detailed study of 27 cases of Edward's syndrome and 27 cases of Patau's syndrome. J Med Genet 5:227, 1968

Yanoff M, Font RL, Zimmerman LE: Intraocular cartilage in a microphthalmic eye of an otherwise healthy girl. Arch Ophthalmol 81:238, 1969

Yanoff M, Frayer WC, Scheie HG: Ocular findings in a patient with 13–15 trisomy. Arch Ophthalmol 70:372, 1963

Trisomy 18

Ginsberg J, Bove K, Nelson R, Englender GS: Ocular pathology of trisomy 18. Ann Ophthalmol 3:273, 1971

Huggert A: The trisomy 18 syndrome: a report of 3 cases in the same family. Acta Ophthalmol 44:186, 1966

Keith CG: The ocular findings in the trisomy syndromes. Proc R Soc Med 61:251, 1968

Mullaney J: Ocular pathology in trisomy 18 (Edwards' syndrome). Am J Ophthalmol 76:246, 1973

Rodrigues MM, Punnett HH, Valdas-Dapena M, Martyn LJ: Retinal pigment epithelium in a case of trisomy 18. Am J Ophthalmol 76:265, 1973

Taylor AI: Autosomal trisomy syndromes: a detailed study of 27 cases of Edwards' syndrome and 27 cases of Patau's syndrome. J Med Genet 5:227, 1968

Trisomy 21

Boué J, Deluchat C, Albert DM, Lahav M: The eyes of embryos with chromosomal abnormalities. Am J Ophthalmol 78:167, 1974

Florey HW (ed): General Pathology. Philadelphia, Saunders, 1970, pp 615–618

Gilbert HD, Smith RE, Barlow MH, Mohr D: Congenital upper eyelid eversion and Down's syndrome. Am J Ophthalmol 75:469, 1973

Hoepner J, Yanoff M: Craniosynostosis and syndactylism (Apert's syndrome) associated with a trisomy 21 mosaic. J Ped Ophthalmol 8:107, 1971

Penrose LS, Smith GF: Down's Anomaly. London, Churchill, 1966

Williams EJ, McCormick AQ, Tischler B: Retinal vessels in Down's syndrome. Arch Ophthalmol 89:269, 1973

Turner's Syndrome

Cameron JD, Yanoff M, Frayer WC: Turner's syndrome and Coats' disease. Am J Ophthalmol 78:852, 1974

Other Trisomies

Boué J, Deluchat C, Albert DM, Lahav M: The eyes of embryos with chromosomal abnormalities. Am J Ophthalmol 78:167, 1974

Hambert G: Males with Positive Sex Chromatin. Göteborg, Akademiförlaget 1966

Peterson RA: Schmid-Fraccaro syndrome ("cat's eye" syndrome). Partial trisomy of G chromosome. Arch Ophthalmol 90:287, 1973

Schwinger E, Wiebusch D: Coloboma of iris and choroid in XYY-syndrome (in German). Klin Monatsbl Augenheilkd 156:873, 1970

Chromosomal Deletion Defects

Florey WH (ed): General Pathology. Philadelphia, Saunders, 1970, pp 606–608

Ginsberg J, Soukup S: Ocular findings associated with ring B chromosome. Am J Ophthalmol 78:624, 1974

Grotsky H, Hsu LYP, Hirschhorn K: A case of cri-du-chat associated with cataracts and transmitted from a mother with a 4/5 translocation. J Med Genet 8:369, 1971

Howard RO: Ocular abnormalities in the cri du chat syndrome. Am J Ophthalmol 73:949, 1972

Saraux H, Réthoré MO, Aussannaire M. Dhermy P, Joly C, LeLoch J, Praud E, Lejeune J: Les anomalies oculaires du phenotype D r (Chromosome D en anneau). Ann Ocul (Paris) 203:737, 1970

Schwartz DE: Noonan's syndrome associated with ocular abnormalities. Am J Ophthalmol 73:955, 1972

Yanoff M, Rorke LB, Niederer BS: Ocular and cerebral abnormalities in chromosome 18 deletion defect. Am J Ophthalmol 70:391, 1970

Mosaicism

Gartler SM, Sparks RS: The Lyon-Beutler hypothesis and isochromosome X patients with Turner's syndrome. Lancet 2:411, 1963

Hoepner J, Yanoff M: Craniosynostosis and syndactylism (Apert's syndrome) associated with a trisomy 21 mosaic. J Ped Ophthalmol 8:107, 1971

Kohn G, Mayall BH, Miller ME, Mellmann WJ: Tetraploid-diploid mosaicism in a surviving infant. Pediatr Res 1:461, 1967

Yanoff M, Rorke LB: Ocular and central nervous system findings in tetraploid-diploid mosaicism. Am J Ophthalmol 75:1036, 1973

INFECTIOUS EMBRYOPATHY

Boniuk M (ed): 1. Rubella and other intraocular viral diseases in infancy. Int Ophthalmol Clin 12:3–166, 1972

Forrest JM, Menser MA, Burgess JA: High frequency of diabetes mellitus in young adults with congenital rubella. Lancet 2:332, 1971

Wolff SM: The ocular manifestations of congenital rubella. A prospective study of 328 cases of congenital rubella. J Ped Ophthalmol 10:101, 1973

Yanoff M: The retina in rubella, in Retinal Diseases in Children. Edited by W Tasman. New York, Harper & Row, 1971, pp. 223–232

Yanoff M, Schaffer DB, Scheie HG: Rubella ocular syndrome—clinical significance of viral and pathologic studies. Trans Am Acad Ophthalmol Otolaryngol 72:896, 1968

Zimmerman LE, Font RL: Congenital malformations of the eye. J Am Med Assoc 196:684, 1966

DRUG EMBRYOPATHY

Apple DJ, Bennett TO: Multiple systemic and ocular malformations associated with maternal LSD usage. Arch Ophthalmol 92:301, 1974

Bogdanoff B, Rorke LB, Yanoff M, Warren WS: Brain and eye abnormalities. Possible sequelae to prenatal use of multiple drugs including LSD. Am J Dis Child 123:145, 1972

Casanovas J, Carbonell M: Malformaciones oculares en la embriopatia thalidomídica. Arch Soc Oftalmol Hisp Am 24:947, 1964

Zimmerman LE, Font RL: Congenital malformations of the eye. J Am Med Assoc 196:684, 1966

OTHER CONGENITAL ANOMALIES

Addison DJ, Font RL, Manschot WA: Proliferative retinopathy in anencephalic babies. Am J Ophthalmol 74:967, 1972

Anderson SR, Bro-Rasmussen F, Tygstrup I: Anencephaly related to ocular development and malformation. Am J Ophthalmol 64:559, 1967

Borit A: Leigh's necrotizing encephalomelopathy: Neuro-ophthalmologic abnormalities. Arch Ophthalmol 85:438, 1971

Duke-Elder S: System of Ophthalmology, Vol III, Part 2, Congenital Deformities. St. Louis, Mosby, 1963, pp 488–495

Haicken BN, Miller DR: Simultaneous occurrence of congenital aniridia, hamartoma and Wilms' tumor. J Pediatr 78:497, 1971

Hirsch SE, Waltman SR, LaPiana FG: Bilateral nanophthalmos. Arch Ophthalmol 89:353, 1973

Howard RO, Albert DM: Ocular manifestations of subacute necrotizing encephalomyelopathy (Leigh's disease). Am J Ophthalmol 74:386, 1972

MacRae DW, Howard RO, Albert DM, Hsia YE: Ocular manifestations of the Meckel syndrome. Arch Ophthalmol 88:106, 1972

Mann I: The Development of the Human Eye. New York, Grune & Stratton, 1964, pp 276–281

Milot J, Demay F: Ocular manifestations in deLange syndrome. Am J Ophthalmol 74:396, 1972

Nicholson DM, Goldberg MF: Ocular abnormalities in the deLange syndrome. Arch Ophthalmol 76:214, 1966

Rosenthal AR, Ryan SJ, Horowitz P: Ocular manifestations of dwarfism. Trans Am Acad Ophthalmol Otolaryngol 76:1500, 1972

Vare AM: Cyclopia. Am J Ophthalmol 75:880, 1973

Yanko L, Zaifrani S: Synophthalmos in a full-term newborn child. An anatomic and pathologic study. J Pediatr Ophthalmol 10:65, 1973

Zimmerman LE, Font RL: Congenital malformations of the eye. J Am Med Assoc 196:684, 1966

chapter 3

Nongranulomatous Inflammation: Uveitis, Endophthalmitis, Panophthalmitis and Sequelae

DEFINITIONS

NONGRANULOMATOUS INFLAMMATION

I. Suppurative inflammation. This is an acute, nongranulomatous, purulent inflammatory reaction in which the predominant cell type is the polymorphonuclear leukocyte. The reaction generally has an acute onset and is characterized by suppuration, i.e., the formation of pus.

This type of inflammation usually is secondary to infection with bacteria that cause a purulent (pus) inflammatory reaction, e.g., *Staphylococcus aureus.*

II. Nonsuppurative inflammation. This may be acute (cellulitis secondary to *Streptococcus hemolyticus*), chronic nongranulomatous (the common type of uveitis) or granulomatous (see Chap. 4). The predominant cell type in nonsuppurative acute inflammation is the polymorphonuclear leukocyte; in chronic nongranulomatous inflammation it is the lymphocyte and plasma cell; and in chronic granulomatous inflammation it is epithelioid cells.

Chronic nongranulomatous inflammation may have an acute, subacute or chronic course.

CLASSIFICATION

TERMINOLOGY

I. If a single tissue is involved, the inflammation is classified according to involved tissue, e.g., cornea-keratitis; retina-retinitis; vitreous-vitritis; optic nerve-optic neuritis (optic disc-papillitis, retroscleral portion of optic nerve-retrobulbar neuritis); sclera-scleritis; and uvea-uveitis (iris-iritis, ciliary body-cyclitis, iris and ciliary body-iridocyclitis, choroid-choroiditis; or anterior uveitis, posterior uveitis and uveitis).

If more than one tissue is involved but not an adjacent cavity (a most unusual occurrence), then the inflammation is classified by the tissues involved with the site of primary involvement first, e.g., retinochoroiditis in toxoplasmosis and chorioretinitis in tuberculosis.

II. Endophthalmitis (Fig. 3–1A) is an inflammation of one or more coats of the eye and adjacent cavities.

Although, by the above definition, a corneal ulcer with a hypopyon or an iritis with aqueous cells and flare would be an endophthalmitis, most clinicians require a significant inflammatory component within the vitreous before they call an ocular inflammation an endophthalmitis.

III. Panophthalmitis (Fig. 3–1B) is usually a suppurative reaction and consists of an endophthalmitis with scleral involvement and spread to orbital structures.

SOURCE OF INFLAMMATION

I. Exogenous sources are those originating outside of the eye and body, e.g., from penetrating and perforating wounds.
II. Endogenous sources are those that originate within the eye, e.g., cellular immunity, necrotic tumor, and blood and lens; spread from contiguous structures, e.g., the sinuses; and spread hematogenously, e.g., rubella ophthalmia.

SUPPURATIVE ENDOPHTHALMITIS AND PANOPHTHALMITIS

CLINICAL FEATURES

I. Severe ocular congestion and haziness of the cornea, aqueous and vitreous are characteristic. A purulent exudate, fre-

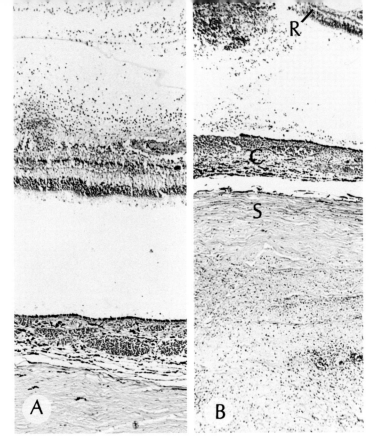

FIG. 3–1. Endophthalmitis and panophthalmitis. **A.** Endophthalmitis consisting of inflammation of artifactitiously detached retina and adjacent vitreous body (if choroid also had been involved, it still would have been considered endophthalmitis). **B.** Panophthalmitis consisting of inflammation of all three coats (necrotic retina, *R*; choroid, *C*; and sclera, *S* as well as adjacent vitreous body and episclera. **A,** H&E, ×35; **B,** H&E, ×35.

quently visible as a hypopyon, may be present in the anterior chamber.

II. Pain is prominent, especially in panophthalmitis, but also in endophthalmitis.

III. With panophthalmitis and extension of the inflammation into Tenon's capsule and orbital tissue, congestion and edema of the lids and even exophthalmos may be seen.

IV. The cause may be infectious or noninfectious.

CLASSIFICATION

I. Exogenous

    A. Keratitis and corneal ulcers secondary to bacteria, fungi or viruses may cause a reflex suppurative iridocyclitis and hypopyon that is often sterile.

    B. Nonsurgical trauma (or rarely, surgical trauma) may lead to the presence of a contaminated intraocular foreign body producing a suppurative infection. A retained sterile foreign body may cause a reactive suppurative inflammation (or a nonsuppurative, nongranulomatous or granulomatous inflammation).

    C. Postoperative suppurative inflammation (Fig. 3–2), if bacterial, usually is manifest within 24 to 48 hours after surgery and frequently follows surgery marked by complications such as lens capsule rupture or loss of vitreous. Postoperative suppurative fungal infections generally have a latent period of several days to a month or more and generally follow uncomplicated surgery.

II. Endogenous

    A. Metastatic septic emboli, especially in children or debilitated persons, may occur in subacute bacterial endocarditis, meningococcemia or other infections associated with a bacteremia, viremia or fungemia.

    B. Necrosis of an intraocular neoplasm, particularly retinoblastoma, rarely may result in a suppurative endophthalmitis or even panophthalmitis.

Histologically necrosis of a malignant melanoma (Fig. 3–3*A*) is more likely to induce an inflammatory reaction (usually lymphocytes and plasma cells) than is

61

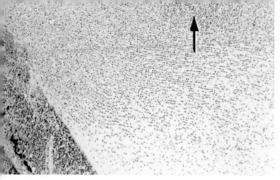

FIG. 3–2. Postoperative (5 days after cataract surgery) suppurative inflammation shows polymorphonuclear leukocytes following natural planes within vitreous below while destruction of framework above (*arrow*) indicates early abscess formation. H&E, ×60.

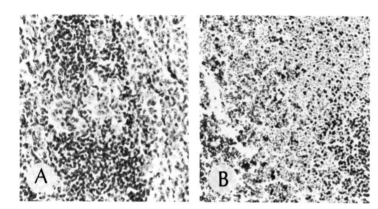

FIG. 3–3. A. Necrotic malignant melanoma shows marked lymphocyte-plasma cell inflammatory infiltrate (small dark cells). **B.** Necrotic retinoblastoma contains no inflammatory cells. Only viable cells at upper right corner; dark material elsewhere, especially lower right, is calcium. **A,** H&E, ×101; **B,** H&E, ×101.

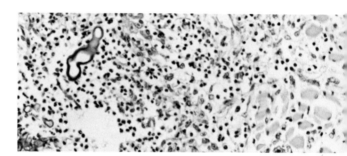

FIG. 3–5. Behcet's disease. Anterior chamber contains exudate and polymorphonuclear leukocytes (hypopyon). **Inset** shows irregular pupil due to posterior synechias at 3 and 5 o'clock positions; hypopyon is present inferiorly (*arrow*). The young woman had bilateral hypopyon, uveitis and aphthous ulcers. **Main figure,** H&E, ×252; **inset,** clinical.

FIG. 3–4. Phycomycosis of orbit. Fungi stain well with hematoxylin and are seen easily toward left. H&E, ×101.

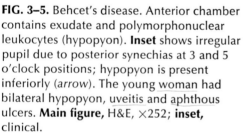
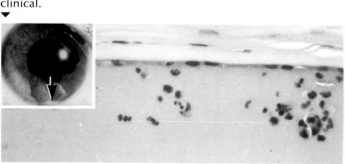

necrosis of a retinoblastoma (Fig. 3–3B). Clinically, however, even though no inflammatory cells are present, the retinoblastoma eye frequently simulates inflammation (in about 8 percent of cases).

C. Inflammation of contiguous or nearby structures, e.g., orbital abscess or cellulitis, meningitis or a nasal phycomycosis (Fig. 3–4), rarely may spread into the eye.

D. Behcet's disease (Figs. 3–5 and 3–6) is an example of a chronic endogenous endophthalmitis. It is a triple-symptom complex consisting of ocular inflammation, oral ulceration (aphthous stomatitis) and genital ulceration. Arthritis or arthralgia, cutaneous lesions, thrombophlebitis, ulcerative colitis, encephalopathy, pancreatitis, central and peripheral neuropathy, subungual infarctions and malignant lymphomas also may be found.

   1. The ocular inflammation is characterized by recurrent iridocyclitis and hypopyon, generally involving both eyes but not necessarily simultaneously. In addition, macular edema, retinal periphlebitis and periarteritis, and retinal and vitreal hemorrhages may occur. Secondary posterior synechias may lead to iris bombé, peripheral anterior synechias and secondary glaucoma.

   2. Biopsy of mucocutaneous lesions shows vasculitis. The serum may show variable increases in polyclonal immunoglobulins and anticytoplasmic antibodies.

   3. Histologically there is a chronic nongranulomatous uveitis and a retinal perivasculitis, vasculitis, hemorrhagic infarction and detachment. An acute, suppurative inflammatory infiltrate with neutrophils in the anterior chamber is seen.

HISTOLOGY

I. Suppurative inflammation is characterized by polymorphonuclear leukocytic infiltration into the involved tissues (Fig. 3–7). There is marked necrosis of tissue so that a suppurative, or purulent, exudate (pus) (Fig. 3–2) is formed.

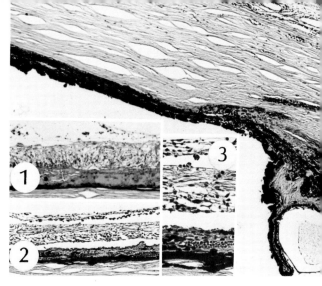

FIG. 3–6. Behcet's disease. Sequelae of disease include peripheral anterior synechia, retinal detachment (**inset 1**), atrophic retina with hemosiderin-pigmented membrane in the vitreous (**inset 2** and in higher magnification in **inset 3**). **Main figure,** H&E, ×40; **inset 1,** H&E, ×28; **inset 2,** H&E, ×40; **inset 3,** H&E, ×101.

II. A secondary chronic nongranulomatous inflammatory infiltrate is seen frequently in adjacent tissues (Fig. 3–7).

NONSUPPURATIVE, CHRONIC, NONGRANULOMATOUS UVEITIS AND ENDOPHTHALMITIS

CLINICAL FEATURES

I. With anterior involvement a severe, acute, "plastic" or exudative recurrent iridocyclitis often is seen, whereas with posterior involvement a choroiditis, or chorioretinitis is noted.

II. In this group is included the "garden-variety" type of uveitis seen in most uveitis patients. This consists of a chronic nongranulomatous uveitis of unknown cause.

CLASSIFICATION

I. Exogenous
   A. Exogenous nonsuppurative, chronic, nongranulomatous inflammation generally is secondary to trauma.

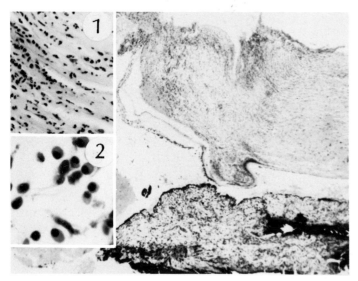

FIG. 3–7. Suppurative inflammation with polymorphonuclear leukocytic infiltration (seen under higher magnification in **inset 1**) is present in area of perforating corneal ulcer. The iris contains a chronic non-granulomatous inflammatory infiltrate of lymphocytes and plasma cells (seen under higher magnification in **inset 2**). **Main figure,** H&E, ×21; **inset 1,** H&E, ×136; **inset 2,** H&E, ×340.

1. The most common type probably is the iridocyclitis (*traumatic* *iridocyclitis*) that follows many injuries to the eye, particulary blunt trauma, alkali burns, and intraocular surgery.
2. Perforating or penetrating injuries to the eye may produce a milieu, in the form of multiple, tiny foreign bodies, degenerating blood, necrotic uvea, etc., which results in a chronic, low-grade, nongranulomatous inflammation.
3. Perforating or penetrating injuries also may introduce viruses into the eye, which could cause a chronic, nongranulomatous inflammation.

II. Endogenous
  A. Idiopathic endogenous, nonsuppurative, chronic nongranulomatous inflammation (Fig. 3–8) is the most common form of endogenous uveitis. The cause is unknown but is probably related to cellular immunity.
  B. Endogenous, nonsuppurative, chronic, nongranulomatous inflammation may be associated with systemic diseases such as rheumatoid arthritis, especially ankylosing spondylitis (10 to 15 percent incidence of uveitis) and Still's disease (15 to 20 percent incidence of uveitis)—see section Scleritis in Chapter 8; Reiter's disease; Behcet's dis-

ease; collagen disease—see section Collagen Diseases in Chapter 6; phaco-anaphylactic endophthalmitis (the uvea usually shows a chronic, nongranulomatous uveitis)—see p. 82 in Chapter 4; regional enteritis and ulcerative colitis; and atopia.
  1. Reiter's syndrome
    a. Reiter's syndrome is characterized by the classic triad of nonbacterial urethritis, conjunctivitis or iridocyclitis and arthritis.
    b. Bilateral mucopurulent conjunctivitis is present in most cases, whereas iridocyclitis generally is seen only in recurrent cases.
    c. Histologically, marked edema along with a lymphocytic and neutrophilic inflammatory infiltrate is noted in the conjunctiva.
  C. Viral infections such as rubella (see p. 48 in Chap. 2), rubeola, herpes simplex (see p. 276 in Chap. 8), subacute sclerosing panencephalitis and others may cause an endogenous nonsuppurative, chronic, nongranulomatous uveitis.
  1. Subacute sclerosing panencephalitis (SSPE) (Figs. 3–9 through 3–12).
    a. SSPE is a chronic, progressive disease of the central nervous system caused by the measles virus, which produces a chronic,

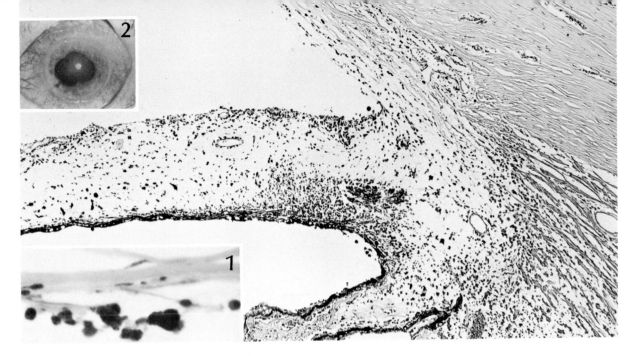

FIG. 3–8. Endogenous uveitis shows chronic nongranulomatous inflammation with lymphocytes and plasma cells in iris root and ciliary body. Note early formation of peripheral anterior synechia. **Inset 1** shows plasma cells, lymphocytes and pigment on posterior corneal surface (fine keratic precipitates). **Inset 2** shows irregular pupil due to posterior synechias in a person with chronic endogenous uveitis. **Main figure, H&E, ×80; inset 1, H&E, ×340; inset 2, clinical.**

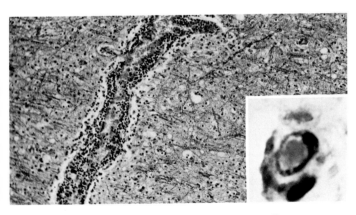

FIG. 3–9. SSPE. Perivascular infiltrate ("cuffing") of lymphocytes and plasma cells in brain of child who died from effects of SSPE. **Inset** is higher magnification of brain to show characteristic intranuclear inclusion body (type A). **Main figure, H&E, ×100; inset, H&E, ×1,000.**

intracellular infection of brain, retina and lymphoid tissue.

b. The ocular findings consist mainly of macular degeneration and peripheral retinochoroidal lesions.

c. Histologically, the retina is necrotic, is infiltrated by lymphocytes and shows conglomerations of multinucleated cells. Intranuclear inclusion bodies within retinal cells can be seen with light and electron microscopy.

D. Nonsystemic syndromes such as uveal effusion, pars planitis, glaucomatocyclitic crisis (Posner-Schlossman) and heterochromic iridocyclitis (Fuchs) may cause a nonsuppurative, chronic, nongranulomatous uveitis.

1. Uveal effusion—see p.351 in Chapter 9.

2. Pars planitis (peripheral uveitis, chronic cyclitis).

a. Pars planitis is a chronic process which consists of vitreous opacities, organization of the vitreous base and retinal edema, especially of the posterior pole.

b. Histologically the few case reports available show a chronic nongranulomatous inflammation of the vitreous base, retinal peri-

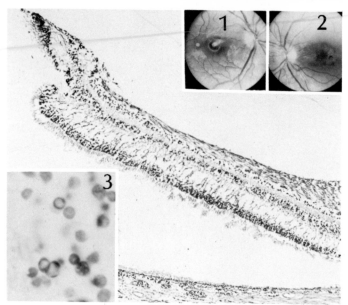

FIG. 3–10. SSPE. Necrotic retina in macular area shows hole formation. **Insets 1** and **2** are clinical appearance of macula in each eye of same child. **Inset 3** is higher magnification of macular retina to show intranuclear inclusions. **Main figure,** H&E, ×50; **inset 1,** clinical; **inset 2,** clinical; **inset 3,** H&E, ×1,000.

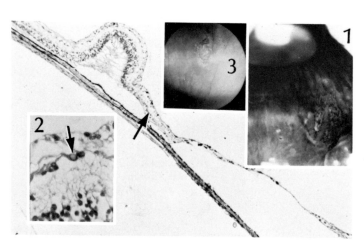

FIG. 3–11. SSPE. Peripheral retina undergoes abrupt necrosis at *arrow* (ora serrata to left). Macroscopic appearance of same lesion (**inset 1**) and higher magnification (**inset 2**) to demonstrate intranuclear inclusion (*arrow*) within same lesion are shown. **Inset 3** shows peripheral lesion of SSPE in fundus of another child. **Main figure,** H&E, ×25; **inset 1,** macroscopic; **inset 2,** H&E, ×800; **inset 3,** fundus.

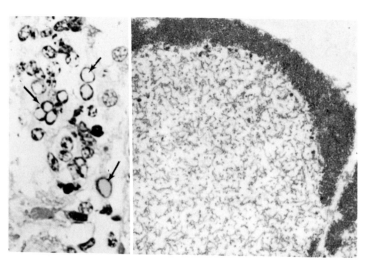

FIG. 3–12. SSPE. Nuclear inclusions (*arrows*) in ganglion cells of macular retina consist of tubular structures of myxovirus, as seen on **right** by electron microscopy. Nuclear chromatin is clumped in the periphery. **Left,** toluidine blue, ×775; **right,** ×27,200.

vasculitis and microcystoid degeneration of the macular retina.

3. Glaucomatocyclitic crisis (Posner-Schlossman syndrome)—see p. 603 in Chapter 16.

4. Fuchs's heterochromic iridocyclitis (Figs. 3–13, 3–14 and 3–24).

   a. Fuchs's heterochromic iridocyclitis consists of a unilateral, chronic, mild iridocyclitis; heterochromia with the involved iris becoming the lighter iris; and cataract and glaucoma developing in the hypochromic eye.

   The hypochromia of the involved eye is due to iris stromal atrophy with loss of stromal pigment. The stromal atrophy may become so severe that the iris pigment epithelium can be observed directly, resulting in a paradoxical or inverse heterochromia with the involved eye becoming the darker eye. The glaucoma probably is due to a combination of rubeosis of the anterior chamber angle, a trabeculitis, and possibly an associated atrophy of the uveal portion of the drainage angle.

   b. In spite of the chronic uveitis characteristically there is a lack of anterior and posterior synechias (even though a cataract forms), and intraocular surgery is tolerated well.

   c. Histologically a chronic nongranulomatous inflammatory reaction is seen within the iris, ciliary body and trabecular meshwork. Inflammatory membranes over the anterior surface of the iris and anterior face of the ciliary body are common. A fine neovascularization of the anterior surface of the iris and anterior chamber angle may be present. The iris stroma and the pigment epithelium show atrophy with loss of pigment, especially in the stroma and the posterior layer of pigment epithelium.

   The rubeosis iridis is quite fine and just within the anterior border layer

of the iris. Clinically observed fine translucent keratic precipitates have their counterpart in small clumps of mononuclear cells, lymphocytes and macrophages on the posterior surface of the cornea.

SEQUELAE OF UVEITIS, ENDOPHTHALMITIS AND PANOPHTHALMITIS

CORNEA

I. Endothelial degeneration or glaucoma may result in chronic stromal and epithelial edema and ultimately in bullous keratopathy (Fig. 3–15). Pannus degenerativus may follow bullous keratopathy. Precipitates (keratic precipitates) of mononuclear cells (mainly lymphocytes and plasma cells) along with pigment (Fig. 3–16) may be found on the endothelium.

II. Ruptured bullae may become infected secondarily (Fig. 3–17) leading to a corneal ulcer.

   Corneal ulceration may lead to corneal perforation. With perforation and resultant abrupt decrease in intraocular pressure a ciliary artery may rupture, producing an expulsive intraocular hemorrhage (Fig. 3–18).

III. Band keratopathy (Fig. 3–19), i.e., calcium deposition, is common beneath the corneal epithelium in chronically inflamed eyes, especially in children with Still's disease.

ANTERIOR CHAMBER

I. Products of inflammation or hemorrhage may become organized, resulting in cicatrization within the anterior chamber (Fig. 3–20).

II. The angle of the anterior chamber may become obliterated from organization of the inflammatory products or hemorrhage or from rubeosis iridis.

IRIS

I. The iris may undergo atrophy and necrosis (Fig. 3–21) with loss of dilator muscle, stroma and even sphincter muscle and pigment epithelium.

II. Neovascularization of the anterior surface

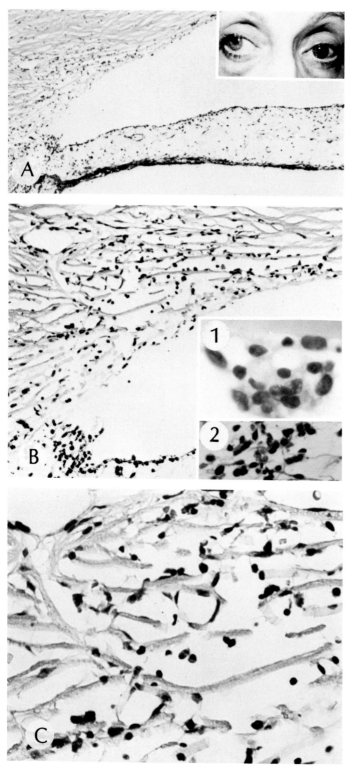

FIG. 3–13. Fuchs's heterochromic iridocyclitis. **A.** Microscopic of exotropic right eye with lighter colored iris (**inset**) shows that iris, anterior face of ciliary body and trabecular meshwork contain chronic, nongranulomatous inflammation. **B.** Higher magnification of **A.** Note inflammatory membrane in anterior chamber angle. **Inset 1** shows keratic precipitate consisting of lymphocytes and histiocytes. **Inset 2** shows nodule of lymphocytes and plasma cells in iris stroma. **C.** Higher magnification of trabecular meshwork to demonstrate chronic trabeculitis with infiltration by lymphocytes and plasma cells. **A,** H&E, ×40; **inset,** clinical. **B,** H&E, ×101; **inset 1,** H&E, ×400; **inset 2,** H&E, ×160. **C,** H&E, ×202.

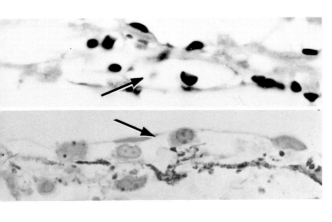

FIG. 3–14. Fuchs's heterochromic iridocyclitis. Thin-walled blood vessels (rubeosis) line anterior chamber surface of trabecular meshwork (*arrow*) in **top** and line (*arrow*) anterior surface of iris (rubeosis iridis) in **bottom. Top,** normal thickness section, H&E, ×400; **bottom,** 1.5 μ thick section, PD, ×400.

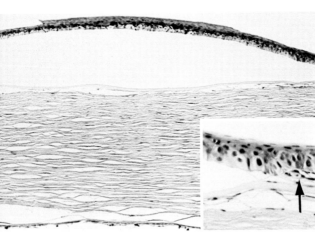

FIG. 3–15. Large bulla consists of epithelium lifted from Bowman's membrane. Basal edema of epithelium is present. **Inset** shows higher magnification of edge of bulla. Just to right of where epithelium (with basal edema) lifts off of Bowman's membrane, fibrovascular tissue (*arrow*) has grown between two structures (early formation of degenerative pannus). **Main figure,** H&E, ×54; **inset,** H&E, ×136.

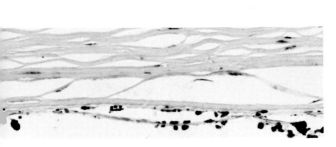

FIG. 3–16. Keratic precipitates (KPs) in form of lymphocytes, plasma cells and pigment on posterior corneal surface form fine KPs seen in chronic, nongranulomatous uveitis. H&E, ×176.

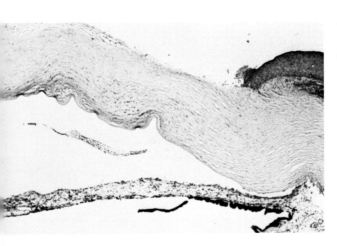

FIG. 3–17. Extensive corneal ulceration from infected bulla secondary to chronic angle closure glaucoma. H&E, ×16.

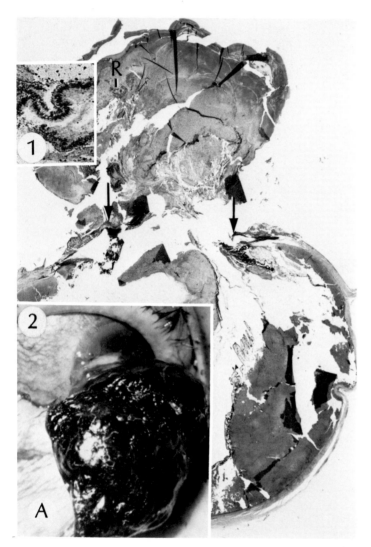

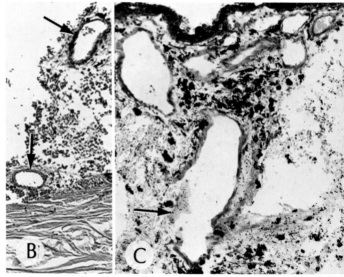

FIG. 3–18. A. Inset 2 shows hemorrhagic, mushroom-shaped mass protruding between lids. Enucleated eye in **main figure** is filled with blood that has ruptured through an extensive corneal perforation (extent of performation between *arrows*). *R*, retina in hemorrhagic mass external to eye, which is shown with higher magnification in **inset 1. B.** Posterior ciliary artery (*arrows*) from same case seems torn as it enters suprachoroidal space. **C.** Posterior ciliary artery as it approaches internal part of massively detached choroid. Wall of artery is ruptured (*arrow*). **A,** H&E, ×4; **inset 1,** H&E, ×75; **inset 2,** clinical; **B,** H&E, ×72; **C,** PAS, ×100.

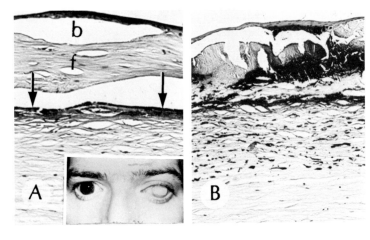

FIG. 3–19. A. Band keratopathy of left eye (**inset**). Microscopic section of left eye in **inset** shows granular deposit of calcium along and under Bowman's membrane (*arrows*). Fibrous tissue (degenerative pannus) is present between epithelium and Bowman's membrane. *b,* bulla between fibrous tissue (*f*) and epithelium. **B.** Stain for calcium shows its presence in Boman's membrane, in underlying stroma and in overlying fibrous tissue. **A,** H&E, ×69; **inset,** clinical; **B,** von Kossa, ×54.

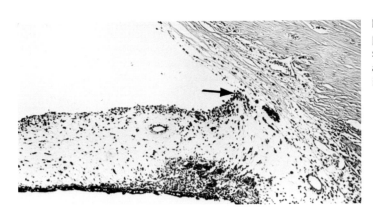

FIG. 3–20. Early organization of inflammatory products (*arrow*) initiates peripheral anterior synechia. Iris is infiltrated by lymphocytes and plasma cells (chronic, nongranulomatous iritis). H&E, ×40.

of the iris (rubeosis iridis) (Fig. 3–21) may cause secondary anterior chamber angle synechias. With contracture (shrinkage) of the fibrovascular membrane on the anterior iris surface the pupillary border of the iris may become everted, termed an *ectropion uveae*.*

III. Inflammatory-fibrous iris membranes may attach the pupillary margin of the iris to the underlying lens (or anterior surface of the vitreous in aphakic eyes), resulting in an immobile pupil, *seclusio pupillae* (Fig. 3–22). The same membrane may grow over the pupil and cover or occlude the area completely, called *occlusio pupillae.*

* An old anatomic term for the pigment epithelium (circa 1850) was pigment epithelium of the uvea. The pigment epithelium is now considered as a neuro-epithelium, separate from uvea, but the term *ectropion uveae* has persisted in clinical usage.

Generally the same membrane that binds the pupil down to surrounding structures grows across the pupil, so that seclusio and occlusio pupillae frequently are found together.

IV. With total (i.e., 360 degrees) posterior synechias a complete pupillary block will prevent aqueous flow into the anterior chamber. The pressure builds up in the posterior chamber bowing the iris forward (iris bombé) (Fig. 3–22). An iris bombé forces the anterior peripheral iris to touch the peripheral posterior cornea, resulting in peripheral anterior synechias and secondary chronic angle closure glaucoma.

LENS

I. Intraocular inflammation frequently induces the lens epithelium to migrate posteriorly. The presence of such aberrant

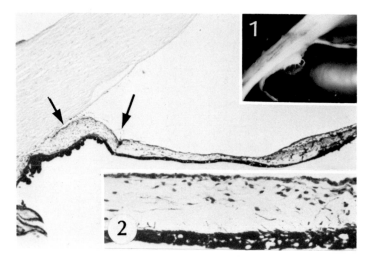

FIG. 3–21. Inset 1 shows macroscopic appearance of peripheral anterior synechia secondary to rubeosis iridis as shown by *arrows* in **main figure. Inset 2** is higher magnification to show loss of dilator muscle (due to necrosis) and stromal atrophy. **Main figure,** H&E, ×21; **inset 1,** macroscopic; **inset 2,** H&E, ×101.

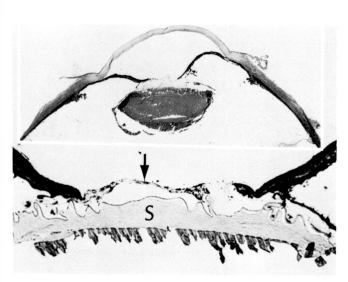

FIG. 3–22. Posterior synechia of pupillary portion of iris to underlying lens in eye with anterior uveitis. Fibrovascular membrane (*arrow*) has grown across pupil (occlusio pupillae), and pupil is immobile (seclusio pupillae). **Inset** shows that total posterior synechia has caused bowing forward of iris (iris bombé). Note anterior subcapsular cataract (S) secondary to anterior uveitis. **Main figure,** H&E, ×16; **inset,** H&E, ×6.

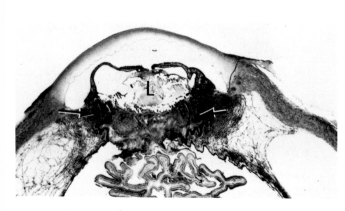

FIG. 3–23. Fibrous membrane extending behind lens (between *arrows*) forming cyclitic membrane has, with shrinkage, pulled ciliary body inwards and detached retina behind it. Massive ciliary body edema ("detachment"), posterior synechias of iris to lens (L) and iris bombé are present. H&E, ×6.

cells under the posterior lens capsule will produce a posterior subcapsular cataract (see p. 368 in Chap. 10).

Although intraocular inflammation present anywhere within the eye can induce posterior subcapsular cataract formation, posterior inflammation (choroiditis) is most likely to cause this type of cataract.

II. Anterior subcapsular cataract (see p. 366 in Chap. 10) frequently results from an anterior uveitis (Fig. 3–22), e.g., iritis or iridocyclitis, especially when posterior synechias are present.

CILIARY BODY

I. With chronic intraocular inflammation the ciliary processes or crests tend to become flattened and attenuated and their cores fibrosed ("hyalinized").
II. The ciliary epithelium (nonpigmented, pigmented or both) may proliferate, sometimes to a remarkable degree, i.e., massive proliferation of ciliary epithelium.
III. Intraocular inflammation may organize and fibrose behind the lens (or behind the pupil in an aphakic eye) between portions of the pars plicata of the ciliary body. Such a fibrous membrane spanning the retrolental space, often incorporating proliferated ciliary epithelium and vitreous base within it, is called a cyclitic membrane (Fig. 3–23).

With shrinkage of a cyclitic membrane the base of the vitreous, pars plana of the ciliary body and peripheral retina can be drawn inward, causing a total ciliary body and retinal detachment (Fig. 3–23). With degeneration of the ciliary body aqueous production is diminished leading to hypotony.

VITREOUS COMPARTMENT

I. Newly formed blood vessels may grow out into the vitreous compartment, generally between the vitreous and internal surface of the retina, along the posterior surface of a detached vitreous or into Cloquet's canal; but almost never do they grow initially into the formed vitreous.
II. The vitreous may "collapse," i.e., become detached posteriorly.

III. Inflammatory products within the vitreous may induce organization of the vitreous, which generally results in fibrous membranes, including a cyclitic membrane with anterior vitreal organization.

CHOROID

I. As an aftermath of choroiditis the choroid may show focal or diffuse areas of atrophy or scarring.
II. With retinochoroiditis or chorioretinitis Bruch's membrane and retinal pigment epithelium may be destroyed, the choroid and retina become fused by fibrosis and a chorioretinal scar or adhesion may result.

Chorioretinal adhesions may result without choroidal involvement. This occurs when proliferated retinal pigment epithelium serves to adhere the underlying choroid to the overlying sensory retina.

RETINA

I. Inflammation anywhere in the eye, even within the cornea, frequently causes a retinal perivasculitis (Fig. 3–24) with lymphocytes surrounding the blood vessels. If extensive, the perivasculitis can be noted clinically as vascular "sheathing."

Permanent vascular sheathing results from organization and cicatrization of a perivascular inflammatory infiltrate or from involution of the blood vessels with thickening of their walls.

II. Intraocular inflammation, especially involving the peripheral retina or ciliary body, may be accompanied by fluid appearing in the macular retina, i.e., macular edema.
III. Retinochoroiditis or chorioretinitis may result in chorioretinal scarring.
IV. The retina may become detached secondary to subretinal exudation or hemorrhage or to organization and formation of vitreal fibrous membranes or a cyclitic membrane.
V. The retinal pigment epithelium is a very reactive tissue and may undergo massive reactive hyperplasia following inflammation, it may show alternating areas of mild hyperplasia and atrophy, or it

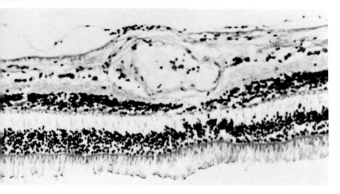

FIG. 3–24. Retinal perivasculitis with lymphocytes surrounding large retinal blood vessel in heterochromic iridocyclitis (Fuchs). Inflammatory membrane is present on inner retinal surface. H&E, ×160.

may be associated with intraocular ossification.

GLAUCOMA

I. Glaucoma may result from inflammatory cells and debris clogging the anterior chamber angle; from peripheral anterior synechias and secondary angle closure; from posterior synechias, pupillary block, iris bombé and secondary angle closure glaucoma; or from trabecular damage (inflammation, i.e., trabeculitis and scarring) (Fig. 3–25).

II. The proper combination of factors must be present for glaucoma to develop; e.g., peripheral anterior synechias may be present, but the inflammation may so damage the capacity for the ciliary body to secrete aqueous that glaucoma does not develop, and in fact hypotony may result.

In the face of peripheral anterior synechias (especially when secondary to iris bombé), chronic uveitis and normal intraocular pressure (or hypotony), intraocular surgery frequently will hasten the development of a phthisical eye.

END STAGE OF DIFFUSE OCULAR DISEASES

I. Atrophy without shrinkage. This refers to atrophy of intraocular structures such as the retina and uvea, but the eye is of normal size or may even be enlarged. The best example is the diffuse atrophy with long-standing glaucoma.

II. Atrophy with shrinkage (Fig. 3–26A, B) (atrophia bulbi). This refers to atrophy of intraocular structures, which remain recognizable, plus atrophy of the globe so that it is smaller than normal. The best example is chronic long-standing uveitis (especially when it starts in childhood) that goes on to hypotony in the face of an anterior chamber angle closed by peripheral anterior synechias.

Clinically the eye is soft and partially collapsed. The pull of the horizontal and vertical rectus muscles causes the shrunken eye to appear cuboid ("squared-off") instead of spherical when viewed with the lids widely separated. A soft, squared-off atrophic eye when seen clinically is called a phthisical eye or a phthisis bulbi. Histologically, however, the eye generally does not show phthisis bulbi but rather atrophia bulbi.

III. Atrophy with shrinkage and disorganization (Fig. 3–26B, C) (phthisis bulbi). This refers to a markedly thickened sclera and a profound atrophy of intraocular structures so that they generally are beyond recognition. The best example of this is the end result of an unchecked purulent endophthalmitis that destroys all the intraocular structures and causes widespread intraocular scarring and shrinkage.

IV. Intraocular ossification. This is common in atrophia bulbi (Fig. 3–26B) and in phthisis bulbi. The bone formation, which is never preceded by cartilage formation, seems to require pigment epithelium for its formation either as an inducer or from actual metaplasia.

A fatty marrow is present frequently within the bone. In younger individuals, generally under 20 years of age, the marrow may possess hematopoietic elements.

V. Calcium may be deposited within a band keratopathy, a cataractous lens, intraocular bone, sclera (see p. 27 in Chap. 1), a gliotic retina or optic nerve.

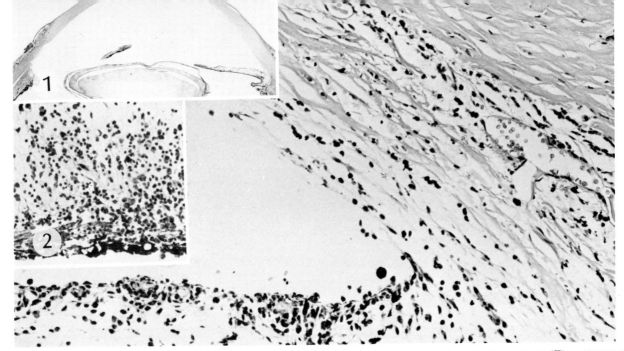

FIG. 3–25. Chronic nongranulomatous uveitis has caused secondary glaucoma, unsuccessfully treated surgically by scleral cautery with peripheral iridectomy, as seen on left side of **inset 1. Inset 2** shows higher magnification of iris root infiltrated extensively by lymphocytes and plasma cells. **Main figure** is high magnification of anterior chamber angle (right side of **inset 1**). Trabecular meshwork and iris stroma are infiltrated by lymphocytes and plasma cells (trabeculitis). Fibrous tissue has increased in amount in trabecular area. **Main figure,** H&E, ×101; **inset 1,** H&E, ×6; **inset 2,** H&E, ×101.

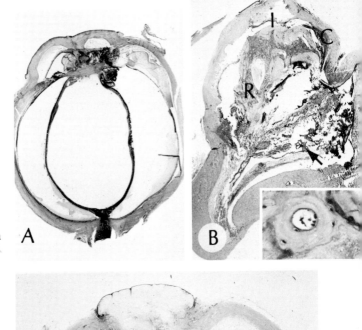

FIG. 3–26. A. Atrophy with shrinkage (atrophia bulbi). Smaller than normal eye has central corneal scar with adherent uveal tissue, cyclitic membrane and retinal and uveal detachment. Although structures are atrophic, they are identifiable. **B.** Globe is smaller than normal and contains bone (*arrow*) (higher magnification in **inset**). Because many structures can be identified, (I, iris; C, ciliary body; R, retina) eye could be called atrophia bulbi. With greater disorganization and intraocular ossification, term phthisis bulbi also is appropriate. **C.** Atrophy with shrinkage and disorganization (phthisis bulbi). Normal intraocular structures are not recognizable within thickened, folded sclera. Purulent endophthalmitis occurred many years previously. **A,** H&E, ×3; **B,** H&E, ×3; **inset,** H&E, ×101; **C,** H&E, ×3.

BIBLIOGRAPHY

SUPPURATIVE ENDOPHTHALMITIS AND PANOPHTHALMITIS

Green WR, Koo BS: Behcet's disease. A report of the ocular histology of one case. Survey Ophthalmol 12:324, 1967

O'Duffy JD, Carney JA, Dendhar S: Behcet's disease: report of 10 cases, three with new manifestations. Ann Intern Med 75:561, 1971

Shimizu K: Harada's, Behcet's, Vogt-Koyanagi syndromes—are they clinical entities? Trans Am Acad Ophthalmol Otolaryngol 77:281, 1973

NONSUPPURATIVE, CHRONIC, NONGRANULOMATOUS UVEITIS AND ENDOPHTHALMITIS

Anderson B Sr: Ocular lesions in relapsing polychondritis and other rheumatoid syndromes. Trans Am Acad Ophthalmol Otolaryngol 71:227, 1971

Font RL, Jenis EH, Tuck KD: Measles maculopathy associated with subacute sclerosing panencephalitis. Arch Pathol 96:168, 1973

Hogan MJ, Kimura SJ: Cyclitis and peripheral chorioretinitis. Arch Ophthalmol 66:667, 1961

Hogan MJ, Thygeson P, Kimura S: Uveitis in association with rheumatism. Trans Am Ophthalmol Soc 54:93, 1956

Hogan MJ, Wood IS, Godfrey WA: Aqueous cytology in uveitis. Arch Ophthalmol 89:217, 1973

Kimura SJ, Hogan MJ: Chronic cyclitis. Arch Ophthalmol 71:193, 1964

Kirpatrick BV, David RB: Subacute sclerosing panophthalmitis: a case report presenting with papilledema. J Pediatr Ophthalmol 10:74, 1973

Levine RA, Ward PA: Experimental acute immunologic ocular vasculitis. Am J Ophthalmol 69:1023, 1970

Marx JL: Slow viruses: role in persistent disease. Science 180:1351, 1973

Maumenee AE: Clinical entities in "uveitis": an approach to the study of intraocular inflammation. Am J Ophthalmol 69:1, 1970

Mills RP, Kalina RE: Reiter's keratitis. Arch Ophthalmol 87:447, 1972

Nelson DA, Weiner A, Yanoff M, and dePeralta J: Retinal lesions in subacute sclerosing panencephalitis. Arch Ophthalmol 84:613, 1970

Obenour LC: Subacute sclerosing panencephalitis. Int Ophthalmol Clin 12:215, 1972

Perry H, Yanoff M, Scheie HG: Fuchs's heterochromic iridocyclitis. Arch Ophthalmol 93:337, 1975

Segawa K, Smelser GK: Electron microscopy of experimental uveitis. Invest Ophthalmol 8:497, 1969

Wirostko E, Johnson LA: Cytology of inflamed aqueous humor in patients with rheumatoid arthritis. Am J Clin Pathol 54:369, 1970

SEQUELAE OF UVEITIS, ENDOPHTHALMITIS AND PANOPHTHALMITIS

Winslow RL, Stevenson W III, Yanoff M: Spontaneous expulsive choroidal hemorrhage. Arch Ophthalmol 92:126, 1974

chapter 4

Granulomatous Inflammation

Posttraumatic
  Sympathetic Uveitis
  Phacoanaphylactic Endophthalmitis
  Foreign Body Granulomas
Nontraumatic Infectious
  Bacterial
  Fungal
  Parasitic
  Viral
Nontraumatic Noninfectious
  Sarcoidosis
  Granulomatous Scleritis
  Chalazion
  Xanthogranulomas
  Granulomatous Reaction to
      Descemet's Membrane
  Chediak-Higashi Syndrome
  Allergic Granulomatosis, Wegener's
      Granulomatosis and Midline Lethal
      Granuloma
  Weber-Christian Syndrome
  Vogt-Koyanagi-Harada Syndrome
  Familial Chronic Granulomatous Disease
      (FCGD) of Childhood

POSTTRAUMATIC

SYMPATHETIC UVEITIS
(Sympathetic Ophthalmia, Sympathetic Ophthalmitis)
(Figs. 4–1 through 4–4)

I. Sympathetic uveitis is a bilateral, diffuse, granulomatous (see p. 14 in Chap. 1) uveitis that occurs from 2 weeks to many years following penetrating or perforating ocular injury to the eye, generally associated with uveal encarceration or prolapse.
   A. Although the uveitis may start as early as 5 days or as late as 50 years following injury, over 90 percent of cases occur after 2 weeks but within 1 year following injury, and most of these (80 percent) within the time period 3 weeks to 3 months post injury.
   B. Removal of the injured eye before sympathetic uveitis develops usually protects completely against future development of the inflammation in the noninjured eye.* Once the inflammation starts, removal of the injured ("exciting") eye does not alter the course of the disease.

   Sympathetic uveitis has been reported in nontraumatized eyes in a few isolated cases. Unless the whole eye is sectioned serially and examined carefully for evidence of perforation, one can never be sure that some long since forgotten penetrating or perforating ocular wound is not present. A diagnosis of sympathetic uveitis in the absence of an ocular injury should be viewed with marked skepticism.

II. The onset of the affliction generally is heralded by the symptoms of blurred vision and photophobia in the noninjured

---

* Rarely sympathetic uveitis has been reported to have developed in the sympathizing eye after the injured eye has been enucleated.

(sympathizing) eye and worsening of vision and photophobia in the injured (exciting) eye, together with the findings of a granulomatous uveitis, especially mutton-fat keratic precipitates, i.e., collections of epithelioid cells plus lymphocytes, macrophages, multinucleated giant cells or pigment on the posterior surface of the cornea.

Glaucoma may develop due to blockage of the angle by cellular debris or peripheral anterior synechias, or hypotony may occur due to a decreased output of aqueous by the inflamed ciliary body.

FIG. 4–1. Sympathetic uveitis. **Inset** shows laceration of inferior-temporal cornea with prolapsed iris (*arrow*). Patient was on steroids from time of injury until enucleation 15 days later. Symptoms of sympathetic uveitis developed in sympathizing eye 14 days after enucleation of exciting eye. **Main figure** shows diffuse chronic granulomatous choroiditis in exciting eye. **Main figure,** H&E, ×101; **inset,** clinical.

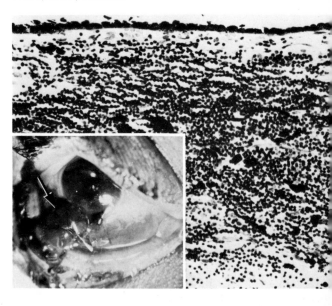

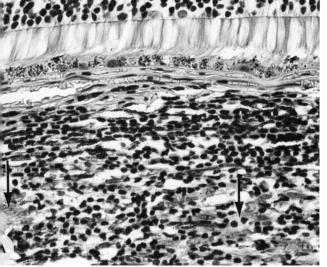

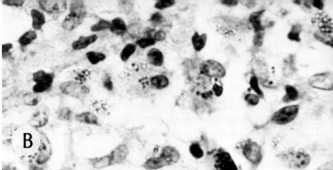

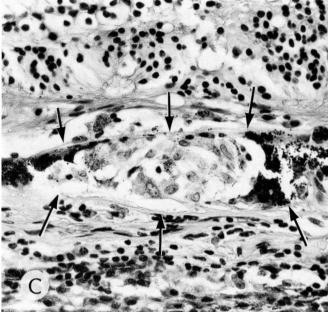

FIG. 4–2. Sympathetic uveitis. **A.** Diffuse, chronic, granulomatous inflammation spares choriocapillaris. *Arrows* show pale areas composed of epithelioid cells. **B.** Many epithelioid cells contain uveal pigment. **C.** Dalen-Fuchs's nodule composed of epithelioid cells present between retinal pigment epithelium (upper *arrows*) and Bruch's membrane (lower *arrows*). Underlying choriocapillaris is spared, and overlying retina is free of inflammatory process. **A,** H&E, ×250; **B,** H&E, ×600; **C,** H&E, ×250.

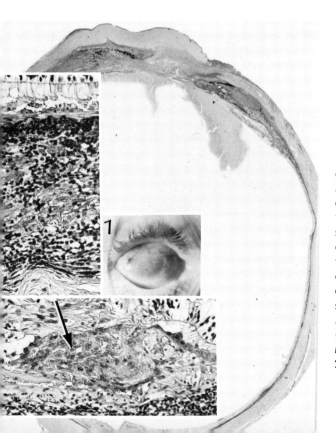

FIG. 4–3. Sympathetic uveitis. **Inset 1** shows opaque, vascularized cornea and iris prolapse at 10 o'clock position 6 months following cataract extraction. Opposite eye had "mutton-fat" keratic precipitates and considerable aqueous flare. **Main figure** demonstrates that anterior segment often is too distorted by injury to see typical reaction of sympathetic uveitis, whereas posterior choroid is diffusely thickened by reaction, seen under higher magnification in **inset 2.** *E,* epithelioid cells. Dalen-Fuchs's nodule (*arrow*) near optic nerve shown in **inset 3.** **Main figure,** H&E, ×3; **inset 1,** clinical; **inset 2,** H&E, ×110; **inset 3,** H&E, ×100.

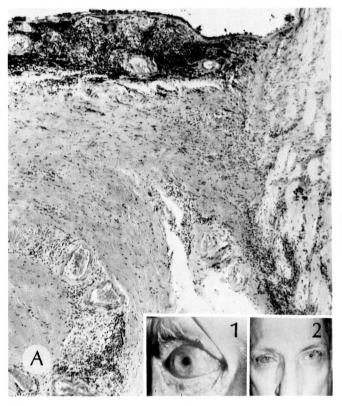

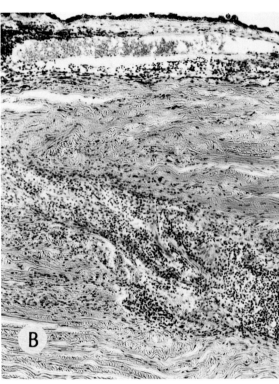

FIG. 4–4. Sympathetic uveitis. **A.** Two to three weeks following cataract extraction of right eye (OD) patient shown in **insets 1** and **2** developed purulent endophthalmitis OD, successfully treated with systemic and local antibiotics and steroids. Next month he suddenly developed sympathetic uveitis. **Main figure** is that of enucleated OD to show diffuse, chronic, granulomatous inflammation involving choroid, scleral canals of short posterior ciliary vessels and meninges around optic nerve. **B.** Scleral canal of long ciliary nerve contains chronic, granulomatous inflammation. **A** and **B** illustrate that evisceration does not prevent sympathetic uveitis, because uveal tissue is still present in scleral canals and around optic nerve. **A**, H&E, ×65; **inset 1**, clinical, OD; **inset 2**, clinical, both eyes; **B**, H&E, ×100.

III. The cause appears to be due to an autosensitivity against uveal protein or perhaps a protein associated closely with uveal pigment. Enhanced lymphocytic transformation occurs in patients with sympathetic uveitis when their peripheral leukocytes are exposed to homologous uveal–retinal antigens in tissue cultures.

> Phacoanaphylactic endophthalmitis, another presumed autosensitivity disease, is found in approximately 25 percent of cases of sympathetic uveitis. The same injury that penetrates the globe and prolapses uvea ruptures the lens capsule and allows lens protein to gain access to the systemic circulation. Because of the possible role of autosensitivity in the cause of the disease, steroids and antimetabolites may be helpful. It has been suggested that sympathetic uveitis represents a forme fruste of Vogt-Koyanagi-Harada disease (see subsection Vogt-Koyanagi-Harada Syndrome below). The relationship between the two entities is still uncertain.

IV. Histologically, sympathetic uveitis has certain characteristics that are suggestive but not diagnostic of the disorder. Sympathetic uveitis is a clinicopathologic diagnosis, never a histologic diagnosis alone.

imp.

A. The following four histologic findings are characteristic and found in both the sympathizing and exciting eyes:
   1. Diffuse granulomatous uveal inflammation composed predominantly of epithelioid cells and lymphocytes—eosinophils may be found but plasma cells and neutrophils typically are rare or absent.
   2. Sparing of the choriocapillaris.
   3. Uveal pigment phagocytosis by epithelioid cells.
   4. Dalen-Fuchs's nodules, i.e., collections of epithelioid cells lying between Bruch's membrane and the retinal pigment epithelium with no involvement of the overlying retina and sparing of the underlying choriocapillaris.*

   Because the signs of the trauma generally are in the anterior portion of the eye, the posterior choroid usually is the best place to look for the granulomatous inflammation. Typically the retina is not involved. If a granulomatous inflammation involves the retina in an area away from the site of trauma, the inflammation most probably is not sympathetic uveitis but more likely one of the other granulomatous diseases such as tuberculosis or syphilis.

B. Other findings:
   1. Tissue damage due to the trauma.
   2. Extension of the granulomatous inflammation into the scleral canals and optic disc.

   Because uveal tissue is found normally in the scleral canals and in the vicinity of the optic disc, evisceration, which does not reach these areas, does *not*

---

* Recent electronmicroscopic study of Dalen-Fuchs's nodule suggests that most of the epithelioid cells occurring within the nodule are derived from retinal pigment epithelial cells.

---

protect against sympathetic uveitis. If surgery is being done to prevent sympathetic uveitis, the procedure must be an enucleation, not an evisceration.

PHACOANAPHYLACTIC ENDOPHTHALMITIS
(Figs. 4–5 and 4–6)

I. Phacoanaphylactic endophthalmitis is a unilateral (sometimes bilateral if the lens capsule is ruptured in each eye), zonal, granulomatous inflammation centered around lens material and dependent for its development on a ruptured lens capsule.

II. The disease is thought to be a result of autosensitization to lens protein liberated through a ruptured capsule and thereby gaining access through the aqueous outflow pathways to the systemic circulation.

A. The lens proteins are isolated from the fetal circulation within the avascular lens by the secretion of an encircling basement membrane (lens capsule) very early in embryologic life.

B. Lens proteins, if liberated into the systemic circulation, are not recognized as "self" and act as antigens, and antibodies are formed against the proteins.

   Lens proteins are organ-specific but not species-specific.

C. The antibodies reach the lens remnants in the eye, and an antibody–antigen reaction takes place (phacoanaphylactic endophthalmitis).

D. Presumably, unlike the lens protein that escapes through a ruptured lens capsule, the type of lens protein that leaks through an intact capsule, e.g., in a mature or hypermature lens, is denatured and incapable of acting as an antigen and eliciting an antibody response.

   The material that leaks through an intact capsule incites a macrophagic response. The macrophages swollen with engulfed denatured lens material may block mechanically the anterior chamber drainage angle and cause an acute secondary open angle glaucoma called *phacolytic glaucoma* (see p. 378 in Chap. 10).

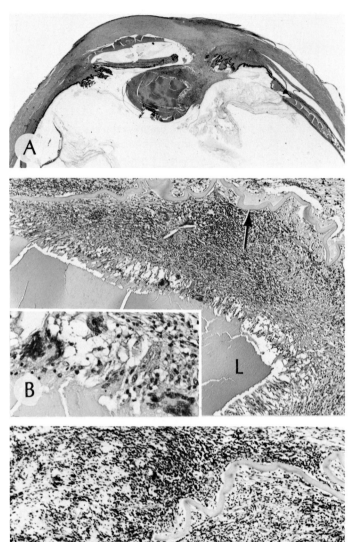

FIG. 4–5. Phacoanaphylactic endophthalmitis. **A.** Zonal granulomatous reaction present around injured lens. **B.** Higher magnification shows epithelioid and giant cells (seen under higher magnification in **inset**) surrounding lens (*L*). *Arrow* shows ruptured, folded lens capsule. **C.** Zonal granulomatous reaction centered around lens remnant (lower right corner), surrounded in turn by granulation tissue containing ruptured capsule. Typically, polymorphonuclear leukocytes (*arrow*) are present between lens and epithelioid cells, seemingly engulfing lens material. **A,** H&E, ×4; **B,** H&E, ×40; **inset,** H&E, ×110; **C,** H&E, ×40.

III. Histologically, in addition to the findings at the site of injury a zonal granulomatous inflammation is found.

    A. Neutrophils surround and seem to "dissolve" or "eat away" lens material.

    B. Epithelioid cells and occasional (sometimes in abundance) multinucleated giant cells are seen beyond the neutrophils.

    C. Lymphocytes, plasma cells and blood vessels, i.e., granulation tissue, surround the epithelioid cells.

    D. Usually the iris is encased in and inseparable from the inflammatory reaction.

    E. The uveal tract generally shows a reactive, chronic, nongranulomatous inflammatory reaction. Sometimes, however, the same trauma that ruptures the lens to set off the phacoanaphylac-

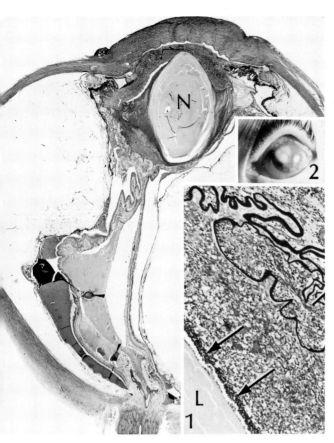

FIG. 4–6. Phacoanaphylactic endophthalmitis. Lens nucleus (N) left behind following extracapsular cataract extraction is surrounded by zonular granulomatous reaction, in which iris is encased. **Inset 1** shows lens (L), surrounded by polymorphonuclear leukocytes (arrows), then by epithelioid and giant cells, which are enclosed by folded, ruptured lens capsule lying within granulation tissue. **Inset 2** shows clinical appearance of eye just prior to enucleation. **Main figure,** PAS, ×5; **inset 1,** PAS, ×40; **inset 2,** clinical.

NONTRAUMATIC INFECTIOUS

BACTERIAL

I. Tuberculosis (*Mycobacterium tuberculosis*) (Figs. 4–7 through 4–10).
  A. The most frequent form of tubercular eye involvement is a cyclitis that rapidly becomes an iridocyclitis—the involvement may also spread posteriorly to cause a choroiditis. Clinically, mutton-fat keratic precipitates are seen on the posterior surface of the cornea.

  The involvement may become massive to form a large tuberculoma involving all the coats of the eye, i.e., a panophthalmitis.

  B. Miliary tuberculosis generally causes a multifocal choroiditis. *"Discrete type*
  C. Histologically the "classic" pattern of caseation necrosis consists of a zonal type of granulomatous reaction around the area of coagulative necrosis. A smooth rod or bacillus can be demonstrated by the Ziehl-Neelsen method.
    1. A diffuse type of granulomatous reaction may be present in areas lacking necrosis.
    2. A discrete (sarcoidal, tuberculoidal) type of granulomatous reaction frequently is seen in miliary tuberculosis.
II. Leprosy (*Mycobacterium leprae*) (Figs. 4–11 through 4–13).
  A. In lepromatous leprosy the lepromin test (analogous to the tuberculin test) is negative, suggesting little or no immunity.

tic endophthalmitis will set off a sympathetic uveitis, i.e., 25 percent of cases of sympathetic uveitis will show an additional phacoanaphylactic endophthalmitis.

FOREIGN BODY GRANULOMAS

I. Foreign body granulomas may develop around exogenous foreign bodies generally introduced into the eye at the time of a penetrating ocular wound, or they may develop around such endogenously produced products as blood in the vitreous or cholesterol (see p. 151 in Chap. 5). Blood in the vitreous on rare occasions incites a foreign body inflammatory response. Almost invariably when this occurs, the intravitreal hemorrhage is traumatic in origin, rather than spontaneous.
II. Histologically a zonal type of granulomatous inflammatory reaction surrounds the foreign body.

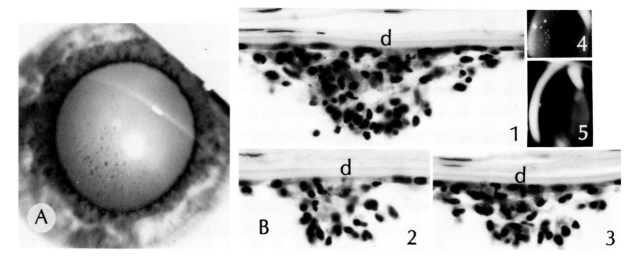

FIG. 4–7. Mutton-fat keratic precipitates (KPs). **A.** Large, "greasy," mutton-fat KPs seen by retroillumination of fundus reflex. **B.** Mutton-fat KPs, shown in **insets 1, 2** and **3,** are composed of collections of epithelioid cells with or without accompanying histiocytes, lymphocytes, plasma cells and pigment. *d,* Descemet's membrane. **Insets 4** and **5** show mutton-fat KPs with wide and narrow beam of slit lamp, respectively. **A,** clinical; **B, inset 1,** H&E, ×252; **inset 2,** H&E, ×252; **inset 3,** H&E, ×252; **inset 4,** clinical; **inset 5,** clinical.

FIG. 4–8. Tuberculosis. Tuberculomatous granulomatous inflammation involves iris, ciliary body, choroid and retina massively. **Inset 1** shows Langhans' giant cell; **inset 2** shows area of caseation necrosis (*N*). **Main figure,** H&E, ×4; **inset 1,** H&E, ×101; **inset 2,** H&E, ×16.

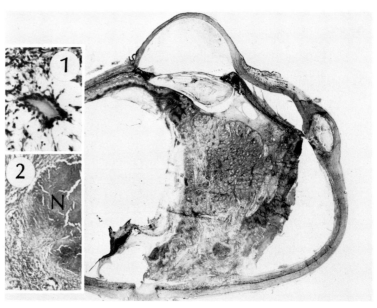

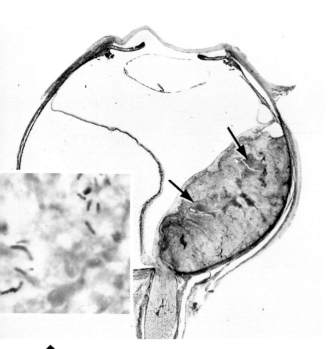

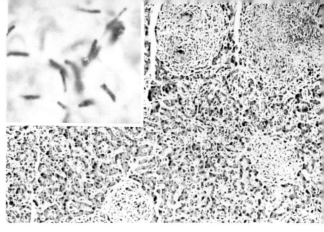

FIG. 4–10. Tuberculosis. Discrete granulomatous inflammation in liver by miliary tuberculosis. **Inset** demonstrates acid-fast bacillae with Ziehl-Neelsen technique. **Main figure,** H&E, ×40; **inset,** Ziehl-Neelsen, ×1,260.

FIG. 4–9. Tuberculosis. Large tuberculoma involves retina and choroid in zonal granulomatous reaction centered around areas of caseation necrosis (*arrows*). **Inset** shows acid-fast organisms by Ziehl-Neelsen method. **Main figure,** H&E, ×5; **inset,** Ziehl-Neelsen, ×1,103.

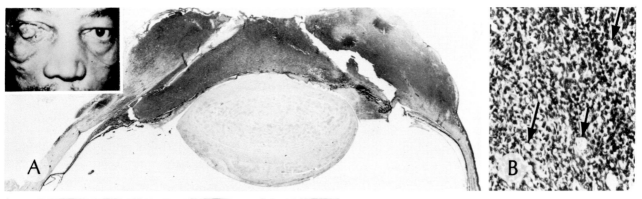

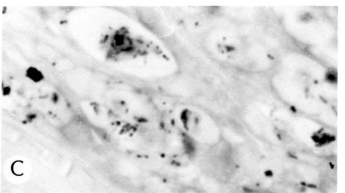

FIG. 4–11. Lepromatous leprosy. **A.** Massive involvement of cornea, limbal area, iris and ciliary body by diffuse granulomatous inflammation (**inset** is eye prior to enucleation). **B.** Higher magnification of inflammation. Large clear cells (*arrows*) contain many organisms, as demonstrated in **C** when stained with special stains. **A,** H&E, ×6; **inset,** clinical; **B,** H&E, ×101; **C,** Ziehl-Neelsen, ×1,103.

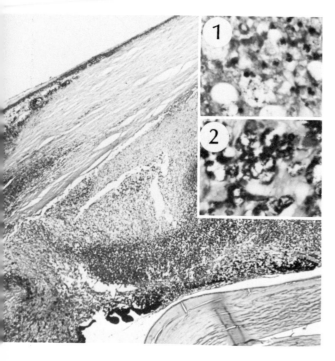

FIG. 4–12. Lepromatous leprosy. Limbal region, iris, ciliary body and anterior chamber show diffuse granulomatous involvement. **Inset 1** demonstrates many "clear" cells as seen with H&E-stained sections. The same cells can be seen teeming with acid-fast leprosy organisms when stained by the Fite method, as noted in **inset 2. Main figure,** H&E, ×21; **inset 1,** H&E, ×252; **inset 2,** Fite, ×252.

FIG. 4–14. Syphilis. Mostly chronic non-granulomatous inflammation, with minor granulomatous component, highly vascular, centered around blood vessels (*arrows*) characterizes gumma of skin seen in **A** and **B.** **A,** H&E, ×54; **B,** H&E, ×69.

FIG. 4–13. Tuberculoid leprosy. **Inset** shows discrete granulomatous inflammation of eyelid with involvement of nerve (*arrow*). Note marked variation in size of granulomas. **Main figure,** H&E, ×40; **inset,** Fite, ×40.

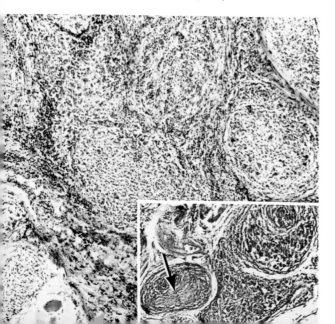

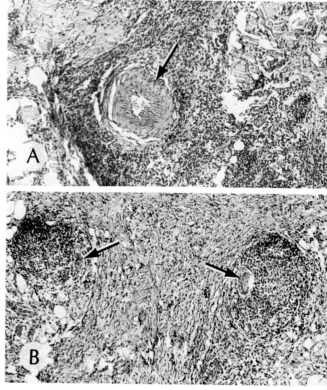

1. The prognosis is poor.
2. Lepromas of the skin result in leonine facies and neurologic changes.
3. The eyeballs are involved, generally in their anterior portions.
4. Histologically a diffuse type of granulomatous inflammatory reaction, known as a leproma, is characterized by the presence of large, pale-staining histiocytes called lepra cells when their cytoplasm is amorphous and Virchow cells when vacuolated.
   a. The lepra cells and Virchow cells teem with bacilli (no immunity), which generally have a beaded appearance with the Ziehl-Neelsen method.
   b. The lepromas involve mainly cornea, anterior sclera and iris; posterior lesions are rare.

   Although lesions have been reported in the posterior portion of the eye, they are quite rare. The bacteria may grow better in the cooler anterior portion of the eye than in the warmer posterior portion, just as they do in the cooler skin rather than in the warmer deeper structures of the body.

B. In *tuberculoid leprosy* the lepromin test is positive, suggesting immunity.
   1. The prognosis is good.
   2. A neural involvement predominates with hypopigmented (vitiligenous), hypoesthetic lesions and thickened nerves.

   The median nerve is particularly vulnerable leading to the characteristic claw hand.

   3. The ocular adnexa and orbital structures are involved, especially the ciliary nerves, but not the eyeballs.
   4. Histologically a discrete (sarcoidal, tuberculoidal) type of granulomatous inflammatory reaction is seen, mainly centered around nerves.
      a. The individual nodules tend to have a much more varied size than in sarcoidosis (see sub-

section Sarcoidosis below) or miliary tuberculosis (see subsection above).
   b. Organisms are extremely hard to find (good immunity) and generally are located in an area of nerve degeneration.
III. Syphilis (*Treponema pallidum*) (Figs. 4–14 through 4–16).
   A. Both the congenital and acquired form of syphilis may produce a nongranulomatous interstitial keratitis or anterior uveitis (see p. 272 in Chap. 8).
   B. The common form of posterior uveitis is a smoldering, indolent, chronic, nongranulomatous inflammatory one characterized by disseminated, large, atrophic scars surrounded by hyperplastic retinal pigment epithelium. A more virulent type of uveitis may occur with a granulomatous inflammation.

   In both the nongranulomatous and granulomatous forms, the overlying retina frequently is involved.

   C. Histologic Findings:
   1. In the chronic nongranulomatous disseminated form of posterior choroiditis:
      a. Within the atrophic scar the outer retinal layers, the retinal pigment epithelium and the inner choroidal layers disappear.
      b. Dehiscences in Bruch's membrane may be present. Retinal elements may "invade" the choroid through the gaps.
      c. Bruch's membrane may be folded into the atrophic, sclerosed choroid.
      d. A chronic, nongranulomatous uveitis may be present with scattered lymphocytes and plasma cells.
      e. The treponema spirochetes can be demonstrated in the ocular tissue with special stains. The organisms frequently are found in areas devoid of inflammatory cells.
   2. In the granulomatous form of posterior chorioretinitis:
      a. Generally the inflammatory

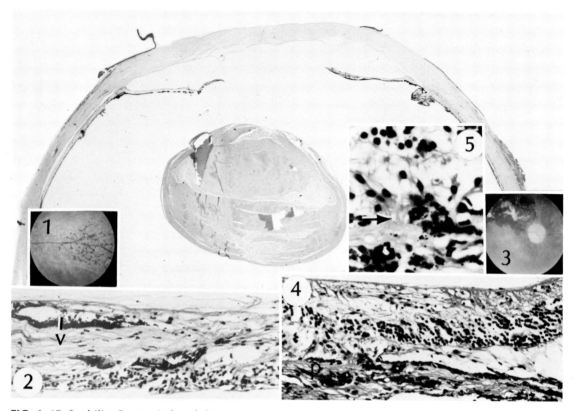

FIG. 4–15. Syphilis. Congenital syphilis (eye from adult) with peripheral anterior synechias, secondary angle closure glaucoma, bullous keratopathy and cataract. **Inset 1** shows fundus with bone corpuscular pigmentation (pseudoretinopathia pigmentosa), due to migration of retinal pigment epithelial cells, and pigment-laden macrophages around retinal blood vessels (v), as shown in **inset 2. Inset 3** shows fundus with coarse pigmentation due to placoid proliferation (p) of retinal pigment epithelium, as shown in **inset 4.** High magnification **inset 5** shows retinal elements (arrow) extending toward choroid through Bruch's membrane. **Main figure,** H&E, ×10; **inset 1,** clinical; **inset 2,** H&E, ×101; **inset 3,** clinical; **inset 4,** H&E, ×101, **inset 5,** H&E, ×252. **Main figure** and **insets 2, 4** and **5** from same case of congenital syphilis; **insets 1** and **3** from two different adult patients, each with positive anterior chamber aqueous sample for spirochetal organisms.

FIG. 4–16. Syphilis. **Inset** shows retinal elements extending through retinal pigment epithelium and Bruch's membrane (between arrows) into choroid (C). **Main figure** is high magnification to demonstrate retinal elements "invading" choroid. **Main figure,** H&E, ×252; **inset,** H&E, ×101.

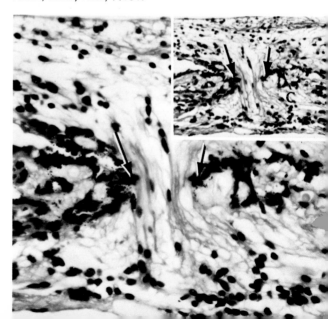

process involves the choroid and overlying retina and is quite vascular.

b. The reaction consists of epithelioid cells along with lymphocytes and plasma cells.

c. Treponemes can be demonstrated in the inflammatory tissue.

3. The above two types of reaction can also involve the anterior uvea.

Spirochetes may be recovered in selected cases by aspiration of aqueous from the anterior chamber.

IV. Tularemia (*Pasturella tularensis*)

A. The common ocular manifestation of tularemia is an oculoglandular involvement, i.e., conjunctivitis and regional (preauricular) lymphadenopathy, which may progress to suppuration.

B. Histologically a granulomatous inflammatory reaction is found in the involved tissue. Organisms have never been demonstrated histologically in the granulomatous tissue.

FUNGAL

I. Blastomycosis (*Blastomyces dermatitidis*) (Fig. 4–17)

A. North American blastomycosis may involve the eyes in the form of an endophthalmitis as part of a secondary generalized blastomycosis that follows primary pulmonary blastomycosis, or it may involve the skin about the eyes in the form of single or multiple, ele-

vated, red ulcers. Cutaneous blastomycosis usually does not become generalized.

B. Histologically, by the use of special stains single budding cells can be demonstrated within a granulomatous reaction.

II. Cryptococcosis (*Cryptococcus neoformans*) (Fig. 4–18)

A. Cryptococcosis also has been called torulosis and the organism's other name is *Torula histolytica*.

B. The fungus has a propensity to spread from its primary pulmonary involvement to central nervous tissue including the optic nerve and retina.

C. Histologically the budding organism is surrounded by a thick, gelatinous capsule and is frequently found within giant cells in a granulomatous reaction. The capsule can be made visible histologically by the use of the "usual" fungus stains (Gridley, periodic acid-Schiff and Gomori's methenamine silver stains) plus stains that demonstrate the thick capsule such as india ink (indirectly) and the mucicarmine stain (directly).

III. Coccidioidomycosis (*Coccidioides immitis*) (Fig. 4–19)

A. Coccidioidomycosis, endemic in the far West and Southwest in the United States, generally starts as a primary pulmonary infection, which may spread to the eyes to cause an endophthalmitis.

B. Histologically, spherules containing multiple spores (endospores) are noted within a granulomatous inflammatory reaction.

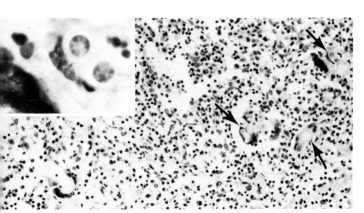

FIG. 4–17. Blastomycosis. Granulomatous process shows individual budding cells (*arrows*) of yeastlike fungus within giant cells. **Inset** is higher magnification of two fungal cells within giant cell. Each yeast is surrounded by its clear capsule. **Main figure,** H&E, ×101; **inset,** H&E, ×504.

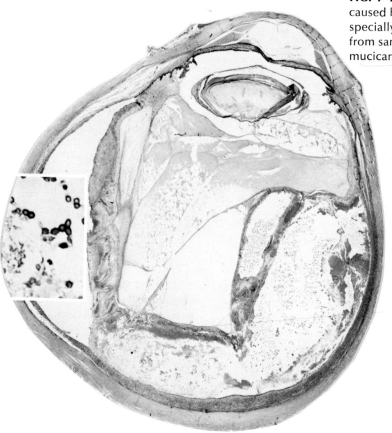

FIG. 4–18. Cryptococcosis. Endophthalmitis caused by *Cryptococcus neoformans*. **Inset** is specially stained to show fungal organisms from same eye. **Main figure,** H&E, ×5; **inset,** mucicarmine, ×400.

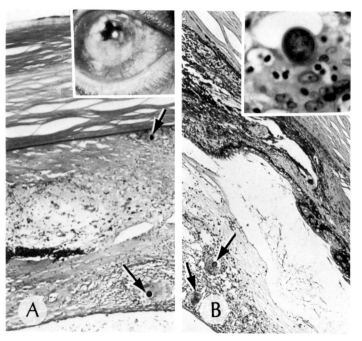

FIG. 4–19. Coccidioidomycosis. **A. Inset** shows clinical appearance of fungal endophthalmitis. Same eye shown in **main figure.** Fungal organisms (*arrows*) seen within fibrogranulomatous anterior chamber reaction. **B.** Same eye. Organisms (*arrows*) present in inflammatory membrane posterior to ciliary body. **Inset** is higher magnification of fungal spherule within giant cell. **A,** PAS, ×40; **inset,** clinical. **B,** H&E, ×40; **inset,** H&E, ×252.

IV. Aspergillosis (*Aspergillus fumigatus*) (Fig. 4–20)
- A. Aspergillosis can cause a painful fungal keratitis or a very indolent, chronic inflammation of the orbit.
- B. Histologically septate, branching hyphae frequently are found within giant cells in a granulomatous reaction.

V. Rhinosporidiosis
- A. Rhinosporidiosis is thought to be a fungus, but the organism has never been grown in culture.
- B. The main ocular manifestation of rhinosporidiosis is lid or conjunctival infection.
- C. Histologically relatively large sacs or spherules (200 to 300 μ in diameter) are filled with spores. The organism may be surrounded by a granulomatous reaction but are more apt to be surrounded by a nongranulomatous reaction of plasma cells and lymphocytes.

FIG. 4–20. Aspergillosis. **Main figure** shows necrotic optic nerve from patient who died from effects of undiagnosed orbital aspergillosis that also involved the brain. **Inset** is specially stained area of optic nerve (from area of *arrow* in **main figure**) to show septate, branching hyphae. **Main figure,** Giemsa, ×16; **inset,** Gridley, ×340.

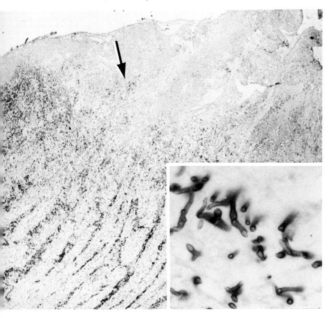

VI. Phycomycosis (Mucormycosis) (Fig. 4–21)
- A. The family Mucoraceae of the class of fungi Phycomycetes contains the two genera, *Mucor* and *Rhizopus*, both of which can cause human infections called phycomycosis.

  Mucormycosis refers only to those infections caused by the genus *Mucor*. Because the hyphae of the two genera of fungi *Mucor* and *Rhizopus* look identical histologically, and because *Mucor* may be difficult to culture, the term phycomycosis is preferred to mucormycosis. Histologically *Mucor* and *Rhizopus* can be separated only by their characteristic sporulation, which is rarely present in sections from infected tissue.

- B. The fungi can infect the orbit or eyeball, typically in patients suffering from acidosis due to any cause but most commonly due to diabetes mellitus (see p. 518 in Chap. 14).
- C. Histologically the hyphae of *Mucor* and *Rhizopus* are nonseptate, very broad (3 to 12 μ in diameter) and branch freely. Unlike most other fungi, which are difficult to identify in routine H&E-stained sections, the Mucoraceae readily take the hematoxylin stain and are identified easily. Typically the hyphae infiltrate and cause thrombosis of blood vessels, leading to infarction. Inflammatory reactions vary from acute suppurative to chronic nongranulomatous to granulomatous.

VII. Candidiasis (*Candida albicans*) (Fig. 4–22)
- A. *Candida albicans* may cause a keratitis or an endophthalmitis.
- B. The endophthalmitis is most likely to occur in patients with an underlying disease that has rendered them immunologically deficient.
- C. Histologically, budding yeasts and pseudohyphal forms are seen surrounded by a chronic nongranulomatous inflammatory reaction but sometimes by a granulomatous one.

VIII. *Streptothrix* (*Actinomyces*) (Fig. 4–23)
- A. The organism responsible for *Streptothrix* infection of the lacrimal sac (see p. 227 in Chap. 6) and for a chronic form of conjunctivitis belongs to the

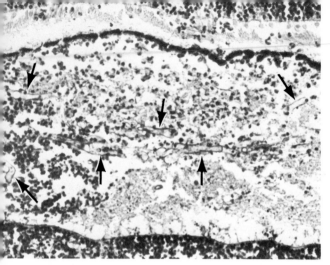

FIG. 4–21. Phycomycosis. Endophthalmitis with large, broad, nonseptate, branching fungi (*arrows*) between retina and choroid. Fungi can be seen even with routinely H&E-stained sections. H&E, ×136.

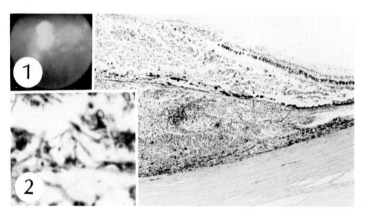

FIG. 4–22. Candidiasis. **Inset 1** shows typical vitreous snowball opacities in patient with *Candida albicans* endophthalmitis. **Main figure** shows granulomatous choroiditis and necrosis of overlying retina due to candidiasis. **Inset 2** is higher magnification to show budding yeasts and pseudohyphal forms. **Main figure,** PAS, ×16; **inset 1,** fundus; **inset 2,** PAS, ×252.

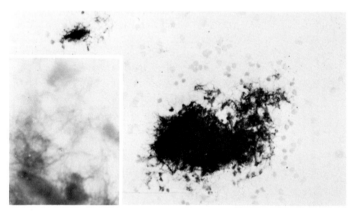

FIG. 4–23. Streptothrix. Smear of lacrimal cast shows large colonies of fungi. **Inset** shows edge of colony at higher magnification to demonstrate delicate, branching, intertwined filaments of fungi. **Main figure,** PAS, ×136; **inset,** PAS, ×504.

class Schizomycetes, which contains the genera *Actinomyces* and *Nocardia*. The organism seems to be transitional between fungi and bacteria.

B. Histologically the fungi are seen in colonies as delicate, branching, intertwined filaments surrounded by necrotic tissue with little or no inflammatory component, e.g., the lacrimal cast from the nasolacrimal system. The fungi are gram-positive.

The colonies can be seen macroscopically as gray or yellow "sulfur" granules. Giant cells are seen on occasion.

IX. Histoplasmosis (*Histoplasma capsulatum*) —see p. 429 in Chapter 11.

FIG. 4–24. Cysticercosis. Various levels of same case. **A. Inset** shows eye enucleated from 6-year-old girl because of suspected retinoblastoma. Cyst (*arrow*), surrounded by granulomatous reaction, is empty in this plane of section. **Main figure** shows scolex area with sucker (*S*) and hooks (*arrows*). **B.** Body of developing cysticercus (*arrow* points to sucker on scolex). **C.** Scolex area with three suckers (*arrows*) and numerous hooks (*h*). **A,** H&E, ×101; **inset,** H&E, ×3; **B,** PAS, ×40; **C,** H&E, ×40.

PARASITIC

I. Cysticercosis (*Cysticercus cellulosae*) (Fig. 4–24)
   A. *Cysticercus cellulosae* is the larval stage of the pork tapeworm *Taenia solium*. The larvae, or bladderworm, hatch in the intestine, and the resultant systemic infestation is called cysticercosis.
   B. The bladderworm has a predilection for the central nervous system and eyes and induces no inflammatory response when alive.
   C. Histologically the necrotic bladderworm is surrounded by a zonal granulomatous inflammatory reaction that generally contains many eosinophils.

II. Toxocariasis (*Toxocara canis*) (Figs. 4–25 and 4–26)
   A. Ocular toxocariasis is a manifestation of visceral larva migrans, i.e., the larvae of the nematode *Toxocara canis*, generally involving children 6 to 11 years of age.

      One is more likely to obtain a history of a puppy in the family rather than an adult dog. Nematodiasis is not an adequate term for the condition, because nematodes other than *Toxocara* also can infest the eye, e.g., *Onchocercus*.

   B. The condition may take two ocular forms:

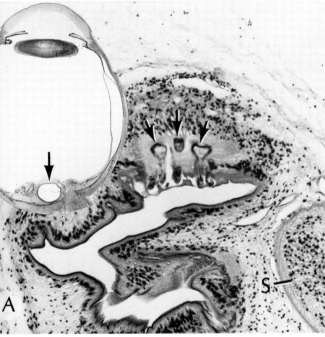

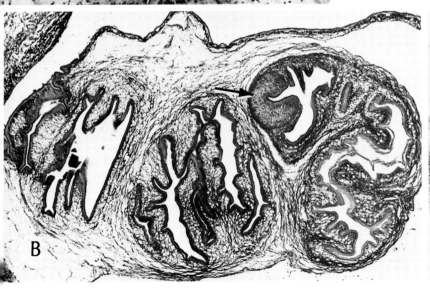

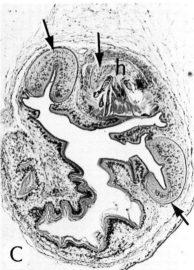

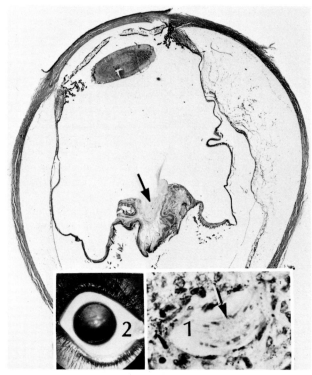

FIG. 4–25. Toxocariasis. Granulomatous inflammatory membrane within retina (*arrow*). **Inset 1** shows *Toxocara canis* (*arrow*) found within membrane. Note tiny nuclei that identify cells of parasite. **Inset 2** shows leukokoria due to toxocariasis. **Main figure,** H&E, ×5; **inset 1,** H&E, ×400; **inset 2,** clinical.

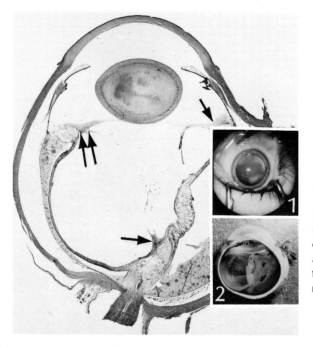

FIG. 4–26. Toxocariasis. Granulomatous inflammation (*double arrow*) with central necrosis surrounded by eosinophils (peripheral retina). Organizing vitreous membranes (*single arrows*) have produced retinal detachment. **Insets 1** and **2** show clinical (leukokoria) and macroscopic appearances of same eye, respectively. **Main figure,** H&E, ×5; **inset 1,** clinical; **inset 2,** macroscopic.

1. Leukokoria with multiple retinal folds radiating out from the necrotic worm, which is generally in the peripheral retina.
2. A discrete lesion usually in the posterior pole and seen through clear media.

C. In both forms the eye is not inflamed externally; the only complaint is loss of vision, and only one eye is involved.

In spite of the fact that the condition presumably follows widespread migration of larvae, only one eye is involved and then only one worm can be found. There is no inflammatory reaction until the worm dies.

D. Histologically a granulomatous inflammatory infiltrate, usually with many eosinophils, surrounds the necrotic worm. The infiltrate is a zonal one with the necrotic worm surrounded by an abscess containing eosinophils, neutrophils and necrotic debris; the abscess is in turn surrounded by granulomatous inflammatory tissue.

III. Toxoplasmosis (*Toxoplasma gondii*) (Figs. 4–27 through 4–30)

A. The definitive host of the intracellular protozoan *Toxoplasma gondii* is the cat, but many intermediate hosts (man, rodents, fowl, etc.) are known.

B. The parasite primarily involves the retina with both congenital and acquired forms recognized:
1. The congenital form is associated with encephalomyelitis, visceral infestation (hepatosplenomegaly) and retinochoroiditis.
2. The acquired form presents usually as a posterior uveitis in an adult.

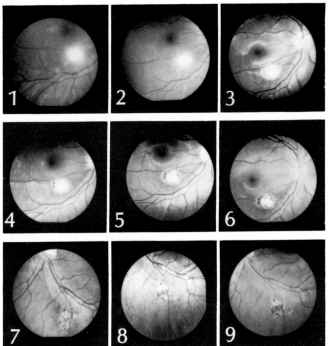

FIG. 4–27. Toxoplasmosis (presumed). **1.** Acute attack in right eye in 12-year-old girl, May 21, 1970 (white spots on blood vessels represent cellular reaction on surface of retina). **2.** June 2, 1970. **3.** September 17, 1970 (early pigmentation present). **4.** March 10, 1971. **5.** March 26, 1973. **6.** December 19, 1973. **7.** Left eye in same girl had old toxoplasmosis lesion inferiorly when first seen May 21, 1970. **8.** March 26, 1973. **9.** December 19, 1973 (note increase in pigmentation over May 21, 1970 in a seemingly inactive lesion). **1** through **9,** fundus.

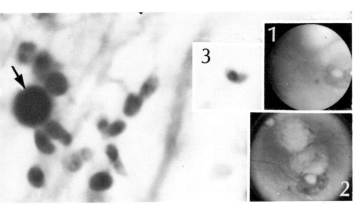

FIG. 4–28. Toxoplasmosis. **Inset 1** shows vitreous reaction overlying acute exacerbation of congenital toxoplasmosis retinal lesion. **Inset 2,** 2 months later following treatment with systemic steroids alone. Lesion is inactive. **Main figure** demonstrates free protozoan organisms of *Toxoplasma gondii* in brain of child who died from effects of congenital toxoplasmosis. Organisms can be differentiated from normal-sized human cell (*arrow*) by their tiny size. **Inset 3** shows one free protozoan in brain. **Main figure,** H&E, ×1,103; **inset 1,** clinical; **inset 2,** clinical; **inset 3,** H&E, ×1,103.

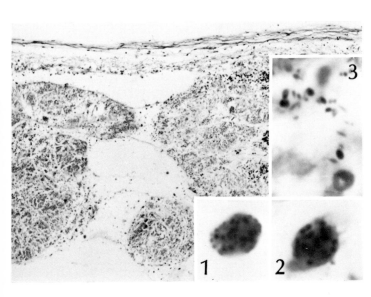

FIG. 4–29. Toxoplasmosis. Necrotic retina from same child as shown in Figure 4–28. Both cyst forms (**insets 1** and **2,** tiny dots represent nuclei of individual organisms) and free forms (**inset 3;** compare tiny size of protozoans to that of plasma cell seen at lower right corner of **inset 3**) are found within necrotic retina. **Main figure,** H&E, ×40; **inset 1,** H&E, ×850; **inset 2,** H&E, ×630; **inset 3,** H&E, ×1,030.

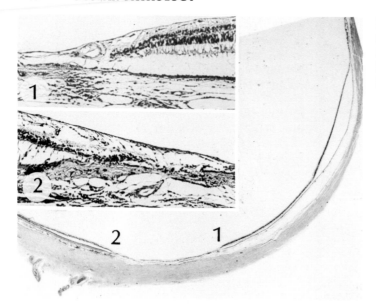

FIG. 4–30. Toxoplasmosis. Healed lesion with sharply demarcated retinochoroidal scar. Higher magnification of 1 and 2 shown in **insets 1** and **2. Main figure,** H&E, ×8; **inset 1,** H&E, ×40; **inset 2,** H&E, ×40.

FIG. 4–31. Trichinosis. **A.** Cyst above shows larva of *Trichinella spiralis* (pork nematode), whereas cyst below is empty. **B.** Higher magnification of larva-containing cyst. **A,** H&E, ×40; **B,** H&E, ×252.

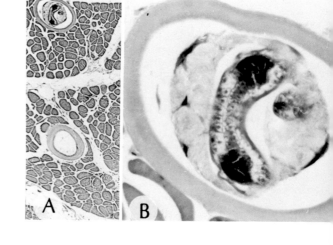

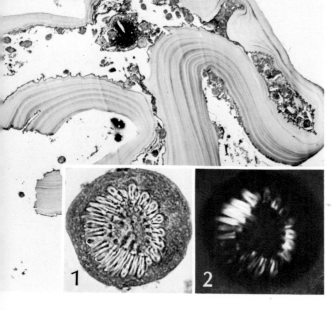

FIG. 4–32. Hydatid cyst. Thick, laminated cyst wall surrounds many larvae of dog tapeworm, *Echinococcus granulosus*. **Insets 1** and **2** show scolex and hooks of tapeworm larva before (**1**) and after (**2**) polarization. **Main figure,** H&E, ×21; **inset 1,** H&E, ×485; **inset 2,** H&E, polarized, ×485.

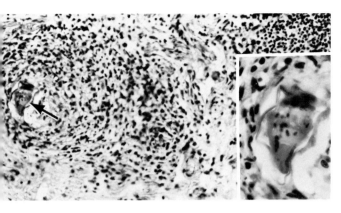

FIG. 4–33. Schistosomiasis. Adult worm (*arrow*) of *Schistosoma mansoni* is present in center of granulomatous reaction. Tiny nuclei identify parasite, as seen in **inset. Main figure,** H&E, ×101; **inset,** H&E, ×252.

C. Histologically the protozoans are found free, in pseudocysts or in true cysts in an area of coagulative necrosis of the retina, which generally is sharply demarcated from the contiguous normal-appearing retina. The underlying choroid, and sometimes sclera, contains a secondary diffuse granulomatous inflammatory infiltrate.

  1. The protozoans may be found rarely free within the retina.

  2. Commonly a protozoan will enter a retinal cell and multiply so that all that is seen histologically is a group of protozoans surrounded by a cell membrane. This is a pseudocyst because the cyst membrane is the cell wall or membrane of the original host cell.

  3. An intracellular protozoan may surround itself by a membrane that it makes, multiply and then form a true cyst. The true cyst, which becomes extruded from the cell and lies free in the tissue, is found in the late stage of the disease when the disease is in remission.

IV. Trichinosis (*Trichinella spiralis*) (Fig. 4–31)

A. The nematode *Trichinella spiralis* is obtained by eating undercooked meat, classically pork, which contains the trichina cysts.

B. Clinically the lids and extraocular muscles may be involved in the systemic migration of the larvae.

C. Histologically the larvae encapsulate or encyst in striated muscle and cause little or no inflammatory reaction. If the larvae die before they encapsulate, a zonal granulomatous inflammatory reaction around the necrotic worm results.

V. Hydatid cyst (*Echinococcus granulosus*) (Fig. 4–32)

A. The onchospheres of the dog tapeworm *Echinococcus granulosus* may enter humans and form a cyst called a hydatid cyst that contains the larval form of the tapeworm represented as multiple scolices provided with hooklets. Each scolex will be the future head of an adult tapeworm.

B. In humans the orbit is the ocular site of predilection.

C. Histologically, multiple scolices are seen adjacent to a thick, acellular, amorphous membrane, which represents the wall of the cyst.

VI. Schistosomiasis (*S. haematobium, S. mansoni* and *S. japonicum*) (Fig. 4–33)

A. The trematode *Schistosoma* can cause a chronic conjunctivitis or blepharitis in endemic areas of the world.

B. The eggs of schistosomas hatch in water into a *miracidium*, which penetrates snails, undergoes metamorphosis and forms *cercariae*. The *cercariae* emerge from the snail and enter the skin of humans as *metacercariae* or *adolescariae*.

C. Histologically the eggs and dead, necrotic, adult worms are seen to incite a marked zonal granulomatous inflammatory response.

VIRAL

I. Cytomegalic inclusion disease (salivary gland disease) (Figs. 4–34 and 4–35)
   A. Cytomegalic inclusion disease is caused by systemic infection with the cytomegalovirus (salivary gland virus). The disease may be on a congenital or acquired basis.
      1. Congenital—characterized by retinochoroiditis, prematurity, jaundice, thrombocytopenia, anemia, hepatosplenomegaly, neurologic involvement and intracranial calcification.
      2. Acquired—found mainly in patients whose immunochemical mechanisms have been modified, as in those with acute leukemia, with malignant lymphomas, having received chemotherapy and with renal transplantation followed by immunosuppressive therapy.
   B. Clinically the picture of a central retinochoroiditis seen in the congenital form is quite similar to that seen in toxoplasmosis. The acquired form starts with scattered white retinal dots or granular patches that may become confluent and are associated with sheathing of adjacent vessels and with retinal hemorrhages.
   C. Histologically a primary coagulative, necrotizing retinitis and a secondary diffuse granulomatous choroiditis is seen. The infected retinal cells show large, eosinophilic intranuclear inclusions and small, multiple, basophilic intracytoplasmic inclusions.

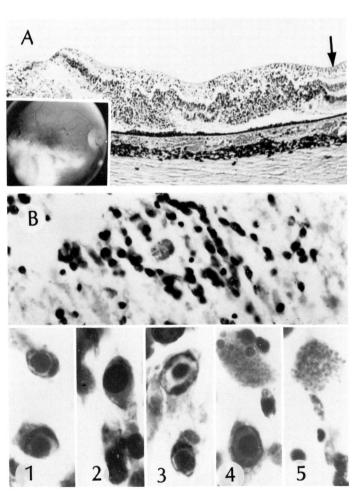

FIG. 4–34. Cytomegalic inclusion disease. **A.** Retina from 32-year-old woman who had undergone bilateral nephrectomy and developed cytomegalic retinitis, as shown in **inset.** Normal retina (*arrow*) suddenly becomes necrotic in area of viral infection. **B.** High magnification of necrotic retina. **Insets 1, 2, 3** and **4** show large eosinophilic intranuclear inclusion bodies, and **insets 4** and **5** show tiny intracytoplasmic basophilic inclusion bodies. **A,** H&E, ×16; **inset,** fundus. **B,** H&E, ×252; **insets 1** through **5,** H&E, ×630.

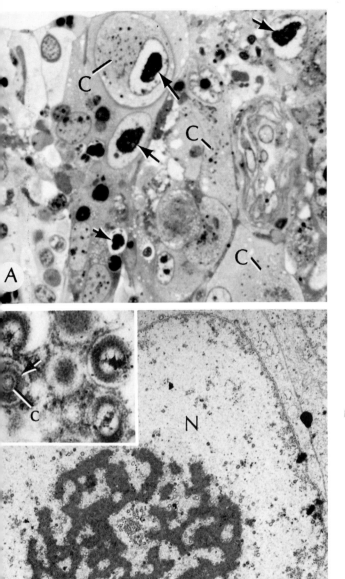

FIG. 4–35. Cytomegalic inclusion disease. Retina obtained from young man who died about 1 year after renal transplantation. **A.** Intranuclear (*arrows*) and intracytoplasmic (c) inclusions present in inner retinal layers. **B.** Virus particles (small spherules) are scattered throughout nucleus (N) and cytoplasm (C). **Inset** shows viruses with envelope (e) surrounding capsid (*arrow*) and core (c). **A,** 1.5 μ section, mallory blue, ×250; **B,** ×3,040; **inset,** ×28,940.

II. Herpes zoster (Fig. 4–36)

— is primarily nongranulomatous — may be zonal granulomatous in sclera

  A. Ocular complications occur in about 50 percent of cases of herpes zoster ophthalmicus:

    1. Cornea—dendritic ulcer (rare), ulceration, perforation, peripheral erosions, bullous keratopathy, epidermidalization (keratinization), band keratopathy, pannus formation, stromal vascularization, hypertrophy of corneal nerves, ring abscess, granulomatous reaction to Descemet's membrane and endothelial degeneration.

    2. Anterior chamber—peripheral anterior synechias, exudate and hyphema.

    3. Iris—patchy necrosis and postnecrotic atrophy, chronic nongranulomatous inflammation, and anterior surface fibrovascular membrane.

    4. Ciliary body—patchy necrosis of anterior portion, especially of circular and radial portions of ciliary muscle. *muscle*

    5. Choroid—chronic nongranulomatous inflammation and less commonly granulomatous inflammation.

    6. Lens—cataract and posterior synechias.

    7. Retina—perivasculitis and vasculitis.

    8. Vitreous—mild mononuclear inflammatory infiltrate.

    9. Sclera—acute or chronic episcleritis and scleritis.

    10. Optic nerve—perivasculitis and chronic leptomeningitis.

    11. Long posterior ciliary nerves and vessels—striking perineural and less commonly intraneural nongranulomatous and occasionally granulomatous inflammation and perivasculitis and vasculitis.

  B. Histologically the most characteristic findings are the lymphocytic (chronic nongranulomatous) infiltration involving the posterior ciliary nerves and vessels, frequently in a segmental distribution, and a diffuse or patchy necrosis involving the iris and pars plicata of the ciliary body. Inclusion bodies have not been demonstrated in the chronic inflammatory lesions.

post ciliary nerve ⊛

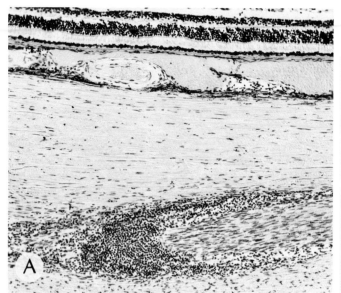

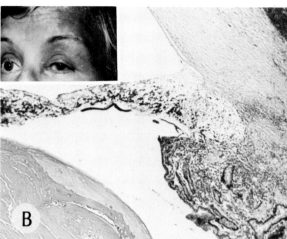

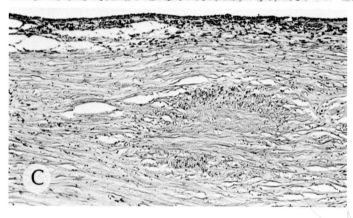

FIG. 4–36. Herpes zoster. **A.** Heavy infiltrate around posterior ciliary nerve as it traverses sclera. Scattered lymphocytic infiltrate present in choroid. **B.** Coagulative necrosis of iris, patchy necrosis of ciliary body, anterior peripheral synechia and marked chronic nongranulomatous inflammation of limbus are seen. Lens is cataractous. **Inset** shows patient with Herpes zoster ophthalmicus involving left eye, causing an iritis. **C.** Nodule consisting of necrotic collagen surrounded by zonal granulomatous reaction of palisading epithelioid cells (reminiscent of rheumatoid scleral nodule, see Figure 4–40) is seen in sclera. **A,** H&E, ×40; **B,** H&E, ×16; **inset,** clinical; **C,** H&E, ×40.

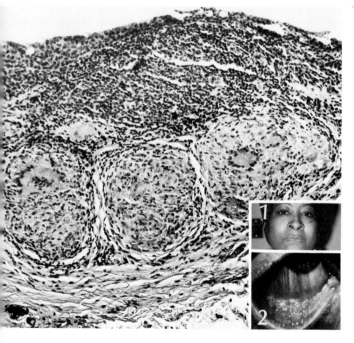

FIG. 4–37. Sarcoidosis. Conjunctival biopsy (from area similar to that shown in **inset 2**) from patient with sarcoidosis shows non-caseating, discrete, granulomatous inflammation in subepithelial area. **Inset 1** shows sarcoid patient with uveitis and involvement of parotid gland (uveoparotid fever, Heerfordt's disease). **Main figure,** H&E, ×110; **inset 1,** clinical; **inset 2,** clinical.

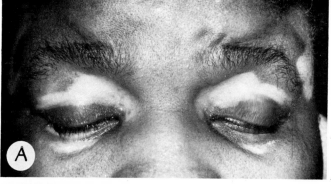

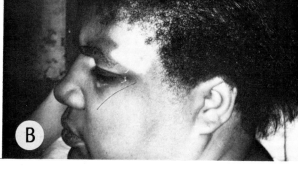

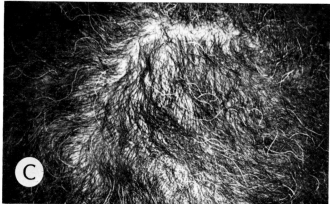

FIG. 4–42. Vogt-Koyanagi-Harada syndrome. (VKH). Patient with VKH shows leukodermia *(vitilig)* (**A**), canities (**B**) and alopecia (**C**). The ocular histology resembles that seen in sympathetic uveitis except that here retina may be involved. */poliosis/*

in abnormal (lessened) degranulation of the neutrophils.

III. Chorioretinitis may be a common finding in these patients.

IV. Histologically, suppurative and granulomatous inflammatory lesions characteristically coexist. The suppurative component may be secondary to infection, whereas the granulomatous component is in response to living or inert intracellular organisms or debris.

BIBLIOGRAPHY

SYMPATHETIC UVEITIS

Blodi F: Sympathetic uveitis as allergic phenomenon. Trans Am Acad Ophthalmol Otolaryngol 63:642, 1959

Brauninger GE, Polack FM: Sympathetic ophthalmitis. Am J Ophthalmol 72:967, 1971

DeVoe AG: Sympathetic ophthalmitis. A case treated by prolonged use of corticotropin and adrenal steroids. Trans Am Ophthalmol Soc 58:75, 1960

Easom HA, Zimmerman LE: Sympathetic ophthalmia and bilateral phacoanaphylaxis. A clinicopathologic correlation of the sympathogenic and sympathizing eyes. Arch Ophthalmol 72:9, 1964

Fine BS, Gilligan JH: The Vogt-Koyanagi syndrome. A variant of sympathetic ophthalmia: report of two cases. Am J Ophthalmol 43:433, 1957

Green WR, Maumenee AE, Sanders TE, Smith ME: Sympathetic uveitis following evisceration. Trans Am Acad Ophthalmol Otolaryngol 76:625, 1972

Hammer H: Lymphocytic transformation test in sympathetic ophthalmitis and the Vogt-Koyanagi-Harada syndrome. Br J Ophthalmol 55:850, 1971

Ishikawa T, Ikui H: The fine structure of the Dalén-Fuchs nodule in sympathetic ophthalmia. Report I. Changes of the pigment epithelial cells within the Dalén-Fuchs nodule. Jap J Ophthalmol 16:254, 1972

Kay ML, Yanoff M, Katowitz JA: Sympathetic uveitis—development in spite of corticosteroid therapy. Am J Ophthalmol 78:90, 1974

Rockliffe WC: Four cases of sympathetic irritation occurring long after injury. Trans Ophthalmol Soc UK 27:88, 1907

Stafford WR: Sympathetic ophthalmia. Report of a case occurring ten and one half days after injury. Arch Ophthalmol 74:521, 1965

Thies O: Gedanken über den Ausbruch der sympathischen Ophthalmie. Klin Monatsbl Augenheilkd 112:185, 1947

Wong VG: Immunosuppressive therapy of ocular inflammatory diseases. Arch Ophthalmol 81:628, 1969

Wong VG, Anderson R, O'Brien PJ: Sympathetic ophthalmia and lymphocytic transformation. Am J Ophthalmol 72:960, 1971

PHACOANAPHYLACTIC ENDOPHTHALMITIS

Chishti M, Henkind P: Spontaneous rupture of anterior lens capsule (phacoanaphylactic endophthalmitis). Am J Ophthalmol 69:264, 1970

Easom HA, Zimmerman LE: Sympathetic ophthalmia and bilateral phacoanaphylaxis. A clinicopathologic correlation of the sympathogenic and sympathizing eyes. Arch Ophthalmol 72:9, 1964

Halbert SP, Manski W: Biological aspects of autoimmune reactions in the lens. Invest Ophthalmol 4:516, 1965

Lemoine AN, Macdonald AE: Observations on phacoanaphylactic endophthalmitis. Arch Ophthalmol 53:101, 1924

Marak GE, Font RL, Czawlytko LN, Alepa FP: Experimental lens-induced granulomatous endophthalmitis: preliminary histopathologic observations. Exp Eye Res 19:311, 1974

Yanoff M, Scheie HG: Cytology of human lens aspirate. Its relationship to phacolytic glaucoma and phacoanaphylactic endophthalmitis. Arch Ophthalmol 80:166, 1968

FOREIGN BODY GRANULOMAS

Ferry AB, Barnet AH: Granulomatous keratitis resulting from the use of cyanoacrylate adhesions for closure of perforated corneal ulcers. Am J Ophthalmol 72:538, 1971

Naumann G, Ortbauer R: Histopathology after successful implantation of anterior chamber acrylic lens. Survey Ophthalmol 15:18, 1970

BACTERIAL

Baghdassarian SA, Zakharia H, Asdourian KK: Report of a case of bilateral caseous tuberculous dacryoadenitis. Am J Ophthalmol 74:744, 1972

Blodi FC, Hervoust F: Syphilitic chorioretinitis: a histologic study. Arch Ophthalmol 79:294, 1968

Hammami H, Faggioni R, Streiff EB, Zellweger JP: Tuberculose miliaire choroididienne disséminée. Ophthalmologica 169:333, 1974

Hanna C, Lyford JH: Tularemia infection of the eye. Ann Ophthalmol 3:1321, 1971

Hornblass A: Ocular leprosy in South Vietnam. Am J Ophthalmol 75:479, 1973

Massaro D, Katz S, Sachs M: Choroidal tubercles. A clue to hematogenous tuberculosis. Ann Intern Med 60:231, 1964

Montenegro ENR, Israel CW, Nicol WG, Smith JL: Histopathologic demonstrations of spirochetes in the human eye. Am J Ophthalmol 67:335, 1969

FUNGAL

Agrawal S, Sharma KD, Shrivastava JB: Generalized rhinosporidiosis with visceral involvement. Arch Dermatol 80:22, 1959

Apostol JG, Meyer SL: Graphium endophthalmitis. Am J Ophthalmol 73:566, 1972

Bell R, Font RL: Granulomatous anterior uveitis caused by Coccidioides immitis. Am J Ophthalmol 74:93, 1972

Bongiorno FJ, Leavell UW, Wirtschafter, JD: The

black dot sign and North American cutaneous blastomycosis. Am J Ophthalmol 78:145, 1974

Chandler JW, Kalina RE, Milam DF: Coccidioidal choroiditis following renal transplant. Am J Ophthalmol 74:1080, 1972

Ferry AP: Cerebral mucormycosis (phycomycosis). Ocular findings and review of literature. Survey Ophthalmol 6:1, 1961

Fine BS: Intraocular mycotic infections. Lab Invest 11:1161, 1962

Gonyea EF, Heilman KM: Neuro-ophthalmic aspects of central nervous system cryptococcosis. Internuclear and supranuclear ophthalmoplegia. Arch Ophthalmol 87:164, 1972

Green WR, Font RL, Zimmerman LE: Aspergillosis of the orbit. Arch Ophthalmol 82:302, 1969

Griffin JR, Pettit TH, Fishman LS, Foos RY: Bloodborne Candida endophthalmitis. A clinical and pathologic study of 21 cases. Arch Ophthalmol 89:450, 1973

Hale LM: Orbit-cerebral phycomycosis. Report of a case and review of the disease in infants. Arch Ophthalmol 86:39, 1971

Jampol LM, Strauch BS, Albert DM: Intraocular nocardiosis. Am J Ophthalmol 76:568, 1973

Michelson PE, Stark W, Reeser F, Green WR: Endogenous candida endophthalmitis. Report of 13 cases and 16 from the literature. Int Ophthalmol Clin 11:125, 1971

Naumann G, Ortbauer R, Witzenhausen, R: Candida albicans-Endophthalmitis nach Kataraktextraktion. Ophthalmologica 162:160, 1971

Ostler HB, Okumoto M, Halde C: Dermatophytosis affecting the periorbital region. Am J Ophthalmol 72:934, 1971

Rainin EA, Little HA: Ocular coccidioidomycosis. Trans Am Acad Ophthalmol Otolaryngol 76:645, 1972

Richards WW: Actinomycotic lacrimal canaliculitis. Am J Ophthalmol 75:155, 1973

Rodrigues MM, Laibson P, Kaplan W: Exogenous mycotic keratitis caused by blastomyces dermatitidis. Am J Ophthalmol 75:782, 1973

Vida L, Moel SA: Systemic North American blastomycosis with orbital involvement. Am J Ophthalmol 77:240, 1974

PARASITIC

Ashton N: Larval granulomatosis of the retina due to toxocara. Br J Ophthalmol 44:129, 1960

Badir G: Schistosomiasis of the conjunctiva. Br J Ophthalmol 30:215, 1946

Baghdassarian SA, Zakharia H: Report of three cases of hydatid cyst of the orbit. Am J Ophthalmol 71:1081, 1971

Hogan MJ, Kimura SG, O'Connor GR: Ocular toxoplasmosis. Arch Ophthalmol 72:592, 1964

Jampol LM, Caldwell JBH, Albert DM: Cysticercus cellulosae in the eyelid. Arch Ophthalmol 89:319, 1973

Massa M, Laurijs L, Wigns L: Lésions parasitaires de la rétine chez une femme bantoue. Bull Soc Belge Ophthalmol 137:412, 1964

Maumenee AE: Clinical entities in "uveitis": an approach to the study of intraocular inflammation. Am J Ophthalmol 69:1, 1970

Perkins ES: Ocular toxoplasmosis. Br J Ophthalmol 57:1, 1973

Segal P, Stanislaw M, Smolarz-Dudarewicz J: Subretinal cysticercosis. Am J Ophthalmol 57:655, 1964

Spaeth GL, Adams RE, Soffe AM: Treatment of trichinosis. Case Report. Arch Ophthalmol 71:359, 1964

Wilder HC: Nematode endophthalmitis. Trans Am Acad Ophthalmol Otolaryngol 54:99, 1950

Wilder HC: Toxoplasma chorioretinitis in adults. Arch Ophthalmol 48:127, 1952

Wilkinson CP, Welch RB: Intraocular toxocara. Am J Ophthalmol 71:921, 1971

VIRAL

Boniuk I: The cytomegaloviruses and the eye. Int Ophthalmol Clin 12:169, 1972

deVenecia G, Rhein GMZ, Pratt M, Kisken W: Cytomegalic inclusion retinitis in an adult. A clinical, histopathologic and ultrastructural study. Arch Ophthalmol 86:44, 1971

Klein S, Roschlau G, Ryssel D: Augenveränderungen bei Zytomegalie. Ophthalmologica 160:209, 1970

Lonn LI: Neonatal cytomegalic inclusion disease chorioretinitis. Arch Ophthalmol 88:434, 1972

Naumann G, Gass JDM, Font RL: Histopathology of herpes zoster ophthalmicus. Am J Ophthalmol 65:533, 1968

Piebenga LW, Laibson PR: Dendritic lesions in herpes zoster ophthalmicus. Arch Ophthalmol 90:268, 1973

Smith ME: Retinal involvement in adult cytomegalic inclusion disease. Arch Ophthalmol 72:44, 1964

Wyhinny GJ, Apple DJ, Guastella FR, Vygantas CM: Adult cytomegalic inclusion retinitis. Am J Ophthalmol 76:773, 1973

SARCOIDOSIS

Chumbley LC, Kearns TP: Retinopathy of sarcoidosis. Am J Ophthalmol 73:123, 1972

Coleman SC, Brull S, Green WR: Sarcoid of the lacrimal sac and surrounding area. Arch Ophthalmol 88:645, 1972

Cook JR, Brubaker RF, Savell J, Sheagren J: Lacrimal sarcoidosis treated with corticosteroids. Arch Ophthalmol 88:513, 1972

Gass JDM, Olson CL: Sarcoidosis with optic nerve and retinal involvement. A clinicopathologic case report. Trans Am Acad Ophthalmol Otolaryngol 77:739, 1973

Israel HL, Goldstein RA: Relation of Kveim-antigen reaction to lymphadenopathy. Study of sarcoidosis and other diseases. N Engl J Med 284:345, 1971

Kelley JS, Green WR: Sarcoidosis involving the optic nerve head. Arch Ophthalmol 89:486, 1973

Laties AM, Scheie HG: Evolution of multiple small tumors in sarcoid granuloma of the optic disc. Am J Ophthalmol 74:60, 1972

Nickerson DA: Boeck's sarcoid; report of 6 cases in which autopsies were made. Arch Pathol 24:19, 1937

Schaumann J: On nature of certain peculiar corpuscles present in tissue of lymphogranulomatosis benigna. Acta med Scand 106:239, 1941

Sieracki JC, Fisher ER: The ceroid nature of the so-called "Hamazaki-Wesenberg bodies." Am J Clin Pathol 59:248, 1973

Somers K: Random biopsies in the diagnosis of sarcoid. Eye Ear Nose Throat Mon 52:369, 1973

GRANULOMATOUS SCLERITIS

Anderson B Sr: Ocular lesions in relapsing polychondritis and other rheumatoid syndromes. Trans Am Acad Ophthalmol Otolaryngol 71:227, 1971

Brubaker R, Font RL, Shepherd EM: Granulomatous sclerouveitis: regression of ocular lesions with cyclophosphamide and prednisone. Arch Ophthalmol 86:517, 1971

Hinzpeter EN, Naumann G, Bartelheimer HK: Ocular histopathology in Still's disease. Ophthalmol Res 2:16, 1971

Jayson MIV, Jones DEP: Scleritis and rheumatoid arthritis. Ann Rheum Dis 30:343, 1971

GRANULOMATOUS REACTION TO DESCEMET'S MEMBRANE

Green WR, Zimmerman LE: Granulomatous reaction to Descemet's membrane. Am J Ophthalmol 64:555, 1967

Wolter JR, Johnson FD, Meyer RF, Watters JA: Acquired autosensitivity to degenerating Descemet's membrane in a case with anterior uveitis in the other eye. Am J Ophthalmol 72:782, 1971

Zimmerman LE: New concepts in pathology of the cornea, in The Cornea World Congress. Edited by JH King, JW McTigue. Washington, DC, Butterworths, 1965, p 30

VOGT-KOYANAGI-HARADA SYNDROME

Fine BS, Gilligan JH: The Vogt-Koyanagi syndrome. A variant of sympathetic ophthalmia: report of two cases. Am J Ophthalmol 43:433, 1957

Hammer H: Lymphocytic transformation test in sympathetic ophthalmitis and the Vogt-Koyanagi-Harada syndrome. Br J Ophthalmol 55:850, 1971

Pattison EM: Uveomeningoencephalitic syndrome (Vogt-Koyanagi-Harada). Arch Neurol 12:197, 1965

Shimizu K: Harada's, Behcet's, Vogt-Koyanagi syndromes—are they clinical entities? Trans Am Acad Ophthalmol Otolaryngol 77:281, 1973

FAMILIAL CHRONIC GRANULOMATOUS DISEASE OF CHILDHOOD

Belcher RW, Czarnetzki B: A simple screening test for chronic granulomatous disease. Am J Clin Pathol 60:450, 1973

Martyn LJ, Lischner HW, Pileggi AJ, Harley RD: Chorioretinal lesions in familial chronic granulomatous disease of childhood. Am J Ophthalmol 73:403, 1972

chapter 5

Surgical and Nonsurgical Trauma

NORMAL WOUND HEALING*

CORNEA†

I. Abrasion (Fig. 5–1)
   A. An abrasion results from an injury that removes some or all of the layers of epithelium but leaves Bowman's membrane intact.
   B. The wound heals by epithelial sliding and mitotic proliferation. If healing is uncomplicated, no scar occurs.
      1. After about an hour lag period the normal epithelium from the edge of the abraded area flattens and so slides inward to cover the gap.

      If the entire corneal epithelium is abraded, the gap can be covered by sliding conjunctival epithelium in 48 to 72 hours. At first the epithelium is thinner than normal, but mitotic cell division restores rapidly the normal thickness. Over a period of weeks to a few months, the conjunctival epithelium takes on completely the morphologic characteristics of corneal epithelium.

      2. Mitotic multiplication of the epithelium restores the normal thickness.

II. Superficial defect (Fig. 5–2)
   A. A superficial defect results from an injury that removes epithelium and Bowman's membrane with or without a few anterior layers of stroma.

B. Healing takes place exactly as in an abrasion except that mitotic multiplication results in a focus of thicker than normal epithelium called an *epithelial facet.*

An epithelial facet can be seen with the slit lamp as a tiny, focal separation of the two anteriormost zones of corneal relucency. This type of lesion results most frequently from a small, superficially embedded foreign body.

C. No attempt is made to repair Bowman's membrane or any superficial stroma that may be involved.

III. Deep defect (Fig. 5–3)
   A. A deep defect results from an injury that removes epithelium, Bowman's membrane and at least the anterior quarter of stroma, i.e., a penetrating injury or avulsion of stromal tissue.
   B. Healing takes place mainly by epithelial sliding, and corneal thinning results.
      1. The epithelium from the edge of the injured area flattens and slides over the wound, thus attempting to fill the gap promptly.
      2. Mitotic multiplication of the epithelium results in a normal thickness or a slightly thicker than normal epithelium but cannot restore the normal curvature of the anterior corneal surface. Thus a concavity of the anterior corneal surface results in corneal thinning.
      3. Bowman's membrane and corneal stroma are not repaired.

      Bowman's membrane and corneal stroma *never* regenerate. When required, they are replaced by scarring.

---

* The example used for the section Normal Wound Healing is a "clean," noninfected, uncomplicated wound as exemplified by the typical, surgical wound.
† The cornea is an unusual tissue because it is avascular. Wound healing, therefore, also is unusual because it does not involve a vascular phase.

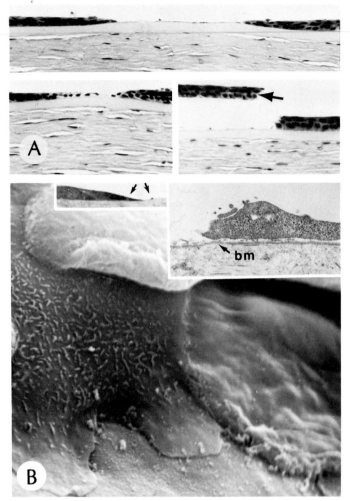

FIG. 5–1. Abrasion. **A.** Epithelial attenuation at edges of abrasion **(upper). Lower left.** Defect is covered by epithelial slide across intact Bowman's membrane. **Lower right.** Artifactitious epithelial break has sharp edges (*arrow*). **B.** Main figure shows advancing cytoplasmic extensions of two epithelial cells, one still covered with microvillae or plicae 6 hours after abrasion. **Inset upper left** shows epithelial attenuation (*arrows*) 4 hours after abrasion of cornea. **Inset upper right** shows advancing cytoplasmic extension of leading epithelial cell along original thin basement membrane (bm) which remained intact. **A, upper,** H&E, ×136; **lower left,** H&E, ×136; **lower right,** H&E, ×136; **B, main figure,** SEM, ×5000; **inset upper left,** TB, ×500; **inset upper right,** TEM, ×15,000.

FIG. 5–2. Epithelial facet. **A.** Superficial defect between cut edges of Bowman's membrane (*arrows*) is filled with hyperplastic epithelium such that smooth topography of epithelial surface is reconstituted. Underlying stroma is normal. **B.** Epithelium occupies defect between cut ends (*arrows*) of Bowman's membrane. Underlying stroma shows scarring here. **A,** Wilder reticulum, ×145; **B,** H&E, ×80.

FIG. 5–3. Deep stromal defect results in corneal thinning. In area of defect (right side) epithelium is hyperplastic, Bowman's membrane is absent and corneal stroma shows thinning; stromal scar formation is noted by increased number and haphazard arrangement of keratocytes. H&E, ×101.

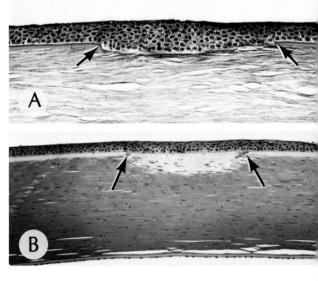

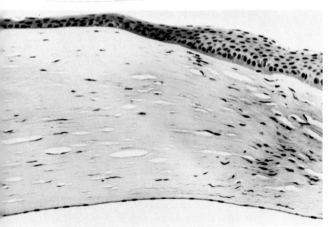

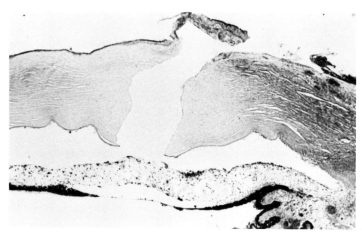

FIG. 5–4. Collagen lamellas retract upon being cut, causing wound to gape when making section for cataract extraction. H&E, ×16.

FIG. 5–5. Descemet's membrane (D) is elastic and curls in area of limbal cataract scar. Note also fibrous overgrowth between cut ends (arrows) of Descemet's membrane. 1.5 μ section, PD, ×101.

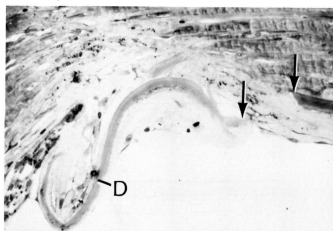

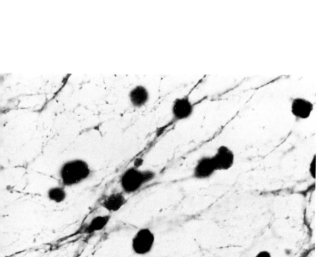

FIG. 5–6. Fibrin is identified by its thin, "cobweblike" appearance. Cells use fibrin as scaffold upon which to migrate and to lay down reparative materials. PAS, ×630.

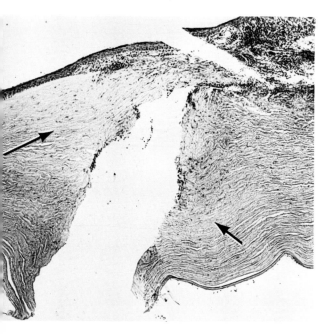

FIG. 5–7. Corneal stromal edema is identified as light-staining areas (arrows) that show loss of normally seen artifactitious clefts between corneal lamellas. Note inflammatory cellular infiltrate at limbus (mainly lymphocytes and plasma cells) and along anterior wound edges (mainly polymorphonuclear leukocytes). Recent cataract surgery. H&E, ×69.

IV. Laceration*—the healing of a laceration of the cornea can be divided into six phases:

A. Immediate phase—initiated immediately following a laceration (Figs. 5–4 through 5–7)

1. Mechanical factors

gaping a. The normal elasticity of the collagen stromal fibers cause them to retract instantly on being cut.

b. Descemet's membrane also has elastic properties and recoils on being cut.

c. The combination of retraction of the stromal fibers and recoiling of Descemet's membrane leads to anterior and posterior gaping of the wound.

2. Fibrin plug

fibrin plug a. When the fibrinogen of the "secondary" aqueous comes into contact with the cut edges of the wound, it precipitates as fibrin, forming a fibrin plug.

b. The fibrin plug helps to seal the wound and also, by acting as a scaffold, aids subsequent fibroblastic reparative stromal processes.

The formation of a fibrin plug can be inhibited by heparin.

edema 3. Corneal stromal edema, although it begins immediately, develops slowly and generally does not become clinically noticeable for a few hours. *mononuclear phase*

B. Leukocytic phase—starts after a lag period of at least 30 minutes (Figs. 5–7 and 5–8).

1. After a delay of about 30 minutes to 5 hours polymorphonuclear leukocytes migrate into the area.

a. Most of the neutrophils come from conjunctival vessels via the tear film; some come from perilimbal vessels, especially in

limbal corneal wounds; and some come from the aqueous.

b. The short-lived neutrophils provide a weak phagocytic function, and supply enzymes, e.g., phosphatase, which aid in the nourishment of the fibroblasts.

2. Mononuclear cells may arrive at the site of the wound after a delay of from 12 to 24 hours.

a. Few mononuclear cells reach clear (central) corneal wounds, except via the aqueous, whereas they are plentiful at the site of limbal wounds (near the perilimbal vessels).

b. The mononuclear cells act as scavengers but also may transform by metaplasia into fibroblasts.

C. Epithelial phase—starts sometime after one hour (Figs. 5–8 through 5–10).

1. By a process of sliding and mitotic multiplication the epithelium grows into the anterior part of a gaping wound.

If there is no gaping anteriorly, the epithelium simply will cover over the wound. With gaping the epithelium grows into the gap so as to completely line the cut ends of the cornea. If the wound perforates the cornea and is not sutured or sutured improperly so that gaping occurs between the cut ends of the cornea, the epithelium will grow inward and completely line the cut edges. If the endothelium is healthy, it inhibits (contact inhibition) the growth of epithelium into the eye, so that the epithelium does not grow beyond the posterior margin of the corneal wound. If the endothelium is unhealthy (e.g., by injury, by iris synechia, or previously diseased by cornea gutatta) or covered by iris, lens remnants or vitreous, it does not inhibit the growth of epithelium and an *epithelial downgrowth (ingrowth)* may result.

2. As the fibroblastic phase progresses, resulting in elaboration of new connective tissue and ground substance, the epithelium slowly "retreats" anteriorly at the same rate that the increased mass of new

* The example used for this section is a laceration through the entire thickness of *clear* cornea. The differences between the healing of clear cornea and of limbal or far peripheral cornea will be pointed out where appropriate. A laceration through the entire thickness of the cornea is a perforating injury of the cornea (through and through) but a penetrating injury of the globe (into but not through).

stroma takes up the volume under it.

3. Ultimately the epithelium recedes completely out of the wound, which becomes filled entirely with the fibroblastic tissue.

4. The epithelium seems to be an important moderator in proper wound healing of underlying structures.

a. It seems to play a key role in the transformation of keratocytes and mononuclear cells into fibroblasts.

b. If the epithelium is prevented from covering the wound, wound healing is delayed markedly.

c. It has the ability to synthesize collagen and may mediate the elaboration of collagen by fibroblasts (keratocytes).

d. It apparently has the ability to secrete enzymes such as a collagenase when the cells have

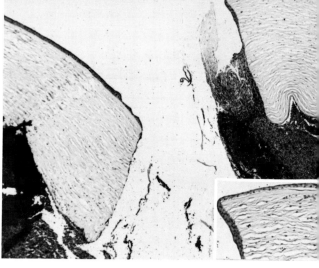

FIG. 5–8. Corneal laceration 1 day old. Epithelium has started to slide over gaping wound edges. Edematous corneal stroma is infiltrated by polymorphonuclear leukocytes. **Inset** shows higher magnification of epithelium sliding over cut edge. **Main figure,** H&E, ×21; **inset,** H&E, ×40.

FIG. 5–9. Organ culture of rabbit corneal button 5 days old. Epithelium grows over cut edge in about 30 hours and then makes contact with endothelium (arrow). No further epithelial growth takes place (contact inhibition). **Insets 1 and 2** show high magnification views of epithelial–endothelial junction (arrows). **Main figure,** H&E, ×101; **inset 1,** 1.5 μ section, azure II, ×176; **inset 2,** 1.5 μ section, azure II, ×252.

been rendered abnormal by disease processes such as infection, chemical burns or desiccation.

The proteolytic enzymes (collagenase and others) released by abnormal epithelial cells and to a lesser extent by neutrophils and keratocytes seem to play a major role in the continued development of corneal ulceration.

D. Fibroblastic phase—starts sometime after 12 hours (Fig. 5–11)

1. In clear corneal wounds fibroblasts are formed mainly from keratocytes, initially from those closest to the wound margin and to the overlying epithelium.

There is evidence to suggest that fibroblasts also may be formed from mononuclear cells that have migrated to the central cornea from the aqueous or perhaps from perilimbal vessels.

2. In limbal corneal wounds fibroblasts are formed from keratocytes and from metaplasia of mononuclear cells that have migrated into the area.

3. However the fibroblasts are derived,

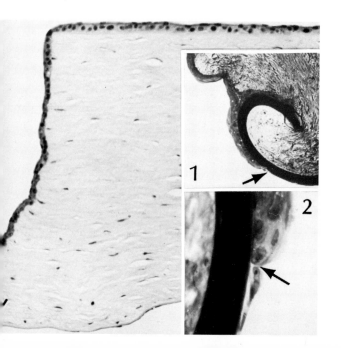

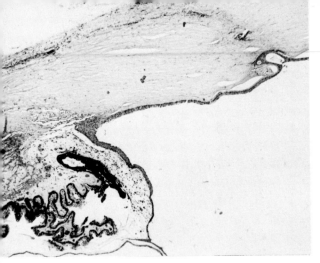

FIG. 5–10. Epithelium has entered surgically aphakic eye, lining posterior cornea, anterior chamber angle and peripheral iris and extending onto vitreous posteriorly. Perhaps endothelium was unhealthy (or covered by iris or vitreous) and could not inhibit ingrowth of epithelium (see Figure 5–39F for higher magnification of same figure). H&E, ×21.

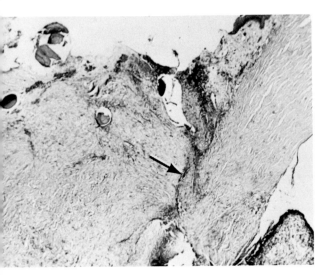

FIG. 5–11. Fibroblastic activity, noted by increased cellularity, results in healing of 19-day-old corneal wound (*arrow*). Round, dark bodies in upper left represent catgut sutures used to close accidental laceration. H&E, ×16.

they enlarge or thicken, multiply and form an active fibroblastic tissue that elaborates collagen and ground substance (acid mucopolysaccharides).

The fibroblastic tissue is similiar to the usual kind of tissue that is involved in wound healing, namely granulation tissue, with one marked exception—absence of a vascular component. The covering epithelium appears to have an effect on the fibroblastic activity. If the epithelium is retarded (by any means) in covering the defect, the fibroblastic activity is greatly delayed. The epithelium probably elaborates a factor that activates stromal cells and attracts mononuclear cells.

FIG. 5–12. Attenuated, advancing edge (*arrow*) of corneal endothelium in rabbit cornea 24 hours after destruction of central endothelial cells by ultraviolet laser. Descemet's membrane was not interrupted. Viable keratocytes (*K*) at edge of stromal injury are enlarged in preparation for reparative activity. 1.5 μ section, PD, ×300.

E. Endothelial phase—starts sometime after 24 hours (Fig. 5–12).
  1. The endothelium heals by endothelial sliding and mitotic and amitotic multiplication.
    a. The endothelium slides over the wound and attempts to cover the gap much as in epithelial sliding.
    b. Initially, in order to cover the defect the endothelial cells enlarge in size. Later, with mitotic division mainly, and perhaps

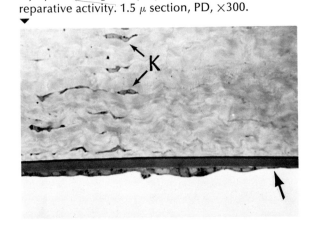

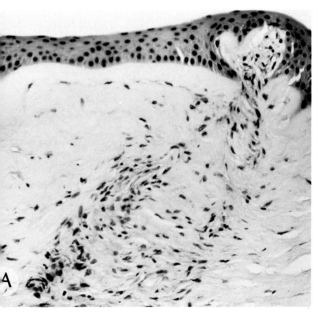

A

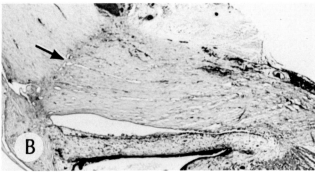

B

FIG. 5–13. A. Young corneal scar has haphazard arrangement of fibroblasts and collagen, although cells on right are assuming orientation more parallel to surface. **B.** Older corneal scar (*arrow*) is less cellular, and lamellas tend to orient more parallel to surface. Iris is adherent to posterior corneal surface at scar (adherent leukoma). **A**, H&E, ×136; **B**, H&E, ×16.

amitosis, the number of endothelial cells increases, so that the original cells can return to their normal size.

  2. A new basement membrane (Descemet's membrane) is produced by the endothelial cells, so that it is regenerated after a few weeks.

F. Late phase—starts sometime after a week (Fig. 5–13).

  1. There is a slow decrease in cellularity along with a reorientation of the nuclei and fibers parallel to the corneal surface.

The fibroblastic tissue at first is highly cellular with the cells and elaborated collagen lying in an apparent haphazard fashion. With time the cellularity decreases and the orientation of the remaining cells and fibrils approaches that of normal cornea, i.e., the normal oblique-to-flattened lamellar arrangement. Not only do the fibroblasts become fewer, but also the remaining ones change from the plump, active fibroblasts to thin resting fibrocytes (the keratocytes).

  2. The fibroblastic tissue shrinks as it becomes less cellular, and with rearrangement of cells and fibrils a thin scar is formed.

The scar is seen much more easily clinically as an opaque area within clear cornea than histologically where it is identified by observing collagen fibers with an orientation somewhat different from the normal corneal lamellae. Thin corneal scars are characteristic of uncomplicated lacerations by a sharp instrument, e.g., a surgical incision, whereas thick corneal scars are characteristic of nonsurgical wounds or complicated surgical wounds, e.g., infected wounds or wounds filled with a material such as uvea or vitreous.

CONJUNCTIVA (Fig. 5–14)

  I. Wound healing in the conjunctiva differs from that in the cornea by the additional presense of a vasculature, a lymphatic system and a reticuloendothelial system.

  A. Because of the vasculature and lymphatics, intracellular and intercellular edema occurs early and rapidly in the conjunctiva, unlike the slow process in the cornea.

  B. The reticuloendothelial system provides a ready source for mononuclear cells in the form of macrophages and fibrocytes, both of which are easily converted to fibroblasts.

  C. Leukocytes, neutrophils and lympho-

117

cytes gain access to the tissue directly from the blood vessels and lymphatics.

D. A laceration, therefore, has an epithelial healing process identical to that of the cornea, but the subepithelial tissue forms granulation tissue, i.e., fibroblasts, inflammatory cells and young capillaries, instead of forming simply fibroblastic tissue.

II. Following the formation of granulation tissue, over a course of 4 to 7 days the vascular and inflammatory components disappear, the fibroblasts become fewer and the remaining ones change into resting fibrocytes, shrinkage takes place and a scar results.

SCLERA (Fig. 5–15)

I. Although the sclera has a vasculature (albeit sparse), it behaves rather inertly with regard to wound healing.

A. If only the outer sclera is wounded or penetrated, the gap in the wound is filled in by a tongue of granulation tissue derived from the overlying vascular episclera.

B. If only the inner sclera is wounded or penetrated, the gap in the wound is filled in by a tongue of granulation tissue derived from the underlying uvea.

C. In a through and through scleral wound, i.e., a perforation of the sclera, the episcleral and uveal tongues of

granulation tissue meet, resulting in "perpendicular" healing.

II. Following the formation of granulation tissue, scar tissue ultimately forms as described above in conjunctival healing.

SURGICAL LIMBAL INCISIONS (Fig. 5–13B)

I. Surgery, such as surgical sections for cataract and glaucoma procedures, generally involves wound healing of all limbal structures, namely cornea, conjunctiva and sclera, as outlined above.

II. With no complications (infection; vitreous loss; incarceration of uvea, lens fragments or vitreous) a fine, hairline scar results.

UVEA

I. Iris

A. Wounds that run perpendicular to the circumferential ridges of the iris (the usual iris wound such as the typical peripheral iridectomy or iridotomy) cause the cut edges to pull apart, gaping the wound.

1. If the iris wound edges gape, they are continuously bathed in flowing aqueous, and little or no wound healing takes place.

2. With complications such as infection or hemorrhage, granulation tissue may bridge the gap, and then wound healing with scar formation will occur.

B. Wounds that run parallel to the circumferential ridges (an extremely rare wound) may not cause the cut edges to pull apart, so that the wound edges remain in apposition.

1. If the wound edges remain in apposition, granulation tissue will form in the anterior stromal part of the wound, which will heal with scar formation.

2. Pigment epithelial cells of the iris migrate over the posterior part of the wound, covering the gap as a

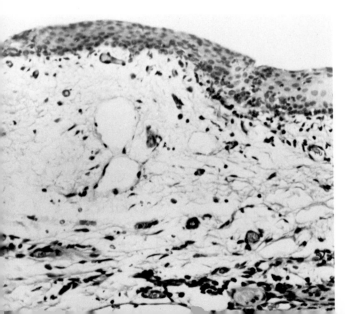

FIG. 5–14. Conjunctiva in area of recent wound shows vascular and lymphatic engorgement. Edema is marked, and numerous inflammatory cells are seen. H&E, ×136.

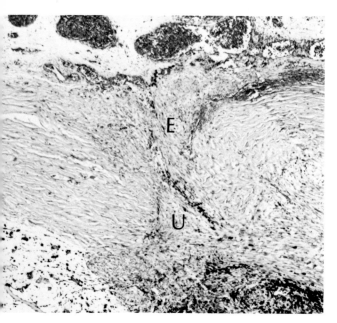

FIG. 5–15. Following scleral laceration, tongues of episcleral (*E*) and uveal (*U*) granulation tissue grow into the wound, producing "perpendicular" healing. H&E, ×28.

single layer. They tend to remain as a single layer rather than to re-establish their normal double-layered structure.

II. Ciliary body and choroid
   A. Both of these tissues tend to heal wounds in the "classic" way, i.e., by the formation of granulation tissue.
   B. The granulation tissue ultimately is supplanted by scar formation.

LENS

I. Tiny wounds to the lens involving a localized capsular rent on occasion may be healed primarily.
   A. The epithelium proliferates to cover the wounded area.
   B. The proliferated epithelium lays down a new basement membrane, i.e., lens capsule (Fig. 10–7).
II. The vast majority of wounds to the lens, however, result in cataract formation.

RETINA AND OPTIC NERVE

I. Injuries to the retina and optic nerve heal by gliosis (see p. 447 in Chap. 11), which involves astrocytes and their filamentous

cytoplasm rather than fibroblasts and their elaboration of collagen.

II. If the injury is complicated by infection or hemorrhage, mesodermal elements can enter the picture with the production of granulation tissue and subsequent collagenous scar tissue formation.

HISTOLOGY OF SOME SPECIFIC TYPES OF ANTERIOR SEGMENT PROCEDURES

CATARACT EXTRACTION

I. See p. 118 in this chapter for histology.
II. The limbal surgical scar is accompanied by aphakia and a sector or peripheral iridectomy.*

SIMPLE IRIDECTOMY OR IRIDOTOMY*

Histologically, peripheral or sector (complete) iridectomy reveals a segment of iris missing with no evidence of healing. An iridotomy shows gaping of the iris in the area of incision with no evidence of healing.

IRIDENCLEISIS (Fig. 5–16)

Iris is prolapsed through a limbal surgical wound and is surrounded by a cystoid scar in the subepithelial conjunctival tissue.

---

* Generally a peripheral iridectomy refers to a removal of full thickness iris peripheral to the sphincter muscle (if it extends peripheral to the iris root, it is a peripheral basal iridectomy). A sector iridectomy refers to a removal of full thickness iris from the pupillary margin extending peripherally (if it extends peripheral to the iris root, it is a sector basal iridectomy). Clinically sector iridectomy and complete iridectomy are used interchangeably. Theoretically, however, sector iridectomy should refer to a segment of full thickness iris being removed (usually by surgery), whereas complete iridectomy should refer to total (360°) removal of the iris (usually as a result of nonsurgical trauma). An iridotomy is a tearing or cutting of the iris without removal of tissue, e.g., a basal iridotomy may be obtained by pulling on the iris and evulsing it for a short distance at the iris root from the anterior face of the ciliary body (synonymous with an iridodialysis), or a sphincterotomy (pupillary iridotomy extending through the sphincter muscle) may be obtained by cutting into the pupillary border of the iris far enough to include the sphincter muscle in the cut.

PERIPHERAL (OR SECTOR) IRIDECTOMY WITH SCLERAL CAUTERY; TREPHINE FILTERING SURGERY (Fig. 5–17)

In both kinds of filtering operations a gaping wound at the limbus is covered by a cystoid scar in the subepithelial conjunctival tissue.

CYCLODIALYSIS (Fig. 5–18)

A cleft is present between the sclera and the meridional muscles of the ciliary body so that the ciliary body is completely freed anteriorly (generally the pars plicata part) from the sclera, generally for a distance of about a quarter of its circumference.

THERMOSCLEROTOMY; CYCLODIATHERMY; CYCLOCRYOTHERMY (Fig. 5–19)

All three techniques produce necrosis and scarring of the pars plicata region of the ciliary body.

TRABECULOCANALECTOMY; SINUSOTOMY; TRABECULOTOMY

All three techniques lead to removal or opening of part of the trabecular meshwork-canal of Schlemm portion of the drainage angle.

KERATOPLASTY

I. A penetrating keratoplasty* consists of a full thickness corneal graft.
II. A lamellar keratoplasty consists of a partial thickness anterior corneal graft.

COMPLICATIONS OF INTRAOCULAR SURGERY†

IMMEDIATE

Complications occurring from the time the decision is made to perform surgery until

---

* Penetrating keratoplasty is confusing terminology. The reference point here is the globe so that when one does a full thickness corneal graft, one penetrates the globe (but perforates the cornea).

† The example used for the section Complications of Intraocular Surgery is the surgical cataract or glaucoma incision (section) that generally involves a wound to the limbal region so that conjunctiva, cornea, sclera and iris all can be considered.

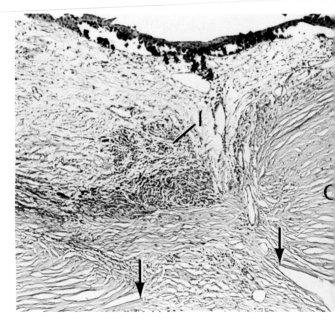

FIG. 5–16. Iris (*I*) projecting through gap (between *arrows*) in Descemet's membrane (iridencleisis). Subconjunctival tissue over exteriorized iris is "spongy" due to filtration of aqueous. *C,* cornea. Eye obtained at autopsy. Successful filtration clinically. H&E, ×40.

FIG. 5–17. Peripheral iridectomy with scleral cautery (**inset**) shown in **main figure** under higher magnification to illustrate "spongy" subconjunctival tissue (*arrows*) in clinically successful filtering bleb. **Main figure,** H&E, ×16; **inset,** H&E, ×4.

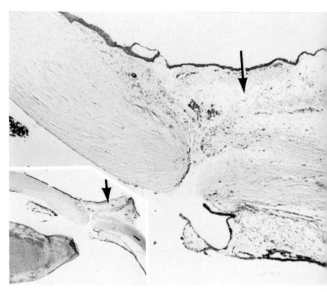

the patient leaves the operating room are considered immediate.

I. "Surgical confusion"
A. Misdiagnosis—not all cataracts are primary, but they may be secondary to such things as trauma, inflammation, neoplasm (Fig. 5–20) or metabolic disease. With opaque media caused by a cataract ultrasound can be helpful in establishing whether or not a neoplasm or a retinal detachment is present behind the cataract.
B. Faulty technique
1. Many complications such as vitreous loss can be avoided (at least some of the time) by an adequate facial and retrobulbar block.
2. Retrobulbar hemorrhage may occur slowly, insidiously collecting behind the eye and bulging the intraocular contents forward as the surgical procedure progresses.
3. In a similar fashion a poorly placed lid speculum can press on the globe, thereby increasing the intraocular pressure.
4. Misplacement of the incision too far anteriorly into clear cornea may make the surgery technically more difficult, whereas misplacement too far posteriorly may cause the incision to enter ciliary body (Fig. 5–21) instead of anterior chamber (especially serious in filtering procedures for the control of glaucoma).
5. Misplacement of corneal sutures may cause anterior gaping or posterior gaping if placed too far posteriorly or anteriorly, respectively; a very deep suture may enter the anterior chamber, leading to "wicking" and a flat chamber postoperatively. If a suture is placed at different depths in the two sides of the wound, faulty apposition of the wound edges results.
6. "Buttonhole" of the conjunctiva is not serious in cataract surgery but may lead to failure in filtering procedures.
7. Splitting off of Descemet's membrane from the posterior cornea can lead to an intractable corneal edema postoperatively.
8. An iridodialysis, although usually innocuous, may lead to anterior

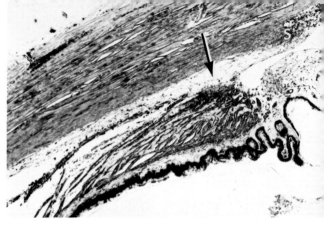

FIG. 5–18. Cyclodialysis. Region of surgical cleft between longitudinal muscle of ciliary body and sclera (arrow) filled with delicate fibrous tissue. Note posterior location of anterior face of ciliary body and angle recess in relationship to scleral spur (s). H&E, ×21.

chamber hemorrhage or problems with pupillary distortion if not taken into account when the iridectomy is performed.

II. Anterior chamber bleeding. This generally occurs from the iridectomy site but may come from the scleral side of the cut edge of the wound. Bleeding will invariably stop in a short time if patience and continuous saline irrigation are used.

III. Rupture of the lens capsule (Fig. 5–22). This makes the surgery technically more difficult and leads to an increased incidence of vitreous loss, complicated wound healing [especially when lens remnants (Fig. 5–23) are caught in the wound], secondary cataracts, phacoanaphylactic endophthalmitis, inflamed eyes, etc.

IV. Vitreous loss. Loss of the vitreous leads to an increased incidence of iris prolapse, bullous keratopathy, epithelial downgrowth, stromal overgrowth, wound infection and endophthalmitis, updrawn or misshapen pupil, vitreous bands, postoperative flat chamber, secondary glaucoma, poor wound healing, retinal detachment, cystoid macular edema, papilledema, vitreous opacities, vitreous hemorrhage, expulsive choroidal hemorrhage and chronic ocular irritability.

The best way to handle vitreous loss is to avoid it!

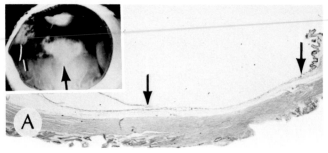

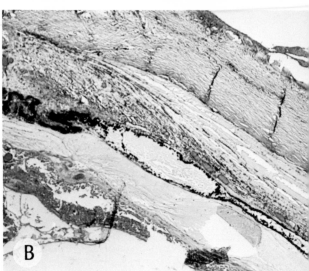

FIG. 5–19. **A.** Cyclodiathermy for treatment of glaucoma produced necrosis in pars plana of ciliary body (between *arrows* in **main figure,** and *arrows* in **inset,** both from same case). **B.** Cyclocryothermy for treatment of glaucoma produced necrosis of ciliary body predominantly in pars plana region. Ciliary pigment epithelium necrotic and cystic. **A,** H&E, ×8; **inset,** macroscopic; **B,** H&E, ×16.

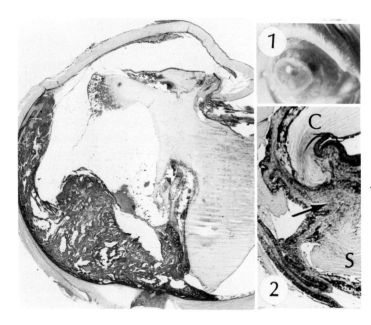

◄ FIG. 5–20. Unsuspected mass was noted in pupil (**inset 1**) following cataract extraction, and eye was enucleated. Metastatic carcinoma is present in choroid. Totally detached retina is herniated through cataract wound, as shown in higher magnification in **inset** (*arrow*) **2.** *C,* corneal side of wound; *S,* scleral side of wound. **Main figure,** H&E, ×5; **inset 1,** clinical; **inset 2,** H&E, ×16.

FIG. 5–21. Ciliary processes (*arrow*) rather than iris in wound placed too far posteriorly in attempted iridencleisis. Persistent flat anterior chamber allowed formation of peripheral anterior synechia (**inset**), producing secondary angle closure glaucoma and subsequent loss of eye. **Main figure,** H&E, ×28; **inset,** H&E, ×28.

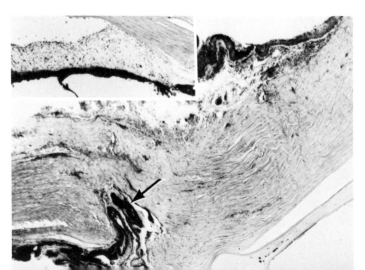

FIG. 5–22. Lens capsule rupture during cataract extraction. Capsule and lens nucleus were removed, but cortical material was left behind. **Insets 1, 2** and **3** show course of events from day 1 following surgery, to 2 weeks later, to 2 months later, respectively. **Main figure** shows lens-filled histiocytes in aqueous aspirated 7 days after needling of congenital cataract. **Main figure,** PAS, ×700; **inset 1,** clinical; **inset 2,** clinical; **inset 3,** clinical.

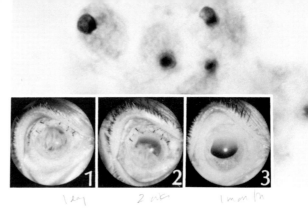

FIG. 5–23. A. Iris (*arrow*) and lens remnants (*L*) caught up in scar of cataract section. **B.** PAS-positive lens capsule caught up in limbal scar of cataract section. **A,** H&E, ×16; **B,** PAS, ×16.

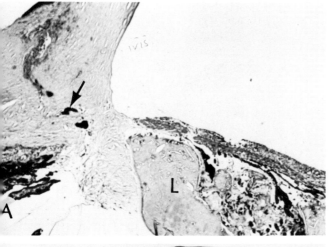

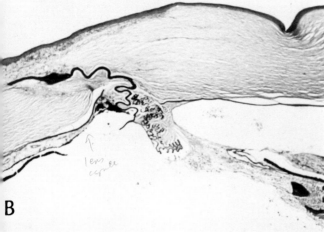

V. Expulsive choroidal hemorrhage (Fig. 5–24*A*). This is a rare, catastrophic complication, which results in total loss of the eye in the majority of cases.

   A. The hemorrhage probably results from rupture of a sclerotic choroidal arteriole as it crosses the suprachoroidal space from its scleral canal, prompted by the sudden hypotony following surgical penetration of the globe.

   B. Although most hemorrhages are massive and immediate, occasionally they are delayed and may not occur for days to weeks following surgery.

   It is difficult to explain a delayed expulsive hemorrhage (Fig. 5–24*B*). Probably there is a small hemorrhage at the time of surgery, which stops spontaneously. At a future date there is a rebleed, i.e., a secondary hemorrhage, which does not stop and becomes massive.

   C. Histologically, massive intraocular hemorrhage associated with a totally detached choroid and retina and a gaping wound is seen. A ruptured ciliary artery may be found.

POSTOPERATIVE

   Postoperative complications may arise from the time the patient leaves the operating room until 3 months following surgery.

   I. Flat anterior chamber*—most chambers refill in 4 to 8 hours.

   * A flat anterior chamber is one in which the iris comes up against the posterior cornea obliterating completely the anterior chamber. This must be differentiated from a shallow chamber in which some space is still present. If the chamber is flat for 5 days or more, peripheral anterior synechias frequently develop well on the posterior surface of clear cornea (i.e., the latter are often called broad-based). With a shallow anterior chamber, however, one can go much longer before synechias form.

A. Secondary to hypotony

   1. Faulty wound closure (Fig. 5–25)

   Faulty apposition of the wound edges
   can lead to poor wound healing and a
   "leaky" wound, which results in
   hypotony and a flat anterior chamber.
   Faulty placement of sutures may cause
   gaping of the wound allowing aqueous
   to leak out, or if the sutures are too
   deep and enter the anterior chamber,
   aqueous can leak out through the
   suture tract ("wicking").

   2. *Choroidal detachment* or *hydrops*
      (Fig. 5–26) ("combined" choroidal
      detachment) is not a true detach-
      ment but rather an effusion or
      edema of the choroid and is always
      associated with a similar process in
      the pars plana (and if extensive in
      the pars plicata) of the ciliary body
      (see p. 351 in Chap. 9).
      a. Rather than the choroidal de-
         tachment causing the flat
         chamber, it generally is sec-
         ondary to a flat chamber caused
         by a "leaky" wound in a hypo-
         tonic eye.
      b. Once a choroidal detachment
         occurs, however, the flat chamber
         and hypotonic eye are compli-
         cated further by a slowing or
         stopping of aqueous production
         by the edematous ciliary body.
      c. Histologically the uveal tissue,
         especially the outer layers, is
         "spread out" like a fan and the
         spaces are filled with an eosino-
         philic coagulum. Frequently the
         edema fluid is "washed out" of
         tissue sections and the spaces
         then appear empty.
   3. *Iris incarceration* (Fig. 5–27) (iris
      within the surgical wound) or iris
      prolapse (Fig. 5–28) (iris through
      the wound into the subconjunctival
      area) acts as a wick through which
      aqueous can escape leading to a flat
      chamber.

   In a similar manner ciliary body incarceration, e.g., following a filtering procedure where the incision is made too
   far posteriorly, can act as a wick leading to a flat chamber. Other ocular

FIG. 5–24. A. Expulsive hemorrhage at time
of cataract extraction. Eye enucleated 3 days
later is full of blood and shows retina
totally detached. **B.** Expulsive choroidal
hemorrhage following flattening of anterior
chamber upon suture removal of otherwise
uneventful cataract extraction (**inset** shows
blood protruding through wound at 1
o'clock). Blood fills the eye and herniates
through corneal wound. **A,** H&E, ×3; **B,**
H&E, ×6; **inset,** clinical.

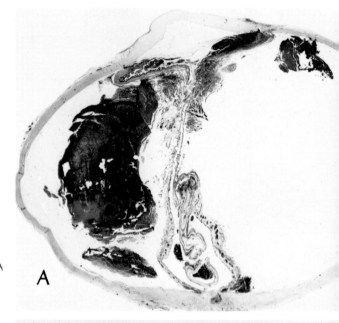

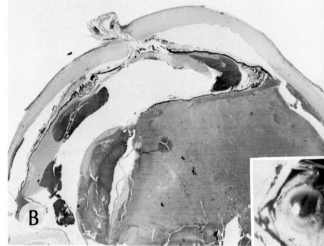

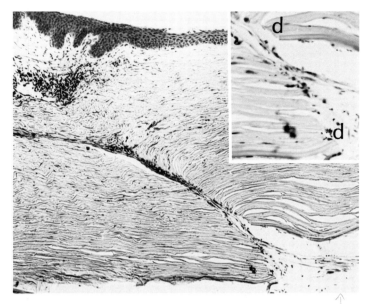

FIG. 5–25. Poor apposition of wound closure following cataract extraction. Vitreous in wound is seen at higher magnification in **inset.** *d,* cut ends of Descemet's membrane. **Main figure,** H&E, ×54; **inset,** H&E, ×101.

FIG. 5–26. Massive edema (hydrops) involving mainly loose outer layers of choroid and ciliary body (*arrows*) produces choroidal detachment. H&E, ×6.

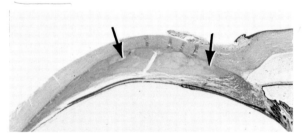

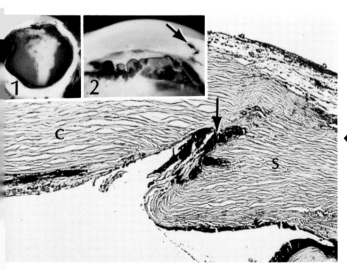

structures such as lens, lens remnants, vitreous or even choroid and retina can become incarcerated in or prolapsed through the wound and lead to a flat chamber. All these structures are more likely to enter the wound following nonsurgical trauma than surgical trauma. The area of involvement may become ectatic resulting in a staphyloma (Fig. 5–29).

Histologically, iris, frequently recognized only by the presence of melanocyte-containing uveal tissue, is present in the limbal scar or in the limbal episclera or in both areas.

4. *Fistulization* of the wound may occur and most of the time is of no clinical significance, but on occasion it may be marked and lead to hypotony, flat chamber, corneal astigmatism and epiphora.
5. *Vitreous wick syndrome* consists of a microscopic wound breakdown with subsequent vitreous prolapse, creating a tiny wick draining to the external surface of the eye.
   a. In some cases severe intraocular inflammation develops and resembles a bacterial endophthalmitis.
   b. Infection can gain entrance into the eye by way of a vitreous wick.
6. *Poor wound healing per se* with no identifiable cause can occur and lead to aqueous leakage and a flat chamber, or it might not become manifest until the sutures are removed postoperatively at which time the wound opens up, aqueous runs out and a flat chamber results.

B. Secondary to glaucoma
   1. *Aphakic glaucoma,* i.e., glaucoma in an aphakic eye, in the postoperative period generally is due to a pupillary block mechanism.

◄ **FIG. 5–27.** Iris (*arrow*) within wound (C, corneal side of wound; S, scleral side of wound) is termed incarceration of iris. **Inset 1** shows iris incarceration (shown by *arrow* in enlargement in **inset 2**) and total retinal detachment following cataract extraction. **Main figure,** H&E, ×40; **inset 1,** macroscopic; **inset 2,** macroscopic.

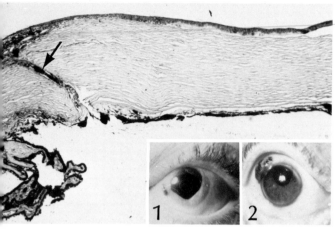

FIG. 5–28. Iris (*arrow*) passing completely through wound into subconjunctival area is termed iris prolapse. **Insets 1** and **2** show clinical appearance of iris prolapse (**inset 1** at 9 o'clock, **inset 2** at 11 o'clock). **Main figure,** H&E, ×21; **inset 1,** clinical; **inset 2,** clinical.

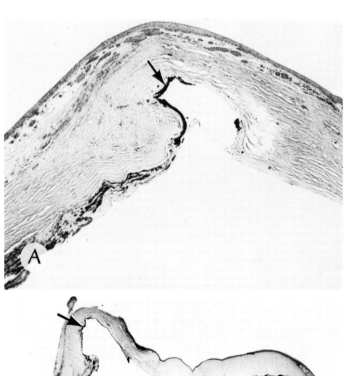

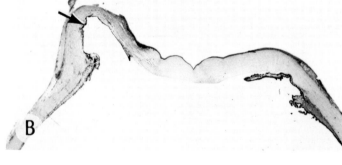

FIG. 5–29. Limbal staphyloma of moderate size (**A**) and large size (**B**) caused by ectatic limbal area lined by iris, with iris incarcerated into limbal wounds (*arrows*). **A,** H&E, ×16; **B,** H&E, ×6.

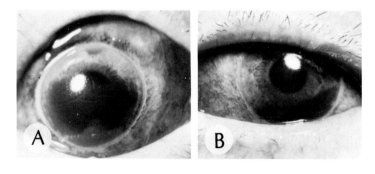

FIG. 5–30. Hyphema, noted on first day after filtering surgical procedure (**A**), had almost cleared 2 days later (**B**) and was completely gone in another 2 days with no treatment. **A,** clinical, 3/15/66; **B,** clinical, 3/17/66.

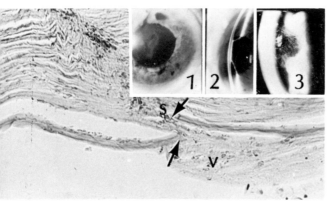

FIG. 5–31. Vitreous (v) adherent to posterior corneal scar (s) between cut ends of Descemet's membrane (*arrows*). **Insets 1** and **2** show two views of same eye to demonstrate vitreous coming through pupil and touching posterior cornea, producing corneal edema. **Inset 3** is another aphakic eye in which vitreous comes through pupil and touches posterior cornea. **Main figure,** H&E, ×69; **insets 1, 2,** and **3,** clinical.

FIG. 5–32. Iris adherent to and partially within posterior aspect of cataract scar (adherent leukoma). H&E, ×21.

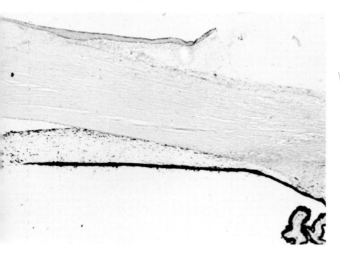

It is important to remember that up to the first 5 days or so following intraocular surgery, the eye is hypotonic. A "normal" intraocular pressure, therefore, during the first few days postoperatively may signify glaucoma.

Histologically a posterior synechia is formed between the posterior pupillary portion of the iris and the anterior vitreous face or lens remnants or both.
2. A *choroidal hemorrhage* can occur slowly rather than abruptly, causing an anterior displacement of the vitreous, resulting in an anterior displacement of the iris diaphragm.
   The hemorrhage may remain confined to the uvea or may break through into the subretinal space, into the vitreous or even into the anterior chamber.

II. Striate keratopathy ("keratitis"). This complication is caused by damage to the corneal endothelium, which results in the appearance of linear striae due especially to posterior corneal edema and folding of Descemet's membrane.
   A. Vigorous bending or folding of the cornea during surgery is the usual cause.
   B. Striate keratopathy generally is reversible completely and disappears within a week.
III. Hyphema (Fig. 5–30)
   A. Most postoperative hyphemas occur 24 to 72 hours following surgery.
   B. They tend not to be as serious as nonsurgical traumatic hyphemas and usually clear with or without specific therapy within 1 week.

IV. Corneal edema may be secondary to:
   A. Glaucoma, generally pupillary block glaucoma (aphakic glaucoma).
   B. Vitreous (Fig. 5–31) or iris (Fig. 5–32) adherent to or within the surgical wound or adherent to the corneal endothelium.
   C. Splitting of Descemet's membrane from posterior cornea—usually occurs when making the cataract section with a scissors.
   D. "Aggravation" of cornea guttata, resulting in a combined endothelial dystrophy and epithelial degeneration.
   E. Idiopathic causes, i.e., unknown.
   F. Histologically (Fig. 5–33), early there is

long term
results
(bullous)
↓
pannus

edema of the basal layer of epithelium. With chronicity subepithelial collections of fluid (bullae or vesicles) may occur. Ultimately, fibrous tissue may grow between epithelium and Bowman's membrane, resulting in a degenerative pannus.

V. Subretinal hemorrhage. This generally is secondary to extension of a choroidal hemorrhage. Hemorrhage frequently is found in the vitreous inferiorly following intraocular surgery. The cause is unknown.

VI. α-Chymotrypsin glaucoma. α-Chymotrypsin glaucoma is caused by an unknown mechanism when α-chymotrypsin is instilled into the anterior chamber prior to cataract delivery.
   A. The glaucoma occurs in about one-third of the patients who receive α-chymotrypsin.
   B. The glaucoma is mild, evanescent and of little clinical importance.

VII. Endophthalmitis (Figs. 5–34 and 5–35). Endophthalmitis in the postoperative stage, especially in the first day or two, generally is purulent, fulminating (i.e., rapid) and caused by bacteria. Although a delayed endophthalmitis is more characteristic of a fungus infection, a bacterial infection is also a possibility even in the later part of the postoperative stage, especially if a leaking wound is present.

VIII. Uveitis. This may occur as an aggravation of a previous uveitis or de novo.
   A. The uveitis that occurs de novo may be chronic granulomatous or nongranulomatous.
   B. The de novo uveitis tends to be recalcitrant to therapy.

IX. Ointment. An ointment (usually antibiotic) may gain access to the anterior chamber especially when applied to the eye immediately after surgery before the first dressing. Generally the ointment incites little or no reaction and can be tolerated by the eye for very long periods of time.

X. "Surgical confusion." Misinterpretation of ocular signs by the clinician constitutes surgical confusion, e.g., a postoperative choroidal detachment misdiagnosed as a uveal malignant melanoma with subsequent enucleation of the eye.

DELAYED

Delayed complications are those which occur after the third month following surgery.

I. Corneal edema secondary to:
   A. The same five entities listed under corneal edema in the subsection Postoperative above.

   B. Peripheral corneal edema
      1. The onset of edema is delayed at least 6 years following surgery.
      2. The edema is bilateral when the surgery is bilateral, occurs mainly in women, generally follows intracapsular cataract extraction and may be associated with peripheral iris atrophy.
      3. The edema involves the stroma and

FIG. 5–33. **A.** Epithelium shows edema of basal cells and is lifted off Bowman's membrane to form a bulla. **B.** Fibrous tissue is present between edematous epithelium and Bowman's membrane (b) in early pannus formation. **C.** Relatively acellular fibrous tissue (f) between epithelium and calcified Bowman's membrane (band keratopathy) constitutes a degenerative pannus. A, H&E, ×136; **B**, H&E, ×136; **C**, H&E, ×176.

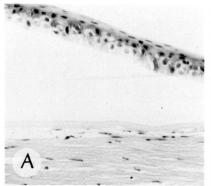
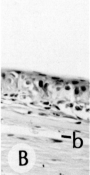
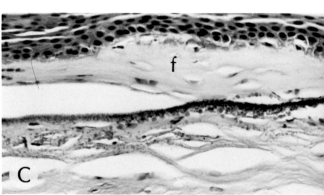

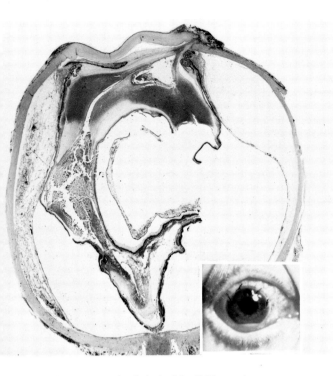

FIG. 5–34. Endophthalmitis. Diffuse vitreous abscess (typical of bacterial infection) has herniated through cataract wound into subconjunctival area; retina is detached completely. **Inset** shows endophthalmitis with hypopyon on second postoperative day following cataract extraction. **Main figure,** H&E, ×5; **inset,** clinical.

epithelium with sparing of the superior and central cornea.

4. Discrete, orange, punctate pigmentation of unknown origin frequently is seen on the endothelial surface behind the edematous areas of the cornea.
5. The cause of the edema is unknown.

II. Cataract

A. Cataracts may be caused or accelerated by glaucoma surgery, even if the lens is in no way damaged physically by the surgery.

The cataract may be a result of "shunting" of the aqueous through the iridectomy, so that the anterior and posterior surfaces of the lens are not nourished properly.

B. Secondary cataract
1. Lens capsule may be left in the pupillary area.
2. *Elschnig's pearls* (Fig. 5–36) result from aberrant attempts by lens cells attached to the capsule to form new lens "fibers."

Histologically, large clear lens cells ("bladder cells") are seen behind the iris, in the pupillary space or in both areas.

3. *Soemmerring's ring* cataract (Fig. 5–36) results from loss of anterior and posterior cortex and nucleus with retention of equatorial cortex so that a "donut" configuration results with apposition of the central portions of the anterior and posterior lens capsule.

Frequently the donut or ring is not complete so that C- or J-shaped configurations result.

Histologically two "balls" of lens cells, degenerated and proliferated, are seen encased in capsule behind the iris leaf, connected by adherent anterior and posterior lens capsule in the form of a dumbbell.

III. Retinal detachment (Fig. 5–37). This occurs in about 2 to 6 percent of aphakic patients (50 percent of these within 1 year following cataract surgery) and in as high as 25 percent of aphakic patients if a retinal detachment had occurred previously in either eye.

Vitreous loss increases the incidence of postoperative detachments. Anterior vitrectomy at the time of vitreous loss, however, does not seem to alter the expected incidence of retinal detachments. In fact, anterior vitrectomy at the time of vitreous loss seems to have little or no effect on any of the expected complications that follow vitreous loss. The damage probably is done at the moment of loss, i.e., the vitreous pulls on the retina at the vitreous base or ora serrata. Subsequent vitrectomy, repair, etc. cannot undo the previous trauma. The best therapy of vitreous loss is prevention.

IV. Aphakic glaucoma. In the delayed phase this glaucoma is due mainly to secondary

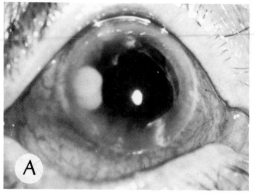

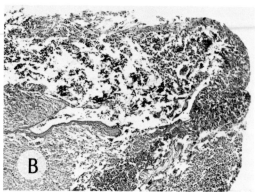

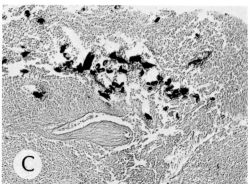

FIG. 5–35. Endophthalmitis. **A.** Localized mass in anterior chamber shortly after cataract extraction. Slow rate of enlargement together with relatively "quiet" eye suggest absence of infective agent. Anterior chamber mass surgically removed. **B.** Histologic examination reveals granulomatous inflammatory reaction. **C.** Special stain for fungi shows positive staining of dark black fibers, which do not morphologically resemble fungi. **D.** Under higher magnification fibers (*arrows*) appear refractile in routine sections. **E.** Fibers, which are birefringent to polarized light, are cotton fibers inadvertently introduced at time of surgery. **A,** clinical; **B,** H&E, ×75; **C,** Gomori methenanine silver, ×75; **D,** H&E, ×300; **E,** H&E, polarized, ×75.

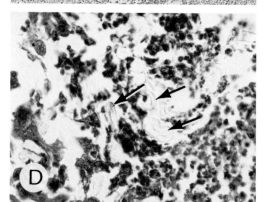

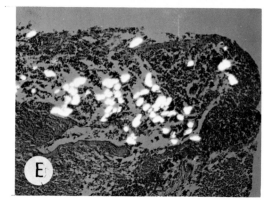

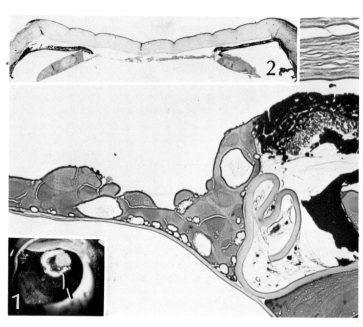

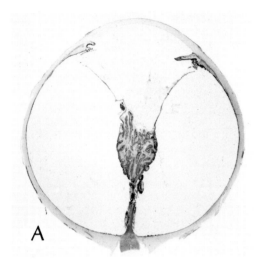

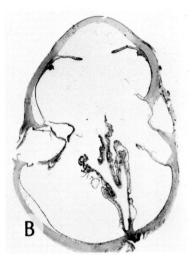

FIG. 5–37. Retinal detachment (RD). **A.** RD noted 4 weeks after cataract extraction; there was no attempt at repair. Secondary chronic angle closure glaucoma necessitated enucleation. **B.** RD noted 5 weeks after cataract extraction; two attempts at repair failed. Large "cystic" spaces within sclera at equator represent areas where scleral silicone implants had been. Note cysts in detached retina, a sign of chronic RD. **A,** H&E, ×3; **B,** H&E, ×3.

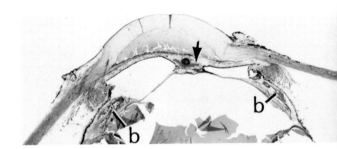

FIG. 5–38. Posterior synechia and iris bombé. Anterior scarred face of vitreous adherent to posterior surface of iris. Section is not quite through pupil, and sphincter muscle (*arrow*) can be seen with dark nodule of lymphocytes and plasma cells in iris stroma just anterior to it. Bone (*b*) present in cyclitic membrane on posterior surface of pars plicata of ciliary body. H&E, ×6.

◄ **FIG. 5–36.** Soemmerring's ring cataract shown in **inset 1** (*arrow*) is incomplete in form of "C." **Inset 2** is microscopic section of same eye in plane of *arrow*. Two "balls" of lens cells encased in lens capsule lie behind iris leaves. Lens remnants peaking out from behind iris are shown with higher magnification in **main figure** and represent aberrant attempts by lens cells to form new lens "fibers," i.e., Elschnig's pearls. **Main figure,** H&E, ×69; **inset 1,** macroscopic; **inset 2,** H&E, ×6.

chronic angle closure glaucoma but may be due to a preexisting simple open angle glaucoma.

A. *Peripheral anterior synechias,* leading to secondary chronic angle closure glaucoma, generally are secondary to persistent postoperative flat chamber (Fig. 5–21).

This type of secondary glaucoma seems to be easier to control medically than other types of secondary angle closure glaucoma.

Histologically the iris is adherent to posterior cornea, frequently central to Schwalbe's ring.

B. *Posterior synechias,* generally the result of posterior chamber inflammation (due to iridocyclitis, endophthalmitis, hyphema, etc.) results in *iris bombé* (Fig. 5–38) and secondary peripheral anterior synechias.

Histologically the posterior pupillary portion of the iris is adherent to the anterior face of the vitreous, to lens remnants or to both. The anterior peripheral iris is adherent to the posterior cornea, frequently central to Schwalbe's ring.

C. *Epithelial downgrowth* (ingrowth) (Fig. 5–39) is more likely to occur with fornix-based conjunctival flaps than with limbus-based flaps; in eyes with problems in wound closure such as vitreous loss, wound incarceration of tissue, delayed reformation of the anterior chamber or frank rupture of the limbal incision; and when instruments such as iridectomy forceps are contaminated with surface epithelium before they are introduced into the eye.*

1. Epithelial downgrowth either causes an anterior chamber angle closure via peripheral anterior synechias or lines an open anterior chamber angle and mechanically obstructs aqueous outflow.

---

* There is good experimental evidence to show that healthy endothelium inhibits the growth of epithelium, i.e., contact inhibition. Epithelium, therefore, probably only grows into the eye if the endothelium is unhealthy, removed by the trauma, or covered, e.g., by iris incarceration, vitreous or lens remnants.

2. Histologically the epithelium is seen to grow most luxuriously and in multiple layers on the iris where there is a good blood supply, whereas it tends to grow sparsely and in a single layer on the posterior surface of the avascular cornea. The epithelium may extend behind the iris, over the ciliary body and far into the interior of the eye through the pupil.

The presence or absence of the lens in the eye has nothing to do with epithelial downgrowth (Fig. 5–40) except that trauma, surgical or nonsurgical, serious enough to cause loss of a lens often is followed by epithelial downgrowth. Most eyes with epithelial downgrowth, therefore, do not contain lenses.

D. *Iris cyst* formation (Figs. 5–41 and 5–42) is caused by implantation of surface epithelium onto the iris at the time of surgery.

1. The cyst generally is slow growing and is accompanied by peripheral anterior synechias, which if extensive may cause a secondary chronic angle closure glaucoma.

2. Histologically the cyst is lined by stratified squamous or columnar epithelium, sometimes containing mucous cells, and is filled with either keratin debris (white cysts) or mucous fluid (clear cysts).

E. *Stromal overgrowth* (Fig. 5–43) is most apt to occur following vitreous loss or tissue incarceration into the surgical wound.

1. The stromal overgrowth may be localized, limited to the area of surgical perforation of Descemet's membrane, or may be quite extensive or anything in between.

2. When extensive, peripheral anterior synechias and secondary angle closure glaucoma result.

3. As with epithelial downgrowth the stromal overgrowth may extend behind the iris, over the ciliary body and far into the interior of the eye.

4. Histologically, fibrous tissue generally extends from or is in con-

F. Histologically, microcystoid spaces are found in the outer retinal layers quite similar in morphologic appearance, if not identical, to peripheral retinal cystoid degeneration (see p. 412 in Chap. 11).

VII. Atrophia bulbi (Fig. 5–48) without or with (phthisis bulbi) disorganization may occur following surgery for no readily apparent clinical or histopathologic reasons.

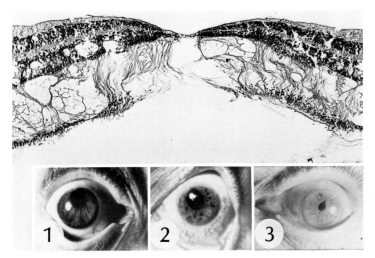

FIG. 5–47. Cystoid macular degeneration following cataract extraction in eye that showed no evidence of vitreous traction. Microcystoid changes mainly in outer retinal layers in section through fovea. **Inset 1** shows updrawn complete sector iridectomy pupil, whereas **insets 2** and **3** show updrawn round pupils with peripheral iridectomies; all followed cataract extraction. Updrawn pupil may or may not be associated with cystoid macular degeneration, and the latter may or may not be associated with updrawn pupil. **Main figure,** H&E, ×40; **inset 1,** clinical; **inset 2,** clinical; **inset 3,** clinical.

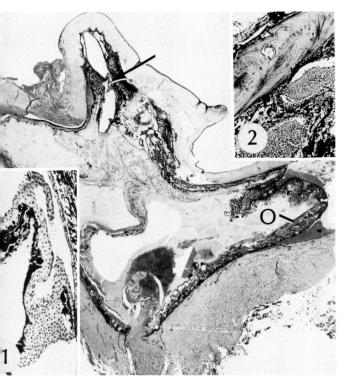

FIG. 5–48. Atrophia bulbi with shrinkage in surgically aphakic eye. Epithelial downgrowth (*arrow*) shown in higher magnification in **inset 1.** Bone spicule within area of intraocular ossification (O) shown in higher magnification in **inset 2. Main figure,** H&E, ×5; **inset 1,** H&E, ×40; **inset 2,** H&E, ×40.

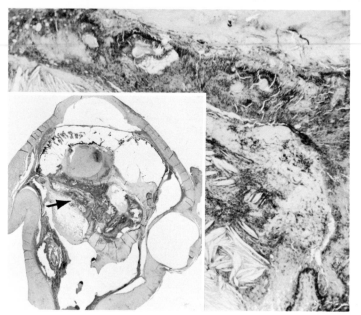

FIG. 5–49. Choroidal detachment secondary to choroidal hemorrhage shown in **inset.** Intrascleral clear space indicates site of silicone implant. Organizing choroidal hemorrhage with cholesterol clefts (*arrow*) shown in higher magnification in **main figure. Main figure,** H&E, ×16; inset, H&E, ×3.

COMPLICATIONS OF RETINAL DETACHMENT SURGERY

IMMEDIATE

I. "Surgical confusion"

    A. Misdiagnosis

        Not all retinal detachments are rhegmatogenous, i.e., primarily due to a retinal hole, but may be secondary to such things as intraocular inflammation or intraocular neoplasm.

    B. Faulty technique

        1. A poor retrobulbar or facial block or retrobulbar hemorrhage may make the surgical procedure more difficult.

        2. Misplacement of the implant or explant or of the scleral sutures can lead to an improper scleral buckle or to premature drainage of subretinal fluid.

        3. Misplacement of, or insufficient or excessive diathermy or cryotherapy can cause unsatisfactory results.

        4. Cutting or obstruction of the vortex veins may lead to choroidal detachment or hemorrhage.

II. Choroidal detachment or hemorrhage (Fig. 5–49)

    A. The most frequent cause of choroidal detachment is hypotony induced by surgical drainage of subretinal fluid. It may also result from overuse of scleral cryotherapy or diathermy.

    B. Choroidal hemorrhage may result from hypotony due to surgical drainage of subretinal fluid, from cutting or obstruction of vortex veins or from incision of choroidal vessels at the time of surgical drainage of subretinal fluid.

    C. Histology—see p. 123 (subsection Expulsive choroidal hemorrhage) and p. 124 (subsection Choroidal detachment) in this chapter.

III. Acute glaucoma

    A. The buckling procedure, especially if unaccompanied by drainage of subretinal fluid or of an anterior chamber paracentesis, may result in acute angle closure glaucoma.

    This should be recognized immediately during the surgical procedure and treated promptly by anterior chamber paracentesis, intravenous diamox, loosening of the buckle, drainage of subretinal fluid or any combination of these. Acute glaucoma, if unrecognized, can cause central retinal artery occlusion with subsequent blindness and optic atrophy.

    B. Histologically the anterior chamber angle is occluded by the peripheral iris.

POSTOPERATIVE

I. The original hole may still be open or a new hole may develop (or be missed preoperatively).

II. Choroidal detachment or hemorrhage—see p. 123 (subsection Expulsive choroidal hemorrhage) and p. 124 (subsection Choroidal detachment) in this chapter.

III. Inflammation

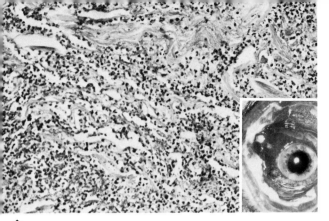

▲
FIG. 5–50. Acute scleral necrosis is characterized by purulent exudate and necrotic scleral debris. Material shown in **main figure** had been obtained from area of scleral necrosis (**inset**) in recent postoperative retinal detachment patient. **Main figure,** H&E, ×101; **inset,** clinical.

FIG. 5–51. Fungal endophthalmitis after retinal detachment surgery. **A.** About 3 weeks after surgical repair of retinal detachment, corneal abscess and scleral thinning (**insets 1** and **2**) developed. Central cornea became necrotic and eye was enucleated (**inset 3** and **main figure**). Areas of scleral thinning (*double arrow*) and intrascleral silicone implant (*arrow*) are shown. **B.** Special stains for fungi show their presence throughout all levels of necrotic cornea, shown under higher magnification in **C. D.** Area of intrascleral implant (*arrow* in **A**) under higher magnification and with special stain shows fungi within implant. **A,** H&E, ×5; **inset 1,** clinical; **inset 2,** clinical; **inset 3,** clinical; **B,** Gomori methenamine silver, ×40; **C,** Gomori methenamine silver, ×101; **D,** Gomori methenamine silver, ×101.

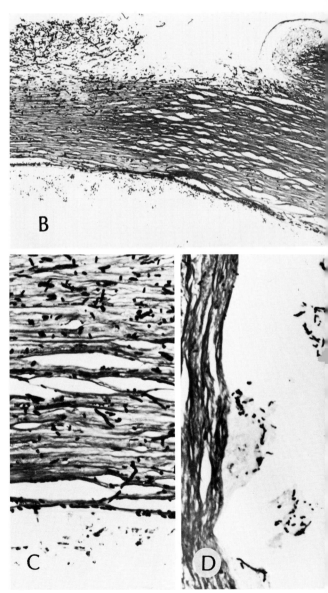

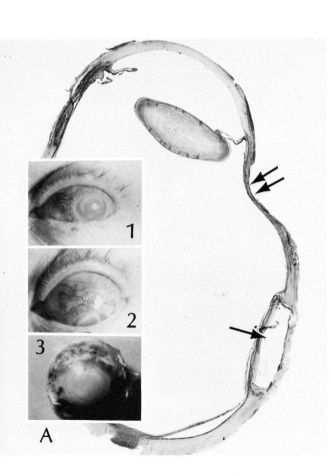

A. *Acute or subacute scleral necrosis* (Fig. 5–50) may follow retinal detachment surgery in days or weeks and is probably due to ischemia rather than infection.
  1. In the acute form the clinical picture starts generally a few days postoperatively and may resemble a true infectious scleritis except that pain is absent.
    a. There is a sudden onset of congestion, edema and a dark red or purple appearance of the tissues over the implant (or explant). Discharge is not marked or is absent.
    b. The vitreous over the buckle generally becomes hazy but may be clear.
    c. The cornea remains clear but the involved area of sclera becomes completely necrotic.
  2. In the subacute form the clinical picture starts with pain generally 2 to 3 weeks postoperatively.
    a. The globe may be congested, but there is no discharge.
    b. The vitreous over the buckle may be hazy or clear.
    c. The sclera in the region of the buckle is necrotic.

B. *Infection* in the form of scleral abscess, endophthalmitis or keratitis may be secondary to bacteria or fungi (Fig. 5–51) and is characterized by redness of the globe, discharge and pain.
    Histology—see section on nontraumatic infections in Chapter 4 and section Suppurative Endophthalmitis and Panophthalmitis in Chapter 3.
C. Anterior segment necrosis (anterior segment ischemic syndrome) (Fig. 5–52)
  1. Anterior segment necrosis is thought to be secondary to interruption of the blood supply to the iris and ciliary body usually by temporary removal of one or more rectus muscles during surgery or to compromising of the blood supply by encircling elements, lamellar dissection, implants or explants and cryotherapy or diathermy.
  2. Clinically, usually in the first week postoperatively, keratopathy and intraocular inflammation develop.
    a. Corneal changes consist of striate keratopathy and corneal edema with epithelial bullae.
    b. Intraocular inflammation is noted clinically by chemosis, anterior chamber flare and cells, large keratic precipitates and white deposits on the necrotic lens capsule. The clinical findings are often mistaken for an infectious endophthalmitis.
    c. Later the pupil becomes irregularly dilated with shrinkage toward the side of the greatest necrosis and hypoxia, and a cataract develops.
    d. Ultimately hypotony, shrinkage of the iris stroma, ectropion uvea and finally phthisis bulbi develop.
  3. A high incidence of the anterior segment ischemic syndrome is seen following scleral buckling procedures in patients with hemoglobin SC disease.

    In hemoglobin SC disease the increased frequency of anterior segment necrosis most likely is related to the increased blood viscosity and tendency toward erythrocyte packing that is found in these patients, especially with a decreased oxygen tension.
  4. Histologically, ischemic necrosis of the iris, ciliary body and lens epithelial cells is present, frequently only on the side of the surgical procedure.
IV. Intraocular hemorrhage
  A. Choroidal hemorrhage may occur for the same reasons as described above (see subsection Immediate).
  B. Hemorrhage in the postoperative period may be due to a delayed expulsive choroidal hemorrhage, most probably due to necrosis of a blood vessel induced by the original diathermy or cryotherapy or to erosion of an implant or explant.
V. Glaucoma
  A. Acute angle closure glaucoma most likely occurs following a retinal detachment procedure in which an encircling element or a very high buckle is created.

1. The buckle decreases the volume of the vitreous compartment, displacing vitreous and lens-iris diaphragm anteriorly.

   Corneal edema on the first postoperative day, especially if accompanied by ocular pain, should be considered glaucomatous in origin until proven otherwise.

2. Histologically the anterior displacement of intraocular structures results in encroachment of the iris on the anterior chamber angle with a resultant angle closure glaucoma.

B. Chronic simple glaucoma may become apparent when the hypotony of a retinal detachment is alleviated by surgical means.

DELAYED

I. Vitreous retraction. This by itself is of little importance; but when it is associated with fibrous or glial membranous connections to the internal surface of the retina, it can result in retinal detachment and new retinal holes (see p. 481 in Chap. 12).

   A. When extensive and causing a total retinal detachment, the process is called *massive vitreous retraction* (*MVR*).

   MVR may occur at any stage following retinal detachment surgery. Ominous preoperative signs of incipient MVR are star-shaped retinal folds, incarceration of retina into a drainage site from previous retinal surgery, fixed folds, fibrous or glial vitreoretinal membranes and "cellophane" retina. All are associated with fibrous or glial membranes lying on the internal surface of the retina.

   B. Histologically, fibroglial membranes are seen on the internal surface of the retina. With shrinkage of the membranes fixed folds of the retina result (see p. 462 in Chap. 11).

II. Migration of implant or explant (Fig. 5–53)

   A. The implant or explant may migrate in its own plane due to loosening of sutures with resultant misplacement of the buckle.

FIG. 5–52. Anterior segment necrosis followed surgical repair of retinal detachment in patient with hemoglobin SC disease. Enucleated eye shows relatively normal area in **A** and area of anterior segment necrosis with necrosis of ciliary body and iris in **B. A,** H&E, ×25; **B,** H&E, ×25.

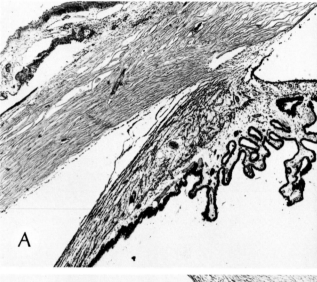

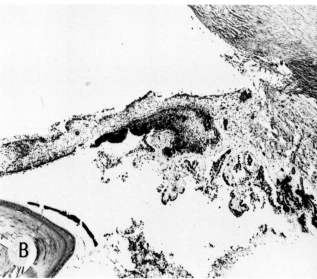

B. Internal migration may result in intraocular penetration with resultant hemorrhage, retinal detachment or infection.

C. External migration results in extrusion.

III. Heterophoria or heterotropia. These conditions most likely result when muscles have been removed temporarily during surgery. In adults when good visual acuity does not return following surgery, exotropia quite commonly occurs.

IV. A new hole. A hole may develop *de novo* or secondary to obvious vitreous pathology, to internal migration of implant or explant or to improper use of cryotherapy or diathermy.

V. Disturbances of lid position and motility are common.

VI. Secondary glaucoma. Glaucoma may be secondary to many causes, e.g., secondary angle closure glaucoma, hemorrhage with hemolytic glaucoma or inflammation with peripheral anterior or posterior synechias.

VII. Macular degeneration or puckering. This can occur even if only cryotherapy or diathermy is used alone without a buckling procedure (see Irvine-Gass-Norton syndrome, p. 136 in this chapter).

VIII. Catgut granulomas (Fig. 5–54). These result when catgut sutures are retained instead of resorbed.

A. The catgut becomes sequestered and acts as a foreign body.

B. Histologically, amorphous, eosinophilic, weakly birefringent material (catgut) is surrounded by a foreign body giant cell granulomatous inflammatory reaction.

Catgut granulomas are most often observed when muscles have been detached during the procedure and then reattached with catgut sutures. They commonly are present following surgery for correction of strabismus. Other complications of strabismus surgery include perforation of the globe, infection, adhesions and "loss" of a muscle.

COMPLICATIONS OF CORNEAL SURGERY

IMMEDIATE

See section Complications of Intraocular Surgery above.

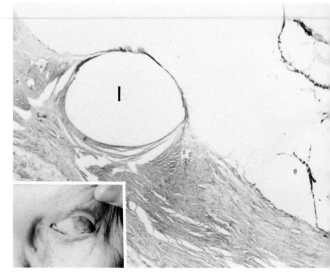

FIG. 5–53. Migration of implant and explant. **Inset** shows external migration of scleral explant resembling lacrimal gland tumor. **Main figure** illustrates internal migration of intrascleral implant (*I*), which has eroded almost completely through sclera into choroid. **Main figure,** H&E, ×16; **inset,** clinical.

Fig. 5–54. **A.** Large dark catgut suture present at top of picture. Catgut material almost completely dissolved in area of foreign body giant cells, lower right corner. **Inset** shows catgut granuloma nasally in left eye following surgery for correction of strabismus. **B.** Large black catgut suture shows little reaction, whereas small lighter suture (*arrow*) surrounded by granulomatous inflammation is almost completely dissolved. **A,** H&E, ×69; **inset,** clinical; **B,** H&E, ×69.

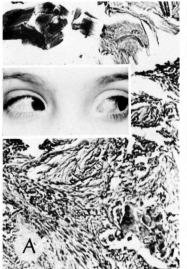 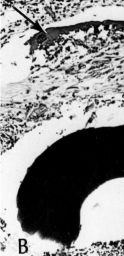

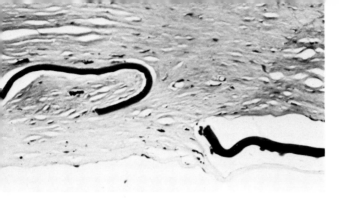

FIG. 5–55. Stromal overgrowth coming through gap between host Descemet's membrane, which shows cornea gutatta on right, and donor Descemet's membrane on left. PAS, ×101.

I. Grafting of vascularized corneas often fail because of the markedly increased incidence of homograft reaction.

II. If the donor cornea is not checked carefully, it may be diseased (e.g., cornea gutatta) and doomed to failure.

III. Poor technique can result in such things as incomplete removal of part or even all of the recipient's Descemet's membrane in removing the recipient's corneal button, or conversely in not removing part or all of Descemet's membrane and endothelium when removing the donor's corneal button; damage to the iris or lens during removal of recipient's corneal button; vitreous loss, especially in aphakic eyes; and so forth.

POSTOPERATIVE

See section Complications of Intraocular Surgery above.

I. Homograft reaction (immune reaction). The reaction generally starts 2 or 3 weeks postoperatively and is characterized by iridocyclitis with fine keratic precipitates, ciliary flush, vascularization of the cornea starting peripherally and then extending into the stroma centrally and epithelial edema followed by stromal edema.

Histologically, polymorphonuclear leukocytes and tissue necrosis are present in a sharply demarcated zone within the donor cornea. Central to the zone the donor cornea is undergoing necrosis. Peripheral to the zone lymphocytes and plasma cells are seen.

II. Defective cicatrization of the stroma. This may result in marked gaping of the graft site and ultimate graft failure.

DELAYED

See section Complications of Intraocular Surgery, this chapter.

I. Stromal overgrowth (Fig. 5–55) (retrocorneal fibrous membrane, postgraft membrane).

A. Stromal overgrowth is apt to follow when there is graft rejection (immune reaction), faulty wound apposition, "poor health" of recipient or donor endothelium or iris adhesions.

B. The fibrous overgrowth may be due to a proliferation of corneal keratocytes, of new mesenchymal tissue derived from mononuclear cells, of endothelial cells that have undergone fibrous metaplasia,* of fibroblastlike cells from the angle tissues or any combination thereof.

C. Histologically a fibrous membrane covers a part or all of the posterior surface of the donor and recipient cornea and may extend over and occlude the anterior chamber angle.

II. Endothelial dystrophy may be present in the donor cornea and lead to graft failure.

COMPLICATIONS OF NONSURGICAL TRAUMA

CONTUSION

Contusion is an injury to tissue caused by an external direct (e.g., a blow) or indirect (e.g., a sound or shock wave) force that usually does not break (lacerate) the overlying tissue surface (e.g., skin, cornea or sclera).

A contusion is the injury that results from a *concussion*, i.e., a violent jar or shake, caused by the external force.

---

* The corneal endothelium is really a mesothelium. Mesothelial cells are derived from mesoderm and have the ability to act like connective tissue in various pathologic conditions. It is not surprising, therefore, that corneal endothelium may undergo fibrous metaplasia under the appropriate stimulus, e.g., inflammation.

I. Cornea
  A. Abrasion—see section Normal Wound Healing above.
  B. Blood staining (a secondary phenomena)—see section Hyphema below and p. 310 in Chapter 8.
  C. Ruptures of Descemet's membrane (see p. 590 in Chap. 16) most commonly occur as a result of birth trauma.
    1. They tend to be unilateral and most frequently in the left eye (most common fetal presentation is left occiput anterior).
    2. They usually run in a diagonal direction across the central cornea.
    3. Histologically, whether the rupture is due to birth trauma, congenital glaucoma or trauma anytime following birth, a gap is seen in Descemet's membrane.
      a. The endothelium may grow over the gap forming a new Descemet's membrane.
      b. The endothelium in its attempt to cover the gap may grow into the anterior chamber over the free, rolled end of the ruptured Descemet's membrane, forming a scroll-like structure.
      c. Combinations of the above two possibilities may occur.
  D. *Keloid* of the cornea (Fig. 5–56) is a hypertrophic scar that occasionally follows ocular injury.
    1. Most appear as a glistening white mass that extends outward from the eye in the region of the cornea, i.e., protuberant white corneal mass.
    2. Histologically, corneal perforation usually is present. There is a haphazard arrangement of fibroblasts, collagen bundles and blood vessels, forming a hypertrophic corneal scar.
II. Conjunctiva may show edema, hemorrhage or laceration.

The conjunctiva always should be carefully explored for lacerations, which may be a clue to a wound of a missile entry into the globe.

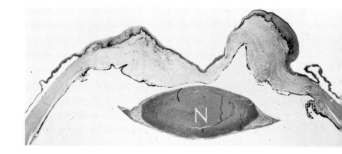

FIG. 5–56. Keloid of cornea is hypertrophic scar that diffusely thickens cornea lined by iris (total anterior synechia). Note nuclear cataract (N); most of cortex has escaped intact through capsule in hypermature cataract (cortex seen only in equatorial region). H&E, ×6.

FIG. 5–57. Blood staining of cornea is noted histologically by presence of hemoglobin particles in corneal stroma. Note size of stromal hemoglobin particles compared to size of anterior chamber erythrocytes in **inset 1. Inset 2** shows hyphema filling almost one-third of anterior chamber and not causing blood staining of cornea. **Insets 3** and **4** show complete or "black ball" hyphema with early blood staining of cornea. **Main figure,** Brenner & Brenn, ×101; **inset 1,** Brenner & Brenn, ×441; **inset 2,** clinical; **inset 3,** clinical; **inset 4,** clinical.

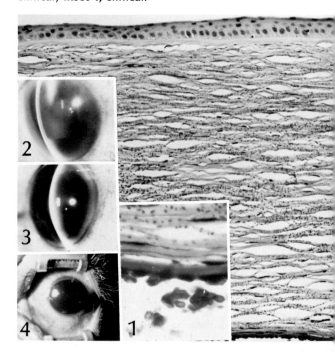

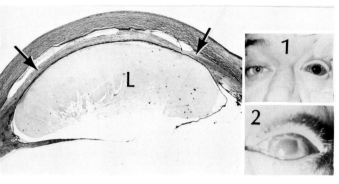

FIG. 5–58. Organization of hyphema has resulted in fibrosis (*arrows*) of anterior chamber. *L,* lens. **Inset 1** shows total anterior chamber hyphema following cataract extraction. **Inset 2** shows same eye 3 weeks later with secondary glaucoma and corneal edema due to fibrosis of anterior chamber angle following organization of hyphema. **Main figure,** PAS, ×6; **inset 1,** clinical, both eyes; **inset 2,** clinical, left eye.

III. Anterior chamber and its angle
   A. *Hyphema* or blood in the anterior chamber angle may lead to a number of secondary complications.
      1. In the face of healthy endothelium blood staining of the cornea (Fig. 5–57 and Color Plate I) (see p. 310 in Chap. 8) may result if elevated intraocular pressure is present uninterrupted for about 48 hours.

      Obviously, excessively high intraocular pressure will cause blood staining of the cornea more rapidly than minimal or intermittently elevated intraocular pressure. If the endothelium is not healthy, blood staining can occur without a rise in the intraocular pressure.

      2. The blood may mechanically occlude the anterior chamber angle and lead to a secondary open angle glaucoma.
      3. Organization of the blood (Figs. 5–40 and 5–58) may result in peripheral anterior synechias and secondary closed angle glaucoma.
      4. The blood may extend posteriorly, especially in an aphakic eye, and result in *hemophthalmos,* i.e., an eye filled completely with blood.
      5. Iron may be deposited in the tissue (hemosiderosis bulbi) and cause heterochromia (the darker iris is the affected iris) and a toxic effect on the retina and trabecular meshwork.
      6. Cholesterolosis of anterior chamber —see p. 151 in this chapter.
   B. *Angle recession (postcontusion deformity of anterior chamber angle)*

(Figs. 5–59 through 5–62) consists of a posterior displacement of the inner part of the pars plicata of the ciliary body (including ciliary processes or crests, circular ciliary muscles and some or all of the oblique ciliary muscles but *not* the meridional ciliary muscle) and the iris root. It is due to a laceration into the anterior face of the ciliary body. Glaucoma may develop in about 6 percent of these eyes, most likely when the recession is 240 degrees or greater.
   1. An injury severe enough to cause a hyphema will cause an angle recession in more than 60 percent of eyes, and if the hyphema fills three-quarters of the volume of the anterior chamber, a traumatic cataract and vitreous hemorrhage will occur in about 50 percent of eyes.

   The size of the hyphema should be judged after the blood has settled.

   2. The acute angle recession probably has little or nothing to do directly with the development of glaucoma, but rather is a sign that indicates damage to the drainage angle.
   3. The glaucoma, if it develops, may be due to a number of factors:
      a. The initial injury may stimulate corneal endothelium to grow over the trabecular meshwork with the formation of a new Descemet's membrane and a secondary open angle glaucoma due to mechanical obstruction of aqueous outflow.

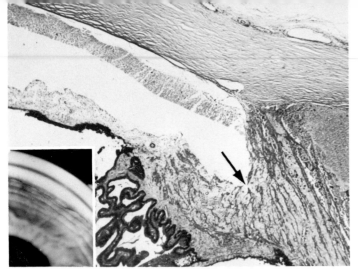

FIG. 5–59. Anterior chamber angle recession follows laceration (*arrow*) into anterior face of ciliary body. Blood is present in anterior chamber and in supraciliary space. Longitudinal muscles of ciliary body still attached to scleral spur. **Inset** shows gonioscopic appearance of angle recession. **Main figure,** PAS, ×16; **inset,** gonioscopy.

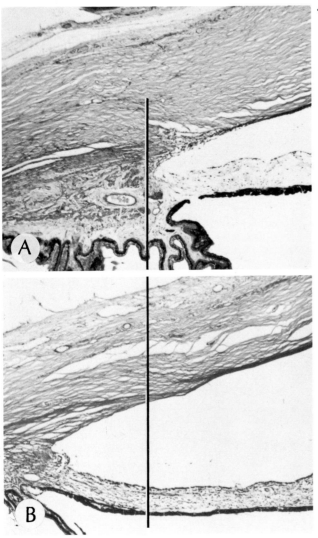

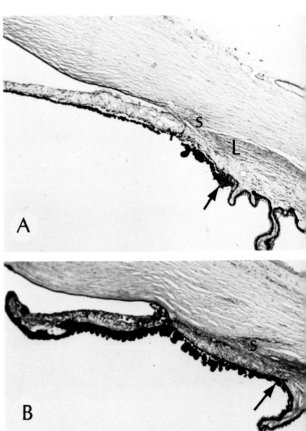

◀ **FIG. 5–60.** Angle recession. **A.** Normal anterior chamber angle. Line parallel to optic axis drawn through scleral spur passes through anterior chamber angle recess, iris root and anterior ciliary process. **B.** Angle recession. Same line drawn through scleral spur passes far anterior to other structures. Trabecular meshwork is sclerosed and unrecognizable. Descemet's membrane extends over trabecular meshwork area and internal sclera far posteriorly. **A,** PAS, ×28; **B,** PAS, ×28.

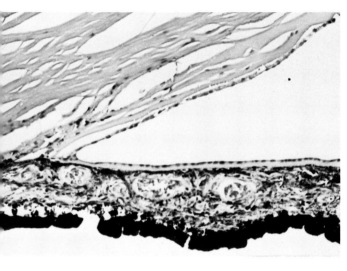

FIG. 5–62. Endothelialization of pseudoangle following contusion and formation of peripheral anterior synechias. Endothelium lines pseudoangle of anterior chamber and continues over anterior surface of iris where it has produced a new Descemet's (i.e., basement) membrane. H&E, ×101.

FIG. 5–63. Cyclodialysis differs from angle recession in that entire ciliary body, including longitudinal muscles, is separated from sclera. **A,** Ciliary body stripped off of scleral spur (S) and sclera and displaced posteriorly. **B.** Ciliary body (arrows) massively stripped off of sclera and present in center of eye. **A,** H&E, ×16; **B,** H&E, ×6.

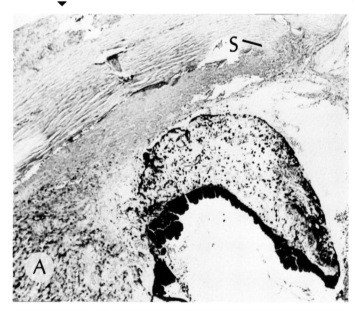

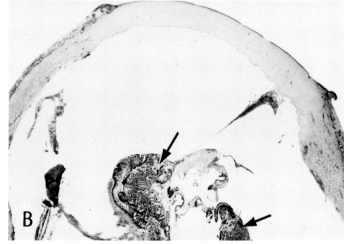

FIG. 5–61. Angle recession with peripheral anterior synechia. **A.** Typical fusiform shape of ciliary body, instead of normal wedge shape, is due to characteristic atrophy of round and oblique muscles of ciliary body with only longitudinal muscles (L) intact. Rubeosis iridis has developed and given rise to secondary anterior peripheral synechia. Iris root (arrow) and anterior ciliary process are displaced posteriorly from scleral spur (s). **B.** Peripheral anterior synechia has developed without rubeosis iridis. Iris root (arrow) and anterior ciliary process displaced posteriorly from scleral spur (s). **A,** PAS, ×16; **B,** PAS, ×21.

b. The initial injury may stimulate fibroblastic activity within the drainage angle leading to sclerosis and a secondary open angle glaucoma.

c. The initial injury may cause hemorrhage or inflammation with subsequent organization, leading to peripheral anterior synechias and a secondary angle closure glaucoma.

The depth of the anterior chamber should be estimated and compared with that of the other eye or another region of the angle in the same eye. An increased depth of the anterior chamber may be a clue to an angle recession, a dislocated lens or a ruptured globe. Sometimes the presence of a ruptured globe may be difficult to prove. Deepening of the anterior chamber associated with a vitreous hemorrhage should be considered to be caused by a ruptured globe until proven otherwise.

4. Histologically the inner part of the pars plicata and the iris root are displaced posteriorly. Frequently a scar extends into the anterior face of the ciliary body.

Complicating factors such as overgrowth of Descemet's membrane, trabecular meshwork sclerosis and peripheral anterior synechias may be seen. Descemet's membrane, produced by endothelium, may be found over the trabecular meshwork and internal sclera (Fig. 5–60) in an anterior chamber angle which is deeply recessed. If a secondary peripheral synechia occurs, a new anterior chamber angle, commonly called a pseudoangle, forms between the posterior cornea and the anterior surface of the pupillary end of the iris synechia. The pseudoangle also may show an overgrowth of endothelium-produced Descemet's membrane, called endothelialization of the pseudoangle. (Fig. 5–62).

C. Cyclodialysis (Fig. 5–63) may be seen and differs from an angle recession in

that the entire pars plicata of the ciliary body *including* the meridional muscles is stripped completely free from the sclera.

D. An *iridodialysis* (Fig. 5–64) or a tear in the iris at its thinnest part (the iris root) may be present and frequently leads to a hyphema.

Other tears in the iris such as sphincter tears and iridoschisis may occur but usually are not serious. They should be noted carefully, however, because they provide a clinical clue of prior trauma.

E. Not only may the trabecular meshwork develop scarring, but also it may be torn and disrupted by the initial injury.

F. Traumatic iridocyclitis is quite common, frequently severe with marked fibrin accumulation, and if untreated may lead to posterior synechias, then peripheral anterior synechias and finally to secondary angle closure glaucoma.

IV. Lens

A. A cataract can result from blunt trauma immediately, in weeks, months or even years later.

B. Anterior subcapsular cataract—see p. 366 in Chapter 10.

C. Posterior subcapsular cataract—see p. 368 in Chapter 10.

A special type of anterior or posterior cataract is seen frequently following trauma. The lens opacities take the form of petals (Fig. 5–65), usually ten, in the anterior or posterior cortex and clinically are called *rosette* or *flowerlike cataracts*.

D. Rupture of the lens capsule (see p. 121 in this chapter), if small, may be sealed by overlying iris or healed in by proliferation of lens epithelium (Fig. 10–7).

1. A small rupture clinically is noted as a small opacity and histologically as a break in the lens capsule associated with contiguous lens epithelial and associated superficial cortical cell changes.

2. A large rupture usually results in the rapid development of a cataract with a great deal of lens material in

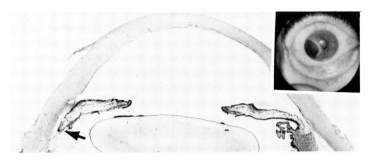

FIG. 5–64. Iridodialysis. Iris torn at its thinnest part, i.e., iris root (*arrow*). **Inset** shows traumatic iridodialysis and cataract. **Main figure,** PAS, ×6; **inset,** clinical.

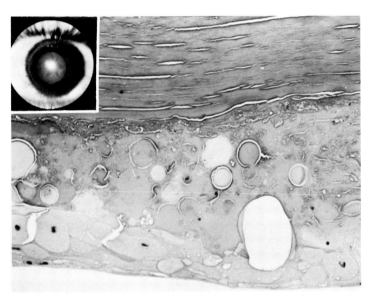

FIG. 5–65. Rosette-shaped traumatic cataract (**inset**) in anterior or posterior cortex. **Main figure** shows posterior cortical degeneration and bladder-cell formation; clinically lens had traumatic posterior rosette cataract. **Main figure,** H&E, ×101; **inset,** clinical.

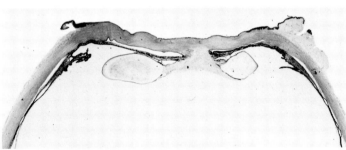

FIG. 5–66. Soemmerring's ring cataract subsequent to traumatic central corneal injury. PAS, ×6.

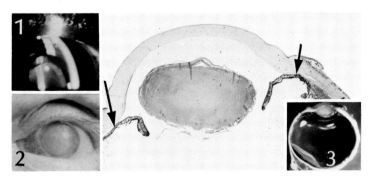

FIG. 5–67. Subluxation of lens, i.e., lens remains in posterior chamber but in abnormal position, shown in **inset 1,** whereas dislocated lens, i.e., lens completely displaced into anterior chamber, is shown clinically in **inset 2,** macroscopically in **inset 3,** and microscopically in **main figure.** Note also peripheral anterior synechias (*arrows*) secondary to pupillary block and iris bombé. **Main figure,** H&E, ×6; **inset 1,** clinical; **inset 2,** clinical; **inset 3,** macroscopic.

the anterior chamber. Histologically this is seen as lens cortex, which after a few days becomes mixed with macrophages. Elschnig's pearls or a Soemmerring's ring (Fig. 5–66) cataract may result.

3. Phacoanaphylactic endophthalmitis (see p. 81 in Chap. 4).

E. Phacolytic glaucoma—see p. 378 in Chapter 10.

F. *Vossius ring*, a pigmented ring on the anterior surface of the lens just behind the pupil, may occur immediately following trauma, and then it probably represents iris pigment epithelium from the posterior iris surface near the pupil deposited as a ring, i.e., iris fingerprints; or if delayed it may represent initial damage to the lens with subsequent deposition of pigment from the aqueous.

G. *Dislocation (luxation)*, i.e., complete zonular rupture with the lens completely out of the posterior chamber (into the anterior chamber or vitreous), and *subluxation*, i.e., incomplete rupture of the zonules with the lens still in the posterior chamber but not in its normal position, can occur following trauma (Figs. 5–67 through 5–69).

The trauma that altered the position of the lens also may cause a cataract. A subluxated lens frequently is suspected because the anterior chamber is obviously deepened by recession of the unsupported iris diaphragm, which tends to undulate with movement of the eye (*iridodonesis* or shimmering iris). A small bead or herniation of vitreous also may be observed in the anterior chamber. Glaucoma may frequently be associated with a posteriorly dislocated lens. The glaucoma generally is a result of the initial blunt trauma to the tissues of the drainage angle. It only is due to the lens secondarily when the lens material itself participates, e.g., phacolytic glaucoma.

V. Vitreous (Fig. 5–70)

A. Blood and inflammatory cells may be seen in the vitreous early and fibrous membranes noted late.

B. The vitreous may become detached, commonly posteriorly, but also its base may detach.

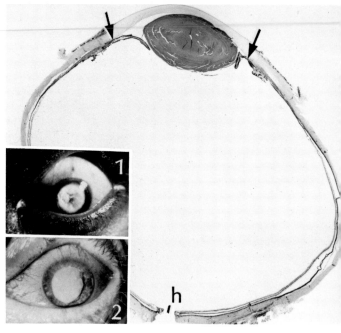

FIG. 5–68. Dislocation of lens into anterior chamber (**insets 1** and **2**) causes pupillary block, iris bombé, peripheral anterior synechias (*arrows*) and secondary angle closure glaucoma. Hole at bottom of eye (*h*) is produced by severing very deep glaucomatous cup on removing the optic nerve from the globe. **Main figure,** H&E, ×5; **inset 1,** clinical; **inset 2,** clinical.

FIG. 5–69. Dislocation of lens into vitreous compartment shown in **insets 1** and **2** and in **main figure.** Main figure, H&E, ×5; **inset 1,** clinical; **inset 2,** macroscopic.

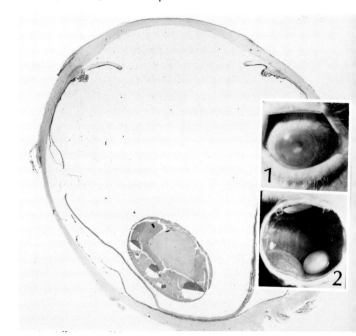

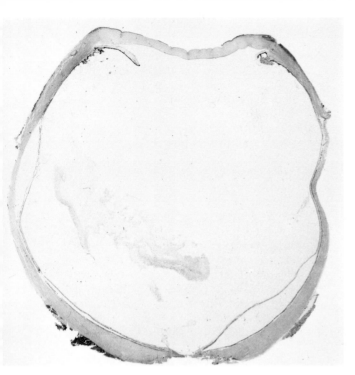

FIG. 5–70. Blood present in vitreous following trauma to eye. H&E, ×5.

Detachment of the vitreous base is almost always caused by severe trauma.

C. *Cholesterolosis (synchisis scintillans)* (Fig. 5–71) most often results following a vitreous hemorrhage.
  1. Cholesterolosis is found mainly in men in their fourth or fifth decade and generally is unilateral.
  2. In aphakic eyes the vitreous-containing cholesterol may pass forward into the anterior chamber so that the patient presents with cholesterolosis (synchisis scintillans) of the anterior chamber.

  Cholesterolosis of the anterior chamber may result from a hyphema without vitreous hemorrhage. The glistening brilliant crystals in the anterior chamber can be dissolved temporarily by applying heat, e.g., as from a hair dryer.

  3. Histologically the cholesterol may be free in the vitreous, may incite a foreign body granulomatous inflammatory reaction, may be phagocytosed by macrophages or may be

surrounded by dense fibrous tissue without any inflammatory reaction. The cholesterol crystals are birefringent to polarized light and stain with fat stains in freshly fixed, frozen-sectioned tissue but are dissolved out by alcohol and xylene in the normal processing of tissue for embedding in paraffin. In processed tissue cholesterol appears as empty spaces, sometimes described as cholesterol clefts.
  D. In aphakic eyes or in eyes with subluxated or dislocated lenses, the vitreous may herniate into the pupil or anterior chamber and may result in pupillary block and iris bombé.
VI. Ciliary body and choroid
  A. Ciliary body and choroidal hemorrhage and detachment may result from trauma—see p. 352 in Chapter 9.

  Hemorrhage and inflammation in the posterior chamber may result in the formation of a cyclitic membrane (Fig. 5–72).

  B. Indirect (posterior) choroidal ruptures (Fig. 5–73), usually crescent-shaped and concentric to the optic disc between fovea and optic disc, and direct or anterior choroidal ruptures at the site of impact may occur following trauma.
    1. The indirect or posterior type is more common than the direct or anterior type.
    2. Most often the overlying retina is intact, but rarely it too is ruptured.
    3. Histologically either Bruch's membrane and choriocapillaris alone or the full thickness of the choroid is ruptured. The overlying retina may be normal, atrophic or ruptured.
  C. *Traumatic chorioretinopathy* (Fig. 5–74) can resemble clinically and histologically retinopathia pigmentosa—see p. 438 in Chapter 11.

Retinitis sclopetaria is a specific type of traumatic chorioretinopathy that results indirectly from blunt injury produced by an orbital missile that richochets off the sclera. The force of the missile (usually a bullet) causes chorioretinal injury in the underlying tissue.

151

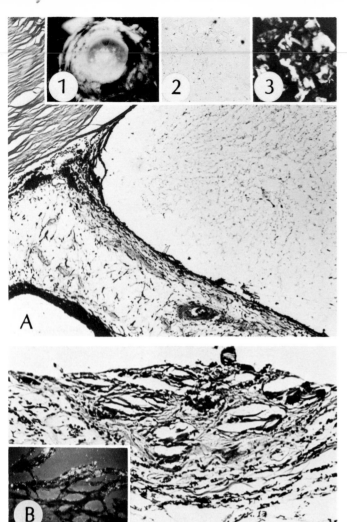

A

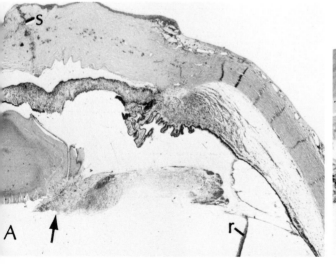

B

FIG. 5–71. Cholesterolosis. **A. Inset 1** shows cholesterolosis of anterior chamber due to cholesterol-filled vitreous (synchisis scintillans) herniating through pupil in aphakic eye. Smear of aqueous aspirate before (**inset 2**) and after (**inset 3**) examination by polarized light; crystals are birefringent. **Main figure** shows delicate vitreous framework in anterior chamber of same eye. **B.** Clear spaces in choroid represent areas where cholesterol had been. Spaces are surrounded by granulomatous inflammation. **Inset** shows frozen section of similar region stained with fat stain and polarized to demonstrate cholesterol crystals. Both from same eye as shown in **A. A,** Wilder reticulum, ×40; **inset 1,** macroscopic; **inset 2,** unstained, ×40; **inset 3,** unstained, polarized, ×101; **B,** H&E, ×69; **inset,** oil red-O, polarized, ×252.

FIG. 5–72. Cyclitic membrane. **A.** Corneal scar (s) of perforating wound. Injury produced hemorrhage and inflammation in posterior chamber. Organization of hemorrhage (arrow) has resulted in early cyclitic membrane formation. Note inward traction of peripheral retina (r) and nonpigmented ciliary epithelium. **B.** Higher magnification of region of arrow in **A** to show fibroblastic proliferation. **A,** H&E, ×11; **B,** H&E, ×28.

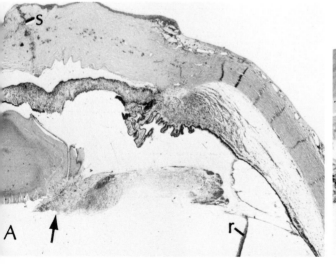

A

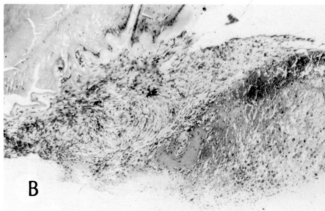

B

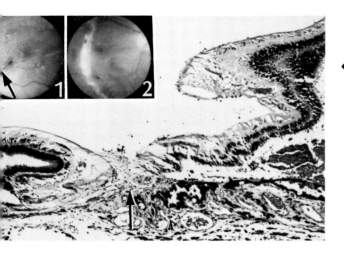

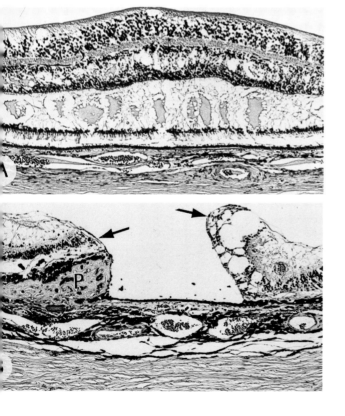

FIG. 5–74. Commotio retinae. **A.** Edema fluid present in outer retinal layers in eye that had recently sustained trauma. **B.** Edema can become massive resulting in retinal macular schisis and even hole formation. Rounded edges (*arrows*) show that hole through macular retina is real, i.e., not an artifact. Note traumatic chorioretinal scarring with marked proliferation of retinal pigment epithelium (*P*) causing adherence of retina to underlying choroid. Most cases of macular holes are accompanied by such chorioretinal scarring and, therefore, do not cause retinal detachments. **A,** H&E, ×40; **B,** H&E, ×40.

◀ FIG. 5–73. Posterior choroidal ruptures. Small rupture (*arrow*) shown in **inset 1** and large rupture in **inset 2**. **Main figure** shows rupture of choroid (*arrow*). Rupture of overlying retina is unusual and is seen here. **Main figure,** H&E, ×28; **inset 1,** fundus; **inset 2,** fundus.

VII. Retina
  A. *Commotio retinae* (Fig. 5–74) (*Berlin's edema*) occurs as a result of a contrecoup effect within 24 hours after blunt injury to the globe (see Table 5–1).
    1. Intraretinal edema, particularly in the macular area, causes the retina to have a pale, white, edematous appearance, which resembles that seen in central retinal artery occlusion.

       Similar patches of edema may be seen in the peripheral retina.

    2. Cystoid degeneration of the macula with cyst and hole formation may occur weeks, months, or years later, or the edema may resolve without sequelae.
    3. Histologically, typical microcystoid degeneration (see p. 412 in Chap. 11) of the macular retina is seen with fluid-filled spaces found mainly in the outer retinal layers.
       a. The fluid may resorb completely or remain. If it remains, the septa between the microcysts may break down, resulting in posterior polar retinoschisis (a macular cyst).
       b. The inner layer of the cyst may develop a hole, or more rarely both inner and outer layers may develop a hole, causing a true through and through retinal hole.
  B. Retinal hemorrhages
    1. Flame-shaped retinal hemorrhages —see p. 404 in Chapter 11 and p. 578 in Chapter 15.
    2. Dot and blot retinal hemorrhages— see p. 404 in Chapter 11 and p. 578 in Chapter 15.
    3. Globular, confluent and massive

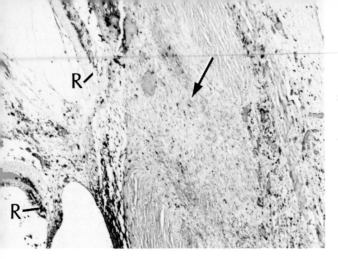

FIG. 5–75. Retinal and choroidal rupture at site of perforating scleral scar (*arrow*) from blunt trauma to the eye. **R,** ruptured ends of retina. *See* Figure 5–83 for lower magnification. H&E, ×21.

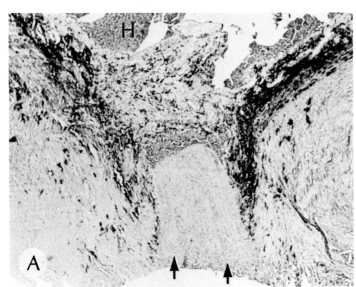

FIG. 5–76. A. Optic nerve shows intrascleral avulsion and inversion. *Arrows* show area of scleral lamina cribosa. Intraocular hemorrhage (*H*) present. **B.** Traumatic avulsion of optic nerve. No tissue present where optic nerve should be. Choroid and retina are detached extensively, and intraocular hemorrhage is present. **A,** H&E, ×16; **B,** H&E, ×5.

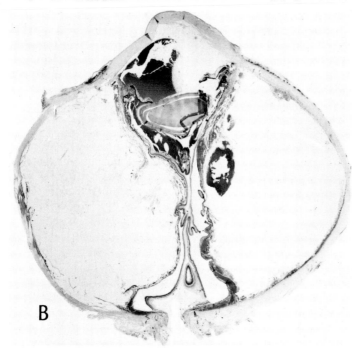

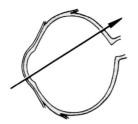
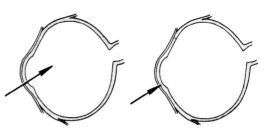

Perforating wound of cornea, sclera and globe.

Perforating wound of cornea, penetrating wound of globe.

Penetrating wound of cornea.

FIG. 5–77. Penetrating and perforating injuries shown diagrammatically. Arrows show direction and extent of injury.

retinal hemorrhages—see p. 578 in Chapter 15.

4. Intraretinal submembranous hemorrhage—see p. 480 in Chapter 12.

Intraretinal submembranous hemorrhage (the clinically so-called pre-retinal or subhyaloid hemorrhage) can occur as a result of direct trauma. It also can be found as a result of sickle cell retinopathy, diabetes mellitus, the blood dyscrasias and, characteristically, following a subarachnoid hemorrhage. The mechanism of hemorrhage within the retina, lying between the internal limiting membrane and the nerve fiber layer of the retina, following or coincidental to a subarachnoid hemorrhage is not known.

C. *Retinal tears* (Figs. 5–73 and 5–75) often irregular with underlying choroidal degeneration and generally located in the superior nasal periphery in the region of the posterior border of the vitreous base, can result from trauma and lead to retinal detachment.

VIII. Optic nerve
   A. A partial or complete rupture or avulsion (Fig. 5–76) may occur.
   B. A hemorrhage may occur into the nerve parenchyma or into the sheaths (meninges) of the optic nerve.
   C. Papilledema may result from ocular trauma.

IX. Sclera—see subsection Penetrating and Perforating Injuries below.

PENETRATING AND PERFORATING INJURIES

I. Penetrating injury. Such an injury is one in which a tissue or structure is partially cut or torn into (Fig. 5–77).

II. Perforating injury. This is an injury in which a tissue or structure is cut or torn completely through (Fig. 5–77).

If a missile goes through the cornea and into but not through the globe, it has caused a perforating injury of the cornea and a penetrating injury of the globe (Fig. 5–78). If a missile goes through the cornea, into the eye and then through the sclera into the orbit, it has caused a perforating injury of the cornea, of the sclera and of the globe.

III. Corneal and scleral rupture due to contusion (Figs. 5–79 through 5–83).
   A. Direct rupture of the globe occurs at the site of impact, most commonly the limbus or cornea, but the sclera also is frequently involved, either alone or due to extension of the cornea or limbal rupture into the sclera.
   B. Indirect rupture of the globe results from force vectors set up at the point of impact on the essentially incompressible globe. The globe tends to rupture at its thinnest parts, i.e., limbus and sclera just posterior to the insertion of the rectus muscles or just adjacent to the optic nerve in a plane in the direction of the force (contre coup) or in a plane perpendicular to the direction of the force.

Because most blows strike the unprotected inferior temporal aspect of the eye, the resultant forces frequently cause a superior nasal limbal rupture. The limbus region is relatively thin (0.8 mm) and is weakened by the internal scleral sulcus, the canal of Schlemm and the collecting

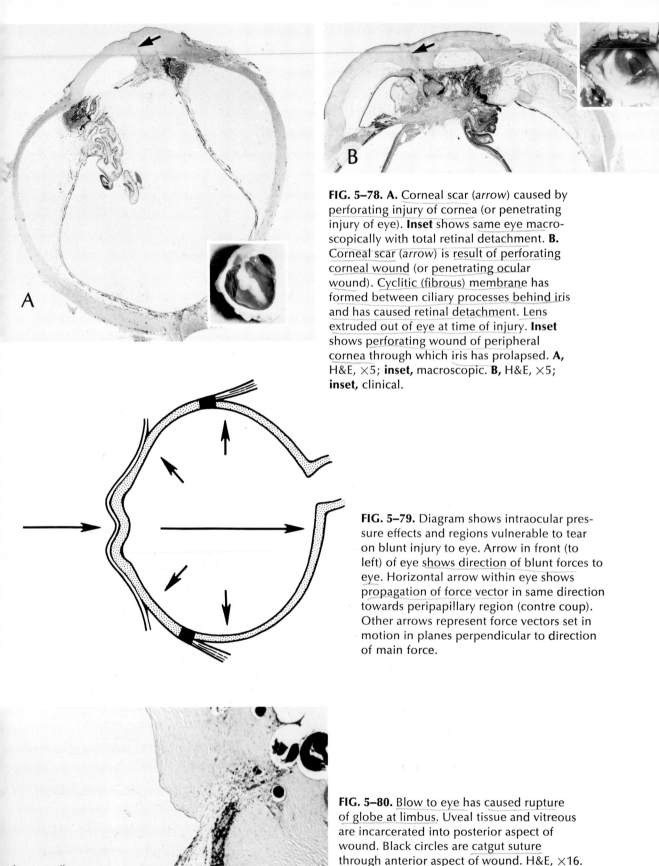

FIG. 5–78. A. Corneal scar (*arrow*) caused by perforating injury of cornea (or penetrating injury of eye). **Inset** shows same eye macroscopically with total retinal detachment. **B.** Corneal scar (*arrow*) is result of perforating corneal wound (or penetrating ocular wound). Cyclitic (fibrous) membrane has formed between ciliary processes behind iris and has caused retinal detachment. Lens extruded out of eye at time of injury. **Inset** shows perforating wound of peripheral cornea through which iris has prolapsed. **A,** H&E, ×5; **inset,** macroscopic. **B,** H&E, ×5; **inset,** clinical.

FIG. 5–79. Diagram shows intraocular pressure effects and regions vulnerable to tear on blunt injury to eye. Arrow in front (to left) of eye shows direction of blunt forces to eye. Horizontal arrow within eye shows propagation of force vector in same direction towards peripapillary region (contre coup). Other arrows represent force vectors set in motion in planes perpendicular to direction of main force.

FIG. 5–80. Blow to eye has caused rupture of globe at limbus. Uveal tissue and vitreous are incarcerated into posterior aspect of wound. Black circles are catgut suture through anterior aspect of wound. H&E, ×16.

aqueous channels. Another frequent site is the superior sclera just behind the insertion of the superior rectus muscle. Both of these positions are ruptured by forces set up in motion perpendicular to the original line of contusion force. A contrecoup effect will result in a posterior scleral rupture, generally just temporal to the optic nerve, in the same directional line as the contusion force.

C. Complications—see sections Complications of Intraocular Surgery and Complications of Nonsurgical Trauma, both in this chapter.

INTRAOCULAR FOREIGN BODIES

I. The amount of damage done by an intraocular foreign body depends upon its size, number, location, composition, path through eye and time retained.

Even if the missile is clean and inert, it may carry passively into the eye fungi, bacteria, vegetable matter, cilia and bone. The missile may be small and leave only a microscopic tract through the cornea, which must be sought after carefully with the slit lamp. Given a history suggestive of the possibility of an intraocular foreign body, any hemorrhagic area in the conjunctiva should be suspected as a possible site of entrance. The examiner should ascertain that such an area does not represent an area of penetration either by clinical examination or surgical exploration. Following ocular trauma an intravitreal hemorrhage, especially if accompanied by a deeper anterior chamber than in the nontraumatized eye, should be considered evidence of a perforated globe until proven otherwise.

II. Inorganic
   A. Gold, silver (see p. 246 in Chap. 7), platinum, aluminum and glass are rather inert and cause little or no reaction.

   Although they cause little or no reaction, they can cause intraocular damage both by their path through the eye and their final position. Glass, for example, lodged in the angle, generally inferiorly, can cause a recalcitrant localized corneal edema months to years following injury. Thus unexplainable, localized corneal edema, especially inferiorly, should arouse

suspicion of glass in the anterior chamber angle. The cornea should be cleared with glycerol and the angle examined by gonioscopy.

   B. Lead and zinc, although capable of causing an inflammatory reaction, generally chronic nongranulomatous, are usually tolerated by the eye with little or no adverse effects except those caused by the initial injury.
   C. Iron can ionize and diffuse throughout the eye, leading to its deposition in many ocular structures, a condition called *siderosis bulbi*.
      1. Bivalent iron (ferrous) is more toxic to ocular tissues than trivalent iron (ferric).
      2. The iron ionizes and spreads to all ocular tissues but is concentrated mainly in epithelial cells (corneal; iris pigmented; ciliary, pigmented and nonpigmented; lens; and retinal pigment epithelia), iris dilator and sphincter muscles, trabecular meshwork and sensory retina (see Color Plate I).
      3. Toxicity due to interference of excess intracellular free iron with some essential enzyme process leads to retinal degeneration and gliosis, anterior subcapsular cataract (*siderosis lentis*) (Fig. 5–84) and trabecular meshwork scarring with secondary chronic open angle glaucoma.

      The structures such as the iris, lens and retina can look "rusty" clinically and macroscopically. The lens frequently is yellow-brown with clumping of rusty material in the anterior subcapsular area. The iris is stained darker so that heterochromia results with the darker iris in the siderotic eye. The iron may be seen clinically in the anterior chamber angle as irregular, scattered, black blotches, which may resemble malignant melanomas and which have caused eyes to be enucleated with the mistaken clinical diagnosis of malignant melanoma.

      4. Histologically the Prussian blue reaction stains the iron blue and shows it to be present in all ocular

epithelial structures, iris dilator and sphincter muscles, sensory retina and trabecular meshwork. In long-standing cases trabecular meshwork scarring and retinal degeneration and gliosis is seen.

Intraocular hemorrhage can produce the same clinical and histopathologic changes as are found with an intraocular foreign body. The iron deposition in tissues that results from an intraocular hemorrhage is called *hemosiderosis bulbi.*

D. Copper can ionize within the eye leading to its deposition in many ocular structures, a condition called *chalcosis* (Fig. 5–85).
  1. Rather than the slowly evolving condition of chalchosis, pure copper tends to cause a violent purulent reaction, usually leading to panophthalmitis and loss of the eye.
  2. Alloy metals with high concentrations of copper tend to cause chalcosis.
  3. The copper has an affinity for basement membranes such as Descemet's and lens capsule and for pseudomembranes such as Bowman's.
  4. Clinically the copper can be seen in the cornea as the Kayser-Fleischer ring (see p. 312 in Chap. 8) and in the anterior area of the lens as a green-gray, almost metallic, disciform opacity, which often has serrated edges with lateral radiations, i.e., a *sunflower cataract* or *chalcosis lentis.*
  5. Histologically there is no adequate stain specific for copper (see p. 312 in Chap. 8).

E. Barium sulfate and zinc disulfide are contained under enormous pressure in the core of golfballs. If cut into, the contents of the core travel at great speed and can penetrate deeply into the tissues of the lids and conjunctiva (Fig. 5–86).

The lids and conjunctiva can be penetrated without the individual realizing it. Also because of the high speed and small size of the particles, no external laceration may be seen at the penetration site.

Histologically a pigmented, amorphous mass without inflammation is present in the tissue. The mass is birefringent to polarized light.

The foreign material is not really pigmented but is white when viewed directly. Because it is opaque to transmitted light, it appears pigmented under the microscope.

III. Organic material. Materials such as cilia, vegetable matter and bone may be carried into the eye. Organic material tends to cause a marked granulomatous reaction. In addition, fungi may accompany the organic material and infect the eye (Fig. 5–87).

CHEMICAL INJURIES

  I. Acid burns (Fig. 5–88)
    A. The tear film can buffer acids unless the amount is excessive or the pH is low, less than 3.0.

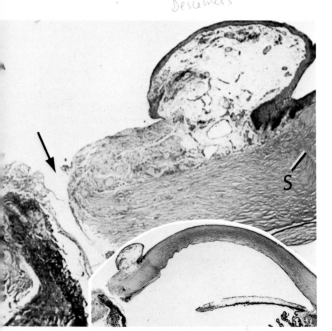

Descemet's

FIG. 5–81. Blow to eye has caused rupture in limbal region (*arrow*) at site of previous filtering surgery. Ciliary body is herniated into wound. Spongy subconjunctival tissue represents filtering bleb. Corneal scar (*S*) is site of previous cataract surgery. **Inset** shows low magnification of anterior segment of same eye. H&E, ×16.

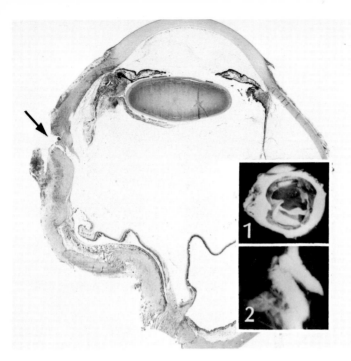

FIG. 5–82. Blow to eye has caused rupture of globe just behind site of insertion of rectus muscle (*arrow*). Sclera, choroid and retina are ruptured in area. **Insets 1** and **2** show macroscopic views of same eye (**inset 2** is higher magnification of ruptured scleral area shown in **main figure** by *arrow* and in **inset 1**). **Main figure,** H&E, ×5; **inset 1,** macroscopic; **inset 2,** macroscopic.

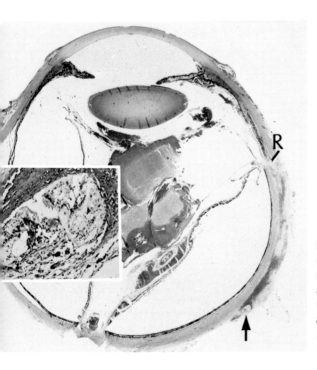

FIG. 5–83. Blow to eye has caused rupture (*R*) of globe just behind site of insertion of rectus muscle (for higher magnification of area see Figure 5–75). Retinal tissue, shown under higher magnification in **inset,** has been avulsed from inside of eye at time of trauma and lies posteriorly in the episclera (*arrow*). **Main figure,** H&E, ×5; **inset,** H&E, ×28.

B. Acid causes an instantaneous coagulative necrosis and precipitation of protein, mainly at the epithelial level, which helps to neutralize the acid and acts to limit the penetrating ability of the acid so that the damage tends to be superficial with intraocular damage slight or nil.

   If the corneal epithelium is defective or the amount of acid is excessive so that the epithelium can no longer act as a protective barrier, the acid can penetrate into the eye and cause extensive damage.

C. Histologically the main finding is a coagulative necrosis of corneal and conjunctival epithelium.

II. Alkali burns (Figs. 5–89 through 5–91)

A. The eye is unable to deal with alkali nearly as effectively as it can deal with acids.

B. Alkali produces an immediate swelling of the epithelium (rather than precipitation of protein as does acid) followed by desquamation, thereby allowing the alkali direct access to the corneal stroma through which it can penetrate rapidly.

C. Alkali coagulates conjunctival blood vessels, and if it gains access to the interior eye, it kills the lens epithelial cells and causes a severe chronic nongranulomatous iridocyclitis.

   Clinically the conjunctiva has a porcelain white appearance due to coagulation of the blood vessels. The effect of alkali on the conjunctiva and lids frequently leads to symblepharon, entropion, etc., as late sequelae.

D. During the healing phase, over the first few weeks enzymes, mainly collagenase, derived from corneal epithelium and to a lesser extent neutro-

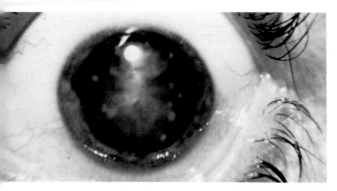

Figure 5–84. Siderosis lentis due to intraocular iron foreign body. Clinical.

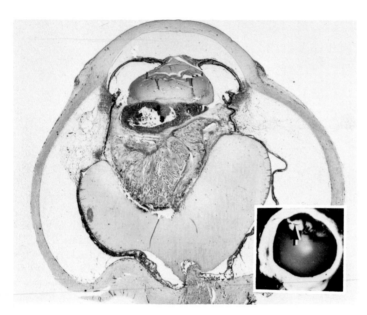

FIG. 5–85. Inset shows brass foreign body (*arrow*) in anterior segment. **Main figure** is same eye showing posterior synechias, iris bombé, retinal detachment and retrolental inflammatory mass where brass foreign body had been. **Main figure,** H&E, ×5; **inset,** macroscopic.

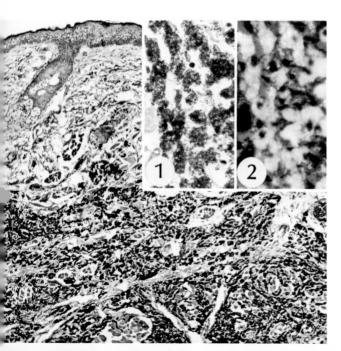

FIG. 5–86. Golfball injury. Dark material in dermis of eyelid appears pigmented; it is shown under higher magnification in **inset 1.** Material is birefringent to polarized light as shown in **inset 2** and represents barium sulfate and zinc disulfide crystals packed tightly within cytoplasm of macrophages. **Main Figure,** H&E, ×70; **inset 1,** H&E, ×395; **inset 2,** H&E, polarized, ×395.

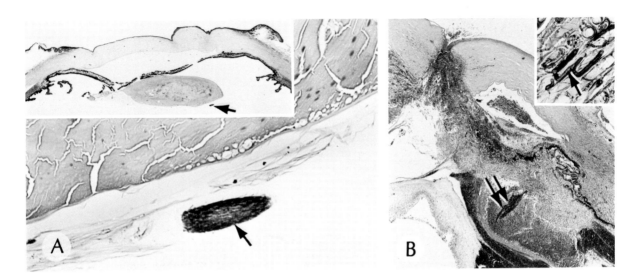

FIG. 5–87. A. Cilia present behind cataractous lens (*arrow*) in eye that had penetrating injury. **Inset** is lower magnification to show cilia (*arrow*), posterior synechias, iris bombé and peripheral anterior synechias (clinically had secondary angle closure glaucoma). **B.** Perforating wound of cornea. Foreign body (*arrows,* piece of wood) lies within abscess overlying ciliary body. Ring of hemorrhage surrounds abscess. Hyphae of pigmented fungus lies within wood as unsuspected potential source of infection (*arrow* in **inset**). **A,** H&E, ×69; **inset,** H&E, ×5. **B,** H&E, ×12; **inset,** iron stain, ×300.

FIG. 5–89. Alkali burn. **Inset 1** shows eye 2 weeks after lye burn. **Inset 2** shows low magnification of anterior segment. Conjunctival flap (*f*) covers cornea. Ciliary body (especially on left side) and iris are necrotic and lens is cataractous (shown under higher magnification in **main figure**; note disappearance of all anterior lens nuclei). **Main figure,** H&E, ×16; **inset 1,** clinical; **inset 2,** H&E, ×6.

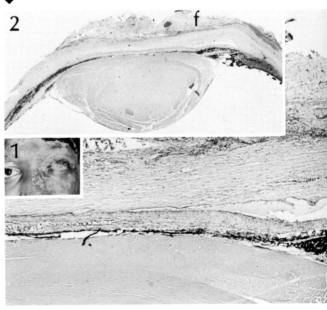

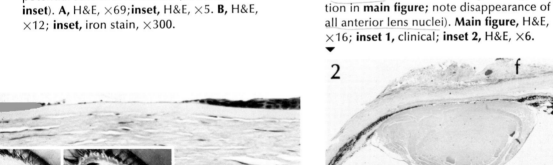

FIG. 5–88. Acid burn. **Insets 1** and **2** show central desquamation of corneal epithelium following accidental splashing of HNO$_3$ solution (**inset 1** in ordinary light; **inset 2** with fluorescein and cobalt blue light). **Main figure** shows analogous microscopic picture with corneal epithelium desquamated from Bowman's membrane centrally. **Main figure,** H&E, ×136; **inset 1,** clinical; **inset 2,** clinical.

philes and keratocytes are released and aggravate the problem by causing keratomalacia.

E. Histologically, widespread necrosis of conjunctiva and cornea is seen, accompanied by a loss of conjunctival blood vessels.

If the alkali has gained access to the inner eye, lens nuclei disappear and cortical degeneration takes place, a chronic nongranulomatous iridocyclitis is found and peripheral anterior synechias frequently result.

Experimental studies have shown that the basal cells at the edge of ulcerating corneas increase in number, have no basement membranes and thrust many cytoplasmic processes into the damaged stroma. The results also suggest that the epithelium produces and secretes a substance into the stroma, probably a collagenase.

III. Tear gas (chloroacetophenone) causes an epithelial exfoliation that heals without sequelae.

IV. Mustard gas (dichlordiethyl sulfide) causes an immediate and sometimes a delayed reaction (Fig. 5–92).

A. The immediate reaction consists of a conjunctivitis that generally is self-limiting and heals without damage.

B. The delayed reaction occurs some decades after the initial injury.

1. The onset is heralded by an attack of conjunctivitis that becomes chronic, followed by corneal clouding (in the area of the interpalpebral fissure) due to stromal keratitis.

2. The entire cornea may be involved, and areas of stromal calcification may develop. The epithelium overlying the calcified areas characteristically breaks down.

3. The conjunctiva develops limbal or perilimbal avascular and calcific patches, producing a "marbling" effect.

4. Aneurysmal dilatations and tortuosity of conjunctival and new corneal vessels complete the picture.

5. Histologically the cornea shows degenerative changes in all layers, consisting of: thinning and atrophy along with areas of thickening of the epithelium; amorphous granular masses beneath the epithelium and sometimes beneath Bowman's membrane; disorganization of the stroma with deposition of hyalin, calcium and crystals; and vascularization.

BURNS

I. Thermal
A. The blink reflex protects the eyes from most burn injuries.
B. The eyes, especially the cornea and conjunctiva, may suffer extensive secondary exposure effects when the lids and face are burned severely.
C. True exfoliation of lens—see p. 360 in Chapter 10.

II. Electric (Fig. 5–93)
A. Electrical injuries, especially if in the area of the head, can cause lens opacities; industrial accidents mainly affect the anterior superficial lens cortex, whereas lightning affects both the anterior and posterior subcapsular areas.
B. The earliest changes are subcapsular vacuoles in the midperiphery of the anterior lens, which can be missed if the pupil is not dilated. The vacuoles form a ring, then they enlarge and coalesce and gradually alter into sunflowerlike anterior subcapsular opacities, which subsequently extend into the visual axis. The latter change may be delayed by several months to over a year.

If the electric energy is close to the eye and intense, an anterior uveitis and even anterior tissue necrosis may result.

C. Histologically the anterior lens opacities are due to a proliferation and abnormal differentiation of lens epithelial cells, whereas the posterior lens opacities are due to faulty formation of lens "fibers."

OCULAR EFFECTS OF INJURIES TO OTHER PARTS OF THE BODY

I. Purtscher's retinopathy—see Table 5–1.
A. Clinically Purtscher's retinopathy gen-

TABLE 5–1
Comparison of Findings in Four Types of Traumatic Retinopathies*

Finding	Purtscher's retinopathy	Traumatic asphyxia	Commotio retinae	Retinal fat embolism
Trauma	Chest compression	Chest compression	Local to eye	Fractures
Vision				
Initially	Variable	Variable	~20/200	Rarely reduced
Duration of loss	Several weeks	Several weeks	Days	Several weeks
Ultimate	Normal	Variable	Normal†	Normal
Systemic signs				
Picture	None	Cyanosis	None	Cerebral and cutaneous
Onset	None	Immediate	None	After 48 hours
Conjunctiva	Normal	Subconjunctival hemorrhages	Variable	None or petechias
Fundus				
Picture	Exudates and hemorrhages	Normal or hemorrhage	Retinal edema	Exudates, hemorrhages and edema
Onset	1 to 2 days	Immediate to a few hours	Few hours	1 to 2 days

* Modified from Kelley, 1972.
† Unless a cystic macula results.

erally follows chest compression and is characterized by superficial white exudates in the retina, frequently accompanied by retinal hemorrhages. Fluorescein angiography shows staining of retinal arteriolar walls and profuse leakage from retinal capillaries in the posterior fundus.

  B. The clinical picture is probably due to damage to retinal vessels secondary to sudden changes in the intraluminal pressure, related directly or indirectly to the compression of the chest; but microemboli cannot be ruled out.

  C. Histologically the retinal changes are probably those of cotton-wool exudates and hemorrhages (see pp. 397, 404 in Chap. 11).

II. Traumatic asphyxia (compression cyanosis)—see Table 5–1.

  A. Clinically traumatic asphyxia generally follows chest compression accompanied by cyanosis and is characterized by retinal hemorrhages.

  B. Histologically hemorrhages are seen in the middle retinal layers.

III. Retinal fat emboli—see Table 5–1

  A. Clinically retinal fat embolization generally follows fractures, frequently of chest bones or long bones of extremities, and is characterized by retinal exudates, edema and hemorrhage after a delay of a day or two.

  B. Histologically fat globules are seen in many retinal and ciliary vessels.

IV. Talc and cornstarch emboli

  A. Talc and cornstarch emboli may occur in drug addicts following intravenous injections of crushed methylphenidate hydrochloride tablets.

  B. Clinically, tiny glistening crystals are found mainly in small vessels around the macula.

  C. Histologically, talc and cornstarch particles are found in the retina and choroid.

V. Caisson disease (barometric decompression)

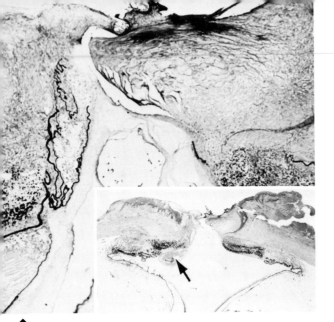

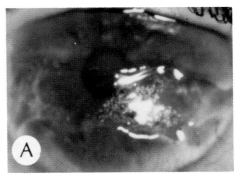

FIG. 5–92. Mustard gas keratopathy. **A.** Band-shaped opacification present in interpalpebral fissure. **B.** Other eye of same patient has thinned apical cornea and vascularized calcified plaque nasally. Patient had been exposed to mustard gas about 50 years previously. Sections of corneal button obtained at time of transplant show in **C** thickened epithelium overlying thinned area of cornea and in **D** a large plaque of calcium (*arrow*) partly replacing Bowman's membrane and superficial stroma. **A,** clinical, right eye; **B,** clinical, left eye; **C,** H&E, ×75; **D,** H&E, ×75.

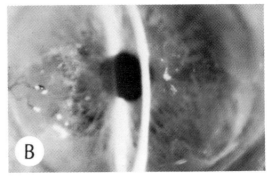

FIG. 5–90. Alkali burn 6 weeks after injury. **Inset** shows central corneal perforation, necrosis of iris and ciliary body and cataractous lens remnant (*arrow*). **Main figure** is higher magnification of necrotic cornea (keratomalacia) with lens capsule in left side of corneal perforation. **Main figure,** PAS, ×16; **inset,** H&E, ×6.

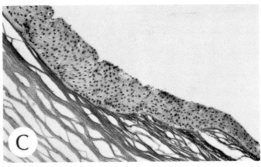

FIG. 5–91. Epithelium at edge of corneal ulcer grows under Bowman's membrane (*b*) into stroma, perhaps secreting collagenase. 1.5 μ section, PD, ×225.

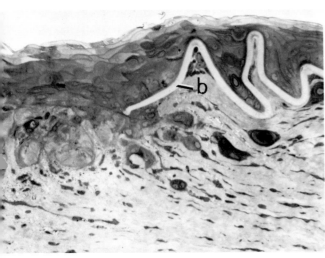

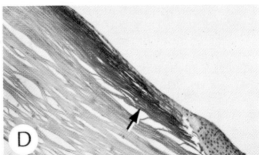

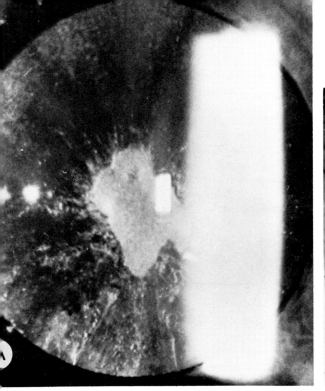

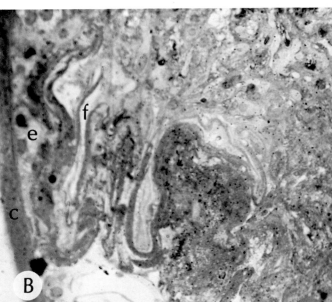

FIG. 5–93. Electric burn. **A.** Retroillumination to show general orientation of fine opacities in anterior midperiphery toward central cataract. Main central cataract located in anterior subcapsular area. **B.** Anterior cataract consists of multiple layers of cells and is thickened at edges by infolding of fibers. Autoradiograph indicates all cells in area have incorporated tritiated leucine into protein. Epithelial cells (e) and extracellular material (f) are covered by lens capsule (c). **A,** clinical; **B,** toluidine blue, ×1,000.

FIG. 5–94. Electromagnetic spectrum with top numbers showing wavelength (meter) and bottom numbers showing frequency (hertz).

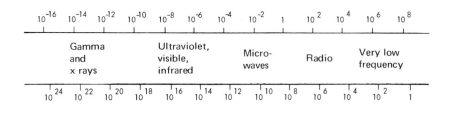

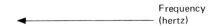

The Electromagnetic Spectrum

A. Caisson disease results from a too sudden decompression, so that nitrogen "bubbles out" of solution in the blood (the bends).

B. The nitrogen bubbles can cause embolization of retinal arterioles leading to ischemic retinal effects (see p. 397 in Chap. 11).

VI. Battered-baby syndrome

A. The most common ocular findings of the battered-baby syndrome include retinal hemorrhages, direct trauma to the eyes and adnexa, retinal tears and retinal detachments.

B. Systemic findings include subdural hematoma, fractures, evidence of sexual molestation, cigarette burns and human bites.

VII. Retinal hemorrhages in the newborn

A. Splinter and flame-shaped hemorrhages are most commonly found in the retina of a newborn, but lake or geographic and dense round "blob" hemorrhages also may be seen.

B. Retinal hemorrhages are present in 20 to 30 percent of newborns.

C. The retinal hemorrhages are probably caused by a mechanical rise in pressure inside the skull during labor; increased blood viscosity and obstetrical instrumentation during delivery may also play a role.

VIII. Carotid-cavernous fistula

A. Traumatic carotid-cavernous fistula causes proptosis, which may be pulsating (but not necessarily), marked chemosis and conjunctival vascular engorgement, frequently glaucoma and in 50 percent of cases abnormal neuro-ophthalmologic signs.

B. The carotid-cavernous fistula may close off spontaneously but generally needs surgical correction.

IX. Acceleration injuries

A. Positive G due to rapid acceleration may force blood downward from the head resulting in arterial pressure reduced below the intraocular pressure, causing collapse of retinal arterioles and retinal ischemia.

B. Negative G (redout), such as occurs in tumbling rotations, forces blood away from the center of rotation toward the head so that arterial and venous pres-

FIG. 5–95. Microwave cataract. **A.** Slit lamp photograph (rabbit eye) of posterior cortical cataract produced by microwaves. **B.** Ring-shaped posterior cortical cataract produced by microwaves. Rabbit lens is viewed from behind. **C.** Edge of cataractous change as seen by electron microscopy. Lens cells are breaking down into globules surrounded by lamellar material. Relatively normal cortical cells are present at upper edge of photo. **A,** clinical; **B,** macroscopic; **C,** ×12,000.

sures may approach each other with cessation of retinal circulation.

C. Transverse G due to rapid deceleration may slam blood from back to front of the head producing subconjunctival and retinal hemorrhages.

RADIATIONAL INJURIES (Electromagnetic)

I. Types of radiation (Fig. 5–94)

A. *Long waves* (30 to 3000 m) are found in radio and diathermy.

B. *Microwaves* (Fig. 5–95) (1 mm to 1 m) are found in radar and rapid-cooking ovens.

C. *Infrared waves* (12,000 to 770 nm*) are found in furnaces, e.g., glass works.

D. *Visible light waves* (770 to 390 nm) are found in sunlight, electric light and nuclear fission.

E. *Ultraviolet waves* (Fig. 5–96) (390 to 180 nm) are found in sunlight and welding arc.

F. *Laser* (light amplification by stimulated emission of radiation) *radiations* are coherent, monochromatic, directional and powerful and currently are produced in the ultraviolet, visible and infrared parts of the spectrum (Figs. 5–97 through 5–99).

G. *Ionizing radiation* is the term applied to those very short waves of the electromagnetic spectrum that disturb the electrical neutrality of the atoms that constitute matter, e.g., x rays and γ rays.

* The old symbol mμ (millimicron) has been replaced by nm (nanometer).

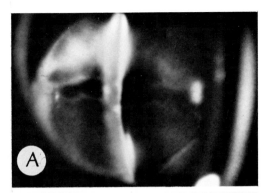

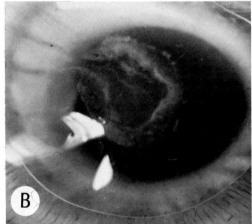

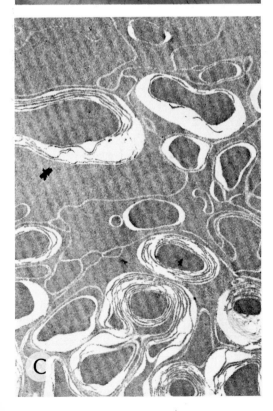

FIG. 5–96. Ultraviolet cataract. **A.** Anterior cortical ring-shaped lamellar cataract (*arrow*) produced in anterior cortex by ultraviolet laser (approximately 600 mw/cm², 6 months) as viewed by slit lamp examination. **B.** Another view of cross section of similar ring-shaped cataract (*arrow*) as viewed by slit lamp. **C.** Cataractous changes deep within anterior cortex 24 hours after irradiation by ultraviolet laser (approximately 375 mw/cm²). Note anteriormost cortical cells appear normal, and there is compression of cells bordering posterior edges of lesions. **A,** clinical; **B,** clinical; **C,** 1.5 μ section, PD, ×300.

▼

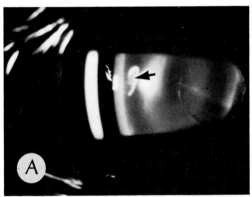

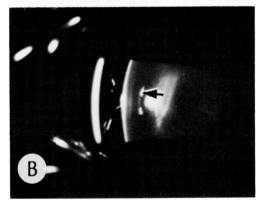

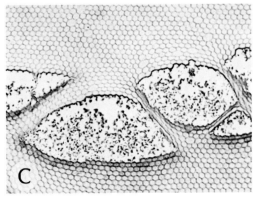

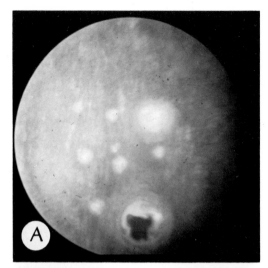

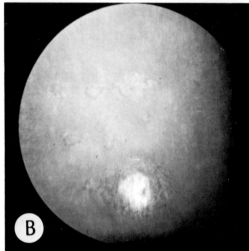

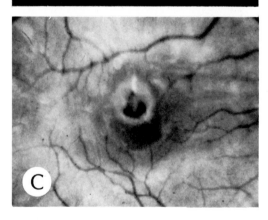

FIG. 5–97. Ruby laser. **A.** Fundus photo of rabbit with fresh lesions of mild, moderate and severe degrees produced by pulsed ruby laser. The last lesion contains fresh hemorrhage from choroidal vasculature. **B.** Lesions are healed by 7 days. **C.** Accidental macular injury from reflected light of pulsed ruby laser. Resultant visual acuity is 20/100. **A,** clinical; **B,** clinical; **C,** clinical.

II. Types of injuries *Not seen in man*

   A. Microwaves can cause cataracts in the experimental animal.

     Although cataracts (posterior cortical) can be produced in animals under severe experimental conditions, it appears highly unlikely that similar changes occur in man exposed to less severe conditions. Microwave-induced cataracts from cumulative exposure in man have yet to be adequately demonstrated.

   B. Infrared waves can cause true exfoliation of the lens (see p. 360 in Chap. 10).

   C. Visible light waves can cause chorioretinal burns if of sufficient intensity.

     This property is used clinically in producing desirable chorioretinal adhesions with the xenon arc photocoagulator.

   D. Ultraviolet waves are generally absorbed by the conjunctiva and cornea and can cause a conjunctivitis and keratitis. The waves can reach the lens if of sufficient power, e.g., ultraviolet laser. *see fig 5-96*

     Superficial punctate keratitis frequently follows overzealous use of sunlamps. The condition, although painful, is self-limiting and heals within 24 hours. A similar picture can be caused by reflected sunlight, e.g., "snow blindness."

   E. Laser radiations can cause chorioretinal injuries (e.g., ruby, argon, krypton and neodymium lasers) or if of longer wavelengths, burns of the cornea and conjunctiva (e.g., CO_2 and erbium lasers).

Ravin JG, Meyer RF: Fluorescein angiographic findings in a case of traumatic asphyxia. Am J Ophthalmol 75:643, 1973

Ring HG: Xenon photocoagulation and the retinal vasculature. Arch Ophthalmol 91:389, 1974

Rodman HI: Chronic open-angle glaucoma associated with traumatic dislocation of the lens. A new pathologic concept. Arch Ophthalmol 69:445, 1963

Rosenthal AR, Appleton B, Hopkins JL: Intraocular copper foreign bodies. Am J Ophthalmol 78:671, 1974

Ruiz RS: Traumatic retinal detachments. Br J Ophthalmol 53:59, 1969

Runyon TE, Levri EA: Vitreous analysis in eyes containing copper and iron intraocular foreign bodies. Am J Ophthalmol 69:1053, 1970

Sezaen F: Retinal hemorrhages in newborn infants. Br J Ophthalmol 55:248, 1971

Smith ME, Zimmerman LE: Contusive angle recession in phacolytic glaucoma. Arch Ophthalmol 74:799, 1965

Spaeth GL: Traumatic hyphema, angle recession, dexamethasone hypertension and glaucoma. Arch Ophthalmol 78:714, 1967

Tso MOM, Fine BS, Zimmerman LE: Photic maculopathy produced by the indirect ophthalmoscope. I. Clinical and histopathologic study. Am J Ophthalmol 73:686, 1972

Verhoeff FM, Bell L: The pathological effects of radiant energy on the eye. Proc Am Acad Arts Sci 51:630, 1916

Wallow IHL, Fine BS, Tso MOM: Morphologic changes in photoreceptor outer segments following photic injury. A comparative study. Ophthalmol Res 5:10, 1973

Wallow IHL, Tso MOM: Repair after xenon arc photocoagulation. 3. An electron microscopic study of the evolution of retinal lesions in rhesus monkeys. Am J Ophthalmol 75:957, 1973

Wallow IHL, Tso MOM, Fine BS: Retinal repair after experimental xenon arc photocoagulation. I. A comparison between rhesus monkey and rabbit. Am J Ophthalmol 75:32, 1973

Walsh FB, Hedges TR: Optic nerve sheath hemorrhage. Am J Ophthalmol 34:509, 1951

Wolff SM, Zimmerman LE: Chronic secondary glaucoma associated with retrodisplacement of iris root and deepening of the anterior chamber angle secondary to contusion. Am J Ophthalmol 54:547, 1962

chapter 6

Skin and Lacrimal Drainage System

SKIN

TERMINOLOGY (Fig. 6–1)

HYPERKERATOSIS (Fig. 6–2)

I. Hyperkeratosis is excessive thickness of the stratum corneum (keratin layer) of the epidermis. The granular layer is thick.

Generally, although exceptions occur, with a slow rate of upward migration of the epidermal cells a thick granular layer is found; with a rapid rate of upward migration few or no granular cells are seen and parakeratosis results.

II. It is seen commonly in verruca and the "scaly" lesions such as actinic and seborrheic keratoses.

PARAKERATOSIS (Fig. 6–3)

I. Parakeratosis is incomplete keratinization in which nuclei are retained in cells of the stratum corneum. The granular layer is absent.
II. It is characteristic of psoriasis and other inflammatory conditions, e.g., seborrheic keratosis.

ACANTHOSIS (Fig. 6–4)

I. Acanthosis consists of an increase in the thickness of the stratum spinosum (squamous or prickle layer) of the epidermis.
II. It is commonly seen in many proliferative epithelial lesions, e.g., papilloma, actinic keratosis and pseudoepitheliomatous hyperplasia.

DYSKERATOSIS (Fig. 6–5)

I. Dyskeratosis consists of keratinization of individual cells within the stratum spinosum where the cells normally are not keratinized.
II. It is characteristic of benign familial intraepithelial dyskeratosis, Darier's disease and Bowen's disease and sometimes is seen in actinic keratosis, in squamous cell carcinoma and after sunburn.

ACANTHOLYSIS (Fig. 6–6)

I. Acantholysis is a separation of epidermal cells due to a dissolution or degeneration of the intercellular cement substance.
II. It is commonly seen in viral vesicles (e.g., herpes simplex), inverted follicular keratosis, pemphigus and Darier's disease.

BULLA (Fig. 6–7)

I. A bulla is a fluid-filled space within or beneath the epidermis.
II. A small bulla arbitrarily is called a *vesicle*.

Vesicles and bullae may arise from primary cell damage or acantholysis. They may be located under the keratin layer (subcorneal), between the epithelium and dermis (junctional) or in the middle layers of epithelium.

ATROPHY (Fig. 6–8)

I. Atrophy consists of 1) thinning of the epidermis (opposite of acanthosis); 2) a smoothing or diminution of rete pegs, resulting in loss of skin markings; and 3) loss of epidermal appendages such as hair.
II. It is commonly seen in aging (e.g., dermatochalasis) or overlying a slow-growing tumor in the corium.

ATYPICAL CELL (Fig. 6–9)

I. An atypical cell is one in which the normal nuclear-to-cytoplasm ratio is altered in favor of the nucleus. Additionally, the nucleus may be hyperchromatic (darker

FIG. 6–1. Normal layers of skin.

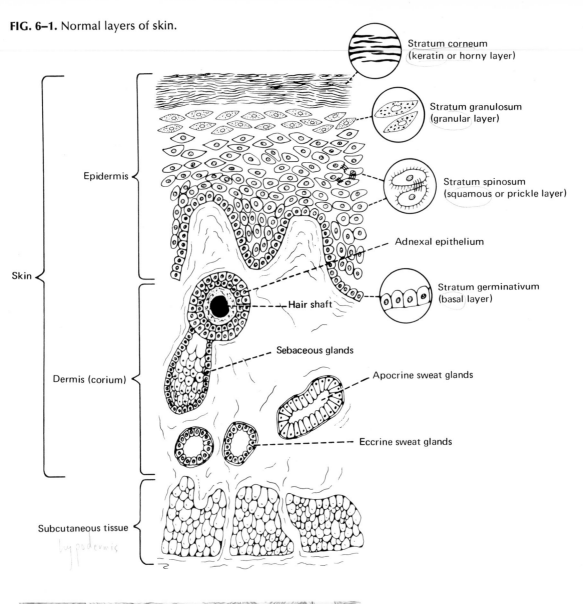

Stratum corneum
(keratin or horny layer)

Stratum granulosum
(granular layer)

Stratum spinosum
(squamous or prickle layer)

Adnexal epithelium

Stratum germinativum
(basal layer)

Epidermis

Hair shaft

Sebaceous glands

Apocrine sweat glands

Eccrine sweat glands

Skin

Dermis (corium)

Subcutaneous tissue

hypodermis

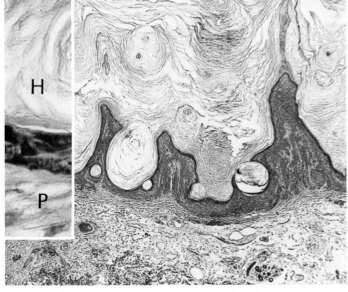

H

P

FIG. 6–2. Hyperkeratosis. Keratin layer is excessively thick. **Inset** is higher magnification to show prominent granular cell layer between prickle cell layer (*P*) and hyperkeratotic layer (*H*). **Main figure**, H&E, ×25; **inset**, H&E, ×400.

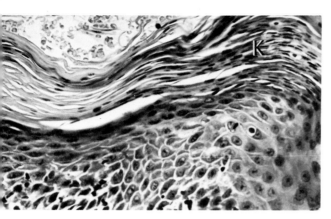

FIG. 6–3. Parakeratosis. Nuclei retained in cells of keratin layer (K) in area of parakeratosis (right side); granular cell layer is not prominent. Where granular cell layer is prominent (arrow), hyperkeratosis, not parakeratosis, is present (left side). H&E, ×176.

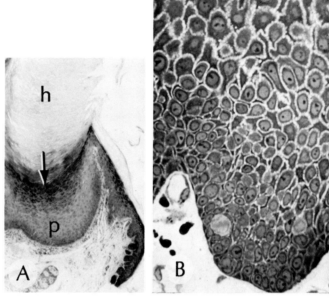

FIG. 6–5. Dyskeratosis. Individual cells are keratinizing (arrows) in prickle cell layer. H&E, ×252.

FIG. 6–4. Acanthosis. A. Prickle cell layer (p) thickened. Granular cell layer is also thickened (arrow), and hyperkeratosis (h) is present. B. Prickle cell layer thickened. Intercellular bridges between cells seen easily. A, H&E, ×28; B, 1.5 μ section, paragon, ×300.

FIG. 6–6. Acantholysis. Epidermal cells in prickle cell layer are separating from each other around small and large squamous eddies (see Figures 6–44 and 6–45). Note diagonal line across larger squamous eddy; line represents scratch in knife blade used to cut tissue. H&E, ×250.

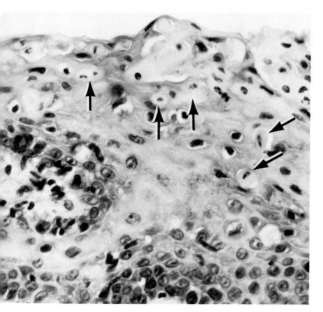

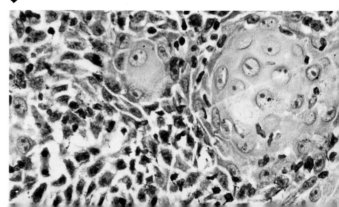

FIG. 6–7. Varieties of bullae encountered in skin.

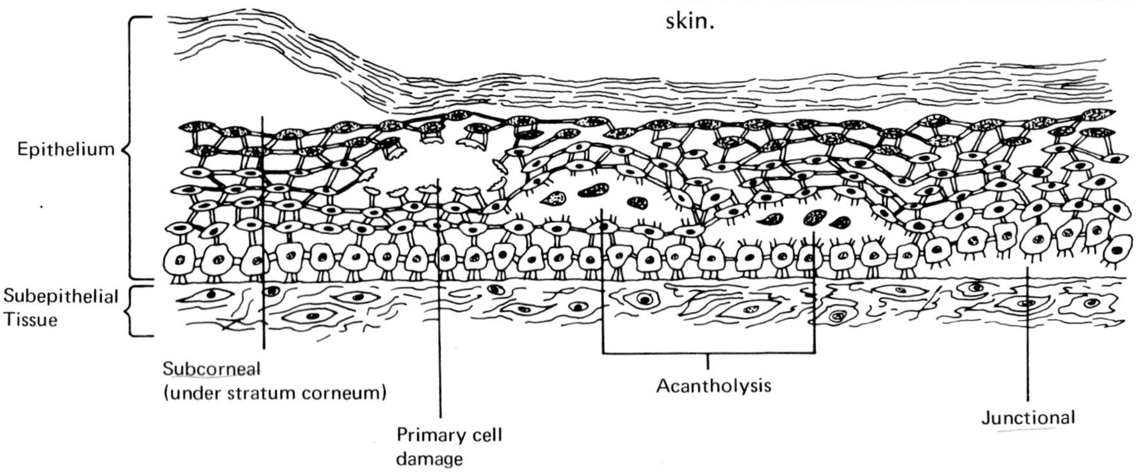

Epithelium

Subepithelial Tissue

Subcorneal (under stratum corneum)

Primary cell damage

Acantholysis

Junctional

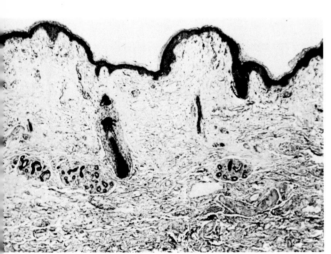

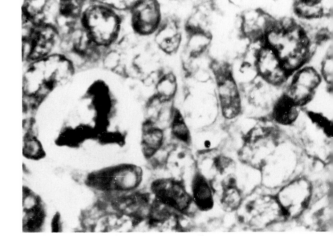

FIG. 6–8. Atrophy. Epidermis and dermis atrophic in area of dermatochalasis (see Figure 6–16). H&E, ×21.

FIG. 6–9. Atypical cell. All cells in field from sebaceous gland carcinoma are atypical. Note abnormal tripolar mitotic figure on left and bipolar mitotic figure on right. H&E, ×850.

FIG. 6–10. Polarity of epidermis is normal in uninvolved area (top left) but is lost in areas of intraepithelial squamous cell carcinoma (arrows). H&E, ×101.

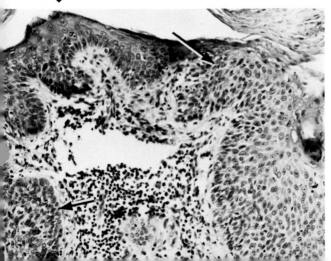

↑ N/C
N hyperchrom
abnormal
mitosis

than normal with the usual stains), may show an abnormal configuration (giant form or multinucleated form) or may contain an abnormal mitotic figure (tripolar metaphase instead of normal bipolar). If sufficiently atypical, according to generally accepted criteria, the cell may be classified as cancerous.

It is the overall pattern of the tissue rather than any one individual cell that aids in the diagnosis of cancer. One dyskeratotic or atypical cell does not necessarily mean the tissue is cancerous.

II. Atypia may be found in an isolated cell or in a few cells in such benign conditions as keratoacanthoma, actinic keratosis and pseudoepitheliomatous hyperplasia, or in abundance in such malignant conditions as carcinoma in situ and squamous cell carcinoma.

LEUKOPLAKIA

I. Leukoplakia is a clinical term (*not* a histopathologic term), which is generally applied to mucous membrane lesions, and means a white plaque. The clinical picture is caused in part by the hyperkeratosis.
II. Clinically any mucous membrane (conjunctival) lesion with hyperkeratosis will appear as a white plaque or leukoplakia, e.g., hyperkeratosis induced by an underlying pinguecula, pterygium, papilloma or carcinoma in situ.

POLARITY (Fig. 6–10)

I. Tissue polarity refers to the arrangement of epithelial cells within the epithelium, i.e., in *normal* polarity (Fig. 6–1) there is an orderly transition from basal cells to squamous (prickle) cells, etc.
II. Complete loss of polarity has occurred when the cells at the surface are indistinguishable from the cells at the base due to loss of normal sequence of cell maturation. Spatial relationships between cells also are disturbed. Disorganized epithelial architecture frequently is a better means of diagnosing epithelial malignancy than individual cell morphology.

CONGENITAL ABNORMALITIES

DERMOID AND EPIDERMOID CYSTS

See p. 526 in Chapter 14.

PHAKOMATOUS CHORISTOMA (Fig. 6–11)

I. Phakomatous choristoma is a congenital choristomatous tumor* of lenticular anlage, usually involving the inner aspect of the lower lid.
II. Histologically, cells resembling lens epithelial cells and lens "bladder cells" (see p. 368 in Chap. 10) along with a PAS-positive membrane closely simulating lens capsule are seen growing in an irregular fashion within a dense fibrous tissue matrix.

* Choristomatous tumor refers to a tumor of tissue not found normally in the area.

FIG. 6–11. Phakomatous choristoma. **A.** Nests of benign cells (*arrows*) resembling lens epithelial cells are present in abnormal (choristomatous) location in dermis of lower lid. **B,** PAS-positive membrane (*arrow*) mimics lens capsule. **A,** H&E, ×101; **B,** PAS, ×101.

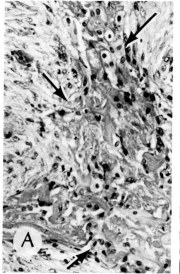
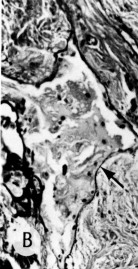

notes nucamch

CRYPTOPHTHALMOS (ablepharon)

I. Cryptophthalmos is a rare condition in which the embryonic lid folds fail to develop.

II. Conjunctiva, cornea and lid folds are replaced by skin that passes smoothly over the orbital margins forming neither palpebral structures nor eyebrows.

Because the cornea is not formed or is rudimentary, an incision through the skin covering the anterior orbit enters directly into the inside of the eye.

MICROBLEPHARON

Microblepharon is a rare condition in which the lids are usually normally formed but shortened; the shortening results in inability to completely close the lids.

COLOBOMA

I. A coloboma of the lid is a defect that ranges from simple notching at the lid margin to complete absence of a segment of lid.

II. Other ocular and systemic anomalies may be found (see *Goldenhar's syndrome*, p. 270 in Chap. 8).

EPICANTHUS

I. Epicanthus consists of a rounded, downward-directed fold of skin covering the caruncular area of the eye. It usually is bilateral and frequently is inherited as an autosomal dominant.

Epicanthus inversus is an upward-directed, rounded fold of skin.

II. Ptosis may be associated with epicanthus.

ECTOPIC CARUNCLE (Fig. 6–12)

Clinically and histologically a normal caruncle may be present in the tarsal area of the lower lid.

LID MARGIN ANOMALIES

I. Congenital entropion. Congenital entropion of the lids may result from an absence of the tarsal plate, hypertrophy of the tarsal plate or hypertrophy of the marginal (ciliary) portion of the orbicularis muscle.

II. Primary congenital ectropion. This is a rare disorder. Most cases are secondary to such conditions as microphthalmos, buphthalmos or an orbitopalpebral cyst.

III. Ankyloblepharon. This defect consists of partial fusion of the lid margins, most commonly the temporal aspects.

IV. Dystichiasis

EYELASH ANOMALIES

I. Hypotrichosis (madarosis)
Primary hypotrichosis or underdevelopment of the lashes is rare. Most cases are secondary to conditions such as chronic blepharitis, any condition that causes lid margin scarring or lid neoplasms.

II. Hypertrichosis—increase in length or number of lashes.
A. *Trichomegaly* is an increase in the length of the lashes.
B. *Polytrichia* is an increase in the number of lashes.
1. Distichiasis—two rows of cilia.
2. Tristichiasis—three rows of cilia.
3. Tetrastichiasis—four rows of cilia.

Distichiasis is the term used for the congenital presence of an extra row of lashes, whereas *trichiasis* is the term used for the acquired condition, which generally is secondary to lid scarring.

PTOSIS

I. Ptosis is a condition in which lid elevation is partially or completely impaired.

II. It may be congenital, associated with other anomalies, caused by trauma, due to third cranial nerve damage or due to many other causes.

III. Histologically the levator muscle may show atrophy or may appear normal.

ICHTHYOSIS CONGENITA (Fig. 6–13)

I. Ichthyosis can be divided into four types:
A. Autosomal dominant ichthyosis vulgaris.
B. Autosomal dominant ichthyosis congenita with a generalized bullous form

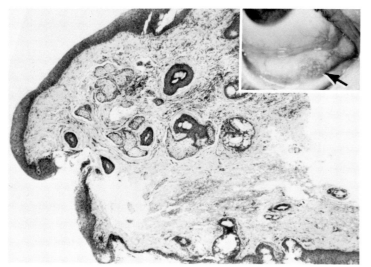

FIG. 6–12. Ectopic caruncle shown in **inset** (*arrow*). Biopsy (**main figure**) shows typical structure of caruncle. **Main figure,** H&E, ×21; **inset,** clinical.

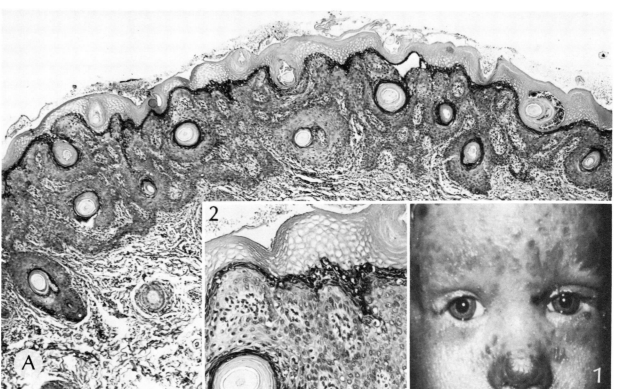

FIG. 6–13. Ichthyosis congenita. **A. Inset 1** shows child with lamellar type, autosomal recessive ichthyosis congenita. **Main figure** is biopsy showing thickened epidermis with very prominent granular cell and keratin layers, shown in higher magnification in **inset 2. B.** Conjunctiva from same child shows papillary reaction with keratinization, shown in higher magnification in **inset. A,** H&E, ×80; **inset 1,** clinical; **inset 2,** H&E, ×200; **B,** H&E, ×40; **inset,** H&E, ×100.

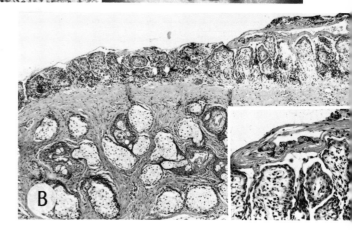

and a localized nonbullous form (ichthyosis hystrix).

C. Sex-linked recessive ichthyosis vulgaris (the most rare).

D. Autosomal recessive ichthyosis congenita with a severe "harlequin" type and a less severe "lamellar" type.

II. All types have in common dryness of the skin with variable amounts of profuse scaling, but only in the autosomal recessive type do ectropion of the lids and conjunctival changes develop.

III. Corneal changes such as gray stromal opacities (*dystrophica punctiformis profunda*) and superficial corneal changes (punctate epithelial erosions, gray elevated nodules and band-shaped keratopathy) occur in ichthyosis vulgaris and autosomal recessive ichthyosis congenita.

IV. The differential diagnosis includes ectodermal dysplasia, poikiloderma congenitale (Rothmund-Thomson syndrome), adult progeria (Werner's syndrome) keratosis palmaris et plantaris, keratosis follicularis spinulosa decalvans (Siemens' disease) and epidermolysis bullosa.

V. Histologically the epidermis is thickened and covered by a thick, dense, orthokeratotic scale.

In the autosomal recessive type the conjunctiva may show a papillary reaction with hyperkeratosis and parakeratosis of the epithelium.

XERODERMA PIGMENTOSUM (Fig. 6–14)

I. Xeroderma pigmentosum is inherited as an autosomal recessive and is characterized by a marked sensitivity of the skin to sunlight.

II. The exposed areas of skin are mainly affected and show three stages of lesions:

A. Mild diffuse erythema associated with scaling and tiny hyperpigmented macules.

B. Atrophy of the skin with mottled pigmentation and telangiectasis—the picture resembles radiation dermatitis.

C. Development of malignant tumors—squamous cell carcinoma, basal cell carcinoma, fibrosarcoma and malignant melanomas.

III. Histologically:

A. Early the epidermis shows hyperkeratotic and atrophic foci associated with pigment phagocytosis by epidermal cells and macrophages. There are perivascular infiltrates of lymphocytes and plasma cells in the corium.

B. Later the hyperkeratosis and pigment deposition become more marked. There is an associated acanthosis of the epidermis and basophilic degeneration of the collagen in the corium.

C. The histopathology of the malignancies is identical to that in individuals not having xeroderma pigmentosum as an underlying predisposing condition.

AGING

ATROPHY (Fig. 6–15)

I. The collagen of the corium has an altered appearance so that it stains basophilic instead of eosinophilic with the H&E stain.

FIG. 6–14. Xeroderma pigmentosum patient (**inset**) developed squamous cell carcinoma of left epibulbar region and right lower lid. Microscopic section shows squamous cell carcinoma. **Main figure,** H&E, ×40; **inset,** clinical.

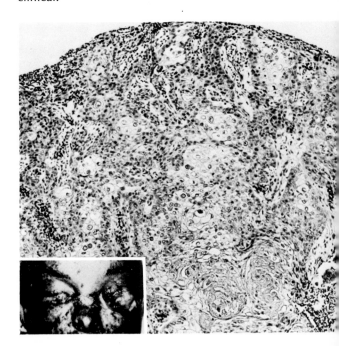

FIG. 6–15. A. Basophilic degeneration (senile elastosis) of dermis (*arrows*). **B.** Same area stains with elastic tissue stain but is resistant to digestion with elastase. **A,** H&E, ×136; **B,** Verhoeff's elastica, ×136.

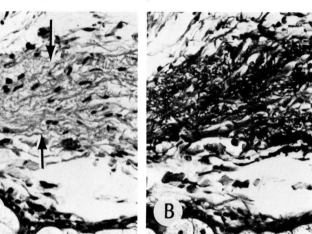

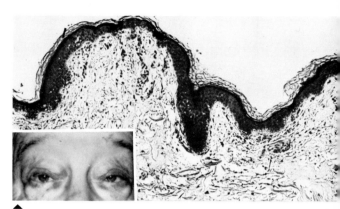

FIG. 6–16. Dermatochalasis. **Inset** shows lax, redundant lid skin hanging in folds. **Main figure** shows atrophic, thin, smooth epidermis with decrease in number and size of rete pegs (see Figure 6–8). Collagen and elastic tissue of dermis are decreased, but vascularity is increased. **Main figure,** H&E, ×40; **inset,** clinical.

The collagen also stains positively for elastin; the positivity is not changed if the tissue is pretreated with elastase.

It is the staining characteristic of the corium that has led to the use of terms such as *basophilic degeneration* and *senile elastosis.*

II. The elastic tissue also may be altered and along with the changed collagen helps to explain the characteristic wrinkling of senile skin.

DERMATOCHALASIS (Figs. 6–8 and 6–16)

I. Dermatochalasis is an aging change characterized by lax, redundant skin of the lids. The folds may even cover the palpebral fissure, thereby impairing vision.

Dermatochalasis should not be confused with *blepharochalasis*, an uncommon condition characterized by permanent changes in the eyelids after recurrent and unpredictable attacks of edema, generally in individuals under 20 years of age.

II. Histologically the epidermis appears thin and smooth with a decrease in or absence of the rete pegs. In the corium there is some loss of elastic and collagen tissue but an increase in capillary vascularity.

HERNIATION OF ORBITAL FAT

I. Defects or dehiscences in the orbital septum produced by aging changes may result in herniation of orbital fat. The herniated fat may simulate an orbital lipoma.
II. Histologically, mature fat is found, which looks quite similar to that found in a lipoma (see p. 532 in Chap. 14).

Frequently the distinction between a primary orbital lipoma and a herniation of orbital fat is more readily made clinically rather than histologically.

INFLAMMATION

TERMINOLOGY

I. Blepharitis
   A. Generally blepharitis means a diffuse inflammation of the lids, which may be acute, subacute or chronic and which has many causes.

   Blepharitis, as it is commonly used today, is synonymous with *dermatitis* (or *eczema*) of the lids.

B. *Seborrheic blepharitis* refers to a specific type of chronic blepharitis primarily involving the lid margins and often associated with dandruff of the scalp. It is characterized by hyperemic inflamed lid margins and yellow, greasy scales on the lashes.

   Histologically the epidermis may show acanthosis, hyperkeratosis or parakeratosis, alone or in combination. There usually is an infiltrate in the corium consisting of lymphocytes and plasma cells. Vascularity may be increased.

C. *Blepharoconjunctivitis* (Fig. 6–17) refers to a specific type of chronic blepharitis involving the lid margins primarily and the conjunctiva secondarily. It is thought to be due to a sensitivity to *Staphylococcus*.

   1. The chronic inflammation frequently results in loss (madarosis) or abnormalities (e.g., trichiasis) of the eyelashes along with secondary phenomena such as hordeolum and chalazion. The lid margins may be thickened and ulcerated with gray tenacious scales at the base of the remaining lashes.
   2. Histologically a chronic, nongranulomatous inflammatory reaction is associated with acanthosis, hyperkeratosis or parakeratosis of the epidermis.

D. *Cellulitis* refers to a specific type of acute blepharitis that involves primarily the subepithelial tissues and frequently is caused by bacteria, especially *Streptococcus*.

   Histologically, polymorphonuclear leukocytes, vascular congestion and edema predominate. Bacteria may be demonstrated with special stains.

II. Hordeolum (Fig. 6–18)

A. An *external hordeolum* (*stye*) results from an acute purulent inflammation of the superficial glands (sweat and sebaceous) and hair follicles of the eyelids. It presents clinically as a discrete, superficial, elevated, erythematous, warm, tender papule or pustule, usually on or near the lid margin.

   Histologically, polymorphonuclear leukocytes, edema and vascular con-

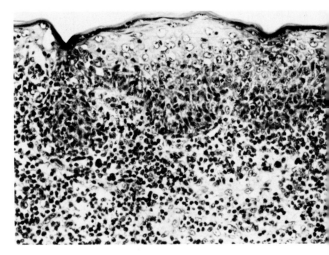

FIG. 6–17. Blepharitis with dermis and epidermis showing chronic nongranulomatous inflammatory infiltrate, predominantly lymphocytes and some plasma cells. H&E, ×136.

FIG. 6–18. Hordeolum. **Inset 1** shows diffuse swelling of both lids of right eye due to external hordeolum at outer aspect of right lower lid. **Inset 2** shows internal hordeolum that has drained internally. **Main figure** shows acute purulent inflammation involving hair follicle and surrounding tissues of eyelid. **Main figure,** H&E, ×40; **inset 1,** clinical; **inset 2,** clinical.

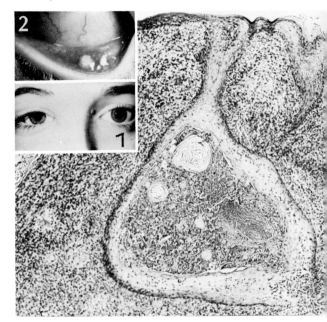

gestion are centered primarily around hair follicles and adjacent structures.

B. An *internal hordeolum* results from an acute purulent inflammation of the meibomian glands within the tarsal plate of the eyelids. It presents clinically as a diffuse, deep, tender, warm erythematous area involving most of the lid.

Hordeolum can be considered simply as an inflammatory papule or pustule ("pimple") of the lid, an external hordeolum being located superficially and an internal hordeolum being deep and internal-pointing.

III. Chalazion (Figs. 6–19 through 6–21)
   A. A chronic inflammation of the meibomian ("deep" chalazion) or Zeis ("superficial" chalazion) sebaceous glands results in a hard, painless nodule in the eyelid.
   B. If the chalazion ruptures through the tarsal conjunctiva, growth of granulation tissue (fibroblasts, young capillaries, lymphocytes and plasma cells) may result in a rapidly enlarging, painless, polypoid mass called a *granuloma pyogenicum*.
   C. Histologically a zonal granulomatous inflammatory reaction is seen centered around clear spaces representing lipid material that filled the spaces but was dissolved out during the processing of the tissue.
   D. In addition to the zonal granulomatous reaction, polymorphonuclear leukocytes, plasma cells and lymphocytes may be found in abundance surrounding the granulomatous reaction.
   E. Not infrequently, multinucleated giant cells (resembling foreign body giant cells or Langhans' giant cells) may be seen, as may asteroid bodies and Schaumann bodies (all nonspecific findings).
IV. Acne rosacea
   A. Acne rosacea affects mainly the face and presents in three patterns, which may occur separately or together: type 1) an erythematous telangiectatic type with follicular pustules and occasional abscesses in addition to erythema and telangiectasis; type 2) a glandular hyperplastic type with enlargement of the nose called rhinophyma; and type 3) the papular type with numerous, moderately firm, slightly raised papules 1 to 2 mm in diameter and generally associated with diffuse erythema.
   B. Histology:
      1. Type 1 shows dilated blood vessels and a nonspecific dermal chronic nongranulomatous inflammatory infiltrate often associated with pustules, i.e., intrafollicular accumulations of neutrophils.
      2. Type 2 shows an increase in size and number (hyperplasia) of sebaceous glands along with the findings seen in type 1.
      3. Type 3 shows papules composed of either a chronic nongranulomatous inflammatory infiltrate or, frequently, a granulomatous inflammatory infiltrate simulating tuberculosis (hence former terms *rosacealike*, *tuberculid* or *lupoid rosacea*).
V. Relapsing febrile nodular nonsuppurative panniculitis (Weber-Christian disease)—see p. 201 in this chapter.

VIRAL DISEASES

I. Molluscum contagiosum (Figs. 6–22 and 6–41)
   A. Clinically a dome-shaped, small, discrete, waxy, papule, often multiple, is seen with a characteristic umbilicated center.
   B. Histologically the presence of large, intracytoplasmic inclusion bodies (*molluscum bodies*) within a markedly acanthotic epidermis characterizes the lesion.
      1. In the deeper layers of the epidermis, near the basal layer, viruses are present as tiny, eosinophilic, intracytoplasmic inclusions.
      2. As the bodies extend toward the surface, they grow enormously so as to exceed the size of the invaded cells.
      3. At the level of the granular layer of the epidermis, the large bodies change their staining characteristics from eosinophilic to basophilic.

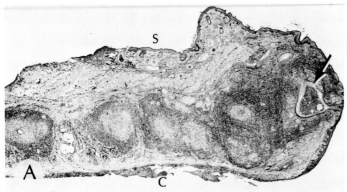

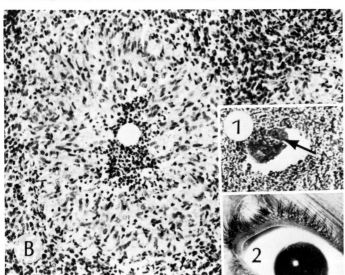

FIG. 6–19. Chalazion. **A.** Whole lid with massive lipogranulomatous inflammation (chalazion) involving tarsal area. Note acute hordeolum (*arrow*) at lid margin. *s*, skin surface; *c*, conjunctival surface. **B.** Clear area in center represents lipid material dissolved out during processing. Chalazion is zonular granulomatous inflammation centered around lipid material. **Inset 1** shows fat-stained, frozen section to demonstrate lipid material (*arrow*) in center of granulomatous reaction. **Inset 2** is clinical appearance of chalazion. **A,** H&E, ×4; **B,** H&E, ×101; **inset 1,** oil red-O, ×69; **inset 2,** clinical.

FIG. 6–20. Granuloma pyogenicum. **A. Inset 1** shows granuloma pyogenicum (*arrow*) of palpebral portion of upper lid conjunctiva. **Main figure** (higher magnification in **inset 2**) demonstrates three main components of polypoid mass: fibroblasts; inflammatory cells, mainly lymphocytes and plasma cells; and capillaries. **B.** Unusually large pyogenic granuloma shown in **inset 1** (same patient in **inset 2** 3 months following surgery). **Main figure** shows microscopic appearance of typical granuloma pyogenicum from same patient. **A,** H&E, ×16; **inset 1,** clinical; **inset 2,** H&E, ×101; **B,** H&E, ×54; **inset 1,** clinical; **inset 2,** clinical.

▼

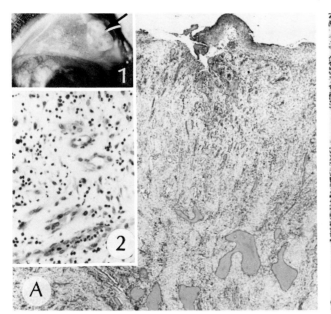

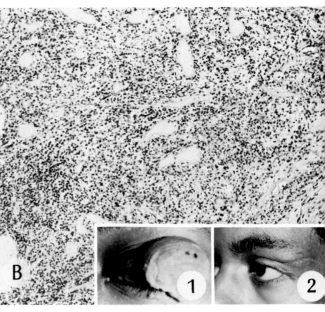

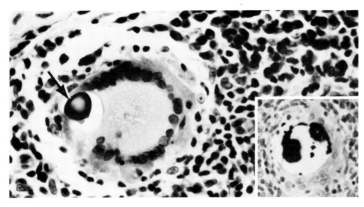

FIG. 6–21. Schaumann body (*arrow*) is seen within giant cell in chalazion. **Inset** shows positive reaction with stain to demonstrate calcium. **Main figure,** H&E, ×252; **inset,** von Kossa, ×176.

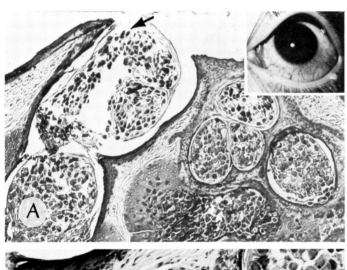

FIG. 6–22. A. Molluscum contagiosum. **Inset** shows molluscum contagiosum at lid margin (outer one-third of lower lid). Microscopic section shows typical molluscum bodies, some of which (*arrow*) appear to be emptying onto surface. **B.** Higher magnification of **A** to show that in deeper layers of epidermis (*D*) intracytoplasmic inclusions are small and eosinophilic. Inward, toward the surface (*arrow*), inclusion bodies become enormous and basophilic. **A,** H&E, ×40; **inset,** clinical; **B,** H&E, ×101.

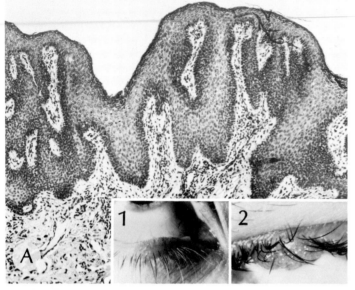

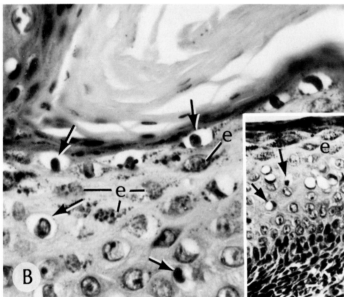

FIG. 6–23. Verruca vulgaris. **A. Insets 1** and **2** show two types of "warty" lesions at lid margins. **Main figure** demonstrates papillomatous lesion with elongated rete ridges typically bent inward, i.e., radiating toward central focus. **B.** Higher magnification shows acanthosis, hyperkeratosis and inclusion bodies (*arrows*). **Inset** shows groups of vacuolated cells, which contain deeply basophilic inclusion bodies (*arrows*). Most of vacuolated cells near surface in **main figure** contain smaller eosinophilic particles (e), probably representing degenerative products. **A,** H&E, ×54; **inset 1,** clinical; **inset 2,** clinical; **B,** H&E, ×441; **inset,** H&E, ×176.

FIG. 6–24. Herpes simplex. Ballooning degeneration in deep epidermis (*arrow*) has resulted in intraepidermal vesicle formation in lesion of tongue. **Inset 1** from same lesion shows eosinophilic intranuclear inclusion bodies in all cells. **Inset 2** shows multiple *Herpes simplex* lesions of eyelids. **Main figure,** H&E, ×69; **inset 1** H&E, ×252; **inset 2,** clinical.
▼

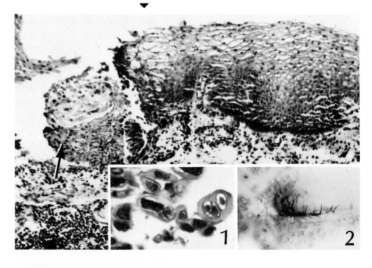

II. Verruca (wart) (Fig. 6–23)
   A. Verruca vulgaris (anywhere on the skin), verruca plana (mainly on face and dorsa of hands), verruca plantaris (soles of feet) and condyloma acuminatum (glans penis, mucosa of female genitalia and around anus) are all caused by the same virus.
   B. Histologically a papillomatous lesion marked by acanthosis, parakeratosis and hyperkatosis is seen.
      1. Characteristically, cells in the upper part of the squamous layer and in the granular layer of epidermis are vacuolated.
      2. Within the vacuolated cells intracellular, round, deeply basophilic bodies represent virus inclusions.

      Previously, round eosinophilic intracellular bodies were thought to represent the virus inclusions, but these have been shown to be degenerative cell products composed principally of keratohyalin.

III. Viral vesicular lesions (Fig. 6–24)
   A. The viruses of variola (smallpox), vaccinia (cowpox), varicella (chicken pox), herpes zoster (shingles) and herpes simplex (cold sore) all have vesicular-pustular eruptions of similar structure.
   B. Histologically all five diseases are characterized by an intraepidermal vesicle (Fig. 6–7).
      1. Ballooning degeneration involves the deep epidermis and results in swollen epidermal cells that lose their intercellular bridges causing acantholysis, i.e., separation of cells and intraepidermal vesicle formation.
      2. Reticular degeneration involves the superficial and peripheral epidermis and results in enormous swelling of the squamous cells (intracellular edema) causing them to burst so that only the resistant parts of cell walls remain as septa forming a multilocular vesicle (Fig. 6–7).

      Ballooning degeneration seems specific for viral vesicles, whereas reticular degeneration may be seen in acute dermatitis (e.g., poison ivy).

      3. Multinucleated epithelial giant cells may be seen with herpes simplex and zoster.
      4. Eosinophilic inclusion bodies are found in all five diseases, mainly in the cytoplasm although occasionally in the nucleus in variola, in the cytoplasm (*Guarnieri* bodies) in vaccinia, exclusively in the nucleus (usually surrounded by a halo or clear zone) in varicella, herpes zoster and herpes simplex.
IV. Trachoma and lymphogranuloma venereum—see pp. 241, 244 in Chapter 7.

BACTERIAL DISEASES

I. Impetigo
   A. Impetigo may be caused by staphylococci (more common) or streptococci (less common), both of which cause a bullous eruption.
   B. Histologically a superficial bulla directly under the keratin layer is filled with polymorphonuclear leukocytes; cocci are found with special stains within neutrophils or free in the bulla.
II. *Staphylococcus*—see under impetigo (above) and blepharoconjunctivitis (p. 186 in this chapter).
III. Parinaud's oculoglandular syndrome—see p. 244 in Chapter 7.

FUNGAL AND PARASITIC DISEASES

See subsections on fungal and parasitic nontraumatic infections pp. 89–97 in Chapter 4.
   I. *Demodex folliculorum* (Fig. 6–25)
      A. The parasitic mite, *Demodex folliculorum*, lives in the hair follicles in humans and certain other mammals, especially around the nose and eyelashes.
      B. Although it is present in almost all middle-aged and elderly people and in a significant percentage of younger people, the mite seems relatively innocuous and only rarely produces any symptoms.
      C. Histologically the mite is seen frequently as an incidental finding in a hair follicle in skin sections. No inflammatory reaction or histopathologic abnormalities are associated with the mite.

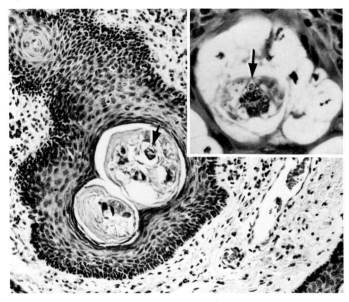

FIG. 6–25. Demodex folliculorum, parasitic mite, seen within hair follicle (*arrow*) in **main figure** and within sebaceous gland of hair follicle (*arrow*) in **inset**; tiny dots represent nuclei of mite. **Main figure,** ×101; **inset,** H&E, ×252.

LID MANIFESTATIONS OF SYSTEMIC DERMATOSES OR DISEASE

ICHTHYOSIS CONGENITA

See section Congenital Abnormalities above.

XERODERMA PIGMENTOSA

See section Congenital Abnormalities above.

PEMPHIGUS

See p. 241 in Chapter 7.

ERYTHEMA MULTIFORME

See p. 246 in Chapter 7.

EHLERS-DANLOS SYNDROME ("Indian Rubber Man")

I. Ehlers-Danlos (E-D) syndrome consists of loose jointedness; hyperextensibility; fragility and bruisability of the skin with "cigarette paper" scarring; generalized friability of tissues; vascular abnormalities with rupture of great vessels; hernias; gastrointestinal diverticula; and friability of the bowel and lungs. There appear to be perhaps six forms of the syndrome with the majority of cases inherited as auto-somal dominants, whereas the others show a sex-linked recessive or autosomal recessive (including one probably distinct "ocular" form) pattern.

The skin in E-D syndrome is hyperextensible but not lax. When it is pulled, it stretches; when let go, it quickly springs to the original position. The skin in cutis laxa (see subsection Cutis Laxa below), on the other hand, tends to return slowly after it is pulled and then let go.

II. The basic defect appears to be an abnormal organization of collagen bundles into an intermeshing network, but this is by no means accepted by all, and the basic defect is still open to question.

III. Ocular findings include epicanthus (the most common finding), hypertelorism, poliosis, strabismus, blue sclera, microcornea, megalocornea, myopia, keratoconus, ectopia lentis, intraocular hemorrhage, retinal abnormalities and angioid streaks (see p. 440 in Chap. 11).

IV. Histologically no eyes have been studied and a conjunctival biopsy studied by light and electron microscopy showed no abnormalities. The pathologic lesions in E-D syndrome are quite controversial with an increase in elastic tissue or a defect in the network of collagen being the proposed cause.

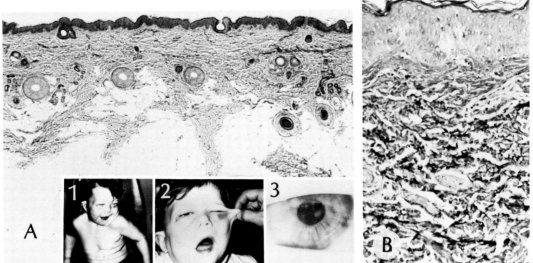

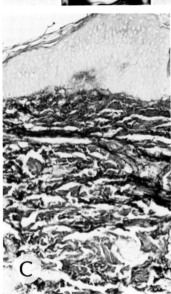

FIG. 6–26. Cutis laxa. **A. Inset 1** shows child with skin hanging in loose folds. **Inset 2** demonstrates extensibility of skin. **Inset 3** shows corneal opacities. **Main figure** is low magnification of skin. **B.** Special stain shows fragmentation and granular degeneration of dermal elastic tissue. **C.** Special stain shows increased amounts of ground substance. **A,** H&E, ×16; **inset 1,** clinical; **inset 2,** clinical; **inset 3,** clinical; **B,** Verhoeff's elastica, ×101; **C,** colloidal iron, ×101.

CUTIS LAXA (Fig. 6–26)

I. In cutis laxa the extensible skin hangs in loose folds over all parts of the body, especially in those areas where it is normally loose, e.g., on the face and around the eyes. The lungs may be involved with emphysema, and cor pulmonale may result in early death. Both autosomal dominant and recessive forms have been reported.

II. The basic defect seems to be in the elastic fibers, which are reduced in number, shortened and show granular degeneration.

III. Ocular findings include hypertelorism, blepharochalasis, ectropion and corneal opacities.

IV. Histologically the skin shows fragmentation and granular degeneration of the dermal elastic tissue along with an increase in the amount of dermal ground substance. The corneal pathology has not been adequately interpreted.

PSEUDOXANTHOMA ELASTICUM (Fig. 6–27)

I. Pseudoxanthoma elasticum (PXE), inherited mainly as an autosomal recessive but also as an autosomal dominant, involves predominantly three areas: the

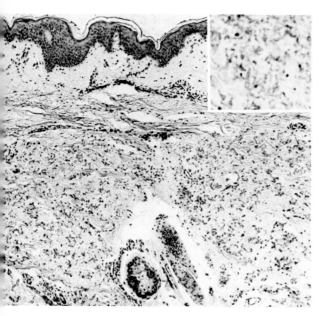

FIG. 6–27. Pseudoxanthoma elasticum. Biopsy is from neck of young woman with typical skin changes. Swollen, fragmented, clumped fibers (elastic fibers? abnormal collagen fibers?) present in middle and lower layers of dermis. **Inset** shows abnormal fibers under higher magnification. **Main figure,** H&E, ×40; **inset,** H&E, ×101.

skin, the eyes and the cardiovascular system.

A. The skin, mainly the face, neck, axillary folds, cubital areas, inguinal folds and periumbilical area, becomes thickened and grooved with the areas between the grooves diamond-shaped, rectangular, polygonal, elevated and yellowish.

1. The skin in the involved areas becomes lax, redundant and relatively inelastic.

2. The skin changes often are not noted clinically until the second decade of life or later.

B. The eyes show angioid streaks.

C. The cardiovascular system manifestations include weak or absent peripheral pulses, intermittent claudication, angina pectoris and internal hemorrhages.

II. The basic defect seems to be related to a

dystrophy of elastic fibers, but some think collagen fibers are at fault.

III. Histologically the skin shows changes in the dermis quite similar to those seen in senile elastosis (basophilic degeneration; see p. 185 in this chapter). Angioid streaks consist of breaks in Bruch's membrane (see p. 440 in Chap. 11).

TOXIC EPIDERMAL NECROLYSIS (Lyell's disease; epidermolysis necroticans combustiformis; acute epidermal necrolysis; scalded skin syndrome)

I. Toxic epidermal necrolysis is an acute disease accompanied by severe malaise and high fever and characterized by exfoliation of large areas of epidermis, so that the denuded areas resemble scalded skin.

II. In most cases the disease is of unknown cause, and in others it is drug related. It generally results in either death or complete recovery.

III. Histologically the changes are limited almost entirely to the epidermis, the dermis being uninvolved or showing only a mild lymphocytic infiltrate.

A. Most cases show a severe degeneration and necrosis of epidermal cells, which results in detachment of the entire epidermis (flaccid bullae).

B. Some cases show involvement of only the upper (outer) portion of epidermis, which results in detachment of only the superficial epidermis.

One theory holds that toxic epidermal necrolysis represents another variant of erythema multiforme (just as Stevens-Johnson syndrome is a variant). The theory has not been substantiated. As in Stevens-Johnson syndrome, the conjunctiva may be involved with ulcerative or pseudomembranous lesions.

CONTACT DERMATITIS

I. An allergenic or irritating substance applied to the skin may result in contact dermatitis.

A. Contact dermatitis is one of the most common abnormal conditions affecting the lids.

B. Such agents as cosmetics and locally applied atropine and epinephrine may produce a contact dermatitis.

C. Contact dermatitis may be present in three forms: 1) an acute form with diffuse erythema, edema, oozing, vesicles, bullae and crusting; 2) a chronic form with erythema, scaling and thick, hard, leathery skin (*lichenification*); and 3) a subacute form showing characteristics of acute and chronic forms.

II. Histology

A. In the acute stage tissue edema involving epidermis (intraepidermal vesicles) and dermis predominates along with a lymphocytic infiltrate.

Spongiosis or intercellular edema between squamous cells contributes to the formation of vesicles (small unilocular bullae). Intracellular edema, on the other hand, results in reticular degeneration and the formation of multilocular bullae.

B. In the chronic stage there is acanthosis, hyperkeratosis and some parakeratosis together with elongation of rete pegs. Mild spongiosis is present, but vesicle formation does not occur. In the dermis lymphocytes are found frequently around blood vessels (eosinophils, histiocytes and fibroblasts also may be seen).

Histologically the distinction between a primary allergic contact dermatitis and an irritant-induced or toxic dermatitis cannot be made except possibly in the early stage. *Atopic dermatitis*, however, does not show vesicles, although it does show lichenified and scaling erythematous areas, which when active may show oozing and crusting but no vesicles.

COLLAGEN DISEASES

I. Dermatomyositis—see p. 525 in Chapter 14.

II. Periarteritis nodosa (Fig. 6–28)

A. Periarteritis nodosa is a fatal disease characterized by a panarteritis of small and medium-sized, muscular-type arteries of kidney, muscle, heart, gastrointestinal tract and pancreas but generally not of the central nervous system or lungs and rarely of the skin.

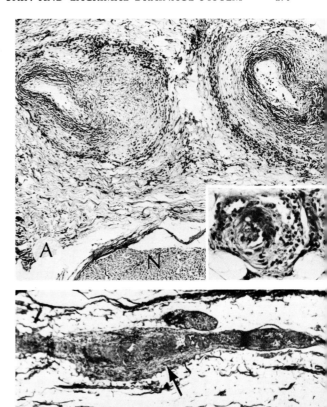

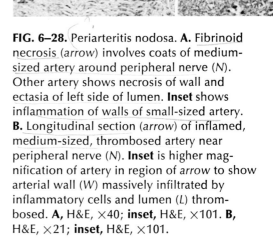

FIG. 6–28. Periarteritis nodosa. **A.** Fibrinoid necrosis (*arrow*) involves coats of medium-sized artery around peripheral nerve (*N*). Other artery shows necrosis of wall and ectasia of left side of lumen. **Inset** shows inflammation of walls of small-sized artery. **B.** Longitudinal section (*arrow*) of inflamed, medium-sized, thrombosed artery near peripheral nerve (*N*). **Inset** is higher magnification of artery in region of *arrow* to show arterial wall (*W*) massively infiltrated by inflammatory cells and lumen (*L*) thrombosed. **A,** H&E, ×40; **inset,** H&E, ×101. **B,** H&E, ×21; **inset,** H&E, ×101.

A benign cutaneous form of periarteritis nodosa exists as a chronic disease limited to the skin and subcutaneous tissue.

B. Histologically, four stages may be seen:
1. The degenerative or necrotic stage —foci of necrosis (fibrinoid necrosis) involve the coats of the artery and may result in localized dehiscences or aneurysms.
2. The inflammatory stage—inflammatory cells, predominantly neutrophils but also eosinophils and lymphocytes, infiltrate the necrotic vascular and perivascular areas.
3. The granulation stage—healing occurs with the formation of granulation tissue (young growing capillaries, fibroblasts, lymphocytes and plasma cells), which may occlude the vascular lumens.
4. The fibrotic stage—healing ends with scar formation.

Allergic granulomatosis (allergic vasculitis), *Wegener's granulomatosis* (Fig. 6–29) and *lethal midline granuloma* of the face may be variants of periarteritis nodosa or independent entities. Allergic granulomatosis involves the same size arteries as periarteritis but differs in having respiratory symptoms, pulmonary infiltrates, systemic and local eosinophilia, granulomatous lesions intra- and extravascularly and frequently cutaneous and subcutaneous nodules and petechial lesions. Wegener's granulomatosis is characterized by necrotizing granulomatous lesions mainly in the upper and lower respiratory tract but also in other viscera, generalized focal necrotizing vasculitis involving both arteries and veins and focal necrotizing glomerulitis. The granulomas in Wegener's granulomatosis have fewer eosinophils and have less of a radial arrangement of epithelioid cells and giant cells around areas of necrosis than do the granulomas in allergic vasculitis. Lethal midline granuloma differs from all three in not having an acute arteritis but rather a bland, vascular necrosis; it also does not have a granulomatous component.

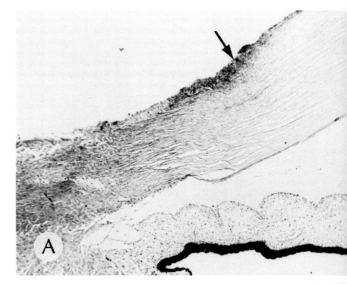
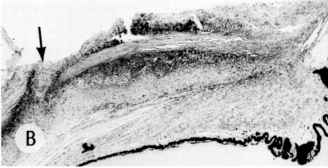
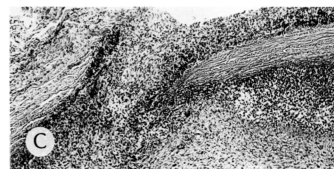

FIG. 6–29. Wegener's granulomatosis. **A.** Peripheral corneal ulcer (*arrow*) is present just anterior to full-thickness limbal necrosis. **B.** Necrotizing granulomatous lesions are destroying scleral collagen and extending through scleral emissary canal (*arrow*). **C.** Higher magnification of **B** in region of *arrow*. **A,** H&E, ×16; **B,** H&E, ×16; **C,** H&E, ×54.

III. Lupus erythematosus (Fig. 6–30) can be subdivided into three types: 1) chronic discoid lupus erythematosus, which is limited to the skin; 2) intermediate, or subacute, lupus erythematosus, which has systemic symptoms in addition to the skin lesions; and 3) systemic lupus erythematosus, which is dominated by visceral lesions with the skin lesions a minor part of the disease.

Transition from the chronic discoid type to the systemic type is rare. Even the intermediate type tends to be a chronic benign disease usually with a negative lupus erythematosus test and only infrequent transition to the systemic type. Fleshy conjunctival lesions may be seen in the systemic type.

A. Histology can be divided into five main findings (when they involve the skin, the three types of lupus erythematosus differ only in degree of involvement with the systemic form being the most severe):
1. Hyperkeratosis with keratotic plugging found mainly in the follicular openings but also found elsewhere.
2. Atrophy of the squamous layer of epidermis and of rete pegs.
3. Liquefaction degeneration of basal cells, i.e., vacuolization and "dissolution" of basal cells (most significant finding).
4. Focal lymphocytic dermal infiltrates mainly around dermal appendages.
5. Edema, vasodilatation and extravasation of erythrocytes in the upper dermis.

All five histologic findings are not necessarily present in each case.

IV. Scleroderma (Fig. 6–31) exists in two forms: 1) a benign circumscribed (morphea) form, which almost never progresses or transforms to the systemic form; and 2) a systemic form (progressive systemic sclerosis), which may prove fatal.
A. The histology of both types is quite similar, if not identical:
1. Early the dermal collagen bundles appear swollen and homogeneous and are separated by edema. Round inflammatory cells, mainly lymphocytes, are found around edematous

FIG. 6–30. Chronic discoid lupus erythematosus. **A.** Note marked hyperkeratosis with keratotic plugging, atrophy of squamous layer of epidermis and rete pegs and focal dermal lymphocytic infiltrates. **B.** Higher magnification to show characteristic liquefaction degeneration of basal cell layer of epithelium. **A,** H&E, ×28; **B,** H&E, ×101.

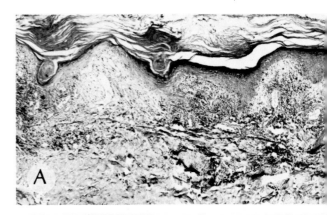

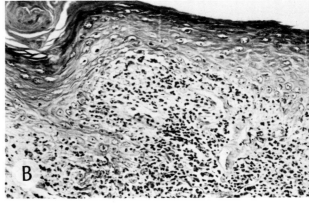

blood vessel walls and between collagen bundles (panniculitis).
2. In the intermediate stages the subcutaneous tissue is infiltrated by round inflammatory cells, dermal collagen becomes further thickened and dermal adnexae are involved in the process. Blood vessel walls show edema with intimal proliferation and narrowing of their lumina.
3. In the late stages the dermis is thickened by the addition of new collagen at the expense of subcutaneous tissue. The subcutaneous

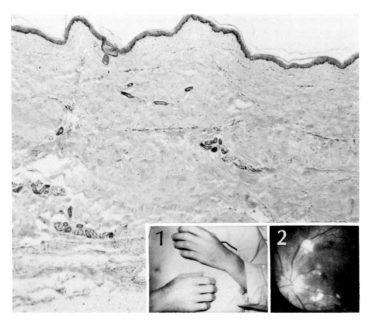

FIG. 6–31. Scleroderma. Dermis is thickened and subcutaneous tissue is replaced to a considerable extent by collagen. Atrophic sweat glands appear "trapped" in midst of collagen bundles. **Inset 1** shows typical changes in hands of patient with scleroderma. **Inset 2** shows appearance of fundus in person with advanced scleroderma. **Main figure,** H&E, ×21; **inset 1,** clinical; **inset 2,** fundus.

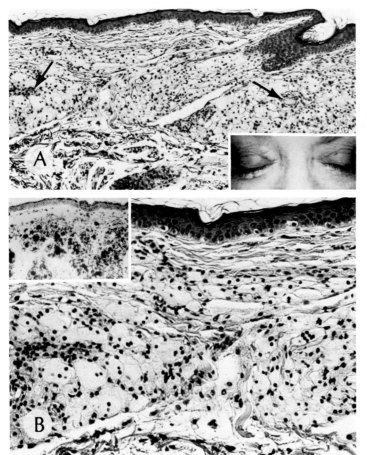

FIG. 6–32. Xanthelasma. **A.** Clusters of lipid-laden foam cells are present in dermis, generally centered around blood vessels (*arrows*). **Inset** shows characteristic clinical appearance of xanthelasma. **B.** Higher magnification of foam cells. **Inset** demonstrates dermal lipid positivity (black globules) with special stain for fat. **A,** H&E, ×54; **inset,** clinical. **B,** H&E, ×101; **inset,** oil red-O, ×20.

fat is replaced by collagen. The thickened dermis contains hyalinized, hypertrophic, closely packed collagen bundles, atrophic sweat glands "trapped" in the midst of collagen bundles and few or no sebaceous glands or hair structures. Inflammation is minor or absent. Blood vessels are narrowed and fibrotic.

4. The overlying epidermal structure, including rete pegs, is rather well preserved except in the late stages of the systemic form when atrophy with disappearance of rete pegs may be seen.

5. The underlying muscle, especially in the systemic form, may be involved and show degeneration, swelling and inflammation early with fibrosis late.

The condition probably starts in the subcutaneous fat tissue.

XANTHELASMA (Fig. 6–32)

I. Xanthelasma most commonly occurs in middle-aged or elderly individuals with normal serum cholesterol. It may occur, however, in primary hypercholesteremia or in individuals who have nonfamilial serum cholesterol elevation.

II. The lesions appear as multiple, soft, yellowish plaques most commonly at the inner aspects of the upper and lower lids.

III. Histologically, clusters of foam cells are found in the superficial dermis. The cells contain a lipid material. The cells generally cluster around blood vessels and may even involve the walls of blood vessels.

JUVENILE XANTHOGRANULOMA

See p. 338 in Chapter 9.

AMYLOIDOSIS

See p. 248 in Chapter 7.

MALIGNANT ATROPHIC PAPULOSIS
(Degos' Syndrome)

I. The syndrome is a rare cutaneovisceral syndrome of unknown cause characterized by the diffuse eruption of asymptomatic, porcelain white skin lesions, followed generally by death within a few months.

II. Ocular lesions other than the porcelain white lid lesions include a characteristic white, avascular thickened plaque of the conjunctiva; telangiectasia of conjunctival blood vessels with microaneurysms; strabismus; choroidal lesions such as peripheral choroiditis, small plaques of atrophic choroiditis, gray avascular areas and discrete loss of peripheral retinal pigment epithelium and choroidal pigment; and intermittent diplopia and papilledema with progressive central nervous system involvement.

III. Histologically, capillaries are occluded by endothelial proliferation and swelling; the endarterioles show endothelial proliferation, swelling and fibrinoid necrosis involving only the intima; artery involvement is greater than vein; thrombosis may occur secondary to endothelial changes and result in ischemic infarction; and no significant inflammatory cellular response is noted.

CALCINOSIS CUTIS (Fig. 6–33)

I. Calcinosis cutis has three forms: 1) *metastatic calcinosis cutis* with calcium deposition secondary to either hypercalcemia (e.g., with parathyroid neoplasm, hypervitaminosis D, excessive intake of milk and alkali and extensive destruction of bone by osteomyelitis or metastatic carcinoma) or hyperphosphatemia (e.g., with chronic renal disease and secondary hyperparathyroidism); 2) *dystrophic calcinosis cutis* with deposition in previously damaged tissue; and 3) *subepidermal calcified nodule* with a single (rarely two), small, raised, hard nodule, occasionally present at birth.

II. Histologically forms 1 and 2 show large deposits of calcium in the subcutaneous tissue and small, granular deposits in the dermis, whereas form 3 shows deposits of irregular granules and globules in the upper dermis. The calcium appears as deep blue or purple granules in sections stained with H&E and stains positively with special stains such as alizarin red and von Kossa stains.

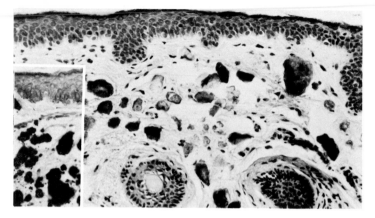

FIG. 6–33. Calcinosis cutis. Subepidermal calcified nodule shows deposits of irregular granules and globules of calcium in upper dermis. **Inset** demonstrates calcium positivity with special stain. **Main figure,** H&E, ×101; **inset,** von Kossa, ×101.

LIPOID PROTEINOSIS (Fig. 6–34)

I. Lipoid proteinosis is a rare condition of the lids and mucous membranes, which has an autosomal recessive inheritance pattern.

II. Multiple, waxy, pearly nodules, about 2 to 3 mm in diameter, cover the lid margins linearly along the roots of the cilia.

III. Whitish, plaquelike lesions are found on mucous membranes.

IV. Histologically there is papillomatosis of the epidermis and large dermal collections of an amorphous, eosinophilic, PAS-positive material with no inflammatory reaction.

Electron microscopy shows large masses of an extracellular, finely granular, amorphous material with no fibrillar structure.

HEMOCHROMATOSIS

See p. 25 in Chapter 1.

I. Brown pigmentation of the lid margin and conjunctiva (near the limbus) and around the disc margin has been described in idiopathic hemochromatosis.

II. Histologically the brown pigmentation of the lid margin and conjunctiva is due to an increased melanin content of the epidermis, especially the basal layer.

A. The peripapillary pigmentation may be due to small amounts of iron in the peripapillary retinal pigment epithelium.

B. Intraocular deposition of iron is most prominent in the nonpigmented ciliary epithelium but also may be found in the sclera, corneal epithelium and peripapillary retinal pigment epithelium.

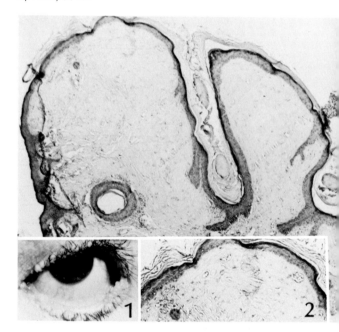

FIG. 6–34. Lipoid proteinosis. **Inset 1** shows clinical appearance of lid margin lesions. Papillomatosis of epidermis with collections of amorphous material is shown in **main figure** and in higher magnification in **inset 2.** **Main figure,** H&E, ×28; **inset 1,** clinical; **inset 2,** H&E, ×40.

FIG. 6–35. Weber-Christian disease. **A.** Nodular lesion of episclera (*arrow*) with shallow ulcer of peripheral cornea. **B.** Photomicrograph to show lesion is located in subepithelial conjunctival tissue and consists of histiocytic granulomatous inflammatory reaction. **C.** Section from subcutaneous skin nodule of same case shows granulomatous reaction to fat necrosis and appears almost identical histologically to conjunctival nodule. **A,** clinical; **B,** H&E, ×101; **C,** H&E, ×240.

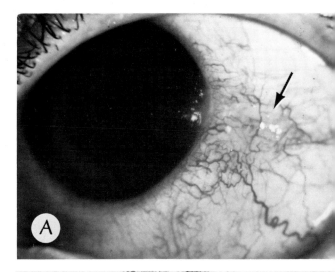

"fat necrosis"
= Lipoid necrosis
see p. 104

p. 197

RELAPSING FEBRILE NODULAR NONSUPPURATIVE PANNICULITIS (Weber-Christian Disease) (Fig. 6–35)

I. The condition, which is of unknown cause, occurs most often in middle-aged and elderly women. It is characterized by malaise and fever and by the appearance of crops of tender nodules and papules in the subcutaneous fat, usually on the trunk and extremities.

II. Ocular findings include ocular nodules of fat necrosis on eyelids, subconjunctiva and, rarely, anterior uveitis and macular hemorrhage.

III. Histologically three stages can be seen:
   A. An early, rapid phase shows fat necrosis and an acute inflammatory infiltrate of neutrophils, lymphocytes and histiocytes.
   B. A second stage shows a granulomatous inflammation with macrophages, many lipid-filled, and some epithelioid cells and foreign body giant cells.
   C. In the third stage fibrosis ensues, which clinically may result in depression of the overlying skin.

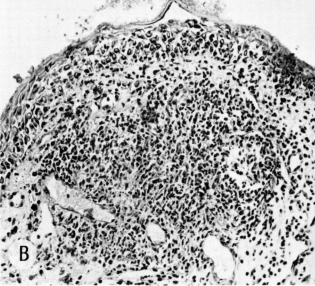

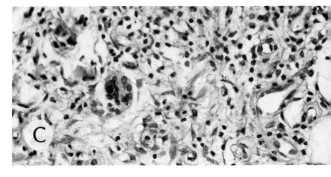

CYSTS, PSEUDONEOPLASMS AND NEOPLASMS

BENIGN CYSTIC LESIONS

I. Epidermoid (Fig. 6–36) and dermoid cysts* (Fig. 6–37) tend to occur at the outer upper portion of the upper lid (see p. 526 in Chap. 14).

II. Epidermal inclusion cysts.* These appear identical histologically to congenital epidermoid cysts; the former, however, are caused by dermal implantation of epidermis following trauma.

Milia are identical histologically to epidermal inclusion cysts; they differ only in size, milia being the smaller; they may represent retention cysts, caused by the occlusion of a pilosebaceous follicle or of sweat pores, or benign keratinizing tumors, or they may have a dual origin.

III. Sebaceous (pilar) cyst* (Fig. 6–38). These cysts may occur by obstruction of the glands of Zeiss, of the meibomian glands or of the sebaceous glands associated with the hair follicles of the lid surface or the brow.

Histologically the cyst is lined by epithelial cells that possess no clearly visible intercellular bridges with the peripheral layer of cells showing a distinct pallisade arrangement and the cells closest to the cavity being swollen without distinct cell borders. The cyst cavity contains an amorphous eosinophilic material.

The lining epithelial cells of the sebaceous cyst are different from the typical cells lining an epidermal inclusion cyst in which the cells are stratified squamous epithelium. The cystic contents of the sebaceous cyst are different from the horny (keratin) material filling the epidermal inclusion cyst. "Old" sebaceous cysts, however, may show stratified squamous epithelial metaplasia of the lining, resulting in keratin material filling the cyst and producing a picture identical to an epidermal inclusion cyst, unless a fortuitous microscopic section passes through the occluded pore of the sebaceous cyst.

*Rupture of any of these cysts results in a marked, granulomatous, foreign body inflammatory reaction in the adjacent tissue (Fig. 6–37).

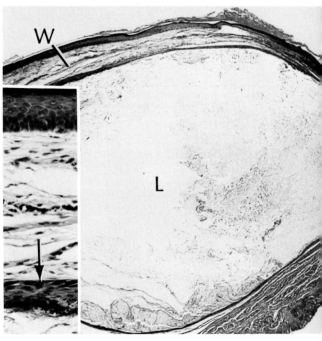

FIG. 6–36. Epidermoid cyst has no skin appendages in cyst wall (*W*), is lined by stratified squamous epithelium (see *arrow* in **inset**) and contains desquamated keratin in its lumen (*L*). **Main figure,** H&E, ×16; **inset,** H&E, ×101.

IV. Comedo (blackhead) is the primary lesion of acne vulgaris.

    A. Histologically the comedo is due to intrafollicular hyperkeratosis, which leads to a cystic collection of sebum and keratin.

        1. The comedo occludes the sebaceous glands of the pilosebaceous follicle, which may undergo atrophy.

        2. With rupture of the cyst wall of the comedo, abscesses develop. These comprise a foreign body giant cell granulomatous reaction to the released sebum and keratin and perhaps to bacteria (especially *Corynebacterium acnes*).

Clinically these are follicular papules and pustules.

        3. Eventually epithelium grows downward encapsulating the inflammatory infiltrate, and the lesion heals by fibrosis.

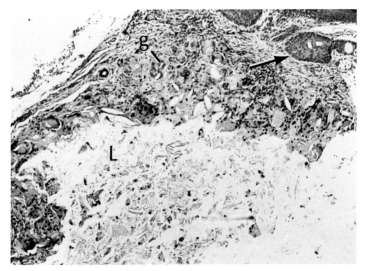

FIG. 6–37. Dermoid cyst has skin appendages in cyst wall (*arrow*), is lined by stratified squamous epithelium and contains desquamated keratin (and sometimes hair shafts) in its lumen (*L*). Dermoid here has ruptured and its contents have incited marked granulomatous inflammatory response (*g*), which has replaced lining epithelium. H&E, ×40.

FIG. 6–38. Sebaceous cyst filled with keratin debris. Section passes through occluded pore of cyst. H&E, ×21.

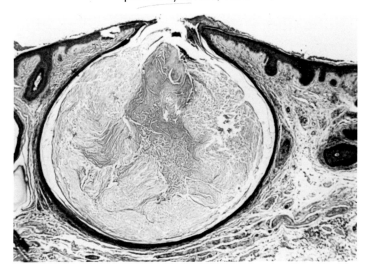

V. Ductal cysts (Fig. 6–39). Ductal cysts of the eyelid generally result from clogging of a sweat gland duct.

Histologically the cysts are lined by a double layer of epithelium, the outer layer being myoepithelium and the luminal layer being cuboidal.

BENIGN TUMORS OF THE SURFACE EPITHELIUM

I. Papilloma is an upward proliferation of skin resulting in an elevated irregular lesion with an undulating surface.
   A. Histologically it generally is character-ized by fingerlike projections or fronds of papillary dermis covered with epidermis showing a normal polarity but some degree of acanthosis and hyperkeratosis along with variable parakeratosis and elongation of rete pegs. The dermal component may have a prominent vascular element.
   B. Five diseases show this type of proliferation: 1) nevus verrucosus (epidermal cell nevus; Jadassohn); 2) actinic keratosis; 3) verruca vulgaris; 4) seborrheic keratosis; and 5) acanthosis nigricans.

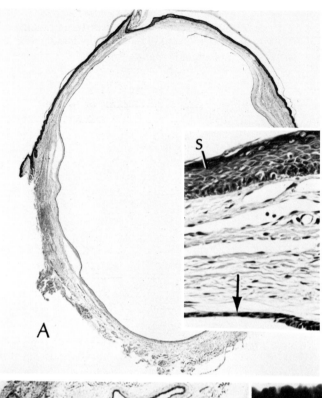

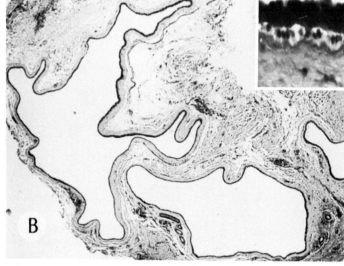

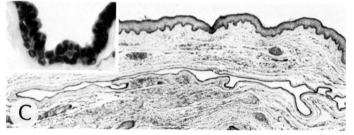

FIG. 6–39. Ductal cyst, due to clogged sweat duct, may take many forms. **A.** Large cyst appears empty. **Inset** shows double layer of lining epithelium (*arrow*); stratified squamous epithelium (s) is surface epidermis. **B.** Multiloculated cyst lined by double layer of epithelium, as shown in **inset. C.** Thin, branching cyst lined by double layer of epithelium, as shown in **inset. A,** H&E, ×4; **inset,** H&E, ×176. **B,** H&E, ×16; **inset,** H&E, ×252. **C,** H&E, ×16; **inset,** H&E, ×252.

hyperkeratosis + acanthosis

1. Nevus verrucosus consists of a single lesion present at birth or appearing early in life. Histologically the lesion consists of closely set, papillomatous, hyperkeratotic papules with marked acanthosis and elongation of rete pegs.
2. Actinic keratosis—see p. 207 in this chapter.
3. Verruca vulgaris—see p. 191 in this chapter.
4. Seborrheic keratosis—see p. 205 in this chapter.
5. Acanthosis nigricans exists in three types, all three presenting papillomatous, verrucous, brownish patches predominantly in the axillae, on the dorsum of fingers, on the neck or in the genital and submammary regions.

   papilloma

   a. Adult (malignant) acanthosis nigricans—the skin lesion occurs in adults and is associated with an internal adenocarcinoma, most commonly of the stomach.
   b. Juvenile (benign) acanthosis nigricans—the skin lesion occurs at birth or at a young age (before 20 years), frequently has a familial tendency and is not associated with an internal adenocarcinoma, with obesity or with endocrinopathy.
   c. Pseudocanthosis nigricans—the skin lesion is associated with obesity or endocrinopathy and tends to clear with reduction of weight.
      Histologically all three are identical and show marked hyperkeratosis and papillomatosis and mild acanthosis (not as marked as in nevus verrucosus) and hyperpigmentation.
C. Usually histologic examination of a papillomatous lesion will indicate one of the above five entities; occasionally, however, no more specific diagnosis than papilloma can be made.

The nonspecific papilloma usually is further subdivided into a type with a broad base and a type with a narrow base. The broad-base type is called a *sessile papilloma* or simply a papilloma. The narrow-base type is called a *pedunculated papilloma*, a *fibroepithelial papilloma* (Fig. 6–40) or simply a *skin tag*.

II. Seborrheic keratosis results from an intraepidermal proliferation of benign basal cells (basal cell acanthoma) (Figs. 6–41 through 6–43).
   A. Seborrheic keratosis increases in size and number with increasing age and is most common in the elderly.
   B. The lesions tend to be sharply defined, brownish, softly lobulated papules or plaques with adherent scale.
   C. Histologically the lesion has a papillomatous configuration, sits as a "button" on the surface of the skin and contains a proliferation of cells closely resembling normal basal cells, called basaloid cells.

   The histologic appearance of seborrheic keratosis is variable. The lesion frequently contains cystic accumulations of horny (keratin) material. It may show marked hyperkeratosis and papillomatosis, or it may be characterized by mainly epithelial thickening or a peculiar adenoid pattern where the epithelium proliferates in the dermis in narrow, interconnecting cords or tracts. It may be deeply pigmented and even confused clinically with a malignant melanoma.

III. Inverted follicular keratosis (basoquamous cell epidermal tumor, basosquamous cell acanthoma, irritated seborrheic keratosis) (Figs. 6–6, 6–44 and 6–45), resembles a seborrheic keratosis but has an additional squamous element.
   A. It generally shows a papillomatous configuration, exists as a solitary lesion and may show rapid growth.
   B. It may be related to, or a variant of, a seborrheic keratosis, or it may be a reactive phenomenon related to pseudoepitheliomatous hyperplasia (see below), or it may be an independent lesion.
   C. Histologically it resembles superficially a seborrheic keratosis with the addition of collections of squamous cells frequently centered around a slightly keratinized focus, which resembles

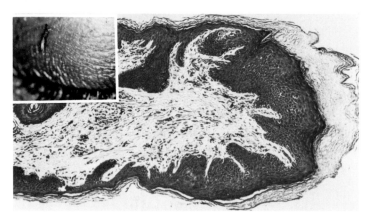

FIG. 6–40. Fibroepithelial papilloma consists of narrow based papilloma covered by acanthotic, hyperkeratotic epithelium and containing fibrovascular core. **Inset** shows same specimen (skin tag) as it looked before removal. **Main figure,** H&E, ×54; **inset,** clinical.

keratin (horn) "pearls." The pearls are surrounded in turn by acantholytic squamous cells, which in turn are surrounded finally by basaloid cells. The entire collection of squamous cells is called a *squamous eddy*.

IV. Pseudoepitheliomatous hyperplasia (Fig. 6–46) (invasive acanthosis, invasive acanthoma, carcinomatoid hyperplasia) consists of a benign proliferation of the epidermis that simulates an epithelial neoplasm.

A. It is seen frequently at the edge of burns or ulcers, near neoplasms such as basal cell carcinoma, malignant melanoma or granular cell myoblastoma, around areas of chronic inflammation such as blastomycosis, scrofuloderma and gumma, or in such lesions as keratoacanthoma and perhaps inverted follicular keratosis.

B. Histologically the usual type of pseudoepitheliomatous hyperplasia, no matter what the associated lesion, if any, has the following characteristics:

1. Irregular invasion of the dermis by squamous cells that may show mitotic figures but do not show dyskeratosis or atypia.

2. Leukocytes that frequently infiltrate the squamous proliferations.

Although an inflammatory infiltrate is seen frequently under or around a squamous cell carcinoma, the inflammatory cells almost never infiltrate the neoplastic cells directly. If one sees inflammatory cells admixed with squamous cells, especially if the inflammatory cells are neutrophils, a reactive lesion such as pseudoepitheliomatous hyperplasia should be considered.

C. *Keratoacanthoma* (Figs. 6–41 and 6–47), a type of pseudoepitheliomatous hyperplasia, consists of a solitary lesion (occasionally grouped lesions) that develops on exposed (usually hairy) areas of skin in middle-aged or elderly people; grows at a rapid rate for 2 to 6 weeks showing a raised, smooth edge and an umbilicated, crusted center; and involutes in a few months to a year, leaving a depressed scar.

Histologically, keratoacanthoma is characterized by its dome- or cup-shaped configuration with elevated wall and central keratin mass under low magnification and by acanthosis with normal polarity under high magnification.

The tumor has in the past been confused frequently with squamous cell carcinoma. The typical noninvasive, elevated, cup shape with a large central keratin core, as seen under low-power light microscopy, along with the benign cytology, as seen under high-power light microscopy, should give the proper diagnosis of keratoacanthoma with no difficulty. If, however, only a small piece of tissue, e.g., a partial biopsy, is available for histopathologic examination, it may be difficult or

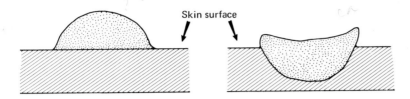

Skin surface

Elevated-umbilicated lesions

Lesion filled with
keratin-keratoacanthoma

Lesion filled with large inclusion
bodies—molluscum contagiosum

FIG. 6–41. Upper left drawing shows elevated lesion that sits as a "button" on surface of skin and is characteristic of benign papillomatous lesions, e. g., seborrheic keratosis. Upper right drawing shows elevated lesion that also invades underlying skin, e. g., basal cell and squamous cell carcinomas. Lower drawing shows how elevated-umbilicated lesions may simulate invasion, but on closer examination they are seen to lie above skin surface with no tendency toward invasion.

impossible to differentiate a keratoacanthoma from a well-differentiated squamous cell carcinoma.

D. *Benign keratosis*, type uncertain, consists of a benign proliferation of epidermal cells, generally acanthotic in form, which does not fit into any known classification.

PRECANCEROUS TUMORS OF THE SURFACE EPITHELIUM

I. Leukoplakia. Leukoplakia is a clinical term that describes a white plaque and gives no information as to underlying cause or prognosis; the term should not be used in histopathology.

II. Xeroderma pigmentosum—see section Congenital Abnormalities above.

III. Radiation dermatosis
   A. The chronic effects of radiation-induced dermatosis include atrophy of epidermis, dermal appendages and noncapillary blood vessels; dilatation or telangiectasis of capillaries; and frequently hyperpigmentation.
   B. Squamous cell carcinoma (most common), basal cell carcinoma or mesenchymal sarcomas such as fibrosarcoma may develop years following skin irradiations, e.g., following radiation for retinoblastoma.

IV. Actinic keratosis (senile keratosis, solar keratosis) occurs generally as multiple lesions on areas of skin exposed to sun (Figs. 6–41 and 6–48).
   A. Fair-skinned people are prone to develop multiple cutaneous neoplasms including solar keratosis and basal and squamous cell carcinomas.
   B. The lesions may be flat and scaly, papillomatous or projecting as a horn, i.e., a cutaneous horn.

   A *cutaneous horn* is a descriptive, clinical term. It has many causes. Solar keratosis frequently presents clinically as a cutaneous horn but so may verruca vulgaris, seborrheic keratosis, inverted follicular keratosis, squamous cell carcinoma (uncommonly) and even sebaceous gland carcinoma (rarely).

   C. Histologically, solar keratosis is characterized by hyperkeratosis, usually parakeratosis, papillomatosis, acanthosis and both cellular atypia and

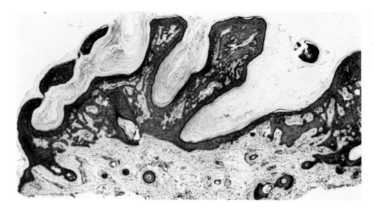

Fig. 6–42. Seborrheic keratosis. Papillomatous lesion above surface of skin shows proliferation of cells resembling normal basal cells, i. e., basaloid cells. H&E, ×16.

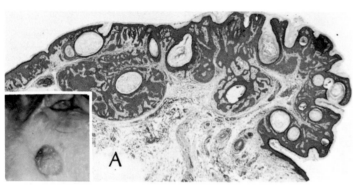

FIG. 6–43. Seborrheic keratosis. **A.** Papillomatous lesion removed from lower lid (**inset**) lies above surface of skin and contains cystic accumulations of horny (keratin) material. **B.** Higher magnification shows proliferated basaloid cells in dermis in narrow, interconnecting cords. **A,** H&E, ×6; **inset,** clinical; **B,** H&E, ×40.

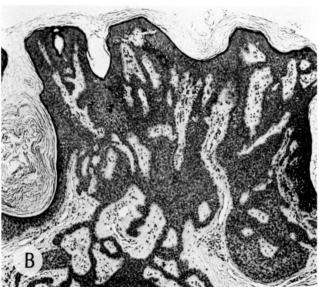

FIG. 6–44. Inverted follicular keratosis. Papillomatous lesion characterized by acanthosis, hyperkeratosis and acantholytic squamous cells surrounding squamous eddies, as shown (*arrows*) in higher magnification in *inset* (see Figure 6–6). **Main figure,** H&E, ×10; **inset,** H&E, ×100.

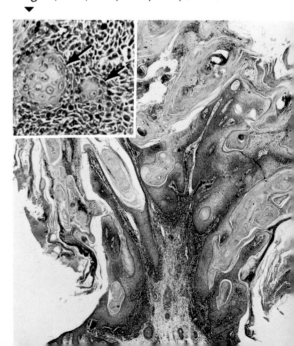

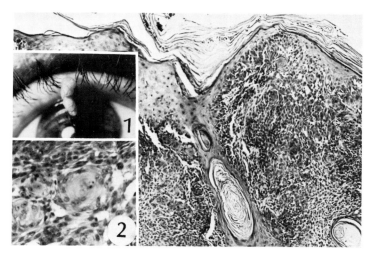

FIG. 6–45. Inverted follicular keratosis. **Inset 1** shows clinical appearance. **Main figure** shows acanthosis, hyperkeratosis and acantholytic squamous cells surrounding squamous eddies, as seen in higher magnification in **inset 2** (see Figure 6–6). **Main figure,** H&E, ×40; **inset 1,** clinical; **inset 2,** H&E, ×101.

mitotic figures in the deeper epidermal layers. The underlying dermis generally shows an inflammatory reaction mainly of lymphocytes and some plasma cells.

Solar keratosis may resemble squamous cell carcinoma or Bowen's disease. It differs from the former in not being invasive and from the latter in not showing total replacement (loss of polarity) of the epidermis by atypical cells. Squamous cell carcinoma infrequently and basal cell carcinoma rarely may arise from solar keratosis.

CANCEROUS TUMORS OF THE SURFACE EPITHELIUM

I. Basal cell carcinoma (Figs. 6–41 and 6–49 through 6–52)

   A. Basal cell carcinoma is by far the most common malignant tumor of the eyelids, occurring most frequently on the lower eyelid, followed by the inner canthus and then the upper eyelid.

   B. The clinical appearance has a great variability, but most present as a painless, indurated, firm, pearly nodule with fine telangiectasia. Ulceration may or may not occur.

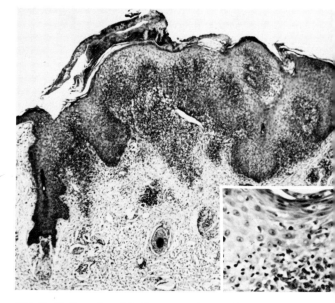

FIG. 6–46. Pseudoepitheliomatous hyperplasia is an inflammatory lesion showing acanthosis, hyperkeratosis and inflammation. Inflammation is present in dermis and in epidermis, as shown in higher magnification in **inset. Main figure,** H&E, ×21; **inset,** H&E, ×101.

   C. These tumors tend to be only locally invasive and almost never metastasize.

   D. Histologically and clinically the tumor has considerable variation, but it can be grouped into two types:

      1. The nodular ("garden variety") type occurs most commonly:

         a. Small, moderate or large-sized groups or nests of cells resembling basal cells show *peripheral palisading.*

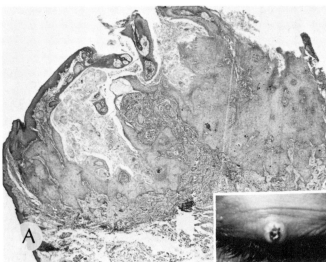

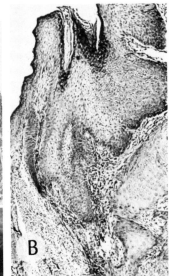

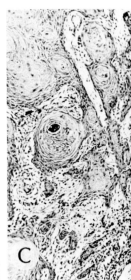

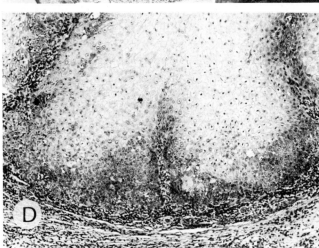

FIG. 6–47. Keratoacanthoma. **A.** Lesion has cup-shaped configuration with central keratin core and involves lid margin (skin surface to left and conjunctival surface to right). **Inset** shows clinical appearance of keratoacanthoma; note elevated lesion with umbilicated center filled with keratin debris. **B** is higher magnification of skin side and **C** is higher magnification of conjunctival side to show acanthotic cells and underlying chronic inflammation of dermis. **D.** Base of another lesion is typically "blunted." **A,** H&E, ×8; **inset,** clinical; **B,** H&E, ×40; **C,** H&E, ×40; **D,** H&E, ×40.

b. Cells within the nests may be pleomorphic and atypical and may contain mitotic figures.

c. In some planes of section the abnormal cells show continuity with the basal layer of epithelium.

d. The neoplasm may show surface ulceration, large areas of necrosis resulting in a cystic structure, areas of glandular formation and squamous or sebaceous differentiation.

Because basal cell carcinomas with areas of squamous differentiation, even if quite large, behave clinically as a basal cell carcinoma, not as a squamous cell carcinoma, there is no clinically useful reason to classify these tumors separately and to call them basal squamous (basalosquamous) cell carcinomas. Similarly, with mature sebaceous differentiation, there is no useful reason to call them sebaceous epithelioma. Some basal cell carcinomas may be heavily pigmented due to melanin deposition and closely simulate clinically malignant melanomas.

e. The surrounding and inter-

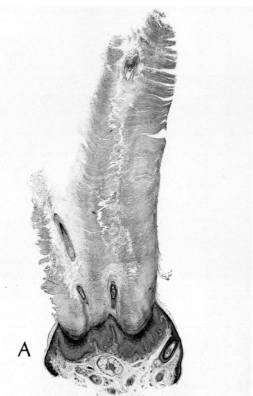

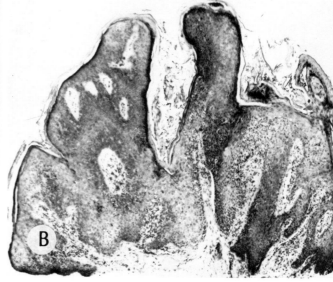

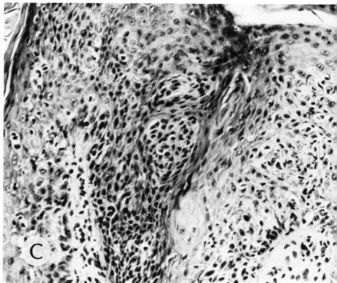

FIG. 6–48. Actinic keratosis. **A.** Papillomatosis, acanthosis and massive hyperkeratosis are present. **B.** Another lesion to show papillomatosis, acanthosis and hyperkeratosis. **C** is higher magnification of **B** to show increased cellularity with "worrisome" cells in deeper epidermal layers. There is no tendency to invade dermis, and surface cells appear quite benign. **A,** H&E, ×6; **B,** H&E, ×28; **C,** H&E, ×136.

vening invaded dermis undergoes a characteristic pseudosarcomatous (resembling a sarcoma) change called *desmoplasia,* i.e., the fibroblasts become large, numerous and often bizarre, and the mesenchymal tissue becomes loose and "juicy" in appearance.

The stromal desmoplastic reaction is quite typical of the basal cell neo-

plasm and helps differentiate the tumor from the similarly appearing adenoid cystic carcinoma (see p. 551 in Chap. 14), which frequently has an amorphous, relatively acellular surrounding stroma.

2. The morphealike or fibrosing type:
   a. Rather than nests of cells with peripheral palisading, the neoplastic, basaloid cells grow in thin strands or cords, often only

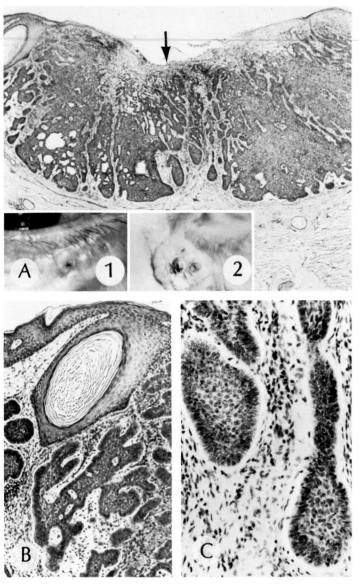

FIG. 6–49. Basal cell carcinoma. **A.** Small, moderate and large-sized nests of cells are originating from epidermis. The surface centrally (*arrow*) shows ulceration. **Insets 1** and **2** show two examples of basal cell carcinomas of lid with central ulceration and crusting. **B** and **C** are higher magnifications to show characteristic peripheral palisading around nests of atypical cells, which resemble epidermal basal cells. Note pseudosarcomatous change, i. e., desmoplasia, of supporting stroma. **A,** H&E, ×16; **inset 1,** clinical; **inset 2,** clinical; **B,** H&E, ×40; **C,** H&E, ×101.

FIG. 6–50. Basal cell carcinoma. **A.** Cystic type. **Inset** shows peripheral palisading. **B.** Pseudoglandular type. **Inset 1** shows structures resembling glands. **Inset 2** shows peripheral palisading. **C.** Basalosquamous type. **Insets 1** and **2** show clinical appearance of nonulcerating basal cell carcinomas of lid margin. **D** is higher magnification of **C** to show area of squamous differentiation (*arrow*) within nest of basal cell carcinoma cells. **A,** H&E, ×16; **inset,** H&E, ×136; **B,** H&E, ×16; **inset 1,** H&E, ×69; **inset 2,** H&E, ×69; **C,** H&E, ×21; **inset 1,** clinical; **inset 2,** clinical; **D,** H&E, ×101.

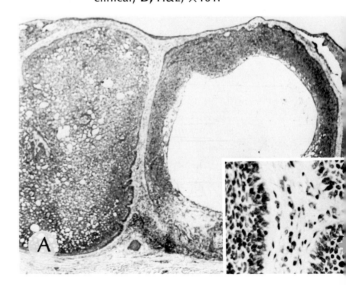

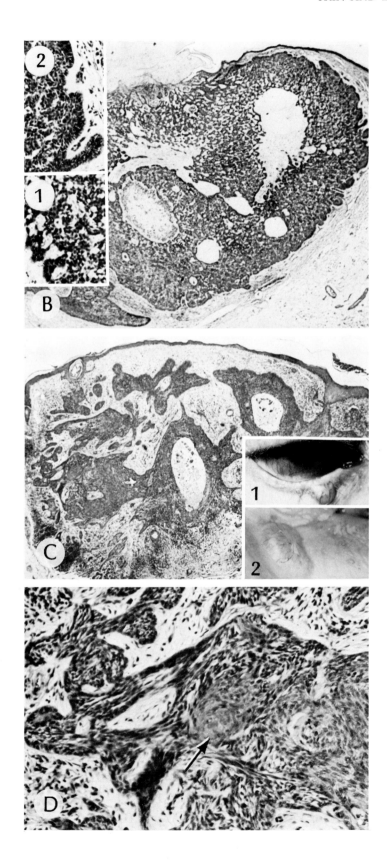

one cell layer in thickness, closely resembling metastatic scirrhous carcinoma of the breast ("indian file" pattern).
    b. The stroma, rather than being juicy and loose (desmoplastic), shows a considerable proliferation of connective tissue into a dense, thick, fibrous stroma.
    c. In this histologic variant it is difficult clinically to determine the limits of the lesion. The tumor tends to be much more aggressive and to invade much deeper into underlying tissue than does the nodular type.

The basal cell nevus syndrome consists of multiple basal cell carcinomas of the skin associated with defects in other tissues such as cysts of the jaw, bifid rib and abnormalities of the vertebrae. It is inherited as an autosomal dominant. Histologically the skin tumors are indistinguishable from the noninherited form of basal cell carcinoma.

II. Intraepidermal squamous cell carcinoma (squamous cell carcinoma in situ) (Fig. 6–53)
  A. Intraepidermal squamous cell carcinoma, the earliest form of squamous cell carcinoma, may arise from the precancerous keratoses (such as actinic keratosis) or may arise de novo.
  B. Histologically the lesion resembles the precancerous keratoses except for more advanced changes.
    1. Marked cellular atypia, dyskeratosis and especially a loss of polarity of the epidermis are important features.
    2. Histologically one cannot distinguish between the clinicopathologic entity of Bowen's disease and intraepidermal squamous cell carcinoma unrelated to Bowen's disease. Bowen's disease is *not* a histopathologic diagnosis but rather a clinicopathologic one.
  C. *Bowen's disease* (intraepidermal squamous cell carcinoma, Bowen type)
    1. Bowen's disease is a clinicopath-

ologic entity that consists of a fairly indolent, solitary (or multiple), erythematous, sharply demarcated, scaly patch, which grows slowly and spreads in a superficial, centrifugal manner, forming irregular, serpiginous borders.

The lesions may remain relatively stationary for up to 30 years.

    2. Bowen's disease is associated with other skin tumors, both malignant and premalignant, in up to 50 percent of cases and with an internal cancer in up to 80 percent of cases.

Arsenic concentration in lesions of Bowen's disease is high and may be of causal significance.

    3. Rarely, Bowen's disease may invade the underlying dermis, and then it behaves like a squamous cell carcinoma.
  D. Histologically the lesion is characterized by a loss of polarity of the epidermis so that the normal epidermal cells are replaced by atypical, sometimes vacuolated or multinucleated, haphazardly arranged cells not infrequently showing dyskeratosis and mitotic figures that are often bizarre. The basal cell layer is intact and the underlying dermis is not invaded.
III. Squamous cell carcinoma (Figs. 6–41 and 6–54)
  A. Squamous cell carcinoma rarely involves the eyelid and is seen about 40 times less frequently than basal cell carcinoma of the lid.

The opposite situation exists in the conjunctiva (see p. 252 in Chap. 7), where squamous cell carcinoma is the most common epithelial malignancy, and basal cell carcinoma almost never occurs.

  B. Histology—see p. 252 in Chapter 7.

Adenoacanthoma may represent a "pseudoglandular" (tubular and alveolar formations within the tumor) form of squamous cell carcinoma, or it may be an independent neoplasm. It is a rare tumor. The prognosis is somewhat more favor-

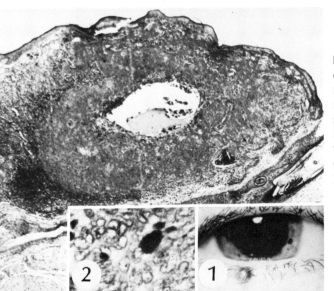

FIG. 6–51. Basal cell carcinoma presented clinically (**inset 1**) as smooth, pigmented mass of lower lid thought to be malignant melanoma. Section of basal cell carcinoma shows cystic center containing pigment. **Inset 2** shows pigment within cells. Pigment within cyst and cells had all histochemical characteristics of melanin. **Main figure,** H&E, ×28; **inset 1,** clinical; **inset 2,** H&E, ×252.

+ desmoplasia

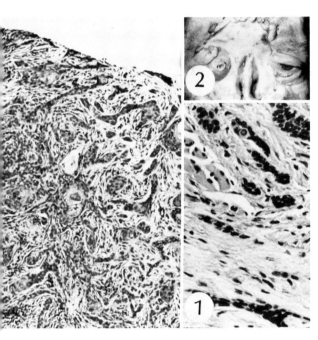

FIG. 6–52. Basal cell carcinoma. Morphea (fibrosing) type shows strands and cords of basaloid cells invading dermis. **Inset 1** is higher magnification to show cords of malignant cells in ''indian file'' pattern between dense, thick fibrous stroma, resembling scirrhous carcinoma of breast. **Inset 2** shows morphealike basal cell carcinoma, which started in the lids and has destroyed most of central face. **Main figure,** H&E, ×54; **inset 1,** H&E, ×136; **inset 2,** clinical.

proliferative fibrosis

FIG. 6–53. Intraepidermal squamous cell carcinoma. Hyperkeratosis, marked cellular atypia in epidermis and loss of polarity are prominent. The neoplastic squamous cells do not invade the underlying dermis. H&E, ×40.

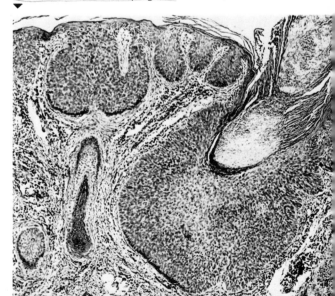

able than the usual squamous cell carcinoma. *Clear cell acanthoma* (Degos' acanthoma) is a benign, solitary, well-circumscribed, noninvasive neoplasm. Histologically there is a proliferation of glycogen-rich, clear, large epidermal cells.

TUMORS OF THE EPIDERMAL APPENDAGES
(Adnexal Skin Structures)

I. Tumors of, or resembling, sebaceous glands
  A. Congenital sebaceous gland hyperplasia (nevus sebaceous of Jadassohn, congenital sebaceous gland hamartoma)
    1. Congenital sebaceous gland hyperplasia consists of a single, hairless plaque, generally on the face or scalp, which usually reaches its full size at puberty.
    2. It seems to be caused by a developmental error, which results in a localized hyperplasia of sebaceous glands frequently associated with numerous imperfectly developed hair follicles and occasionally apocrine glands. The tumor can be considered hamartomatous.
    3. Histologically a group or groups of mature sebaceous gland lobules with or without hair follicles and frequently with underlying apocrine glands are present just under the epidermis, which generally shows papillomatosis.

    Basal cell carcinoma may develop in up to 20 percent of the lesions, and much more rarely other tumors may develop (e.g., syringocystadenoma papilliferum and sebaceous carcinoma).

  B. Acquired sebaceous gland hyperplasia (senile sebaceous gland hyperplasia, senile sebaceous nevi, adenomatoid sebaceous gland hyperplasia) (Fig. 6–55)
    1. Acquired sebaceous gland hyperplasia consists of one or more small, elevated, soft, yellowish, slightly umbilicated nodules occurring on the face (especially the forehead) in the elderly.

also seen in acne rosacea

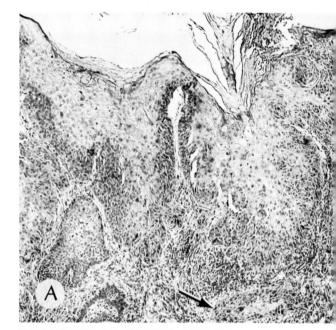

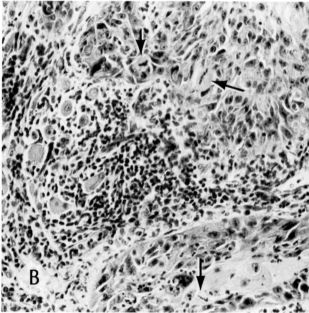

FIG. 6–54. Squamous cell carcinoma. **A.** Epidermis shows hyperkeratosis, acanthosis, marked cellular atypia and invasion (*arrow*) of underlying dermis. **B.** Higher magnification to show atypical squamous cells invading dermis. Mitotic figures (*arrows*) are prominent. **A,** H&E, ×40; **B,** H&E, ×136.

FIG. 6–55. Acquired sebaceous gland hyperplasia. **A.** Sebaceous gland greatly enlarged and grouped around large, central sebaceous duct. **B.** Higher magnification to compare hyperplastic sebaceous cells (*arrow*) to adjacent normal sebaceous gland cells (*N*). **A,** H&E, ×54; **B,** H&E, ×69.

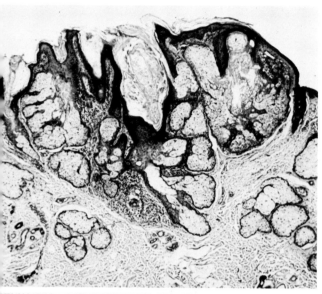

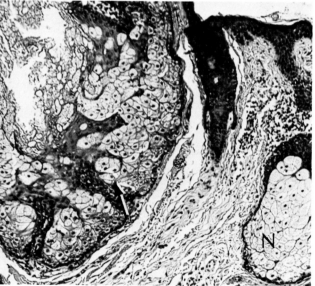

2. Histologically there is a greatly enlarged sebaceous gland composed of numerous lobules grouped around a central, large sebaceous duct.

Sebaceous gland hyperplasia may follow chronic dermatitis, especially acne rosacea and rhinophyma (see p. 187 in this chapter).

C. Adenoma sebaceum of Pringle (angiofibromas of face) (Fig. 6–56)
  1. The small, reddish, smooth papules seen on the nasolabial folds, on the cheeks and on the chin in people with *tuberous sclerosis* (see p. 36 in Chap. 2) have been called adenoma sebaceum (Pringle) but are truly angiofibromas.
  2. Histologically the sebaceous glands generally are atrophic, and in the smaller lesions dilated capillaries and fibrosis are seen, whereas in the larger lesions, capillary dilatation is minimal or absent and markedly sclerotic collagen is arranged in thick concentric layers around atrophic hair follicles.
D. Sebaceous adenoma (Fig. 6–57)
  1. Although rare, sebaceous adenoma has a predilection for the eyebrow and eyelid and appears as a single, firm, yellowish nodule.
  2. Histologically the irregularly shaped lobules are composed of three types of cells:
     a. Generative or undifferentiated cells identical in appearance to the cells present at the periphery of normal sebaceous glands—these cells are increased in number and allow the diagnosis to be made.
     b. Mature sebaceous cells.
     c. Transitional cells between the above two types.
E. Sebaceous gland carcinoma (Figs. 6–58 through 6–60)
  1. Sebaceous gland carcinoma generally arises from the meibomian glands but may arise from the glands of Zeis, or from both.
  2. Clinically, most of the time

sebaceous gland carcinoma is mistaken for a chalazion, but it may present as a diffuse blepharitis or a cutaneous horn.

Any recurrent chalazion should be submitted for histologic study, and any chronic, recalcitrant, atypical blepharitis should be biopsied.

3. Histologically the tumor resembles sebaceous adenoma but tends to be more bizarre and to show distinct invasiveness.
   a. Fat stains of frozen sections of fixed tissue show that many of the cells are lipid-positive.
   b. The malignant epithelial cells may invade the epidermis producing an overlying change that resembles Paget's disease and is called *pagetoid change.*

   Pagetoid change of the epidermis resembles intraepidermal squamous cell carcinoma. In the former, however, the intervening epidermal cells are benign, whereas in the latter all the cells are malignant.

II. Tumors of, or resembling, hair follicles
   A. Trichoepithelioma (epithelioma adenoides cysticum, benign cystic epithelioma) (Fig. 6–61)
      1. The tumor may occur as a single nodule, as a few isolated nodules or

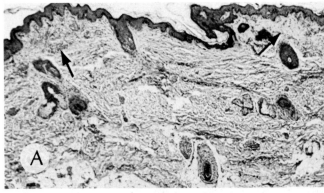
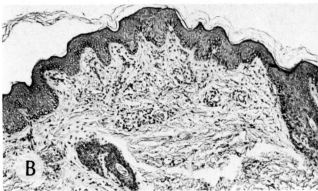

FIG. 6–56. Adenoma sebaceum of Pringle. **A.** Capillary dilatation (*arrows*) and fibrosis prominent in typical facial lesion removed from patient with tuberous sclerosis. **B.** Higher magnification of area near arrow on left to show capillary dilatation and fibrosis. **A,** H&E, ×21; **B,** H&E, ×192.

FIG. 6–57. Sebaceous adenoma. Irregular lobules composed (see **inset**) of mature sebaceous cells, undifferentiated (generative) cells and transitions between two. **Main figure,** H&E, ×16; **inset,** H&E, ×101.

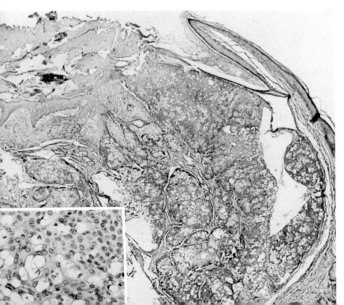

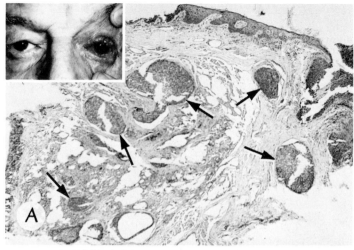

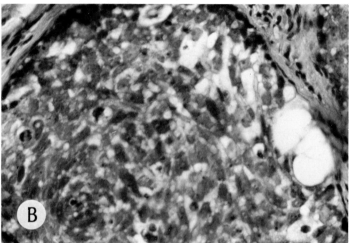

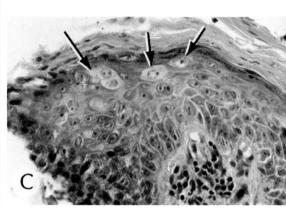

FIG. 6–58. Sebaceous gland carcinoma. **A.** Patient shown in **inset** had been treated for chronic blepharitis. Biopsy of lids shows sebaceous gland carcinoma (*arrows*) arising from meibomian and Zeis glands. **B.** Higher magnification shows poorly differentiated, atypical cells showing tendency to form sebaceous cells. **C.** Surface epidermis is invaded by sebaceous gland carcinoma cells (*arrows*) simulating Paget's disease, i.e., pagetoid change. **A,** H&E, ×32; **inset,** clinical; **B,** H&E, ×400; **C,** H&E, ×275.

as multiple symmetrical nodules with its onset at puberty. It occurs predominantly on the face and is inherited as an autosomal dominant (*Brooke's tumor*).

2. The isolated nodule (or the nodules of Brooke's tumor) is small, rosy yellow or flesh colored and tends to grow to several millimeters or occasionally to a centimeter or more.

3. Histologically, multiple squamous cell cysts, i.e., *horn cysts*, consisting of a completely keratinized center surrounded by basaloid cells, are the characteristic finding and represent immature hair structures.

a. Cells indistinguishable from the cells that constitute basal cell carcinoma (basaloid cells) are present around the horn cysts and in the surrounding tissue as a lacework network or as solid islands.

b. Occasionally the cysts have openings to the surface and resemble abortive hair follicles.

c. The cysts may rupture and induce a granulomatous, foreign body giant cell reaction, or they may become calcified.

The horn cyst shows complete and abrupt keratinization thereby dis-

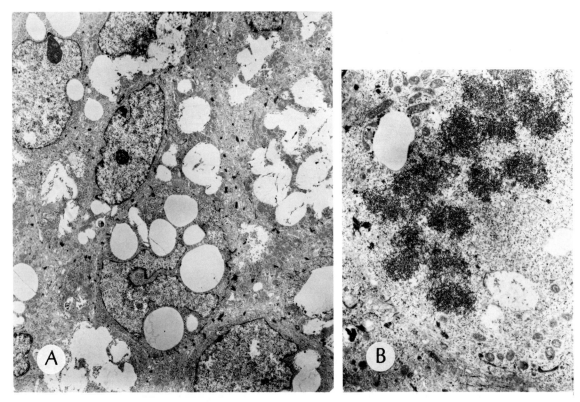

FIG. 6–59. Sebaceous gland carcinoma. **A.** Electron micrograph shows vacuolated cells; presumably vacuoles represent areas where lipid had been. **B.** Large dark areas represent clumped chromatin in cell undergoing mitosis. **A,** ×4500; **B,** ×8500.

FIG. 6–60. ▶

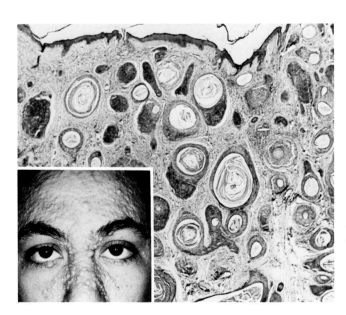

FIG. 6–61. Trichoepithelioma. Patient with Brooke's tumor, i.e., multiple facial tricho-epitheliomas inherited as autosomal dominant, is shown in **inset.** Multiple squamous cell cysts, i.e., horn cyst, repre-senting immature hair structures are present in dermis. **Main figure,** H&E, ×16; **inset,** clinical.

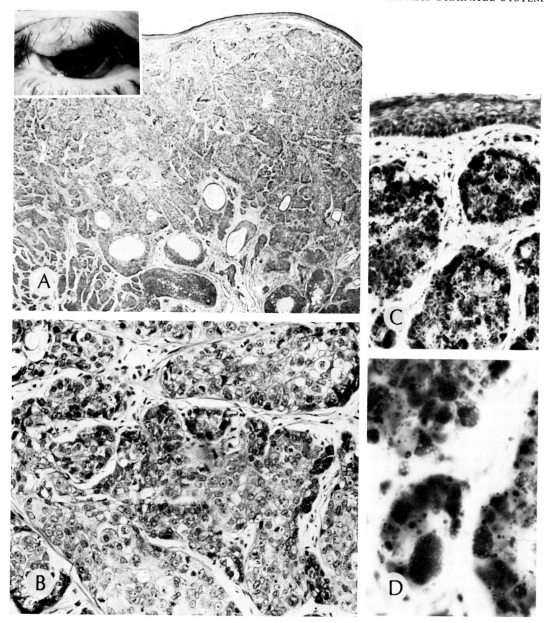

FIG. 6–60. Sebaceous gland carcinoma. **A.** Patient shown in **inset** had lesion of upper lid resembling chalazion. Excisional biopsy shows nests of atypical cells forming gland-like spaces. **B.** Higher magnification shows nests of atypical, large, undifferentiated cells showing tendency to form sebaceous cells. **C.** Fat stain shows mark positivity within cytoplasm of abnormal cells. **D.** Higher magnification to show cytoplasmic positive fat staining. **A,** H&E, ×16; **inset,** clinical; **B,** H&E, ×101; **C,** oil red-O, ×136; **D,** oil red-O, ×340.

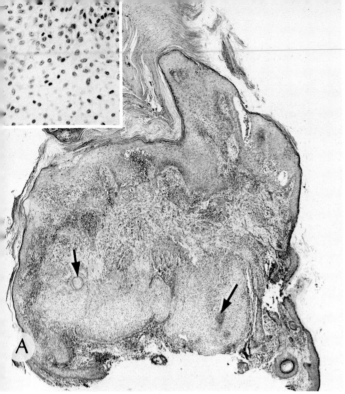

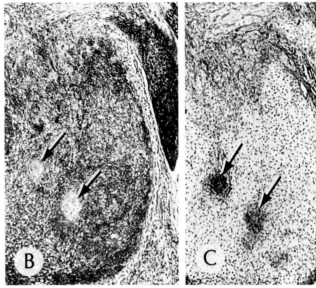

FIG. 6–62. Trichilemmoma. **A.** Lobular acanthosis composed of clear cells is oriented around hair follicles (*arrows*). Overlying epidermis shows acanthosis and marked hyperkeratosis. **Inset** is higher magnification of clear cells as shown in H&E stain. **B.** Periodic acid—Schiff (PAS) stains cytoplasm of "clear" cells. **C.** Pretreatment of sections with diastase eliminates PAS staining. PAS-positive diastase-labile cytoplasmic material is glycogen. Note clear cells oriented around follicles (*arrows* in **B** and **C** show follicles through edge). Also note similarity to clear cell hidradenoma (Figure 6–67). **A,** H&E, ×6; **inset,** H&E, ×101; **B,** PAS, ×40; **C,** diastase-PAS, ×40.

FIG. 6–63. Pilomatrixoma. **A.** Low power shows large areas of necrosis (*N*) containing shadow cells and basophilic cells. Areas of calcification (*arrow*) are present. **B.** Higher magnification (near *N* in **A**) of dark basophilic cells and pale shadow cells. **A,** H&E, ×3; **B,** H&E, ×101.

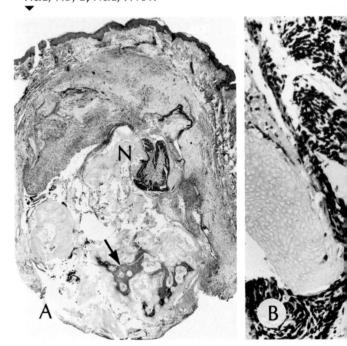

tinguishing it from the *horn pearl* of the squamous cell carcinoma, which shows incomplete and gradual keratinization.

B. Trichofolliculoma
1. Trichofolliculoma consists of a small, solitary lesion frequently with a central pore and is found in adults.
2. Histologically a large cystic space lined by squamous epithelium and containing keratin and hair shaft fragments is seen in the dermis surrounded by smaller, well-differentiated, "secondary" hair follicles.

C. Trichilemmoma (Fig. 6–62)
1. Trichilemmomas tend to be solitary, asymptomatic lesions located on the face and found mainly in middle-aged men.
2. Histologically, lobular acanthosis of glycogen-rich cells is oriented about hair follicles. The edge of the lesion usually shows a palisade of columnar cells that resemble the outer root sheath of a hair follicle and rest on a well-formed basement membrane.

D. Calcifying epithelioma of Malherbe (*pilomatrixoma*) (Fig. 6–63)
1. Calcifying epithelioma of Malherbe can occur at any age and presents as a solitary tumor, firm and deep-seated and covered by normal skin. The tumor seems to originate from hair root matrix.
2. Histologically the tumor is sharply demarcated and composed of two types of cells, basophilic and shadow cells.
   a. Basophilic cells closely resemble the basaloid cells of a basal cell carcinoma.
   b. Shadow cells stain faintly, have distinct cell borders and show no nuclei but rather show central, unstained "shadows" where the nuclei should be.

Older tumors may show complete disappearance of the basophilic cells so that only shadow cells remain.

c. Areas of keratinization and calcification frequently occur.

E. Adnexal carcinoma (Fig. 6–64)
The term adnexal carcinoma should be restricted to those tumors that histologically are identical to basal cell carcinoma but in which the site of origin (e.g., epidermis, hair follicle, sweat gland, sebaceous gland) cannot be determined.

III. Tumors of, or resembling, sweat glands

Apocrine sweat glands are represented in the eyelids by the glands of Moll; eccrine sweat glands are present in the lids both at the lid margin and in the dermis over the surface of the eyelid.

A. Syringoma (Fig. 6–65)
1. Syringoma represents an adenoma of eccrine sweat structure that occurs mainly in young women and consists of small soft papules, usually only 1 or 2 mm, found predominantly on the eyelids.
2. Histologically, dermal epithelial strands of small basophilic cells and cystic ducts lined by a double-layered epithelium and containing a colloidal material are characteristic. The ducts often have comma-like tails, appearing like tadpoles.

B. Syringocystadenoma papilliferum (papillary syringadenoma) (Fig. 6–66)
1. Syringocystadenoma papilliferum represents an adenoma of apocrine sweat structures, which differentiates toward apocrine ducts.
2. Generally the lesion is solitary and occurs in the scalp as a hairless, smooth plaque until puberty, after which it becomes raised, nodular and verrucous.
3. Histologically there is papillomatosis of the epidermis; one or more cystic invaginations (frequently forming villus-like projections) extending into the dermis and lined by a double layer of cells consisting of luminal high columnar cells and outer myoepithelial cells; and deep, dermal apocrine gland structures.

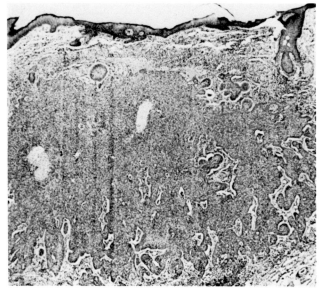

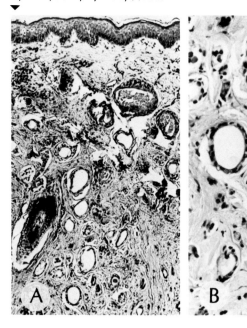

FIG. 6–64. Adnexal carcinoma. Neoplasm in dermis is identical to basal cell carcinoma except serial sections failed to reveal any connection to overlying epidermis. H&E, ×21.

FIG. 6–65. Syringoma. A. Proliferated eccrine sweat structures form dermal epithelial strands and cystic spaces. B. Higher magnification shows epithelial strands and cystic spaces lined by double-layered epithelium; some cystic spaces contain colloidal material. A, H&E, ×54; B, H&E, ×136.

FIG. 6–66. Syringocystadenoma papilliferum. A. There is papillomatosis of epidermis and multiple cystic invaginations in dermis. B. Cystic structures lined by double layer of cells, showing areas of proliferation (arrow). A, H&E, ×16; B, H&E, ×101.

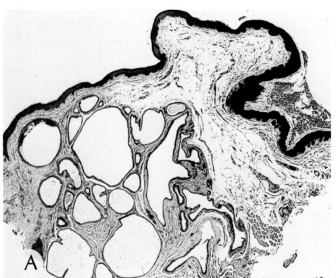

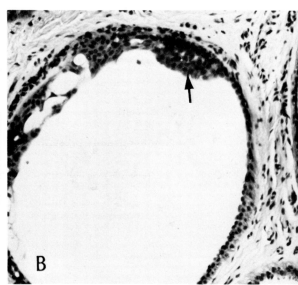

Frequently a heavy plasma cell inflammatory infiltrate is present. Also quite often congenital abnormalities of sebaceous glands and hair follicles are present. One-third of the cases are associated with congenital sebaceous hyperplasia, and in one-tenth of cases a basal cell carcinoma develops. A similar tumor, *hidradenoma papilliferum,* occurs only in women on the labia majora or in the perineal or perianal region. Like syringocystadenoma papilliferum it represents an adenoma of apocrine sweat glands, but it differentiates toward apocrine glands rather than ducts.

C. Eccrine spiradenoma (nodular hidradenoma, clear cell hidradenoma, clear cell carcinoma, clear cell myoepithelioma, myoepithelioma)

1. Eccrine spiradenomas generally occur as deep, solitary, dermal nodules, which occasionally are painful and arise from eccrine structures.
2. Histologically the tumor is composed of one or more lobules arranged in intertwining bands and tubules containing two types of cells and surrounded by a connective tissue capsule.
   a. Small dark cells with dark nuclei and scant cytoplasm are present toward the periphery of the bands and tubules.

   These undifferentiated basal cells were previously incorrectly thought to be myoepithelial cells.

   b. Cells with large pale nuclei and scant cytoplasm are present in the center of the bands and tubules and line the few small lumina usually present.

   A possible variant of the eccrine spiradenoma is a tumor composed primarily of cells with clear cytoplasm called a *clear cell hidradenoma* (Fig. 6–67) (eccrine acrospiroma, clear cell myoepithelioma, clear cell papillary carcinoma, porosyringoma, nodular hidradenoma).

It is more likely, however, that the tumor is of apocrine gland origin. The clear cytoplasm of the component cells usually contains diastase-sensitive, PAS-positive material (glycogen). It may, however, sometimes contain diastase-resistant, PAS-positive material, thereby helping to differentiate these cells from clear cells in squamous cell carcinoma, which contain diastase-sensitive, PAS-positive material (glycogen) in the cytoplasm and from the large, foamy cells of sebaceous gland carcinoma, which are PAS-negative but lipid-positive (positive fat stains on frozen sections of "wet" fixed tissue). A more probable variant is the eccrine hidrocystoma (Fig. 6–68), which consists of a dilated sweat duct lined by two rows of flattened epithelium and sometimes containing papillary projections into the lumen of the cysts. A further variant of the clear cell hydradenoma is the *apocrine mixed tumor.* The histology is the same as the lacrimal gland mixed tumor (see p. 549 in Chap. 14).

D. *Eccrine mixed tumor* is rarer than the apocrine mixed tumor and is histologically similar—eccrine mixed tumor has tubular lumina lined by a single layer of flat epithelial cells, whereas the tubular lumina of apocrine mixed tumors are larger, more irregularly shaped and lined by at least a double layer of epithelial cells (see p. 549 in Chap. 14).
E. Cylindroma (turban tumor)
1. Cylindroma probably is of apocrine origin, is almost always benign, frequently has an autosomal dominant inheritance pattern and has a predilection for the scalp.

   Cylindromas and trichoepitheliomas frequently are associated together.

2. Histologically, islands of two types of cells, irregular in size and shape, are separated from each other by an amorphous, hyalinelike stroma.
   a. Cells with small, dark nuclei and

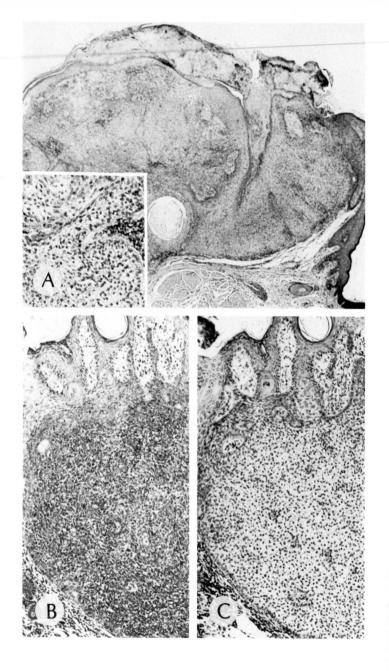

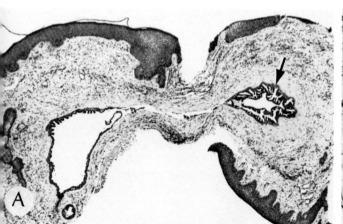

FIG. 6–67. Clear cell hidradenoma. A. Intertwining bands of lobules are composed (**inset**) primarily of large clear cells. B. Periodic acid-Schiff (PAS) stains cytoplasm of "clear" cells. C. Pretreatment of sections with diastase eliminates PAS staining. PAS-positive diastase-labile cytoplasmic material is glycogen. Note similarity to trichilemmoma (Figure 6–62). **A,** H&E, ×16; **inset,** H&E, ×69; **B,** PAS, ×54; **C,** diastase-PAS, ×54.

FIG. 6–68. Eccrine hidrocystoma. **A.** Probable variant of clear cell hidradenoma consists of dilated sweat ducts lined by two rows of flattened epithelium, which have undergone papillary proliferation (*arrow*). **B.** Higher magnification of area near *arrow*. **A,** H&E, ×21; **B,** H&E, ×101.

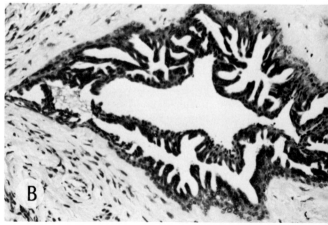

scant cytoplasm are found in the periphery of the island.

   b. Cells with large, pale nuclei and scant cytoplasm are present in the center of the island and also line tubular lumina, which usually are present.

F. *Eccrine poroma* generally occurs on the soles of the feet but may occur elsewhere and consists of intraepidermal masses of cells that thicken the epidermis and extend down into the dermal area.

   1. The cells are connected by intercellular bridges, resemble squamous cells, but are smaller.

   2. Small ductal lumina usually are present and are lined by a PAS-positive, diastase-resistant cuticle.

G. Sweat gland carcinomas are rare.

   1. Eccrine sweat gland carcinomas have a tubular structure.

   2. Apocrine sweat gland carcinoma (from glands of Moll in the eyelid) are adenocarcinomas.

PIGMENTED TUMORS

See Chapter 17.

MESENCHYMAL TUMORS OF THE EYELID

The same mesenchymal tumors that may occur in the orbit also may occur in the eyelid and are histopathologically identical (see subsection Mesenchymal Tumors in Chap. 14).

LACRIMAL DRAINAGE SYSTEM

CONGENITAL ABNORMALITIES

ATRESIA OF THE NASOLACRIMAL DUCT

  I. The nasolacrimal duct generally becomes completely canalized and opens into the nose by the eighth month of fetal life.

  II. The duct may fail to canalize (generally at its lower end) or may be clogged by epithelial debris.

 III. Most ducts not open at birth will open spontaneously during the first six months postpartum.

ATRESIA OF THE PUNCTUM

  I. Atresia of the punctum may occur alone or associated with atresia of the nasolacrimal duct.

  II. An acquired form may result secondarily to scarring from any cause.

The punctum may be absent or multiple, both as congenital anomalies.

CONGENITAL FISTULA OF LACRIMAL SAC (minimal facial fissure)

  I. An opening of the lacrimal sac directly into the nose (internal fistula) or out onto the cheek (external fistula and most common of the two) is a not uncommon finding.

  II. The opening, which may be unilateral or bilateral, usually is quite fine and may be overlooked.

There are many other anomalies of the lacrimal puncta, canaliculus, sac and nasolacrimal duct, but these are beyond the scope of this book.

INFLAMMATION—DACRYOCYSTITIS (Fig. 6–69)

See Chapters 3 and 4.

BLOCKAGE OF TEAR FLOW INTO THE NOSE

  I. Most inflammations and infections of the lacrimal sac are secondary to a blockage of tear flow at the level of the sac opening into the nasolacrimal duct or distal to that point.

  II. A cast of the lacrimal sac (Fig. 4–23) may be formed by a proliferation of the fungus *Streptothrix* (*Actinomyces*), which also can cause a secondary conjunctivitis.

TUMORS

EPITHELIAL (Figs. 6–70 through 6–72)

  I. The epithelial lining of the lacrimal sac is the same as that which lines the rest of the upper respiratory tract, i.e., pseudostratified columnar epithelium. Tumors, there-

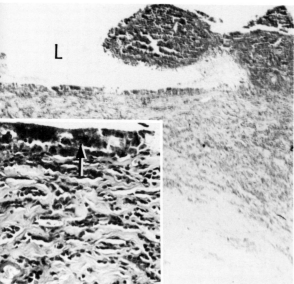

FIG. 6–69. Dacryocystitis. Lumen (*L*) and wall of lacrimal sac contain purulent exudate. Wall of sac lined by partially necrotic pseudocolumnar epithelium, shown (*arrow*) with higher magnification in **inset. Main figure,** PAS, ×28; **inset,** PAS, ×101.

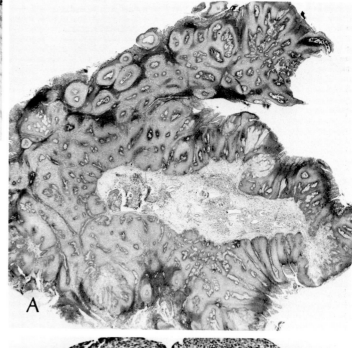

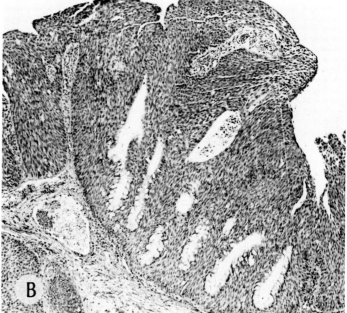

FIG. 6–70. Papillomas. **A.** Squamous cell papilloma showing epidermal papillomatosis and acanthosis. **B.** Transitional cell papilloma showing glandlike structures containing goblet cells within proliferated, thickened epithelium. **A,** H&E, ×10; **B,** H&E, ×70.

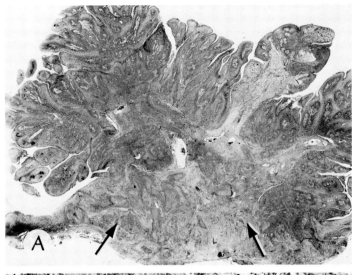

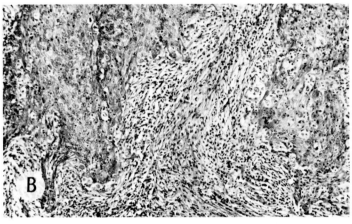

FIG. 6–71. Papillary squamous cell carcinoma. **A.** Frank invasion (between *arrows*) present at base. **B.** Higher magnification shows invasion of subepithelial tissue by nests of squamous cell carcinoma. **A,** H&E, ×6; **B,** H&E, ×90.

FIG. 6–72. Papillary transitional cell carcinoma. **A.** Papillary carcinoma protrudes into lumen (*L*) of lacrimal sac. **B.** Higher magnification shows papillary transitional cell carcinoma quite similar to type seen in urinary bladder. Note fibrovascular core in center of each papilla. **A,** H&E, ×19; **B,** H&E, ×100.

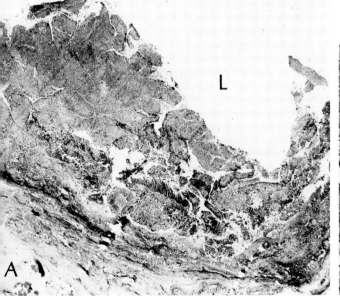

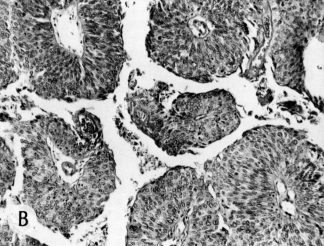

fore, are similar to those found elsewhere in the upper respiratory system, namely "papillomas," squamous cell carcinomas, transitional cell carcinomas and adeno-carcinomas.

II. Tumors are relatively rare and generally cause symptoms of epiphora early.

III. Histology

A. The papillomas may be squamous (see p. 252 in Chap. 7), transitional or may be a proliferation of benign, glandular tissue, i.e., adenoma.

Rarely, a lacrimal sac papilloma may undergo "onkocytic" metaplasia, i.e., an eosinophilic cystadenoma.

B. Squamous cell carcinomas are the most common carcinomas and are identical to those found elsewhere (see p. 257 in Chap. 7).

C. Transitional cell carcinomas are composed of transitional cell epithelium showing greater or lesser degrees of differentiation.

D. Adenocarcinomas are composed of malignant glandular elements.

MELANOTIC

Melanotic tumors arising from the lacrimal sac (i.e., malignant melanomas) are quite rare and are identical histologically to those found in the lid (see section Melanotic Tumors of Lids in Chap. 17).

MESENCHYMAL

The same mesenchymal tumors that may involve the lids and orbit may involve the lacrimal sac (see subsection Mesenchymal Tumors in Chap. 14).

BIBLIOGRAPHY

SKIN

Terminology

Graham JH, Johnson WC, Helwig EB (eds): Dermal Pathology. Hagerstown, Harper & Row, 1972

Lever WF: Histopathology of the Skin, 4th ed. Philadelphia, Lippincott, 1967

Congenital Abnormalities

Bellows RA, Lahav M, Lepreau FJ, Albert DM: Ocular manifestations of xeroderma pigmentosum in a black family. Arch Ophthalmol 92:113, 1974

Bronner MA, Buck P: L'agénésie bilatérale et symétrique des paupiéres supérieures. Bull Soc Ophtalmol Fr 61:689, 1961

Filipic M, Silva M: Phakomatous choristoma of the eyelid. Arch Ophthalmol 88:172, 1972

Gupta SP, Saxena RC: Cryptophthalmos. Br J Ophthalmol 46:629, 1962

Hadida E, Marill FG, Sayag J: Xeroderma pigmentosum. Ann Dermatol Syphiligr (Paris) 90:467, 1963

Katowitz JA, Yolles EA, Yanoff M: Ichthyosis congenita. Arch Ophthalmol 91:208, 1974

Orth DH, Fretzin DF, Abramson V: Collodion body with transient bilateral upper lid ectropion. Review of ocular manifestations in ichthyosis. Arch Ophthalmol 91:206, 1974

Otradovec J, Janovsky M: On cryptophthalmos (in Czechoslovakian). Cesk Oftalmol 18:128, 1962

Scheie HG, Albert DM: Distichiasis and trichiasis: Origin and management. Am J Ophthalmol 61:718, 1965

Wilson FM, Grayson M, Pieroni D: Corneal changes in ectodermal dysplasia. Case report, histopathology, and differential diagnosis. Am J Ophthalmol 75:17, 1973

Zimmerman LE: Phakomatous choristoma of the eyelid: a tumor of lenticular anlage. Am J Ophthalmol 71:169, 1971

Aging

Gillman T, Penn J, Brooks D, Roux M: Abnormal elastic fibers—appearance in cutaneous carcinoma, irradiation injuries, and arterial and other degenerative connective tissue lesions in man. Arch Pathol 59:733, 1955

Klintworth GK: Chronic actinic keratopathy—a condition associated with conjunctival elastosis (pingueculae) and typified by characteristic extracellular concretions. Am J Pathol 67:327, 1972

Lund HZ, Sommerville RL: Basophilic degeneration of the cutis: data substantiating its relation to prolonged solar exposure. Am J Clin Pathol 27:183, 1957

Stieglitz LN, Crawford JS: Blepharochalasis. Am J Ophthalmol 77:100, 1974

Inflammation

Jacobson JH: *Demodex follicularum*. Infestation of the eyelids. Trans Am Acad Ophthalmol Otolaryngol 75:1242, 1971

Ketel, WG van: Rosacea-like tuberculid of Lewandowsky. Dermatologica 116:201, 1958

Lever WF: Histopathology of the Skin, 4th ed. Philadelphia, Lippincott, 1967, pp. 365–389

Lutzner MA: Molluscum contagiosum, verruca and zoster viruses: electron microscopic studies in skin. Arch Dermatol 87:436, 1963

MacVicar DN, Graham JH: Pathodynamics of sub-epidermal bullous dermatoses: basement membrane studies. Am J Pathol 48:52, 1966

Michelson HE: Does the rosacea-like tuberculid exist? Arch Dermatol 78:681, 1958

Middelkamp JN, Munger BL: Ultrastructure and histogenesis of molluscum contagiosum. J Pediatr 64:888, 1964

Nauheim JS, Sussman W: Herpes simplex of the eyelids and adjacent areas. Trans Am Acad Ophthalmol Otolaryngol 75:1236, 1971

Norm MS: The follicle mite (Demodex folliculorum). Eye Ear Nose Throat Mon 51:187, 1972

Pinkus H, Mehregan AH: The primary histologic lesion of seborrheic dermatitis and psoriasis. J Invest Dermatol 46:109, 1966

Prose PH, Sedlis E: Morphologic and histochemical studies of atopic eczema in infants and children. J Invest Dermatol 34:149, 1960

Thygeson P: Complications of staphylococcic blepharitis. Am J Ophthalmol 68:446, 1969

Lid Manifestations of Systemic Dermatoses or Disease

Davies G, Dymock I, Harry J, Williams R: Deposition of melanin and iron in ocular structures in haemochromatosis. Br J Ophthalmol 36:338, 1972

Farkas TG, Sylvester V, Archer D: The choroidopathy of progressive systemic sclerosis (scleroderma). Am J Ophthalmol 74:875, 1972

Flax MH, Caulfield JB: Cellular and vascular components of allergic contact dermatitis. Am J Pathol 43:1031, 1963

Frayer WC: The histopathology of perilimbal ulceration in Wegener's granulomatosis. Arch Ophthalmol 64:58, 1960

Frayer WC, Wise RT, Tsaltas TT: Ocular and adnexal changes associated with relapsing febrile non-suppurative panniculitis (Weber-Christian disease). Trans Am Ophthalmol Soc 66:233, 1968

Freedman J: Ocular pathology associated with the Weber Christian syndrome. Br J Ophthalmol 56:896, 1972

Gold DH, Morris DA, Henkind P: Ocular findings in systemic lupus erythematosus. Br J Ophthalmol 56:800, 1972

Green WR, Friedman-Kien A, Banfield WG: Angioid streaks in Ehlers-Danlos syndrome. Arch Ophthalmol 76:197, 1966

Harrison SM, Frenkel M, Grossman BJ, Matalon R: Retinopathy in childhood dermatomyositis. Am J Ophthalmol 76:786, 1973

Helwig EB: Diseases of elastic tissue, in Dermal Pathology. Edited by JH Graham, WC Johnson, EB Helwig. Hagerstown, Harper & Row, 1972, pp 741–756

Helwig EB: Disorders of connective tissue and mucinoses, in Dermal Pathology. Edited by JH Graham, WC Johnson, EB Helwig. Hagerstown, Harper & Row, 1972, pp 757–790

Howard RD, Klaus SN, Savin RC, Fenton R: Malignant atrophic papulosis (Degos' syndrome). Arch Ophthalmol 79:262, 1968

Jensen AD, Khodadoust AA, Emery JM: Lipoid proteinosis. Arch Ophthalmol 88:273, 1972

Katowitz JA, Yolles EA, Yanoff M: Cutis laxa (in preparation)

Lever WF: Histopathology of the Skin. Philadelphia, Lippincott, 1967, pp. 164–187, 451–481

Lichtenstein JR, Martin GR, Kohn LD, Byers PH, McKusick V: Defect in conversion of procollagen to collagen in a form of Ehlers-Danlos syndrome. Science 182:298, 1973

McKusick VA: Heritable Disorders of Connective Tissue, 4th ed. St. Louis, Mosby, 1972

Ostler HB, Conant MA, Groundwater J: Lyell's disease, the Stevens-Johnson syndrome and exfoliative dermatitis. Trans Am Acad Ophthalmol Otolaryngol 74:1254, 1970

Rohmer F, Kurtz D, Malleville J, Batzenschlager A, Held N, Paul C: Neurologic complication in Degos' disease (in French). Rev Neurol (Paris) 124:531, 1971

Roth AM, Foos RY: Ocular pathologic changes in primary hemochromatosis. Arch Ophthalmol 87:507, 1972

Verhoeff FH: Histologic findings in a case of angioid streaks. Br J Ophthalmol 32:531, 1948

Cysts, Pseudoneoplasms and Neoplasms

Aurora AL, Blodi FC: Lesions of the eyelids: a clinicopathological study. Survey Ophthalmol 15:94, 1970

Aurora AL, Blodi FC: Reappraisal of basal cell carcinoma of the eyelids. Am J Ophthalmol 70:329, 1970

Boniuk M, Halpert B: Clear cell hidradenoma or myoepithelioma of the eyelid. Arch Ophthalmol 72:59, 1964

Boniuk M, Zimmerman LE: Eyelid tumors with reference to lesions confused with squamous cell carcinoma. II. Inverted follicular keratosis. Arch Ophthalmol 69:698, 1963

Boniuk M, Zimmerman LE: Eyelid tumors with reference to lesions confused with squamous cell carcinoma. III. Keratoacanthoma. Arch Ophthalmol 77:29, 1967

Boniuk M, Zimmerman LE: Sebaceous gland carcinoma of the eyelid, eyebrow, caruncle, and orbit. Trans Am Acad Ophthalmol Otolaryngol 72:619, 1968

Brownstein MH, Fernando S, Shapiro L: Clear cell adenoma: clinicopathologic analysis of 37 new cases. Am J Clin Pathol 59:306, 1973

Brownstein MH, Shapiro L: Trichilemmoma: analysis of 40 new cases. Arch Dermatol 107:866, 1973

Einaugler RB, Henkind P: Basal cell epithelioma of the eyelid: apparent incomplete removal. Am J Ophthalmol 67:413, 1969

Feman SS, Apt L, Roth AM: The basal cell nevus syndrome. Am J Ophthalmol 78:222, 1974

Fisher ER, Horvat BL, Wechsler HL: Ultrastructural features of mycosis fungoides. Am J Clin Pathol 58:99, 1972

Forbis R Jr, Helwig EB: Pilomatrixoma (calcifying epithelioma). Arch Dermatol 83:608, 1961

Graham JH, Helwig EB: Bowen's disease and senile keratosis: relationship to arsenic, in Excerpta Medica Foundation International Congress Series No. 55, 1962 p 316

Graham JH, Johnson WC, Helwig EB (eds): Dermal Pathology. Hagerstown, Harper & Row, 1972

Hall TE, Tappan WM, Decker JW: Metastasis of basal cell carcinoma. Rocky M Med J 67:39, 1970

Haslam RHA, Wirtschafter JD: Unilateral external oculomotor nerve palsy and nevus sebaceous of Jadassohn. Arch Ophthalmol 87:293, 1972

Kierland RR: Cutaneous signs of internal cancer. CA 22:365, 1972

Kwitko ML, Boniuk M, Zimmerman LE: Eyelid tumors with reference to lesions confused with squamous cell carcinoma. I. Incidence and errors in diagnosis. Arch Ophthalmol 69:693, 1963

Lever WF: Histopathology of the Skin, 4th ed. Philadelphia, Lippincott, 1967

Markovits AS, Quickert MH: Basal cell nevus. Arch Ophthalmol 88:397, 1972

Mason JK, Helwig EB: Nevoid basal cell carcinoma syndrome. Arch Pathol 79:401, 1965

Nover A von, Korting GW: Zur Kenntnis des familiären Basalzellnaevus. Klin Monatsbl Augenheilkd 156:621, 1970

Payne JW, Duke JR, Butner R, Eifrig DE: Basal cell carcinoma of the eyelids. A long term follow-up study. Arch Ophthalmol 81:553, 1969

Rodrigues MM, Lubowitz RM, Shannon GM: Mucinous (adenocystic) carcinoma of the eyelid. Arch Ophthalmol 89:493, 1973

Scheie HG, Yanoff M, Frayer WC: Carcinoma of sebaceous glands of the eyelid. Arch Ophthalmol 72:800, 1964

Schuster SAD, Ferguson EC III, Marshall RB: Alveolar rhabdomyosarcoma of the eyelid. Arch Ophthalmol 87:646, 1972

Wolken SH, Spivey BE, Blodi FC: Hereditary adenoid cystic epithelioma. Am J Ophthalmol 68:26, 1969

LACRIMAL DRAINAGE SYSTEM

Congenital Abnormalities

Duke-Elder S: System of Ophthalmology, Vol III, Normal and Abnormal Development, Part 2, Congenital Deformities. St. Louis, Mosby, 1963, pp. 911–941

Grossman T, Putz R: Anatomy, consequences and treatment of congenital stenosis of lacrimal passage in newborn infants. Klin Monatsbl Augenheilkd 160:563, 1972

Tumors

Aurora AL: Oncocytic metaplasia in a lacrimal sac papilloma. Am J Ophthalmol 75:466, 1973

Gurney N, Chalkley T, O'Grady R: Lacrimal sac hemangiopericytoma. Am J Ophthalmol 71:757, 1971

Harry J, Ashton N: The pathology of tumors of the lacrimal sac. Trans Ophthalmol Soc UK 88:19, 1969

Ryan SJ, Font RL: Primary epithelial neoplasms of the lacrimal sac. Am J Ophthalmol 76:73, 1973

Sen DK, Mohan H: Neurilemmoma of the lacrimal sac. Eye Ear Nose Throat Mon 50:179, 1971

Conjunctiva

Cysts, Pseudoneoplasms and Neoplasms
   Choristomas
   Hamartomas
   Cysts
   Pseudocancerous Epithelial Lesions
   Potentially Precancerous Epithelial
     Lesions
   Cancerous Epithelial Lesions
   Pigmented Lesions of the Conjunctiva
   Stromal Neoplasms

CONGENITAL ANOMALIES

CRYPTOPHTHALMOS (ABLEPHARON)

See p. 182 in Chapter 6.

EPITARSUS

I. Epitarsus consists of a fold of conjunctiva that is attached to the palpebral surface of the lid or lids of one or both eyes.
II. The conjunctival fold has a free edge with both surfaces (front and back) covered by conjunctival epithelium.
III. Histologically, folded conjunctival tissue is seen. The tissue looks like normal conjunctiva except that occasionally islands of cartilage may be present within the folded tissue.

HEREDITARY HEMORRHAGIC TELANGIECTASIA (Rendu-Osler-Weber Disease)

I. The condition, characterized by multiple telangiectases in the skin and mucous membranes (including conjunctiva), has an autosomal dominant inheritance pattern. Occasionally, similar telangiectases can be observed in the retina.
II. Dilated conjunctival blood vessels, frequently in a star or sunflower shape, may appear at birth but usually are not fully developed until late adolescence or early adult life.
III. Histologically, abnormal, dilated blood vessels are seen in the substantia propria of the conjunctiva.

ATAXIA TELANGIECTASIA (Louis-Bar Syndrome)

See p. 37 in Chapter 2.

CONGENITAL CONJUNCTIVAL LYMPHEDEMA (Nonne-Milroy-Meige Disease)

I. The condition, characterized by massive edema mainly of the lower extremities and rarely of the conjunctiva, has a sex-linked recessive inheritance pattern.
II. The disease is thought to be due to a congenital dysplasia of the lymphatics, resulting in chronic lymphedema.
III. Histologically, dilated lymphatic channels and edematous tissue are seen (Fig. 7–1).

DERMOIDS, EPIDERMOIDS AND DERMOLIPOMAS

See p. 251 in this chapter and p. 526 in Chapter 14.

VASCULAR DISORDERS

HEREDITARY HEMORRHAGIC TELANGIECTASIA

See section Congenital Anomalies above.

ATAXIA TELANGIECTASIA

See p. 37 in Chapter 2.

SICKLE CELL ANEMIA

See p. 407 in Chapter 11.

I. In homozygous sickle cell disease conjunctival capillaries may show widespread sludging of blood, and the venules may show saccular dilatations, but the characteristic findings (marked in SS disease, mild in SC disease and equivocal in the trait) are multiple, short, comma-shaped or curlicued capillary segments often seemingly isolated from the vascular network.

Similar conjunctival capillary abnormalities may be seen occasionally in the nasal and temporal conjunctiva in nonsickle cell patients. When found in the inferior conjunctiva, however, they are almost exclusively in sickle cell patients. The vessel abnormalities seem positively related to the presence of sickled erythrocytes and may be useful in gauging the severity of the systemic disease. Observation of the comma-shaped capillaries is enhanced following local application of neosynephrine. Occasionally momentary pressure on the conjunctival vessels with an applicator may be followed by vasodilatation. The blood stream then may appear to be slowed when examined by slit lamp biomicroscopy. Such a finding of slowed blood flow may be a clinical manifestation of sickle cell disease or trait.

II. Histologically the capillary lumen is irregular and filled with sickled erythrocytes.

DIABETES MELLITUS

See section Conjunctiva and Cornea in Chapter 15.

CONJUNCTIVAL HEMORRHAGE (Subconjunctival Hemorrhage) (Fig. 7–2)

I. Intraconjunctival hemorrhage into the substantia propria, or hemorrhage between conjunctiva and episclera, most often occurs as an isolated finding without any obvious cause.

II. The condition on occasion may result from trauma; severe conjunctival infection, e.g., leptospirosis and typhus; local vascular anomalies; sudden increase in venous pressure, e.g., after a paroxysm of coughing; local manifestation of such systemic diseases as arteriolarsclerosis, nephritis, diabetes mellitus, chronic hepatic disease, etc.; blood dyscrasias, especially when anemia and thrombocytopenia coexist; acute febrile systemic infection, e.g., subacute bacterial endocarditis; spontaneously during menstruation; and in trichinosis.

III. Histologically, blood is seen in the substantia propria of the conjunctiva, an observation that also is made readily by biomicroscopy.

LYMPHANGIECTASIA

I. Abnormal diffuse enlargement of lymphatics appears clinically as chemosis. Localized, dilated lymphatics appear

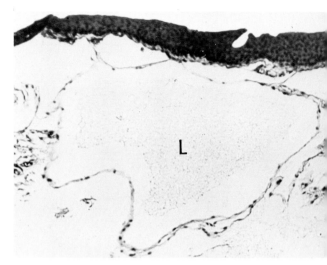

FIG. 7–1. Dilated lymphatic channels (L) and edema present in conjunctiva. H&E, ×69.

FIG. 7–2. Conjunctival hemorrhage. Blood present in substantia propria of conjunctiva. **Inset 1** shows spontaneous conjunctival hemorrhage in seemingly healthy man. Within 2 years patient had died from acute leukemia. **Inset 2** shows massive conjunctival hemorrhage following trauma. **Main figure,** H&E, ×101; **inset 1,** clinical; **inset 2,** clinical.

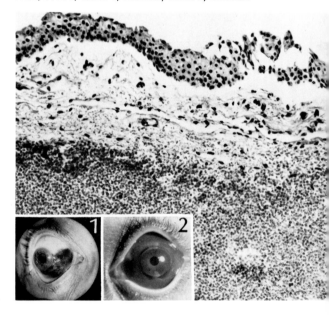

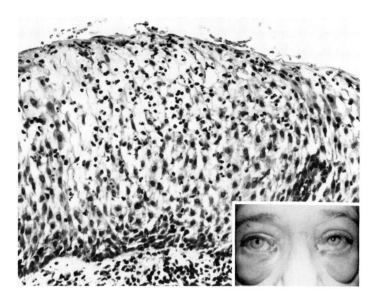

FIG. 7–3. Acute conjunctivitis. Epithelium edematous and infiltrated by polymorphonuclear leukocytes. **Inset** shows bilateral acute conjunctivitis with purulent exudate. **Main figure,** H&E, ×136; **inset,** clinical.

clinically as a cyst or a series of cysts, the latter commonly in the area of the interpalpebral fissure.

II. With diffuse involvement the cause generally is not known.

III. In the localized variety the dilated lymphatics generally are obstructed secondarily by an old scar, a pinguecula or some other conjunctival pathology.

IV. Histologically the lymphatic vessels are dilated abnormally.

LYMPHANGIECTASIA HEMORRHAGICA CONJUNCTIVAE

I. The condition is characterized by a connection between a blood vessel and a lymphatic so that the latter is permanently or intermittently filled with blood.

II. The cause is not known.

LYMPHANGIOMA AND HEMANGIOMA

See p. 528 and 532 in Chapter 14.

INFLAMMATION

BASIC HISTOLOGIC CHANGES

I. Acute conjunctivitis (Fig. 7–3)
   A. Edema (chemosis), hyperemia and cellular exudates are characteristic of acute conjunctivitis.

Cellular Exudate (Fig. 7–4)	Type of Conjunctivitis
Neutrophils	Bacterial
Eosinophils	Allergic, especially vernal catarrh
Basophils	Allergic
Mononuclear cells (especially lymphocytes)	Viral
Multinucleated cells	Herpes, rubella, tuberculosis

   B. Inflammatory membranes
      1. A *true membrane,* as may be seen in epidermic keratoconjunctivitis, *Corynebacterium diphtheriae* infection, Stevens-Johnson syndrome, pneumococcus and *Staphylococcus aureus* infections, consists of an exudate of fibrin-cellular debris firmly attached to the underlying epithelium by fibrin. Characteristically, when the true membrane is removed, the epithelium also is stripped off, leaving a raw, bleeding surface.
      2. A *pseudomembrane,* as may be seen in epidermic keratoconjunctivitis,

Corynebacterium diphtheriae infection, Stevens-Johnson syndrome, *Streptococcus hemolyticus* infection, pharyngoconjunctival fever, vernal conjunctivitis, ligneous conjunctivitis and chemical burns (especially alkali), consists of a loose fibrin-cellular debris exudate not adherent to the underlying epithelium from which it is stripped off easily.

3. *Ligneous conjunctivitis* (Fig. 7–5)

   a. Ligneous conjunctivitis is an unusual type of bilateral, chronic, recurrent membranous or pseudomembranous conjunctivitis of childhood of unknown etiology, which persists for months to years and may become massive.

   b. Histologically the conjunctival epithelium frequently is thickened and may be dyskeratotic. The subepithelial tissue consists of an enormously thickened membrane composed primarily of fibrin and amorphous eosinophilic material containing a sprinkling of lymphocytes and plasma cells.

C. *Ulceration*, i.e., loss of epithelium with or without loss of subepithelial tissue associated with an inflammatory cellular infiltrate, may occur during the course of acute conjunctivitis.

D. A *phlyctenule* generally starts as a localized, acute inflammatory reaction, followed by central necrosis and then replacement of acute inflammatory cells by lymphocytes and plasma cells.

II. Chronic conjunctivitis (Figs. 7–6 through 7–8)

A. With chronic conjunctivitis the epithelium and its goblet cells may increase in number, i.e., become hyperplastic.

Infoldings of the proliferated epithelium and goblet cells may resemble glandular structures in tissue section and have been called *pseudoglands* (Henle). Commonly the surface openings of the pseudoglands may become clogged by debris, especially in the inferior palpebral conjunctiva,

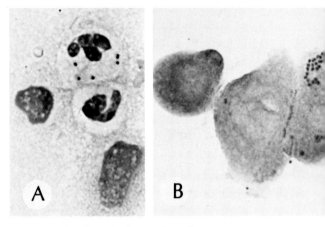

FIG. 7–4. Conjunctival scrapings from purulent conjunctivitis stained with gram stain. Bacteria (cocci) are present in polymorphonuclear leukocyte (*A*) and in large (epithelial?) cell (**B**). **A,** gram, ×1,000; **B,** gram, ×1,000.

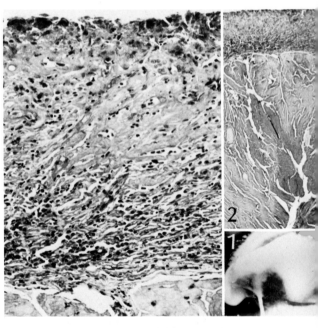

FIG. 7–5. Ligneous conjunctivitis. **Inset 1** shows membrane covering upper palpebral conjunctiva. Biopsy of same case (**inset 2**) shows thick, amorphous material covered (**main figure**) by inflammatory membrane composed of fibrin, amorphous material, lymphocytes, plasma cells and polymorphonuclear leukocytes. **Main figure,** H&E, ×101; **inset 1,** clinical; **inset 2,** H&E, ×16.

forming clear or yellow cysts called *pseudoretention cysts*.

B. The conjunctiva may undergo *papillary hypertrophy*, which is caused by the conjunctiva's being thrown into folds. The folds or projections are covered by hyperplastic epithelium and contain a core of vessels surrounded by edematous subepithelial tissue infiltrated with chronic inflammatory cells (lymphocytes and plasma cells predominate). Papillary hypertrophy basically is a vascular response with secondary lymphocyte and plasma cell infiltration.

Clinically the small (0.1 to 0.2 mm) hyperemic projections are fairly regular, are most marked in the upper palpebral conjunctiva and contain a central tuft of vessels. The valleys between the projections are pale and relatively vessel-free. Papillae characterize the subacute stage of many inflammations, e.g., vernal catarrh.

C. The conjunctiva may undergo *follicular formation* as a response to chronic irritation. Follicular hypertrophy is basically lymphoid hyperplasia with secondary vascularization.

At birth lymphoid tissue is not present in the conjunctiva, but it develops normally within the first few months of life. In inclusion blenorrhea of the newborn, therefore, a papillary reaction develops, whereas the same infection in adults may cause a follicular reaction. Lymphoid hyperplasia develops in such diverse conditions as drug toxicities (e.g., atropine, pilocarpine, eserine), allergic conditions and infections (e.g., trachoma) and from idiopathic causes. Clinically lymphoid follicles are smaller and paler than papillae and lack the central tuft of vessels.

D. With vitamin A deficiency or with drying the conjunctiva may undergo *keratinization*, e.g., as in chronic exposure with an ectropion of the lid.

E. Chronic inflammation during healing may cause an overexuberent amount of granulation tissue to be formed, i.e., granuloma pyogenicum (Fig. 7–9).

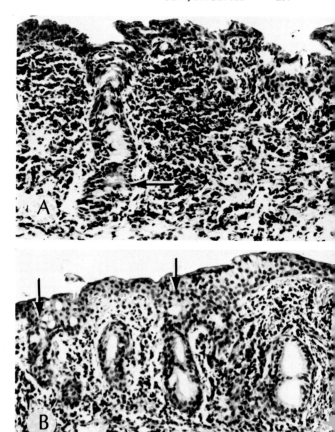

FIG. 7–6. Chronic conjunctivitis. **A.** Infoldings of proliferated epithelium and goblet cells (*arrow*) are called pseudoglands (Henle). Subepithelial tissue infiltrated by lymphocytes and plasma cells. **B.** Surface openings of pseudoglands (*arrows*) may become clogged leading to formation of pseudoretention cysts. Again note chronic, nongranulomatous inflammation in substantia propria. **A,** H&E, ×101; **B,** H&E, ×101.

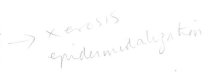

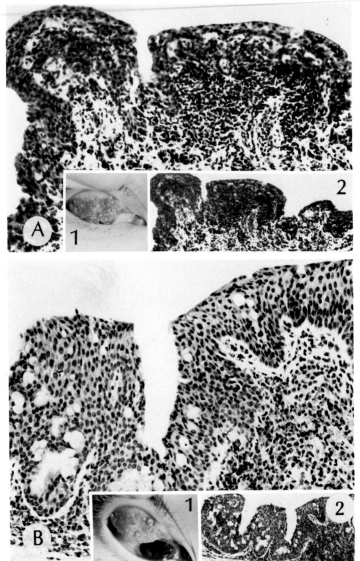

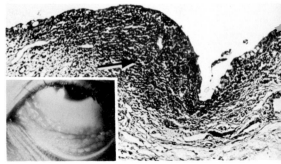

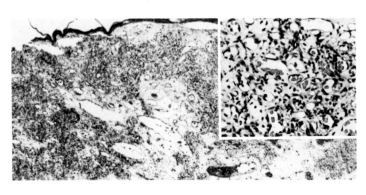

FIG. 7–7. Papillary hypertrophy in chronic conjunctivitis. **A. Inset 1** shows papillary ("cobblestone") hypertrophy in patient with vernal catarrh. Conjunctiva is thrown into folds (**main figure** and **inset 2**); folds are covered by hyperplastic epithelium and contain vascular core and edematous subepithelial tissue infiltrated with lymphocytes and plasma cells. **B. Inset 1** shows papillary hypertrophy in patient with vernal catarrh. Low (**inset 2**) and high (**main figure**) magnifications show same type of histologic changes demonstrated in **A. A,** H&E, ×101; **inset 1,** clinical; **inset 2,** H&E, ×40; **B,** H&E, ×101; **inset 1,** clinical; **inset 2,** H&E, ×28.

FIG. 7–8. Follicular formation (**inset**) consists of benign lymphoid hyperplasia in sub-epithelial tissue (*arrow*) and secondary vascularization. **Main figure,** H&E, ×54; **inset,** clinical.

FIG. 7–9. Granulation tissue may form during healing; if overexuberant, it is called granuloma pyogenicum (**main figure**). **Inset** is higher magnification to show three components: capillaries, fibroblasts and inflammatory cells. **Main figure,** H&E, ×28; **inset,** H&E, ×101.

F. The conjunctiva may be the site of granulomatous inflammation, e.g., sarcoid—see p. 101 in Chapter 4.

III. Scarring of conjunctiva

A. *Ocular pemphigoid* (benign mucous membrane pemphigoid, cicatricial pemphigoid, pemphigus conjunctivae, chronic cicatrizing conjunctivitis, essential shrinkage of conjunctiva (Fig. 7–10)

1. Ocular pemphigoid is a rare, bilateral (one eye may be involved first) conjunctival disease. It may involve the conjunctiva alone or, more commonly, also other mucous membranes and skin in elderly individuals.

   The conjunctiva is the only site of involvement in about 1 out of 30 cases. It may precede involvement of other sites by 2 months to 10 years.

2. The disease is chronic, but usually the general health is not impaired.

3. The chronic conjunctival disease results in primary conjunctival scarring and secondary corneal scarring.

4. Histology:
   a. Subepithelial conjunctival bullae rupture and are replaced not by epithelium but by fibrovascular tissue containing lymphocytes and plasma cells.
   b. The vascular and inflammatory components lessen with chronicity, resulting in contracture of the fibrous tissue with subsequent shrinkage, scarring, symblepharon, ankyloblepharon, etc.

   Pemphigus, unlike pemphigoid, is characterized histologically by acantholysis resulting in intraepidermal vesicles and bullae rather than subepithelial vesicles and bullae. Also, the bullae of pemphigus, unlike pemphigoid, tend to heal without scarring. In pemphigus the conjunctiva, especially the bulbar portion, rarely is involved and even then scarring is not a prominent feature.

B. Secondary scarring

Many conditions, e.g., chemical burns, erythema multiforme (Stevens-Johnson), may result in secondary conjunctival scarring.

SPECIFIC INFLAMMATIONS

I. Infection

A. Bacteria (Fig. 7–3)—see section Phases of Inflammation in Chapter 1 and section Suppurative Endophthalmitis and Panophthalmitis in Chapter 3.

B. Virus—see subsection on chronic nongranulomatous inflammation in Chapter 1.

1. Trachoma (Figs. 7–11 and 7–12)
   a. Trachoma, one of the world's leading causes of blindness, is a disease primarily affecting the conjunctival and corneal epithelium and caused by the virus *Chlamydia trachomatis*. Healing is marked by scarring or cicatrization.
   b. Histology of MacCallan's four stages:
      1) Stage I—the stage of early formation of conjunctival follicles, subepithelial conjunctival infiltrates, diffuse punctate keratitis and early pannus. The conjunctival epithelium undergoes a marked hyperplasia, and its cytoplasm contains minute elementary bodies and large basophilic initial bodies forming the conjunctival and corneal epithelial cytoplasm *inclusion bodies* of Halberstaedter and Prowazek. The subepithelial tissue is edematous and infiltrated by round inflammatory cells, mainly lymphocytes and plasma cells. Fibrovascular tissue in the substantia propria proliferates and starts to grow into the cornea under the epithelium, destroying Bowman's membrane. The corneal epithelium simultane-

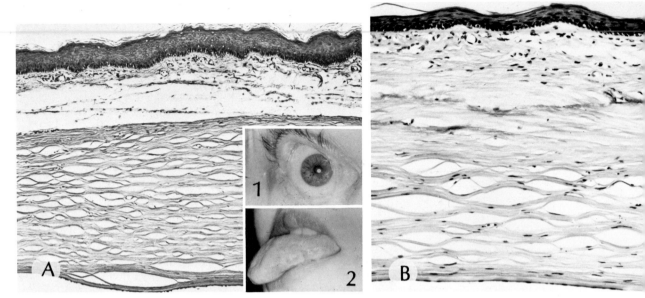

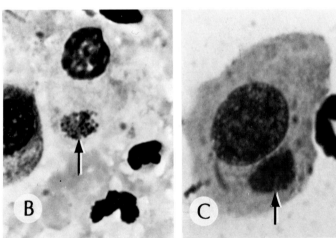

FIG. 7–10. Ocular pemphigoid. **A. Insets** show conjunctival (**inset 1**) and tongue (**inset 2**) changes. Cornea from same patient shows epidermidalization of epithelium and subepithelial fibrovascular pannus. **B.** Another section of cornea from same patient shows epidermidalization of epithelium, destruction of Bowman's membrane and scarring of superficial corneal stroma. **A,** H&E, ×54; **inset 1,** clinical; **inset 2,** clinical; **B,** H&E, ×101.

FIG. 7–11. Trachoma produced experimentally in monkeys. **A.** Early pannus formation (stage I) involving about 1 mm of peripheral cornea. **B** and **C** show cytoplasmic (elementary bodies in **B** and large basophilic initial bodies in **C**) inclusions (*arrows*). **D.** Pannus formation is more marked, and numerous large follicles can be seen (stage II). **A,** clinical; **B,** H&E, ×950; **C,** H&E, ×950; **D,** clinical.

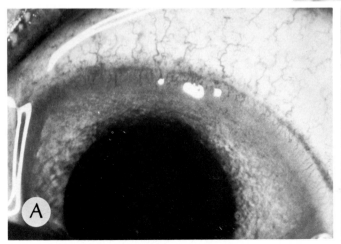

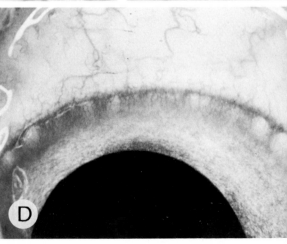

ously undergoes necrosis with minute areas of punctate erosions. Polymorphonuclear leukocytes infiltrate corneal and conjunctival epithelium.

2) Stage II—the stage of florid inflammation mainly of the upper tarsal conjunctiva with the formation of follicles early (see p. 239 in this chapter) and then of papillas (see p. 239 in this chapter) with the follicles appearing like sago grains. The corneal pannus increases. Large macrophages with phagocytized debris (*Leber cells*) appear in the conjunctival substantia propria along with an increase in the epithelial hyperplasia, subepithelial edema and round cell infiltrate. The follicles cannot be differentiated histologically from lymphoid follicles secondary to other causes, e.g., allergic.

3) Stage III—the stage of scarring and cicatrization. In the peripheral cornea follicles disappear and the area is filled with thickened, transparent epithelium (*Herbert's pits*); the palpebral conjunctiva scars with the formation of a white linear horizontal line or scar near the upper border of the tarsus (*von Arlt's line*). Cicatricial entropion and trichiasis may result. Along with the subepithelial scar tissue, scattered lymphocytes and plasma cells may be found.

4) Stage IV—the stage of arrest of the disease.

2. Inclusion conjunctivitis (inclusion blennorrhea)

a. The disease caused by *Chlamydia oculogenitale* is an acute contagious disease of newborns quite similar clinically and histologically to trachoma with the main difference being a predilec-

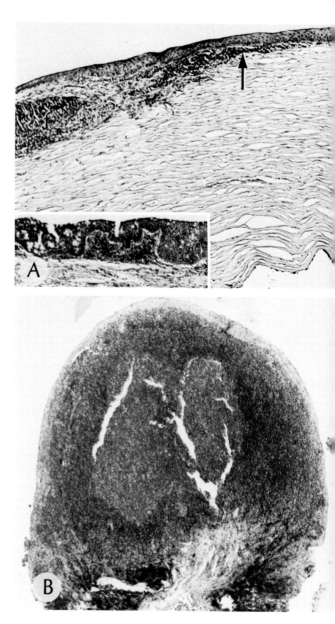

FIG. 7–12. Trachoma. **A.** Early formation of inflammatory pannus (*arrow*) destroys Bowman's membrane as it grows into cornea under epithelium. Lymphoid follicle (*f*) is present. **Inset** shows later stage with epithelium thrown into folds, i.e., papillary formation (both **main figure** and **inset** from nontrachomatous chronic conjunctivitis). **B.** Case of trachoma with enormous conjunctival papilla shown. **A,** H&E, ×40; **inset,** H&E, ×28; **B,** H&E, ×16.

243

tion for the lower palpebral conjunctiva and fornix rather than the upper.

b. Histologically, mainly a follicular reaction is present quite similar to the early stages of trachoma, with epithelial cytoplasmic inclusion bodies indistinguishable from those found in trachoma.

3. Lymphogranuloma venereum (inguinale)

a. Lymphogranuloma venereum, caused by a virus belonging to the lymphogranuloma-psittacosis group (*Miyagawanella lymphogranulomatosis*), is characterized by a follicular conjunctivitis or a nonulcerating conjunctival granuloma usually near the limbus and is associated with a nonsuppurative regional lymphadenopathy.

b. Histologically there is a granulomatous conjunctivitis and lymphadenitis, the latter containing stellate abscesses. Organisms, in the form of either elementary bodies or inclusion bodies, cannot be identified in histologic sections.

C. Fungal—see section Fungal Nontraumatic Infectious in Chapter 4.

D. Parasitic—see section on parasitic nontraumatic infections in Chapter 4 and p. 273 in Chapter 8.

E. Rickettsial

F. *Parinaud's oculoglandular syndrome* (Fig. 7–13)—all basically are granulomatous inflammations (see p. 12 in Chap. 1) and may be caused by tuberculosis, sarcoidosis, syphilis, tularemia, cat scratch disease, leptothrix, soft chancre (chancroid—*H. ducreyi*), pasteurellosis, glanders and fungi.

II. Noninfection

A. Physical—see sections on burns and on radiational injuries in Chapter 5.

B. Chemical—see section Chemical Injuries in Chapter 5.

C. Allergic

1. Vernal keratoconjunctivitis (vernal catarrh, spring catarrh) (Fig. 7–7)

a. Vernal keratoconjunctivitis tends to be a bilateral, recurrent, self-limited, conjunctival disease occurring mainly in warm weather and affecting young people (mainly boys). It is of unknown etiology but is presumed to be an immediate hypersensitivity reaction to exogenous antigens. It may be associated with, or accompanied by, keratoconus.

b. The involvement may be limited to the tarsal conjunctiva (palpebral form), the bulbar conjunctiva (limbal form) or the cornea (vernal superficial punctate keratitis form) or combinations of all three.

c. Histology:

1) The tarsal conjunctiva may undergo hyperplasia of its epithelium and proliferation of fibrovascular connective tissue along with an infiltration of round inflammatory cells, especially eosinophils and basophils, resulting in the formation of papillas (see section Inflammation above). The papillas can become quite large, clinically resembling cobblestones.

2) The epithelium and subepithelial fibrovascular connective tissue of the limbal conjunctival region may undergo hyperplasia along with round cell inflammatory infiltration producing limbal nodules. Concretions, containing eosinophils, within the larger yellow or gray vascularized nodules appear clinically as white spots (*Horner-Trantas' spots*).

3) Degeneration and death of corneal epithelium results in punctate epithelial erosions, especially prone to occur in the upper part of the cornea.

2. Hay fever conjunctivitis

3. Contact blepharoconjunctivitis

4. Phlyctenular keratoconjunctivitis

5. *Neoplastic processes* (Fig. 7–14) (e.g., sebaceous gland carcinoma) can cause a chronic, nongranulomatous blepharoconjunctivitis with cancerous invasion of the epithelium and subepithelial tissues.

INJURIES

See Chapter 5.

CONJUNCTIVAL MANIFESTATIONS OF SYSTEMIC DISEASE

DEPOSITION OF METABOLIC PRODUCTS

   I. Cystinosis (*Lignac's disease*)—see p. 306 in Chapter 8.
  II. Ochronosis—see p. 315 in Chapter 8.
 III. Hypercalcemia—see p. 285 in Chapter 8.
  IV. Addison's disease—melanin is deposited in the basal layer of the epithelium.
   V. Mucopolysaccharidoses—see p. 302 in Chapter 8.
  VI. Lipoidosis—see pp. 440–441 in Chapter 11.
 VII. Dysproteinemias
VIII. Porphyria
  IX. Jaundice—bilirubin salts are deposited diffusely in the conjunctiva and episclera but generally not in the sclera unless the jaundice is chronic and excessive.
   X. Malignant atrophic papilosis (Degos' syndrome)—see p. 199 in Chapter 6.

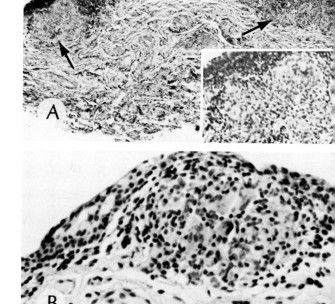

FIG. 7–13. Sarcoidosis. **A.** Patient had known sarcoidosis. Conjunctival biopsy (inferior cul-de-sac) shows subepithelial granulomatous inflammatory infiltrate (*arrows*), shown with higher magnification in **inset. B.** Conjunctival biopsy from another sarcoid patient again shows subepithelial granulomatous inflammatory infiltrate. **A,** H&E, ×28; **inset,** H&E, ×69; **B,** H&E, ×101.

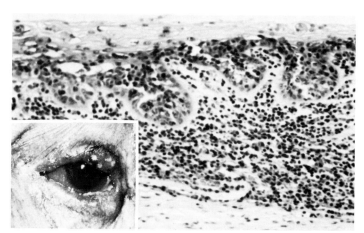

FIG. 7–14. Chronic conjunctivitis (**inset**) due to sebaceous gland carcinoma of upper and lower lids. Marked lymphocytic and plasma cell infiltration in subepithelial tissue. Malignant sebaceous gland carcinoma cells invading conjunctival epithelium (pagetoid change). **Main figure,** H&E, ×101; **inset,** clinical.

DEPOSITION OF DRUG DERIVATIVES

I. Argyrosis (Fig. 7–15)
   A. Chronic use of silver-containing medications may result in a slate gray discoloration of the mucous membranes, including the conjunctiva, and of the skin, including the lids. The discoloration also may involve the nasolacrimal apparatus.
   B. Histologically the silver is deposited in the reticulin (i.e., loose collagenous) fibrils of the subepithelial tissue and in basement membranes of epithelium, endothelium (e.g., Descemet's membrane) and blood vessels.
II. Chlorpromazine—see p. 313 in Chapter 8.
III. Atabrine
IV. Epinephrine (Fig. 7–16)—see p. 312 in Chapter 8.
V. Mercury
VI. Arsenicals (also in Bowen's disease) p. 214

VITAMIN A DEFICIENCY AND BITOT'S SPOT

See p. 279 in Chapter 8.

SJÖGREN'S SYNDROME

See p. 279 in Chapter 8 and p. 552 in Chapter 14.

SKIN DISEASES

I. Erythema multiforme (Stevens-Johnson syndrome) (Fig. 7–17)
   A. Erythema multiforme is an acute, self-limited dermatosis with multiform lesions of macules, papules (most common lesion), vesicles and bullae.

   Severe erythema multiforme, starting suddenly with high fever and prostration and showing predominantly a bullous eruption of the skin and mucous membranes, is referred to as Stevens-Johnson syndrome.

   B. Histologically the conjunctival bullae, formed by detachment of the entire epithelium from the subepithelial tissue, heal by cicatrization, leading to symblepharon and entropion.
      1. Frequently the conjunctival epithelial goblet cells and openings of the accessory lacrimal glands are destroyed, leading to marked drying of the conjunctiva with subsequent epidermidalization.
      2. The conjunctiva may undergo extensive necrosis with a purulent inflammatory reaction or may show only a chronic, nongranulomatous inflammatory reaction.
II. Atopic dermatitis
III. Rosacea—see p. 187 in Chapter 6.
IV. Xeroderma pigmentosum—see p. 184 in Chapter 6.
V. Ichthyosis congenita—see p. 182 in Chapter 6.
VI. Molluscum contagiosum—see p. 187 in Chapter 6.
VII. Dermatitis herpetiformis, epidermolysis bullosa, erythema nodosum and many others may show conjunctival manifestations.

DEGENERATIONS

XEROSIS (Fig. 7–18)

I. Xerosis or dry eyes due to conjunctival disease may result from keratoconjunctivitis sicca (Sjögren's syndrome), ocular pemphigoid, trachoma, vitamin A deficiency, proptosis with exposure, familial dysautonomia, chemical burns, erythema multiforme (Stevens-Johnson) and so forth.
II. Histologically the epithelium undergoes epidermidalization with keratin formation, and the underlying subepithelial tissue frequently shows cicatrization.

PTERYGIUM

See p. 281 in Chapter 8.

PINGUECULA (Fig. 7–19)

I. Pinguecula is a localized, elevated, yellowish white area near the limbus, generally found nasally and bilaterally, seen predominantly in middle and late life.

   Pigmented, triangular, brown "pingueculae" may appear during the second decade of *Gaucher's disease*. The lesions on biopsy contain Gaucher cells.

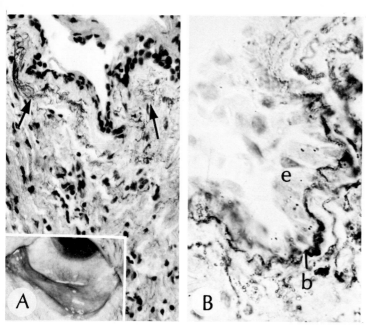

FIG. 7–15. Argyrosis. **A.** Dense deposition of silver granules along elastic fibers (*arrows*). **Inset** shows conjunctival staining following prolonged use of silver-containing drops. **B.** Lacrimal sac with silver deposited in epithelium (*e*) and in mucosal basement membrane (*b*). **A,** H&E, ×280; **inset,** clinical; **B,** H&E, ×900.

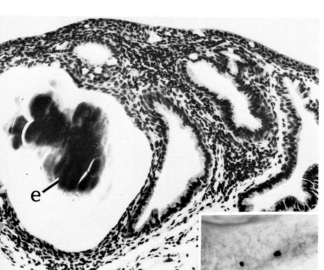

FIG. 7–16. Epinephrine deposits in conjunctiva (two black spots in **inset**) following long-term use of epinephrine drops for treatment of glaucoma. Material in conjunctival cyst (*e*) is epinephrine derivative, which stains like melanin, i.e., bleaches and reduces silver salts. **Main figure,** H&E, ×101; **inset,** clinical.

FIG. 7–17. Stevens-Johnson syndrome. Section of skin shows retention of epidermis and accumulation of inflammatory cells within dermis. **Inset** shows conjunctival involvement. **Main figure,** H&E, ×154; **inset,** clinical.

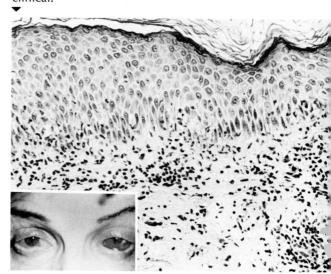

II. Histologically it appears identical to a pterygium (see p. 281 in Chap. 8) except that there is no corneal involvement. The subepithelial tissue shows senile elastosis (basophilic degeneration) due to a breakdown in the collagen. The subepithelial abnormal material stains for elastin but is not sensitive to elastase (*elastotic degeneration*).

AMYLOIDOSIS

I. Classification as to eye involvement
   A. Primary
      1. Systemic (primary familial amyloidosis) (Figs. 7–20 and 12–13)— vitreous opacities are the most important finding but ecchymosis of lids, proptosis, ocular palsies, internal ophthalmoplegia, neuroparalytic keratitis and glaucoma may result from amyloid deposition in tissues (see p. 480 in Chap. 12).
         a. Amyloid deposition is found around and in walls of ocular blood vessels, especially retinal and uveal.
         b. Skin and conjunctiva may be involved, but this is not so important as involvement of other ocular structures.
      2. Localized (Fig. 7–21) (localized nodular amyloidosis)—small and large, brownish red nodules may be found in the conjunctiva and lids. The intraocular structures are not involved.

   Lattice corneal dystrophy, one of the inherited corneal dystrophies, is considered by some to be a primary, localized amyloidosis of the cornea (see p. 301 in Chap. 8). Rarely, a localized amyloidosis of the cornea, unrelated to lattice corneal dystrophy also can occur idiopathically. Conversely, lattice corneal dystrophy, on rare occasions, can occur in primary systemic amyloidosis.

   B. Secondary
      1. *Systemic*—secondary systemic amyloidosis may result from such chronic inflammatory diseases as leprosy, osteomyelitis or rheumatoid arthritis, or it may be part of multiple myeloma. The ocular structures including eyes, eyelids, conjunctiva and adnexa generally are spared.
      2. *Local*—secondary localized amyloidosis may result from such chronic local inflammations of the conjunctiva and lids as trachoma and chronic, nongranulomatous, idiopathic conjunctivitis and blepharitis. This is not as common as primary local amyloidosis.

II. Histology
   A. Amyloid appears as amorphous, eosinophilic, pale, hyaline deposits free in the connective tissue or around or in blood vessel walls. A nongranulomatous inflammatory reaction or, rarely, a foreign body giant cell reaction or no inflammatory reaction may be present.
   B. The material demonstrates metachromasia (polycationic dyes such as crystal violet and toluidine blue change color from blue to purple), positive staining with Congo red, dichroism (change in color that varies with the plane of polarized light, usually from green to orange with rotation of polarizer), birefringence (double refraction with polarized light) of Congo red-stained material and fluorescence with thioflavine-T.
   C. Electron microscopically, amyloid has a fine, filamentous structure.
   D. Amyloid is believed to be composed of a variety of immunoglobulins.

FIG. 7–18. Xerosis. Conjunctival epithelium has undergone epidermidalization, and substantia propria (s) shows cicatrization. H&E, ×54.

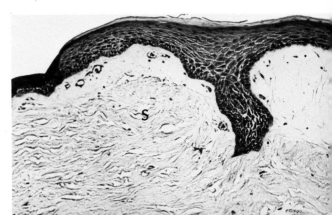

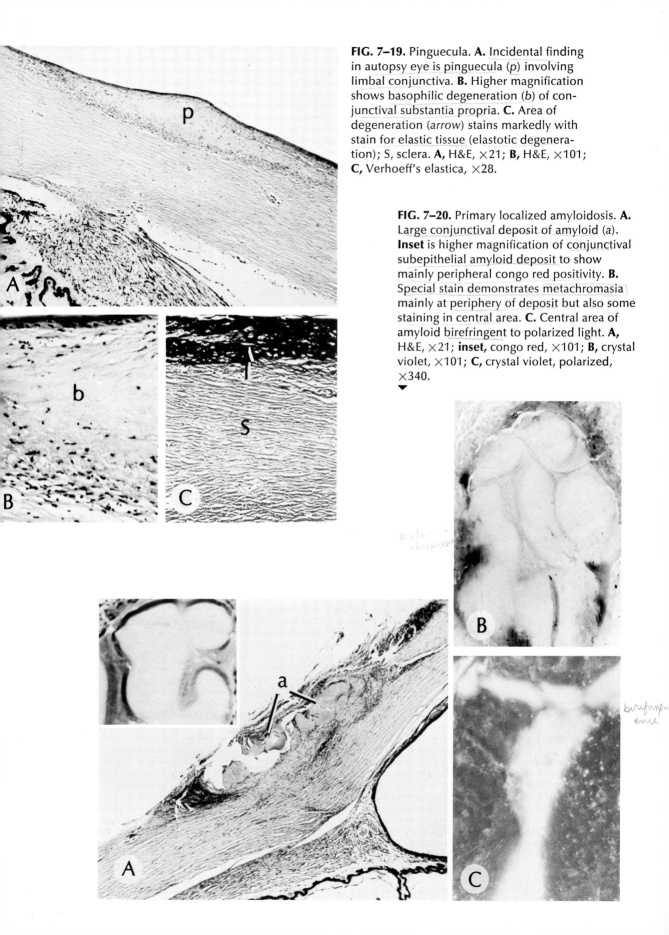

FIG. 7–19. Pinguecula. **A.** Incidental finding in autopsy eye is pinguecula (*p*) involving limbal conjunctiva. **B.** Higher magnification shows basophilic degeneration (*b*) of conjunctival substantia propria. **C.** Area of degeneration (*arrow*) stains markedly with stain for elastic tissue (elastotic degeneration); S, sclera. **A,** H&E, ×21; **B,** H&E, ×101; **C,** Verhoeff's elastica, ×28.

FIG. 7–20. Primary localized amyloidosis. **A.** Large conjunctival deposit of amyloid (*a*). **Inset** is higher magnification of conjunctival subepithelial amyloid deposit to show mainly peripheral congo red positivity. **B.** Special stain demonstrates metachromasia mainly at periphery of deposit but also some staining in central area. **C.** Central area of amyloid birefringent to polarized light. **A,** H&E, ×21; **inset,** congo red, ×101; **B,** crystal violet, ×101; **C,** crystal violet, polarized, ×340.

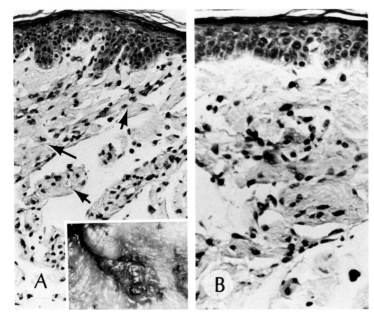

FIG. 7–21. Secondary systemic amyloidosis. **A. Inset** shows purpuric skin lesion (patient had multiple such lesions over lids of both eyes with tendency toward spontaneous bleeding) of eyelid. Photomicrograph is biopsy of skin, which shows numerous, dermal vascular channels surrounded by fibrillar substance (*arrows*). **B.** Perivascular substance stains positively with congo red. Multiple myeloma was diagnosed 6 months later. **Main figure,** H&E, ×101; **inset,** clinical; **B,** congo red, ×176.

FIG. 7–22. Cysts. **A.** Large, sausage-shaped cyst fills inferior cul-de-sac in young woman. **B.** Epithelial inclusion cyst is lined by conjunctival epithelium and appears empty. **C.** Limbal lesion at 5 o'clock position was thought clinically to be lymphoid lesion. **D.** Same lesion as **C** shown to be ductal cyst lined by double layer of epithelium and containing periodic acid-Schiff positive material. **A,** clinical; **B,** H&E, ×40; **C,** clinical; **D,** PAS, ×28.

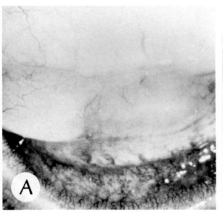

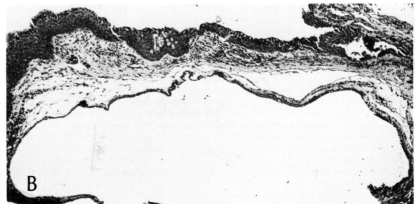

(continued)

CYSTS, PSEUDONEOPLASMS AND NEOPLASMS

CHORISTOMAS

I. Epidermoid cyst—see p. 526 in Chapter 14.
II. Dermoid cyst—see p. 526 in Chapter 14.
III. Dermolipoma. A dermolipoma, encountered as a bilateral large yellowish white, soft tumor near the temporal canthus and extending backward and upward, is a form of solid dermoid composed primarily of fatty tissue.

Frequently, serial sections of the tumor have to be made to find nonfatty elements such as stratified squamous epithelium and dermal appendages.

HAMARTOMAS

I. Lymphangioma—see p. 532 in Chapter 14.
II. Hemangioma—see p. 528 in Chapter 14.
III. Phakomatoses—see Chapter 2.

CYSTS (Fig. 7–22)

I. Cysts of the conjunctiva may be congenital or acquired, with the latter predominating.
II. Acquired conjunctival cysts are mainly implantation cysts of surface epithelium, resulting in an *epithelial inclusion* cyst. Other cysts may be ductal (e.g., from accessory lacrimal glands) or inflammatory.
III. Histologically the structure depends on the type of cyst.

A. Epidermoid and dermoid cyst—see p. 526 in Chapter 14.
B. Epithelial inclusion cyst is lined by conjunctival epithelium and contains a clear fluid.
C. Ductal cysts are lined by a double layer of epithelium and contain a periodic acid-Schiff positive material.
D. Inflammatory cysts contain polymorphonuclear leukocytes and cellular debris.

PSEUDOCANCEROUS EPITHELIAL LESIONS

I. Hereditary benign intraepithelial dyskeratosis (HBID) (Fig. 7–23)
A. HBID is a bilateral dyskeratosis of the conjunctival epithelium associated with comparable lesions of the oral mucosa and inherited as an autosomal dominant.

The disease is indigenous to family members of a large triracial (Indian, black and white) isolate in Halifax County, North Carolina. Members of the family now live in other parts of the United States, so that the lesion may be encountered outside of North Carolina.

B. Clinically, raised, horseshoe-shaped plaques, granular appearing, richly vascularized, gray in color, are present at the nasal and temporal limbus in each eye. Additionally there generally is a whitish placoid lesion of the mucous membrane of the mouth (tongue or buccal mucosa).

(continued)

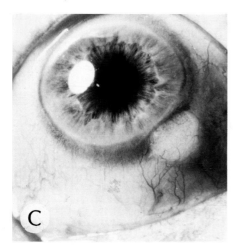

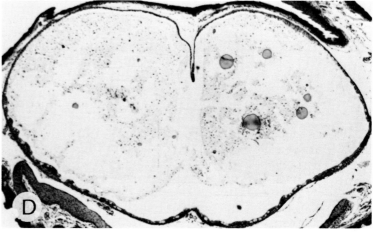

C. Histologically, considerable thickening of the epithelium with acanthosis and dyskeratosis, the latter especially prominent in the superficial layers, is present along with a chronic non-granulomatous inflammatory reaction and increased vascularization of the subepithelial tissue.

II. Pseudoepitheliomatous hyperplasia (PEH) —see p. 206 in Chapter 6.

A. PEH may mimic clinically and microscopically a neoplasm.

B. The epithelial hyperplasia and chronic nongranulomatous inflammatory reaction, frequently along with neutrophilic infiltration of the hyperplastic epithelium, of the subepithelial tissue are characteristic of PEH.

PEH may occur within a pinguecula or pterygium, causing sudden growth and clinically (and sometimes histologically) simulating a neoplasm.

C. Keratoacanthoma (see p. 206 in Chap. 6) is a specific variant of PEH, perhaps caused by a virus.

III. Papilloma (Fig. 7–24)

A. Conjunctival papillomas tend to be predunculated when they arise at the lid margin or caruncle, sessile with a broad base at the limbus and rare in other locations.

B. Histologically the fronds or fingerlike projections are covered by acanthotic epithelium lined by a core of fibrovascular tissue. Generally there is a tendency to slight or moderate keratinization.

Goblet cells are common within the papillomas, except within those arising at the limbus. Although the vast majority of papillomas are infectious or irritative in origin and have no malignant potential, an occasional one may develop into a squamous cell carcinoma.

IV. Eosinophilic cystadenoma (apocrine cystadenoma, oncocytoma) (Fig. 7–25)

A. Eosinophilic cystadenoma is a rare tumor of the caruncle, probably of apocrine origin.

B. Histologically one or more cystic cavities are lined by proliferating epithelium, resembling apocrine epithelium (hence, apocrine cystadenoma).

POTENTIALLY PRECANCEROUS EPITHELIAL LESIONS

I. Xeroderma pigmentosa—see p. 184 in Chapter 6.

II. Other actinic keratoses—see p. 207 in Chapter 6.

III. Dysplasia (Figs. 7–26 and 7–27)

A. Clinically dysplasia may appear as leukoplakia* (white plaque) or as a fleshy lesion, generally located at or near the limbus.

B. Histologically atypical epithelial cells are present, sometimes accompanied by dyskeratotic epithelial cells.

1. The normal polarity (from basal cell to surface cell) is retained.

2. The full thickness of the epithelium is *not* involved, generally only the deeper layers.

CANCEROUS EPITHELIAL LESIONS

All may appear clinically as leukoplakia.*

I. Carcinoma in situ (intraepithelial carcinoma, intraepithelial epithelioma) (Fig. 7–28)

A. Clinically it may appear as leukoplakia* or a fleshy mass.

B. Histologically:

1. The full thickness of the epithelium is replaced by atypical, often bizarre and pleomorphic, epithelial cells.

2. The epithelial area of involvement is thickened and characteristically sharply demarcated from the contiguous, normal appearing conjunctival epithelium.

The thickening generally ranges about two to five times normal thickness but may be greater in malignant transformation of papillomas.

3. Polarity of the epithelium is lost.

* Leukoplakia is a clinical, descriptive term and neither a clinical nor a microscopic diagnosis. Clinically leukoplakic lesions run the gamut from pinguecula to frank squamous cell carcinoma. The leukoplakic or white, shiny appearance is due to keratinization of the normally nonkeratinized conjunctival epithelium.

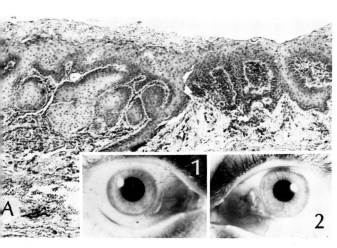

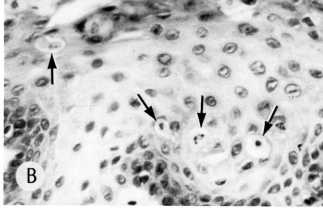

FIG. 7–23. Hereditary benign intraepithelial dyskeratosis (HBID). **A. Insets 1** and **2** show right and left eyes of young girl with HBID; note typical limbal lesions. Acanthotic epithelium and dermal chronic nongranulomatous inflammation are prominent in lesion from same girl. **B.** Higher magnification to show characteristic dyskeratotic cells (*arrows*). **A,** H&E, ×40; **inset 1,** clinical; **inset 2,** clinical; **B,** H&E, ×252.

FIG. 7–24. Papilloma. **A.** Sessile papilloma of limbal conjunctiva shows typical "strawberry" pattern with dark areas representing vascular cores. **B.** Acanthotic epithelium covers fibrovascular core. **A,** clinical; **B,** H&E, ×40.

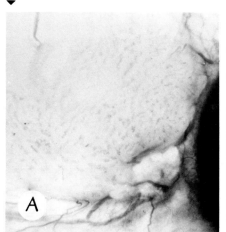

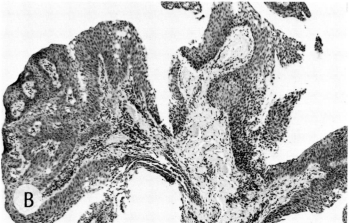

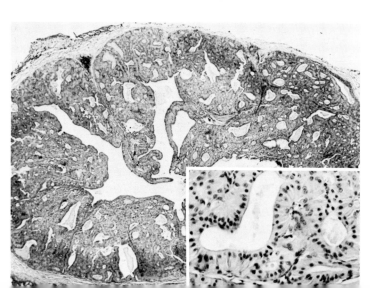

FIG. 7–25. Eosinophilic cystadenoma. Cystic cavity is filled with proliferating epithelium. **Inset** shows large, eosinophilic cells, resembling apocrine cells, forming glandlike spaces. **Main figure,** H&E, ×16; **inset,** H&E, ×101.

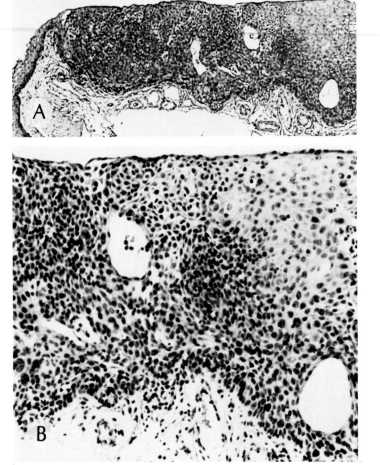

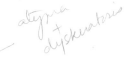
atypia + dyskeratosis

FIG. 7–26. Dysplasia. **A.** Characteristically epithelium is thickened and contains atypical cells, but normal polarity is preserved. **B.** Higher magnification shows almost complete replacement of epithelial cells on left half of figure, but still not quite enough to be termed carcinoma in situ. **A,** H&E, ×40; **B,** H&E, ×101.

FIG. 7–27. Dysplasia. **A. Inset** shows clinical appearance of limbal lesion. Although almost complete replacement of epithelium is present in different areas (see **B** and **C**), enough polarity remains and typical cells are not quite "bad" enough so that diagnosis of dysplasia, rather than carcinoma in situ, was made. **A,** H&E, ×101; **inset,** clinical; **B,** H&E, ×101; **C,** H&E, ×101.
▼

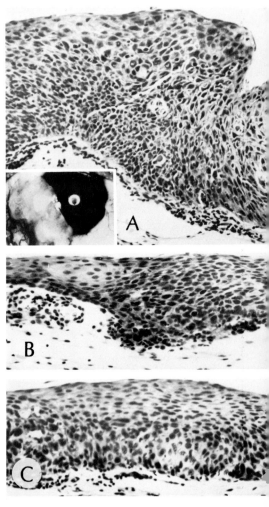

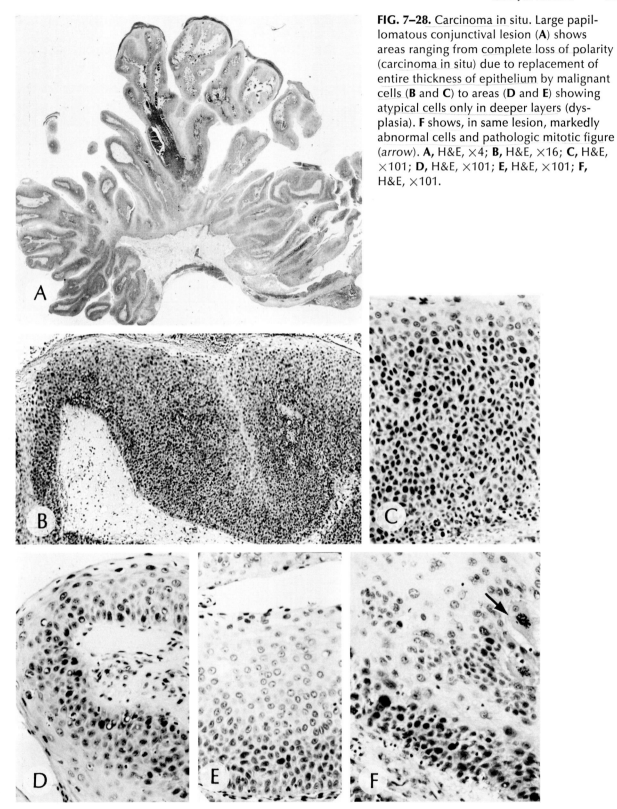

FIG. 7–28. Carcinoma in situ. Large papillomatous conjunctival lesion (**A**) shows areas ranging from complete loss of polarity (carcinoma in situ) due to replacement of entire thickness of epithelium by malignant cells (**B** and **C**) to areas (**D** and **E**) showing atypical cells only in deeper layers (dysplasia). **F** shows, in same lesion, markedly abnormal cells and pathologic mitotic figure (*arrow*). **A**, H&E, ×4; **B**, H&E, ×16; **C**, H&E, ×101; **D**, H&E, ×101; **E**, H&E, ×101; **F**, H&E, ×101.

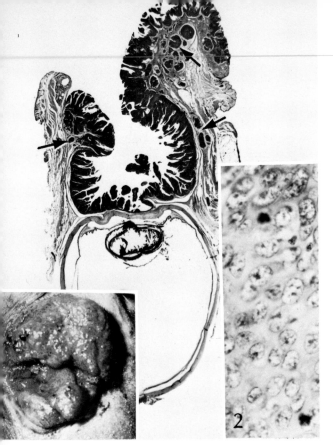

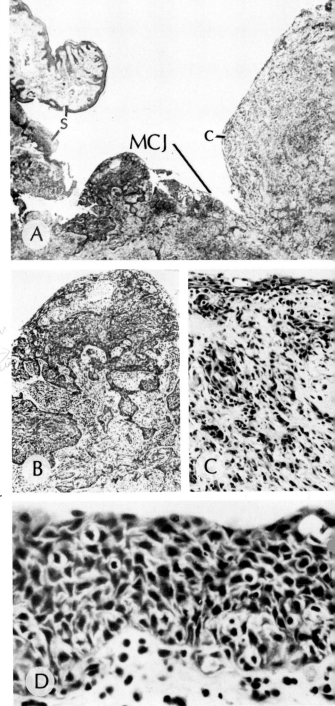

FIG. 7–29. Squamous cell carcinoma arising in papillary form from conjunctival epithelium shows deep invasion into lids (*arrows*). **Inset 1** clinical picture same case. **Inset 2** higher magnification to show two mitotic figures in poorly differentiated squamous cell carcinoma. **Main figure,** H&E, ×3; **inset 1,** clinical; **inset 2,** H&E, ×252.

nodular
desmoplastic

FIG. 7–30. Basal cell and squamous cell carcinoma. **A.** Section from lid margin showing skin surface (*s*) and conjunctival surface (*c*). *MCJ*, mucocutaneous junction. **B.** Higher magnification of surface just to skin side of MCJ shows primary basal cell carcinoma of skin of lid. **C.** Higher magnification of conjunctival side of MCJ shows primary squamous cell carcinoma of conjunctiva with deep invasion of subepithelial tissue. **D.** Conjunctival epithelium away from MCJ shows complete replacement by markedly atypical cells, i.e., carcinoma in situ. Basal cell carcinoma remained localized, whereas squamous cell carcinoma invaded into orbit and into bones of nose and maxillary sinus. **A,** H&E, ×16; **B,** H&E, ×40; **C,** H&E, ×101; **D,** H&E, ×101.

Carroll JM, Kuwabara T: A classification of limbal epitheliomas. Arch Ophthalmol 73:545, 1965

Dykstra PC, Dykstra BA: The cytologic diagnosis of carcinoma and related lesions of the ocular conjunctiva and cornea. Trans Am Acad Ophthalmol Otolaryngol 73:979, 1969

Irvine AR Jr: Epibulbar squamous cell carcinoma and related lesions. Int Ophthalmol Clin 12:71, 1972

Linwong M, Hermann SJ, Rabb MF: Carcinoma in situ of the corneal limbus in an adolescent girl. Arch Ophthalmol 87:48, 1972

Stafford WR: Conjunctival myxoma. Arch Ophthalmol 85:443, 1971

von Sallman L, Paton D: Hereditary benign intraepithelial dyskeratosis. I. Ocular manifestations. Arch Ophthalmol 63:421, 1960

Yanoff M: Hereditary benign intraepithelial dyskeratosis. Arch Ophthalmol 79:291, 1968

chapter 8

Cornea and Sclera

Inflammations

    Episcleritis

    Scleritis

Injuries

Tumors

    Fibromas

    Nodular Fasciitis

    Hemangiomas

    Neurofibromas

    Contiguous Tumors

    Episcleral Osseous Choristoma

    Aberrant Lacrimal Gland

CORNEA

CONGENITAL DEFECTS

ABSENCE OF CORNEA

Absence of cornea is a very rare condition usually associated with absence of other parts of the eye derived from primitive invaginating ectoderm, e.g., lens.

ABNORMALITIES OF SIZE

I. Microcornea (<11 mm in greatest diameter).
   A. The eye usually is structurally normal.

   Microcornea may be associated with other ocular anomalies such as are found in microphthalmos with cyst or 13–15 trisomy.

   B. The condition may be inherited as an autosomal dominant.
   C. Histologically the cornea generally is normal except for its small size.
II. Megalocornea (>13 mm in greatest diameter) (Fig. 8–1).
   A. Most megalocorneas are bilateral, non-progressive and do not in themselves produce symptoms (except for refractive error).

   Cataract and subluxated lens commonly develop in adulthood. Glaucoma may develop secondary to the dislocated lens.

   B. Associated congenital anomalies are rare.
   C. The condition usually has a recessive sex-linked inheritance pattern but may be autosomal dominant or recessive.
   D. Histologically the cornea generally is normal except for its large size.

ABERRATIONS OF CURVATURE

I. Astigmatism
II. Cornea plana

A. Frequently cornea plana is associated with other ocular anomalies, e.g., posterior embryotoxon, colobomas of iris and choroid and congenital cataract.
B. Both recessive and autosomal dominant inheritance patterns have been reported.
C. Histologically the cornea generally is normal except for its flattened anterior curve.
III. Keratoconus—see section Dystrophies below.

CONGENITAL CORNEAL OPACITIES

The two main theories of causation are arrested development during embryogenesis and intrauterine inflammation.

   Similar changes also can be on an acquired basis due to trauma or inflammation.

FIG. 8–1. Megalocornea. **A.** Corneal diameter measures 15 mm; rest of eye seems normal. **B.** Megaloglobus shows enlarged cornea and enlarged globe. **C.** Brother of patient shown in **A** (third brother also had megalocornea). Corneal diameter measures 16 mm, and lens is dislocated, as shown in **D.** Secondary chronic open angle glaucoma is present. **A–D,** clinical.

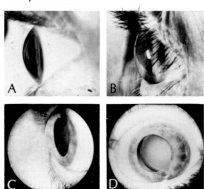

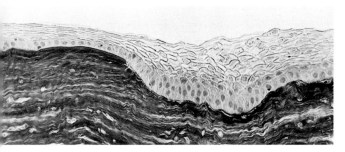

FIG. 8–2. Facet. Loss of Bowman's membrane and superficial stroma is compensated for by thicker layer of epithelium. 1.5 μ section, PD, ×150.

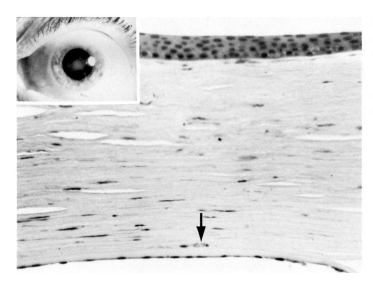

FIG. 8–3. Nebula. Blood vessel (*arrow*) just anterior to Descemet's membrane and diffuse stromal scarring present in cornea from patient with luetic (congenital) interstitial keratitis. **Inset** shows diffuse, cloudlike clinical appearance of similar lesion. **Main figure,** H&E, ×176; **inset,** clinical.

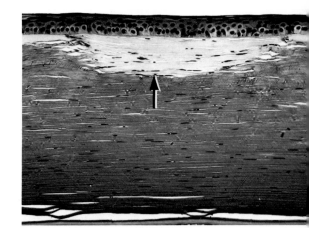

FIG. 8–5. Leukoma. Cornea thinned and scarred. Overlying epithelium hyperplastic. Bowman's membrane shows fold (*f*), breaks (*arrows*) and large gap (*g*). H&E, ×101.

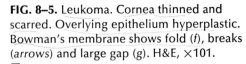

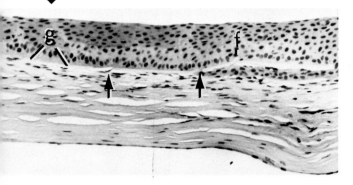

FIG. 8–4. Macula. Dense scar present (*arrow*) in area of interruption of Bowman's membrane. H&E, ×145.

CLINICOPATHOLOGIC TYPES—GENERAL

I. Facet (Fig. 8–2)
  A. A facet is a small, superficial spot seen clinically by focal illumination as a distortion of the corneal light reflex or by slit lamp as a focal increased separation of the anteriormost two lines of corneal relucency.
  B. Histologically epithelium that is thicker than normal fills in the gap of previously abraded epithelium, Bowman's membrane and sometimes the very anterior corneal stroma; no scar tissue is present.
II. Nebula (Fig. 8–3)
  A. A nebula is a slight, diffuse, cloudlike opacity with indistinct borders.
  B. Histologically scar tissue is found predominantly in the superficial stroma.
III. Macula (Fig. 8–4)
  A. A macula is a moderately dense opacity with a circumscribed border.
  B. Histologically the scar is dense and involves the corneal stroma.
IV. Leukoma (Figs. 8–5 and 8–6)
  A. A leukoma is a white, opaque scar (e.g., see section Peters' anomaly below).
  B. Histologically a large area of stromal scarring, often with overlying epithelial change, is present.

When iris is adherent to the posterior surface of the cornea under an area of corneal scarring, the resulting condition is called an *adherent leukoma.*

CLINICOPATHOLOGIC TYPES—SPECIFIC

I. Anterior embryotoxon (Fig. 8–7)
  A. Anterior embryotoxon is synonymous with *arcus juvenilis.*
  B. It may be present at birth or develop in early life and clinically appears identical to an *arcus senilis (gerontoxon)* (see p. 281 in this chapter).
  C. The condition may be associated with elevated serum lipids or cholesterol.
  D. Histology—see arcus senilis p. 281 in this chapter.
II. Corneal keloid (Fig. 5–56)
  A. Corneal keloid presents clinically as a hypertrophic scar generally involving the entire cornea.

B. Overabundant stromal corneal reparative processes following trauma seems to be the cause of corneal keloid.
  C. Although frequently noted at birth, probably secondary to intrauterine trauma, corneal keloids can develop at any age following trauma.
  D. Histologically, abundant scar tissue in disarray replaces most or all of the cornea.
III. Mesodermal-ectodermal dysgenesis of cornea
  A. Peters' anomaly (Figs. 8–8 and 8–9)
    1. Peters' anomaly consists of bilateral central corneal opacities with abnormalities of the deepest corneal stromal layers and local absence of endothelium and Descemet's and usually Bowman's membrane.
    2. It usually is associated with anomalies of the anterior segment structures (corectopia, iris hypoplasia, anterior polar cataract, iridocorneal adhesions) and may be due to a defect of mesodermal and ectodermal origin with failure or delay in separation of the lens vesicle from surface epithelium.
    3. It usually is inherited as autosomal recessive, but autosomal dominance or no inheritance also may occur.
    4. *Internal ulcer of von Hippel* is probably the same anomaly, although some think of the latter as being of inflammatory origin.

Perhaps the term internal ulcer of von Hippel should be reserved for those cases that show the typical corneal abnormalities of Peters' anomaly but which have no lens abnormalities.

    5. Histologically, endothelium and Descemet's and Bowman's membranes are absent from the cornea centrally. Lens, iris and other abnormalities may or may not be present.
  B. Localized posterior keratoconus
    1. Localized posterior keratoconus consists of central or paracentral, craterlike corneal depressions associated with stromal opacity.

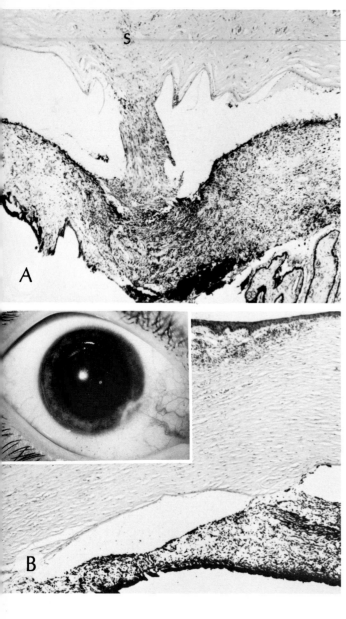

FIG. 8–6. Adherent leukoma. **A.** Fibroblastic proliferation attaches iris to cornea through a gap in Descemet's membrane in 3-week-old wound. Overlying scar (s) present through full thickness of cornea. With organization and shrinkage of fibroblastic membrane scar will look much like scar of adherent leukoma in **B. B.** Peripheral iris adherent to corneal stroma through gap in Descemet's membrane. Overlying stroma scarred. **Inset** shows peripheral adherent leukoma in 12-year-old girl who had accidental perforation of globe (scissors) 5 weeks previously; perforation of cornea repaired same day of injury. Sympathetic uveitis developed 2 days before picture was taken. **A,** H&E, ×21; **B,** H&E, ×28; **inset,** clinical.

FIG. 8–7. Anterior embryotoxon, i.e., arcus juvenilis shown in **inset** in **A.** Patient (28-year-old black woman) had familial hyper-cholesterolemia. Subcutaneous nodule of elbow (xanthoma tuberosum) was biopsied (low magnification in **A**). **B.** Higher magnification of xanthoma tuberosum to show lipid-laden histiocytes (foam cells) and cholesterol clefts. **A,** H&E, ×7; **inset,** clinical; **B,** H&E, ×252.

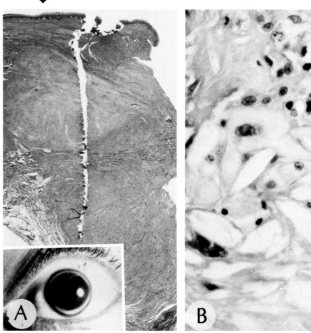

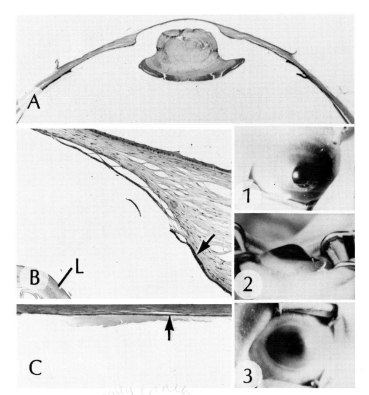

FIG. 8–9. Peters' anomaly. **A. Inset** shows dense leukoma produced by corneal scarring and extensive adherence of iris leaf. Photomicrograph shows central replacement of Bowman's membrane and anterior stroma by scar tissue (*S*). There is continuity between collagenous tissue of iris stroma and posterior corneal stroma (*arrows*), better seen in **B** in enlargement of another section. **B.** Discontinuity of endothelium and Descemet's membrane (*arrows*) is clear. Blending of iris and corneal stroma is seen on left. Sphincter muscle (*SP*) is cut here along its length. **A,** 1.5 μ section, PD, ×50; **inset,** macroscopic; **B,** 1.5 μ section, PD, ×100.

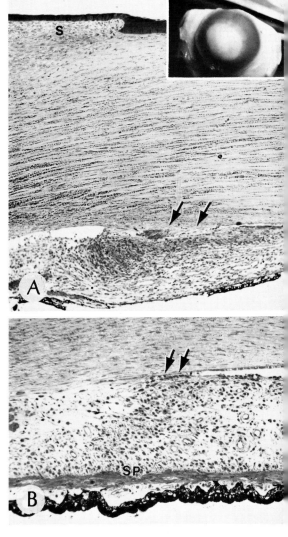

FIG. 8–8. Peters' anomaly. **A.** Anterior segment showing posterior corneal defect, "top hat" appearance of lens and total anterior synechias. **B.** Higher magnification to show termination of endothelium and Descemet's membrane (*arrow*), corneal thinning and localized absence of Bowman's membrane. Lens (*L*) is artifactitiously separated from cornea. **C.** PAS-positive membrane on posterior corneal surface (*arrow*) is lens capsule with underlying adherent cortex, artifactitiously separated from rest of lens (see **B**). Insets **1** and **2** clinical appearance of same eye. Inset **3** shows other eye (OS) of same child with bilateral Peters' anomaly. **A,** H&E, ×5; **B,** H&E, ×21; **C,** PAS, ×130; **inset 1,** clinical, right eye; **inset 2,** clinical, right eye; **inset 3,** clinical, left eye.

The depression involves the posterior corneal surface.

2. Unlike Peters' anomaly, endothelium and Descemet's membrane are present.

3. Typically no other ocular anomalies are present.

4. Mesodermal maldevelopment, infection and trauma all are proposed causes.

5. Histologically the posterior curve of the cornea is abnormal, and the overlying collagen of the corneal stroma is in disarray.

IV. Mesodermal dysgenesis of the cornea and iris includes a wide spectrum of developmental abnormalities ranging from posterior embryotoxon (Axenfeld's anomaly) to extensive anomalous development of the cornea, iris and anterior chamber angle (Rieger's syndrome).* There may be an associated congenital glaucoma, but the presence or absence of glaucoma does not necessarily depend on the degree of malformation. The abnormalities may be congenital, noninfectious and noninherited (e.g., as part of trisomy 13–15); congenital and inherited (e.g., Rieger's syndrome); or congenital and infectious (e.g., rubella syndrome).

A. Posterior embryotoxon or *embryotoxon corneae posterius* (Axenfeld's anomaly) (Fig. 8–10)

* The differentiation of Axenfeld's anomaly and Rieger's syndrome is one of degree and therefore subject to a host of interpretations and classifications. The classification used here is chosen for its simplicity and because it is as close as possible to what Axenfeld and Rieger described originally. Axenfeld in 1920 described a boy with a white annular corneal line about 1.0 mm from the limbus, at the level of Descemet's membrane. At this level a semitransparent opacity was observed between the line and the limbus. From the anterior layer of the poorly developed iris stroma (partial iris coloboma) a number of delicate fibrillae traversed the anterior chamber toward this line. He called the abnormality *embryotoxon corneae posterius*. Axenfeld's patient did not have glaucoma. Rieger in 1935 described a more marked iridocorneal defect in a mother and her two children, showing an autosomal dominant inheritance pattern. In 1941 Rieger showed an association of dental abnormalities, particularly oligodontia or anodontia. Because of the overlapping descriptions of the iridocorneal defect given by Axenfeld and Rieger, Kolker and Hetherington in *Becker-Shaffer's Diagnosis and Therapy of the Glaucomas* suggest not using eponyms, but using the term mesodermal dysgenesis or goniodysgenesis.

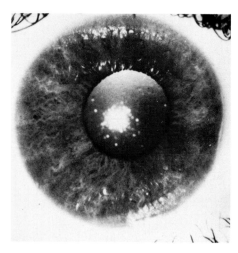

FIG. 8–10. Axenfeld's anomaly (posterior embryotoxon). "Ropy" corneal opacity seen from 2 to 4 o'clock adjacent to limbus. No iris processes or glaucoma present. Other eye was normal. Clinical.

1. Posterior embryotoxon is an enlarged and more centrally located than normal ring of Schwalbe, which is recognized clinically as a bow or ring-shaped opacity in the peripheral cornea.

2. It usually is observed in an otherwise normal eye, or one that shows only a few mesodermal strands of iris tissue bridging the chamber angle to become attached to the "displaced" Schwalbe's ring.

3. Posterior embryotoxon may be accompanied by glaucoma.

4. Dominant autosomal pedigrees, especially with iris involvement, have been reported, but autosomal recessive inheritance also may occur; or it may not be inherited (commonest type).

B. Mesodermal dysgenesis of the iris and cornea (Rieger's syndrome) (Figs. 8–11 and 8–12)

1. The syndrome includes Axenfeld's anomaly together with more marked anomalous development of the iris mesoderm (ectopia of the pupil, dyscoria, slit pupil, severe hypo-

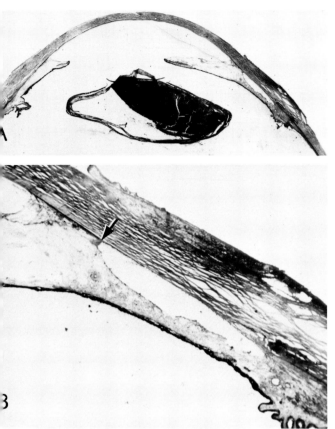

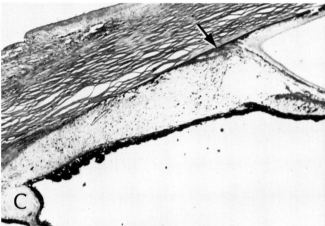

FIG. 8–11. Rieger's syndrome. **A.** Posterior embryotoxon (see *arrows* pointing to central location of Schwalbe's ring in **B** and **C**), iridocorneal processes (marked on left side) and iris hypoplasia are seen. **A,** trichrome, ×6; **B,** trichrome, ×16; **C,** trichrome, ×21.

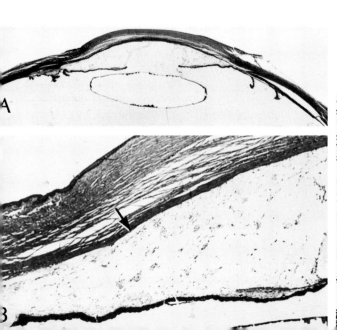

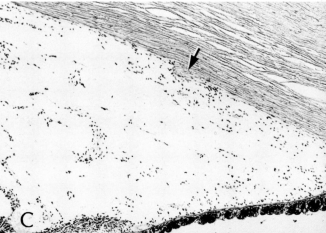

FIG. 8–12. Rieger's syndrome. **A.** Posterior embryotoxon (see *arrows* pointing to central location of Schwalbe's ring in **B** and **C**), marked iridocorneal processes and iris hypoplasia are present. **A,** H&E, ×6; **B,** H&E, ×16; **C,** H&E, ×40.

plasia of the anterior layer of the iris, iris strands bridging the anterior chamber angle, etc.), anterior chamber angle and the limbus generally.
  2. Glaucoma may be present.
  3. Facial, dental, and osseous abnormalities may be present.
  4. It is inherited as an autosomal dominant.
V. Sclerocornea (Fig. 8–13)
  A. The condition, usually bilateral, may involve the peripheral cornea or the whole cornea, with superficial or deep vascularization. The cornea appears white and is difficult to differentiate from sclera.
  B. Nystagmus, strabismus, aniridia, cornea plana, horizontally oval cornea, glaucoma and microphthalmos may be present.
  C. Congenital cerebral dysfunction, deafness, cryptorchism, pulmonary disease, brachycephaly and defects of the face, ears and skin may coexist with sclerocornea.
  D. The cause is unknown.
  E. Histologically the most frequent findings are increased numbers of collagen fibrils of variable diameters, a decrease in diameters of collagen fibrils from the anterior to the posterior layers and a thin Descemet's membrane.

  Sclerocornea is mainly a clinical descriptive term, and it is doubtful if a distinct clinicopathologic entity of sclerocornea exists as a single entity.

VI. Goldenhar's syndrome (Figs. 8–14 and 8–15)
  A. Goldenhar's syndrome is a bilateral condition characterized by epibulbar dermoids, accessory auricular appendages and aural fistulas.
  B. Sometimes it is associated with mandibulofacial dysostosis, phocomelia and renal malformations.
  C. Generally the condition is not inherited and on occasion may be related to first trimester maternal intake of a teratogenic agent.
  D. Histologically the epibulbar dermoids appear the same as when found elsewhere (see p. 526 in Chap. 14).

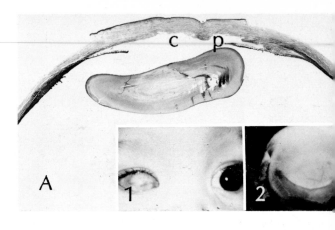

INFLAMMATIONS–NONULCERATIVE

EPITHELIAL KERATITIS

I. Punctate epithelial erosions and keratitis.
  A. Epithelial erosion may be secondary to traumatic, toxic or inflammatory keratitis or to inherited corneal dystrophies such as lattice and Reis-Bücklers and is characterized by damage to the corneal epithelial cells best seen after staining the cornea with fluorescein.
  B. Epithelial keratitis may be caused by the same entities that cause epithelial erosions and is characterized by large areas of epithelial damage that can be seen grossly without the aid of fluorescein.
  C. Histologically, basal cell edema of the epithelium is prominent along with an absence of hemidesmosomes and a separation of the cells from their basement membrane.

SUBEPITHELIAL KERATITIS

I. Epidemic keratoconjunctivitis (Fig. 8–16) is a combined epithelial and subepithelial punctate keratitis caused by adenovirus type 8.

The subepithelial opacities, unlike the fine- or medium-sized ones with adenoviruses types 3, 4 and 7, tend to be coarse like a cluster of tiny bread crumbs. The epithelial component is evanescent. There are many other causes of subepithelial keratitis such as nummular (Dimmer's) keratitis, rosacea, pharyngokeratoconjunctivitis and onchocerciasis.

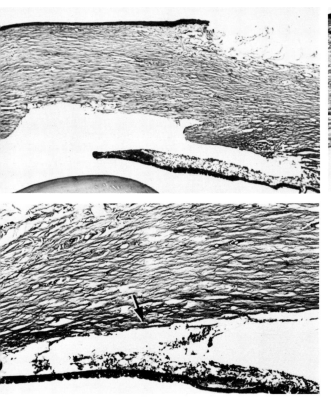

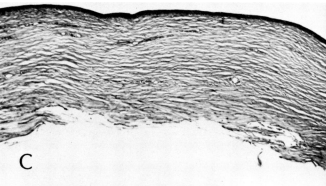

FIG. 8–13. Sclerocornea. **A.** Paracentral (*p*) (see **B**) and central (*c*) (see **C**) absence of endothelium and Descemet's and Bowman's membranes is reminiscent of Peters' anomaly. Peculiar shape of lens due to coloboma of zonules on right side producing notched appearance macroscopically (see Figure 10–1) and "blunted" appearance microscopically (see also Figure 9–4). **Inset 1** shows clinical appearance of right eye before enucleation, and **inset 2** shows eye after enucleation. Sclera and cornea are indistinguishable (sclerocornea). **D.** Iridocorneal processes are present, iris is hypoplastic and Schwalbe's ring (*arrow*) is displaced centrally; findings suggestive of Rieger's syndrome. **A**, PAS, ×6; **inset 1**, clinical; **inset 2**, macroscopic; **B**, PAS, ×21; **C**, PAS, ×28; **D**, PAS, ×40.

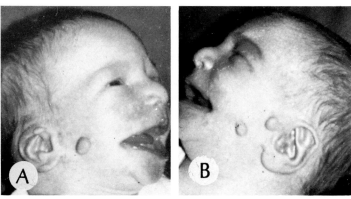

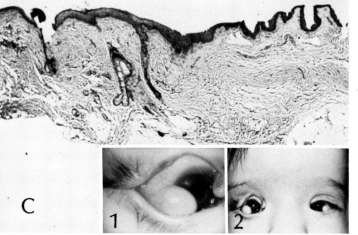

FIG. 8–14. Goldenhar's syndrome. **A** and **B.** Accessory auricular appendages and aural fistulas are shown. **C.** Dermoid composed of epidermis, dermis, epidermal appendages and adipose tissue present in limbal dermoid OD, seen in **insets. Insets 1** and **2** show bilateral dermoids and coloboma of right upper lid. **A,** clinical; **B,** clinical; **C,** H&E, ×16; **inset 1,** clinical, right eye; **inset 2,** clinical, both eyes.

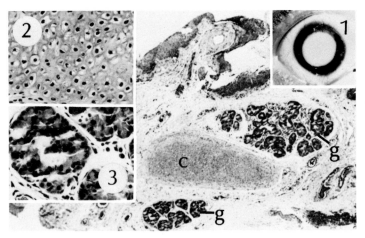

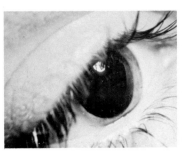

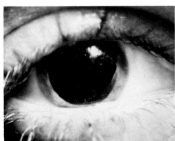

FIG. 8–15. Corneal dermoids unassociated with Goldenhar's syndrome. **Inset 1** shows rare central corneal dermoid. **Main figure** demonstrates cartilage (c) and lacrimal glandlike tissue (g) in corneal limbal dermoid (shown with higher magnification in **insets 2** and **3**). **Main figure,** H&E, ×21; **inset 1,** clinical; **inset 2,** H&E, ×101; **inset 3,** H&E, ×101.

FIG. 8–16. Epidemic keratoconjunctivitis in both eyes with typical subepithelial opacities. Both pictures here are different views of right eye.

II. Trachoma (see p. 241 in Chap. 7).

III. Leprosy (see p. 83 in Chap. 4).

STROMAL (INTERSTITIAL) KERATITIS

I. Syphilis (Fig. 8–17)

   A. Widespread inflammatory infiltrate of the corneal stroma, especially of the deeper layers, is characteristic of luetic keratitis.

   B. An associated anterior uveitis is present in the early stages.

   C. The congenital form:

      1. Generally it is bilateral and develops in the second half of the first decade or in the second decade of life.

      It is rare for it to occur under 5 years of age, but the keratitis may be present even at birth.

      2. Initially the cloudy cornea is a result of inflammatory cell infiltration associated with an anterior uveitis; this is followed by ingrowth of blood vessels just anterior to Descemet's membrane.

Sarcoidosis, tuberculosis, leprosy, syphilis and Cogan's syndrome all can produce a deep interstitial keratitis with deep stromal blood vessels.

      3. The acute inflammation may last 2 to 3 months followed by a regression over many months.

      4. The corneal changes are frequently associated with Hutchinson's teeth and deafness, i.e., *Hutchinson's triad.*

      5. Histologically the cornea is edematous and infiltrated by lymphocytes and plasma cells. Blood vessels are present just anterior to Descemet's membrane. With healing the edema and inflammatory cells disappear, but the blood vessels persist.

D. The acquired form:
1. Generally it is a late manifestation with an average time of appearance of 10 years following the primary luetic infection.
2. Usually it is unilateral and frequently is limited to a sector-shaped area of the cornea.
3. Histologically it has the same appearance as the congenital form.

II. Tuberculosis—see p. 83 in Chapter 4.
III. Sarcoidosis—see p. 101 in Chapter 4.
IV. Nematode-Onchocerciasis (Figs. 8–18 and 8–19)
A. Onchocerciasis is one of the leading causes of blindness in the world.
B. In the acute phase of the infestation there are nummular or snowflake corneal opacities forming a superficial punctate keratitis. A stromal punctate "interstitial" keratitis also may occur.
C. With healing, scar tissue forms in the corneal stroma along with a corneal pannus; the cornea can become completely opaque.
D. Secondary glaucoma with uveitis and peripheral anterior and posterior synechias is a common complication and the main cause of blindness.
E. The disease, which is endemic in Africa and Central America, mainly affects children and young adults.
F. The adult nematode worms, *Onchocerca volvulus*, produce microfilaria, which migrate through skin and subcutaneous tissue (not blood) to reach ocular tissue. The small, black Simulian fly ingests the microfilaria from an in-

fected individual and transmits them to the next human he bites.
G. Histologically the tiny worm is found along with an infiltrate of lymphocytes and plasma cells.

V. Protozoal
A. Leishmaniasis
B. Trypanosomiasis

VI. Viral
A. Herpes simplex (see p. 277 in this chapter).
B. Herpes zoster (see p. 99 in Chap. 4).

VII. Cogan's syndrome
A. Cogan's syndrome consists of non-syphilitic interstitial keratitis and vestibuloauditory involvement.

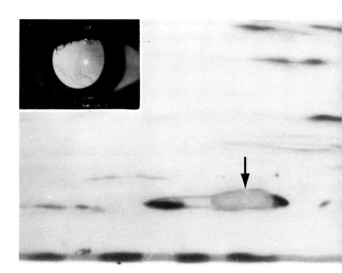

FIG. 8–17. Syphilis. Blood vessel present anterior to Descemet's membrane (*arrow*). **Inset** shows corneal ghost vessel as viewed by fundus reflex in patient with interstitial keratitis and congenital syphilis. **Main figure,** H&E, ×882; **inset,** clinical.

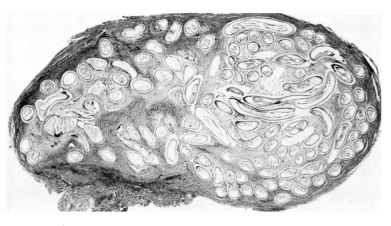

FIG. 8–18. Onchocerciasis. Adult worm of *Onchocerca volvulus* in skin nodule removed from eyelid. H&E, ×6.

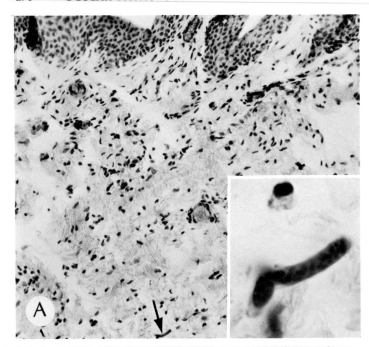

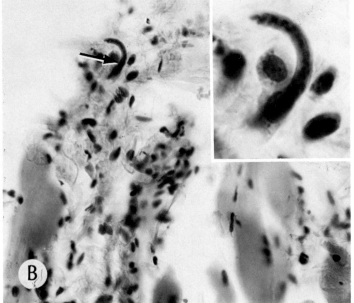

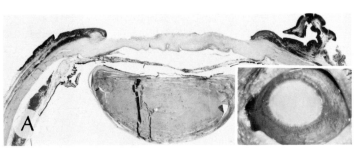

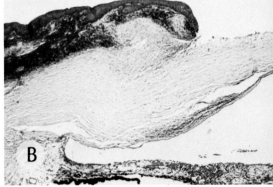

FIG. 8–19. Onchocerciasis. **A.** Microfilaria of *Onchocerca volvulus* (*arrow*) present deep in substantia propria of conjunctiva (seen in **inset** with higher magnification; note tiny size of onchocercal nuclei). **B.** Microfilaria (*arrow*) in orbicularis muscle of upper lid (note tiny size of onchocercal nuclei in higher magnification in **inset**). **A,** H&E, ×180; **inset,** H&E, ×1,100. **B,** H&E, ×360; **inset,** H&E, ×1,100.

FIG. 8–20. Ring ulcer. **A. Inset** shows that spread of ring ulcer in debilitated patient involves most of cornea. Eye removed at autopsy next day. Corneal ulcer involves almost entire surface of cornea. **B.** Higher magnification to show peripheral edge of corneal ulcer. **A,** H&E, ×6; **inset,** clinical; **B,** H&E, ×16.

B. It may be associated with periarteritis nodosa.

VIII. Many other entities such as *Hodgkin's disease*, *lymphogranuloma venereum* and *mycosis fungoides* may cause a secondary stromal keratitis.

INFLAMMATION–ULCERATIVE*

PERIPHERAL

I. Primary

    A. Ring ulcer (Fig. 8–20)

        1. A ring ulcer, i.e., a superficial ulcerated area involving the corneal limbus, most frequently develops in the evolution of superficial marginal keratitis. It may result from coalescence of several marginal ulcers.

        2. A ring ulcer may be associated with acute systemic diseases such as influenza, bacillary dysentery, acute leukemia, scleroderma, systemic lupus erythematosus, periarteritis nodosa, rheumatoid arthritis, Sjögren's syndrome, Wegener's granulomatosis, porphyria, brucellosis, gonococcal arthritis, dengue fever, tuberculosis, hookworm infestation and gold poisoning.

        3. Histologically the corneal area of involvement is infiltrated with neutrophils, lymphocytes and plasma cells.

    B. Ring abscess (Fig. 8–21)

        1. Generally a ring abscess follows trauma to the eye (accidental or surgical). The cornea may not be the initial site of ocular injury.

        2. It starts with a 1 to 2 mm purulent corneal infiltrate in a girdle about 1 mm within clear cornea. A peripheral zone of clear cornea always remains. The central cornea rapidly becomes necrotic and may slough; a panophthalmitis ensues. The eye usually is lost.

        3. An infectious etiology, bacteria or fungus, is the most common cause. It may also occur with collagen disease.

---

* An ulcer is characterized by loss of tissue, inflammation, necrosis, progression and chronicity.

FIG. 8–21. Ring abscess. **A.** Patient had retinal detachment procedure (see Figure 5–51) about 3 weeks previously; corneal ring abscess developed. **B.** Cornea central to ring abscess became necrotic and eye was enucleated. **C.** Ring abscess (*arrows*) with central corneal necrosis and ulceration. **Inset** shows high magnification of cornea specially stained to show myriad fungi. **A,** clinical; **B,** macroscopic; **C,** H&E, ×6; **inset,** Gomori's methenamine silver, ×101.

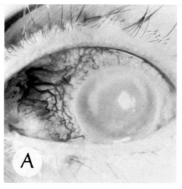

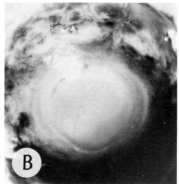

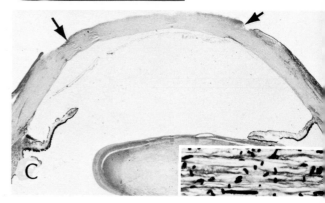

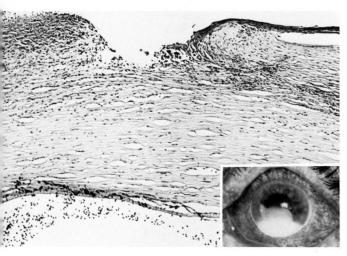

FIG. 8–22. Central corneal ulcer filled with necrotic debris. Polymorphonuclear leukocytes infiltrate cornea and are present in anterior chamber (hypopyon). **Inset** shows corneal ulcer (outlined by fluorescein) and large hypopyon. **Main figure,** H&E, ×40; **inset,** clinical.

FIG. 8–23. Herpes simplex. **A.** Light micrograph of corneal epithelium near edge of ulcer. Note many intranuclear inclusions (*arrows*). **Inset** shows typical dendritic ulcer as delineated by fluorescein. **B.** By electron microscopy virus particles (*arrows*) identical with those of Herpes simplex are present in nucleus (*N*) as well as within cytoplasm (in **C**). Some particles are empty capsids, while others are complete, containing nucleoids. Note the larger size of the cytoplasmic virions. **A,** H&E, ×350; **B,** ×44,000; **C,** ×40,000.
▼

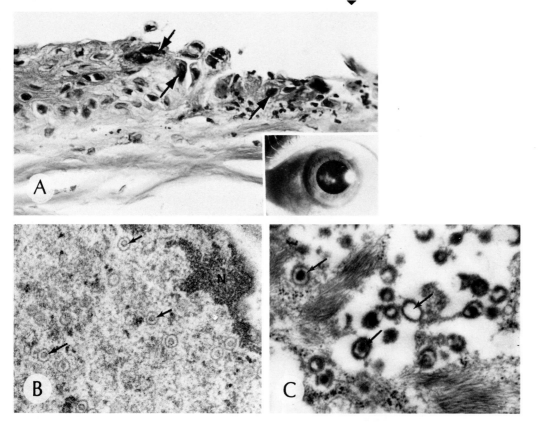

4. Histologically the cornea is infiltrated with polymorphonuclear leukocytes and contains necrotic debris.

II. Secondary *allergic*
  A. Marginal (catarrhal) ulcer
    1. Marginal ulcer usually is superficial, single and localized at the limbus or just within the clear cornea. It may become circumferential to form a superficial marginal keratitis or even a ring ulcer.
    2. Generally it is a secondary allergic reaction to toxins or allergens of bacterial conjunctival infections, especially staphylococcus, i.e., an endogenous sensitization to bacterial protein.
    3. It may occur secondary to such systemic diseases as Wegener's granulomatosis, periarteritis nodosa, systemic lupus erythematosis, scleroderma or bacillary dysentery.
    4. Histologically lymphocytes and plasma cells predominate.
  B. Phlyctenular ulcer
    1. A phlyctenular ulcer appears early as a whitish elevation within a hyperemic limbus. The elevation then develops a central, gray crater.
    2. It occurs mainly in children in the first and second decades of life.
    3. Generally it is a secondary allergic reaction to toxins or allergens of conjunctival infections, especially tuberculosis and staphylococcus, i.e., an endogenous sensitization to bacterial protein.
    4. Histologically lymphocytes and plasma cells predominate.

CENTRAL

I. Bacterial (Fig. 8–22)—cause a purulent infiltrate of polymorphonuclear leukocytes.
  A. Pneumococcus
  B. *β-Hemolytic streptococcus*
  C. *Pseudomonas aeruginosa*
  D. *Klebsiella pneumoniae* (Friedlander)
  E. Petit's diplobacillus
  F. *Staphylococcus aureus*
    G. Hemophilus
II. Viral
  A. Herpes simplex (Figs. 8–23 and 8–24)
    1. Herpes simplex is the most common cause of central corneal ulcer. Clinically it presents with a characteristic dendritic ulcer.

    Dendritic keratitis also may occur rarely with Herpes zoster.

    2. It is an epithelial infection caused by the Herpes simplex virus and is characterized by intranuclear epithelial inclusion bodies.
    3. Complications—spread to stroma, especially with recurrence:
      a. Disciform keratitis is a chronic, localized, discoid opacity.
      b. Bullous keratopathy (*metaherpetic phase*)—see p. 278 in Chapter 8.
      c. Virus may or may not be responsible for stromal phase. It may be an allergic reaction although virus particles within keratocytes, compatible with those of Herpes simplex, have been found electron microscopically.
    4. Histologically lymphocytes and plasma cells predominate along with intranuclear epithelial inclusion bodies. By electron microscopy viral particles are found in the epithelial nucleus and cytoplasm. With deep involvement multinucleated giant cells may be found within the corneal stroma or even in the anterior chamber or iris.
  B. Vaccinia
  C. Trachoma (see p. 241 in Chap. 7).
III. Mycotic (Fig. 8–25)
  A. Mycotic keratitis is characterized clinically by a "dry" main lesion, which may be accompanied by satellite lesions. Hypopyon is common.
  B. Fungus is most readily found in scrapings from viable tissue at the margin and depths of the ulcer rather than in the necrotic central debris.
  C. The keratitis may be caused by molds (e.g., *Aspergillus*) or yeasts (e.g., *Candida*).
  D. Generally fungal keratitis is a complication of trauma with contamination by plant or animal matter, e.g., as in farmers and fruit pickers.
  E. Histologically the inflammatory infil-

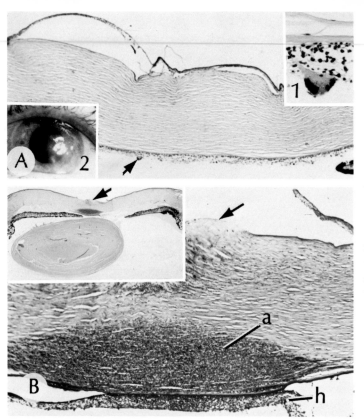

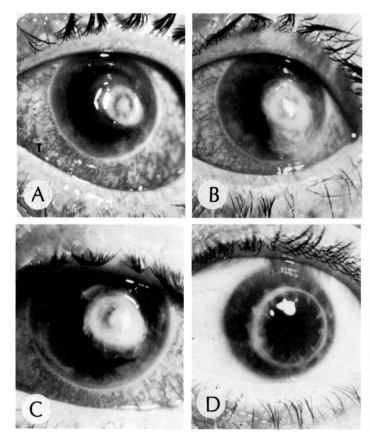

FIG. 8–24. Herpes simplex. **A.** Chronic condition with development of bullous keratopathy (metaherpetic phase). Anterior chamber inflammatory reaction contains multinucleated inflammatory giant cells (*arrow*), shown with higher magnification in **inset 1. Inset 2** shows clinical appearance of metaherpetic lesion. **B.** Bullous keratopathy has ulcerated (*arrow* in **main figure** and in **inset.**) Corneal abscess (a) and hypopyon (h) are present. Note in **inset** that lens is subluxated to left due to loss of zonula-lens attachments on right, resulting in "blunted" appearance of right side of lens. **A,** H&E, ×16; **inset 1,** H&E, ×101; **inset 2,** clinical; **B,** PAS, ×28; **inset,** H&E, ×4.

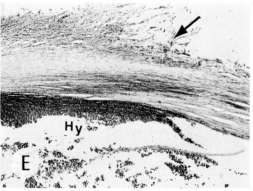

FIG. 8–25. Myotic ulcer. **A, B** and **C** show progression of fungal corneal ulcer; **D** shows same eye after penetrating graft. **E.** Edge of mycotic ulcer. Note ragged appearance of the stromal lamellas (*arrow*) and heavy infiltration with cells (polymorphs). Organism is most easily found and is generally viable (i.e., proper location to obtain scraping for culture) in area of ulcer periphery. *Hy,* hypopyon. **F.** Higher power of ulcer edge seen in **E** and stained with PAS. Stromal lamellas are infiltrated with polymorphs and widely invaded by branching, septate hyphae of mold. **A,** clinical; **B,** clinical; **C,** clinical; **D,** clinical; **E,** H&E, ×35; **F,** PAS, ×400.

trate may be granulomatous, chronic nongranulomatous, or, rarely, purulent.

SEQUELAE

  I. Descemetocele (Fig. 8–26)
  II. Ectasia, i.e., thinned, protruding area.
 III. Staphyloma, i.e., ectasia lined by uveal tissue, usually iris.
 IV. Cicatrization, i.e., scarring.
  V. Adherent leukoma, i.e., corneal perforating scar with iris adherent to posterior corneal surface.

INJURIES

See Chapter 5.

DEGENERATIONS

Degenerations may be unilateral or bilateral and are secondary phenomena following, or resulting from previous disease, i.e., ocular "fingerprints" left by a prior disease.

EPITHELIAL

  I. Keratitis sicca—see p. 522 in Chapter 14.
   A. The watery part of the tear secretion is lacking, and widespread corneal epithelial punctate erosions develop in exposed areas.
   B. Epithelial filaments (*filamentary keratitis*) (Fig. 8–27) may develop.

     Filamentary keratitis may be found in such conditions as Sjögren's syndrome, superior limbic keratoconjunctivitis and viral infections (adenovirus; Herpes simplex, vaccinia) and following cataract extraction.

   C. Keratitis sicca may be related to *Sjögren's syndrome*, which consists of keratoconjunctivitis sicca, xerostomia and rheumatoid arthritis.
   D. Histologically filaments composed of degenerated epithelial cells and mucus are seen.
 II. Recurrent erosion
   A. In recurrent erosion the epithelium forms small blebs and then desquamates in recurring cycles.

     Frequently the blebs rupture on opening the eyelids in the morning. This leads to the common complaint of sharp, severe pain on awakening with the pain subsiding as the day progresses.

   B. Generally the condition follows "incomplete" healing of traumatic corneal abrasion.
   C. It may be inherited as an autosomal dominant, but most are not inherited.
   D. The cause is uncertain but seems to be due to a defect in the epithelium producing a "proper" basement membrane.
 III. Keratomalacia
   A. Keratomalacia is characterized by night blindness and diffuse, excessive keratinization of mucous membrane epithelia including the cornea and conjunctiva (*xerophthalmia*).
   B. It occurs most commonly in children.
   C. The condition may proceed to hypopyon ulcer, corneal necrosis and panophthalmitis.
   D. It is due to a deficiency of vitamin A.
   E. Bitot's spot (Fig. 8–28)
     1. Bitot's spot is a localized form of keratomalacia, usually involving the limbus, with a thickened, bubbly appearance to the involved area.
     2. It may or may not be associated with a vitamin A deficiency.
     3. Young male children are most commonly affected.
     4. Bacteria of *Corynebacterium xerosis* are found in great numbers on the lesion.

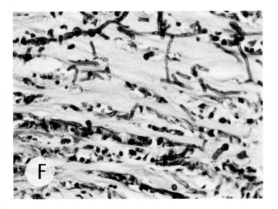

(handwritten note) (hypervitaminosis A : pseudotumor & optic atrophy

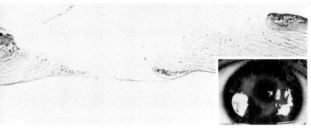

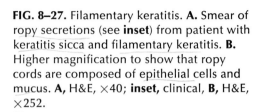

FIG. 8–26. Descemetocele shown in **inset.** Photomicrograph shows corneal ulcer eroded completely through stroma so that only Descemet's membrane is left. Intraocular pressure will cause Descemet's membrane to balloon forward, forming a descemetocele. **Main figure,** PAS, ×21; **inset,** clinical.

FIG. 8–27. Filamentary keratitis. **A.** Smear of ropy secretions (see **inset**) from patient with keratitis sicca and filamentary keratitis. **B.** Higher magnification to show that ropy cords are composed of epithelial cells and mucus. **A,** H&E, ×40; **inset,** clinical, **B,** H&E, ×252.

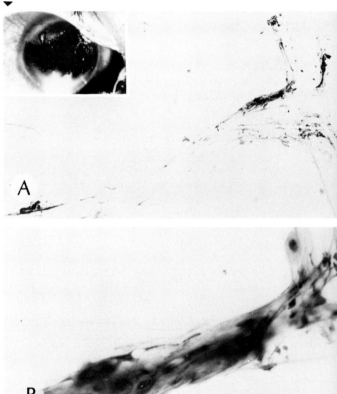

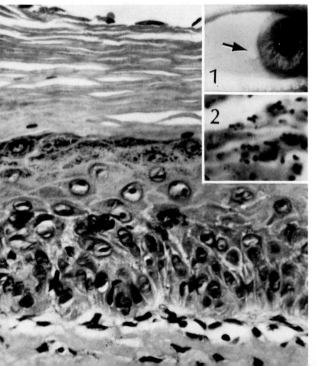

FIG. 8–28. Bitot's spot. Conjunctival epithelium shows hyperkeratosis. Note prominent granular cell layer. **Inset 1** shows clinical appearance (*arrow*). **Inset 2** demonstrates pleomorphic gram-positive rods, compatible with diphtheroids, clustered around keratin debris. **Main figure,** H&E, ×200; **inset 1,** clinical; **inset 2,** Mac Callum-Goodpasture, ×400.

5. Histologically the epithelium is thickened and keratinized, in extreme cases appearing as skin epithelium with rete pegs.

IV. Neuroparalytic keratopathy
   A. Early neuroparalytic keratopathy may resemble recurrent erosion, but generally it progresses to almost total corneal epithelial desquamation.
   B. Frequently it is complicated by secondary infection leading ultimately to perforation.
   C. The condition is due to a lesion anywhere along the course of the ophthalmic division of the 5th cranial nerve. It generally runs a chronic, slow course.

V. Exposure of the cornea due to any cause can lead to epidermidalization (Fig. 8–29) and scarring.

STROMAL

I. Arcus senilis (Gerontoxon) (Fig. 8–30)
   A. Lipid deposit is limited to the peripheral cornea.
      1. Although annular in the late stage, it starts earliest at the inferior, then the superior, pole of the cornea.
      2. The lipid first concentrates in the area of Descemet's membrane, then in the area of Bowman's, forming

two triangles apex to apex (both clinically and histologically).

Rarely lipid accumulates in such large quantities that it may extend into the visual axis ("primary lipoidal dystrophy" of the cornea), a condition that appears to be related to the corneal dystrophy of Schnyder (see p. 302 in this chapter).

   B. Arcus senilis may have a recessive inheritance pattern and is not generally related to serum lipids or cholesterol.
   C. Histologically (and clinically) a narrow, peripheral ring of lipid deposit with a more peripheral, clear corneal area is characteristic. The peripheral margin of the arcus is sharply defined, whereas the central margin is less discrete. Histologically (and clinically) it appears identical to an arcus juvenilis (see p. 265 in this chapter).

Histologically a similar concentration of lipid is demonstrable in the superficial and deep layers of the sclera posterior to the vascular limbal region, which is free of lipid. The retrolimbal zone of fatty infiltration, being present in sclera, is of course not visible clinically.

II. Pterygium (Figs. 8–31 and 8–32)
   A. The conjunctival component is identical histologically to *pinguecula* (see p. 246 in Chap. 7).
   B. Generally it develops nasally, rarely temporally, and is most often bilateral. The cause is unknown.
   C. Histologically the characteristic feature is the invasion of superficial cornea preceded by dissolution of Bowman's membrane.

III. Senile marginal degeneration of Fuchs (Terrien's ulcer; chronic peripheral furrow-keratitis; symmetric marginal dystrophy; gutter degeneration) (Fig. 8–33)

   A. The lesion, a limbal depression or gutter, starts superiorly and spreads circumferentially, rarely reaching inferiorly, and develops very slowly, often taking 10 to 20 years.

FIG. 8–29. Epidermidalization of cornea in patient with exposure keratitis is characterized by rete peg formation and keratinization of corneal epithelium. H&E, ×69.

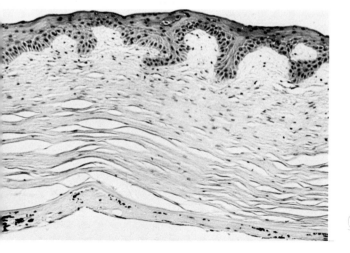

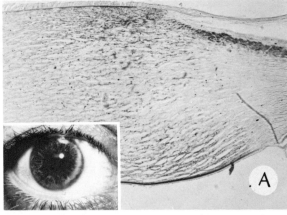

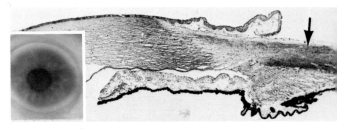

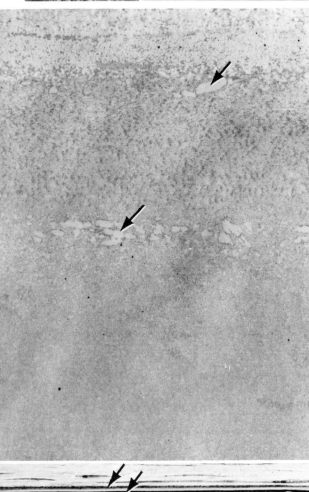

FIG. 8–30. Arcus senilis. A. Inset shows segment of whitish ring in corneal periphery separated from limbus by clear cornea. Photomicrograph stained for fat shows lipids concentrated in anterior and posterior stroma as two triangles apex to apex toward midstroma. Bowman's and Descemet's membranes are infiltrated heavily. **B.** Similar lipoidal infiltration occurs within sclera (*arrow*) posterior to vascular limbal region, which is relatively free of lipoidal infiltration. **Inset** shows arcus senilis in autopsy eye from which main section was made. **C. Inset** shows dual line (*arrows*) of lipoidal infiltration often found in Descemet's membrane. Larger micrograph is equivalent view as seen by electron microscopy. *Arrows* indicate sites of lipoidal deposits in two appropriate planes. **A,** oil red-O, ×35; **inset,** clinical. **B,** oil red-O, ×8; **inset,** macroscopic. **C,** ×16,500; **inset,** oil red-O, ×30.

FIG. 8–31. Pterygium. A. Inset shows typical clinical appearance of pterygium. Photomicrograph demonstrates basophilic degeneration of subepithelial tissue and "dissolution" of Bowman's membrane (*arrow*). **B.** Area of basophilic degeneration stains deeply with stain for elastic tissue. **A,** H&E, ×101; **inset,** clinical; **B,** elastica, ×101. ▶

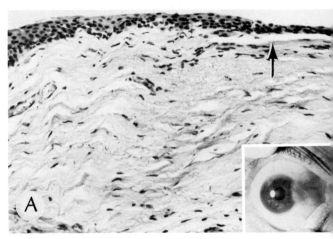

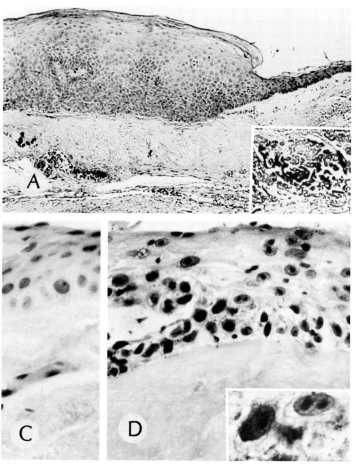

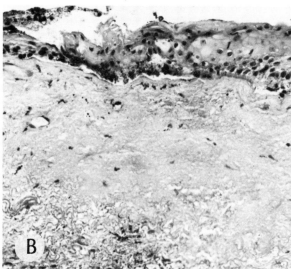

FIG. 8–32. Pterygium with associated changes. **A.** Overlying epithelium shows mild dysplastic changes. **Inset** shows positive staining of subepithelial tissue with stain used to demonstrate elastic tissue. **B.** Typical basophilic degeneration (senile elastosis) in subepithelial tissue of pterygium. Overlying epithelium appears normal in **C** but contains intracellular inclusions (viral?) in **D,** shown at higher magnification in **inset. A,** H&E, ×40; **inset,** elastica, ×69; **B,** H&E, ×136; **C,** H&E, ×252; **D,** H&E, ×252; **inset,** H&E, ×630.

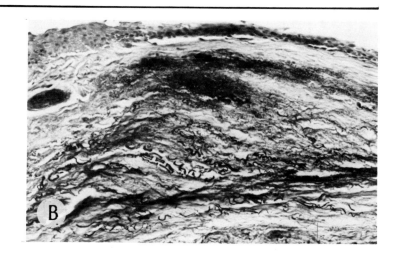

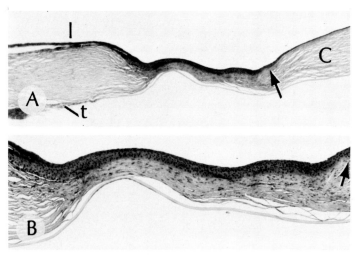

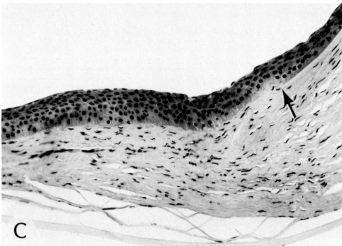

FIG. 8–33. Senile marginal degeneration of Fuchs (Terrien's ulcer). **A, B** and **C** show different magnifications of Terrien's ulcer to show stromal thinning near limbus (**l**), thickened epithelium and loss of Bowman's membrane (*arrows* show end of membrane): *t*, trabecular meshwork; **C,** cornea. **A,** H&E, ×16; **B,** H&E, ×40; **C,** H&E, ×101.

FIG. 8–34. Band keratopathy. Bowman's membrane (*b*) shows deposit of granular material (calcium). Pannus (*P*) present between Bowman's membrane and epithelium. Clinical **insets 1** and **2** show early band keratopathy and posterior synechias (before, **1,** and after, **2,** dilatation) in patient with chronic uveitis. **Insets 3** (enucleated eye) and **4** (clinical) show advanced band keratopathy. **Main figure,** H&E, ×252; **inset 1,** clinical before dilatation; **inset 2,** clinical after dilatation; **inset 3,** macroscopic; **inset 4,** clinical.
▼

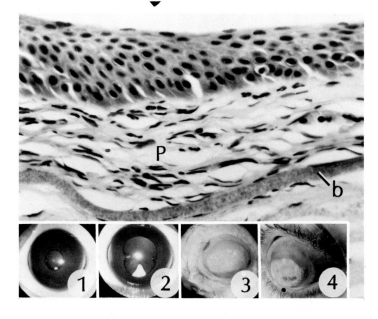

B. The peripheral involvement is similar in location to an arcus senilis.

C. The central wall is very steep, and the peripheral wall slopes gradually.

D. The epithelium remains intact, but the underlying stroma thins and the gutter widens. The base of the gutter later becomes vascularized.

E. The floor may become so thin that the intraocular pressure produces an ectasia instead of a gutter. Rarely the lesion may perforate.

F. The cause is unknown, but degenerative and hypersensitivity causes have been proposed.

Similar lesions may be seen in rheumatoid arthritis and Sjögren's syndrome, but differ from senile marginal degeneration in that they usually are located inferiorly, are not vascularized and rarely encircle the cornea.

G. Histologically the main feature is a peripheral corneal stromal thinning. When inflammatory cells are present, they are lymphocytes and plasma cells.

IV. Band keratopathy (Figs. 8–34 and 8–35)

A. Band keratopathy generally starts in the nasal and temporal periphery with a translucent area at the level of Bowman's membrane; the semiopaque area contains characteristic circular clear areas.

B. The extreme peripheral cornea remains clear, but the central cornea ultimately may become involved.

C. A deposition of calcium salts on and in Bowman's membrane is apparently related to abnormal epithelial activity.

D. Band keratopathy may be secondary to primary hyperparathyroidism; increased vitamin D absorption; chronic renal failure; ocular disease, especially uveitis and particularly uveitis associated with Still's disease; long-standing glaucoma; and some forms of nonspecific superficial injury, e.g., experimental laser injury.

E. Histologically, in H&E-stained sections a blue, granular material (calcium salts) is seen in and around Bowman's membrane.

V. Elastotic degeneration (Labrador keratopathy; Bietti's nodular hyaline band-shaped keratopathy; chronic actinic keratopathy; climatic droplet keratopathy; proteinaceous corneal degeneration) (Fig. 8–36)

A. "Oil droplet" or "hyalinelike" deposits may occur in the superficial corneal stroma, usually bilaterally, in a variety of chronic ocular and corneal disorders having in common a relationship to climate, i.e., outdoor exposure.

B. The condition may result from the cumulative effect of chronic actinic irradiation, presumably ultraviolet irradiation.

C. Histologically, granules and concretions of variable size and shape are located in the superficial stroma and in and around Bowman's membrane. The deposits resemble most the degenerated connective tissue of pingueculas and are considered a form of elastotic degeneration of collagen.

VI. Salzmann's nodular degeneration

A. The condition, an elevated white or yellow corneal area, is unilateral, occurs mainly in women and is superimposed on an area of old corneal injury, especially on the edge of an old pannus.

B. Histologically the epithelium shows areas of both hypertrophy and atrophy with a marked increase of subepithelial basement membrane material.

VII. Lipid keratopathy (Fig. 8–37)

A. Lipid keratopathy may be unilateral or bilateral and follows old injury, especially surgical. It appears as a nodular yellow, often elevated, corneal infiltrate.

B. Histologically the lipid deposition is located mainly in a thick pannus between Bowman's membrane and epithelium.

Lipid keratopathy and primary lipoidal degeneration (Fig. 8–38) are related. Primary lipoidal degeneration seems to be an exaggeration of an arcus senilis.

VIII. Amyloid (Fig. 8–39)—see p. 248 in Chapter 7.

A. Secondary amyloidosis is found rarely as an isolated corneal degeneration.

B. It has been described as secondary to

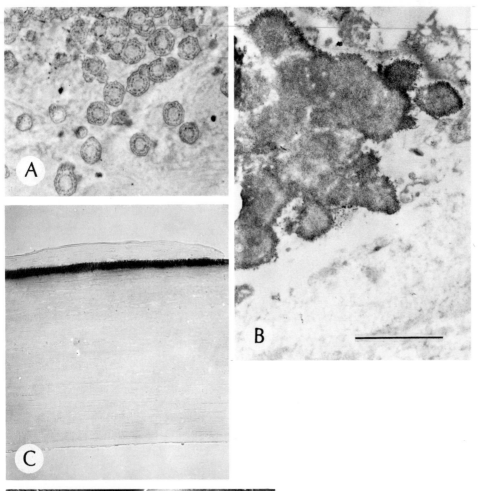

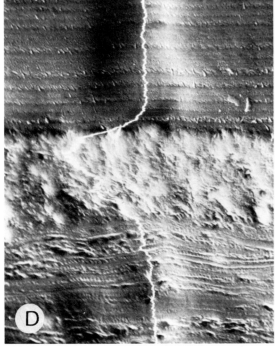

FIG. 8–35. Band keratopathy. **A.** Numerous small calcific spherules produced beneath corneal epithelium in rabbit eye with mild injury from CO_2 laser. **B.** Sample of calcified Bowman's membrane in human band keratopathy. Spherules have coalesced into conglomerate or mass of calcific material. **C.** Band keratopathy stained to demonstrate calcium. **D.** Human band keratopathy. Calcium line scan (i.e., calcium concentration line) across scanning electron micrograph of specimen. Epithelium (missing) is on top, superficial stromal lamellas on bottom. Section is oriented to correspond with **C.** **A,** ×16,500; **B,** ×24,000; **C,** alizarin red, ×145; **D,** ×2,150.

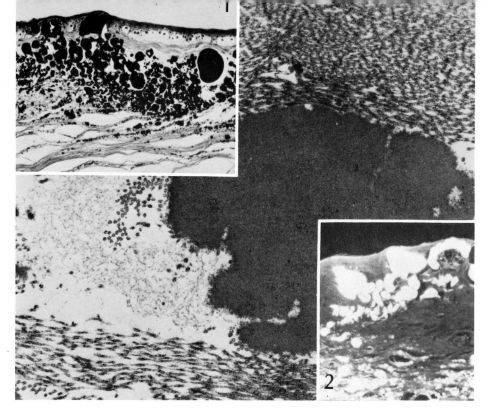

FIG. 8–36. Elastotic degeneration. **Inset 1** shows that granules, whether in epithelium, Bowman's membrane or stroma, stain well with stains that demonstrate elastic tissue. **Inset 2** shows that corneal deposits produce bright yellow autofluorescence when stimulated with blue or near ultraviolet light. Electron micrograph shows that single granule is dense with a suggestion of blending with some of adjacent collagen fibrils. Application of silver tetraphenylporphine sulfonate (Ag-TPPS) stain did not enhance the density, nor does the granule digest with elastase in such "elastotic" degenerations. **Main figure,** ×15,750; **inset 1,** elastica, ×85; **inset 2,** unstained, ×160.

FIG. 8–37. Lipid keratopathy. **A.** Patient (**inset**) had pterygium surgery on both eyes about 30 years previously. Both eyes developed *secondary* lipid degeneration, and corneal graft was performed on the right eye. Lipid in form of globules and cholesterol clefts present in thick pannus between Bowman's membrane (*arrows*) and epithelium. Corneal stroma normal (folding is artifact). **B** and **C** are higher magnifications to show lipid-containing pannus (*p*) anterior to Bowman's membrane (*b*) and normal appearing corneal stroma (*s*). **A,** H&E, ×16; **inset,** clinical; **B,** trichrome, ×40; **C,** trichrome, ×101.

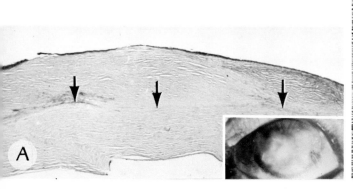

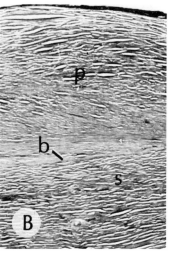

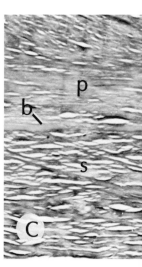

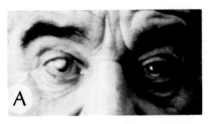

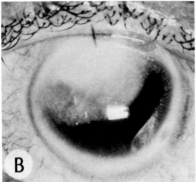

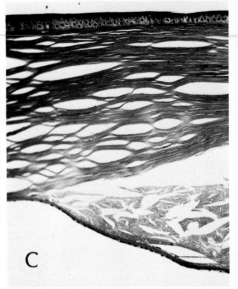

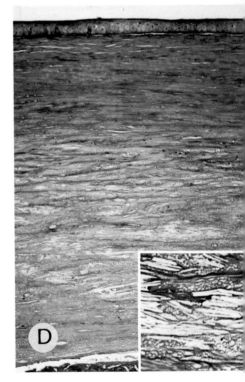

FIG. 8–38. *Primary* lipoidal degeneration of cornea. **A.** Note corneal opacity in right eye and dense arcus senilis in left cornea. **B.** Continuity of dense yellowish white mass with very dense arcus senilis is more clearly seen in enlarged photo of right eye. **C.** Histologically mass of material containing clefts (cholesterol crystals) has dissected Descemet's membrane from stroma. **D.** Less severely involved portion of corneal stroma shows lack of vascularization and accumulation of cholesterol crystal clefts in deeper stromal layers (see enlarged view in **inset**). **A,** clinical, both eyes; **B,** clinical, right eye; **C,** H&E, ×100; **D,** 1.5 μ section, PD, ×110; **inset,** 1.5 μ section, PD, ×530.

different ocular diseases, e.g., retrolental fibroplasia and penetrating injury.

C. Histology—see p. 248 in Chapter 7.

IX. Limbus girdle of Vogt

    A. The limbus girdle of Vogt appears as a symmetrical, yellowish white, corneal opacity forming a half-moonlike arc running concentrically within the limbus superficially in the interpalpebral fissure zone, most commonly nasally.

    B. Histologically Bowman's membrane and superficial stroma are replaced largely by basophilic, granular deposits.

X. Mooren's ulcer (chronic serpiginous ulcer)

    A. About 25 percent of the cases are bilateral. The cause is unknown.

    B. The ulcer starts in the peripheral cornea and spreads in three directions:

        1. Most rapid movement is centrally with the leading edge both de-epithelialized and undermined.

        2. Moves circumferentially

        3. Slowest movement toward sclera

    C. It may be relentlessly progressive or self-limiting.

    D. Histologically the cornea is infiltrated by lymphocytes and plasma cells, and there is a loss of stroma corresponding to the clinical configuration.

XI. Dellen

    A. A delle is a reversible, localized area

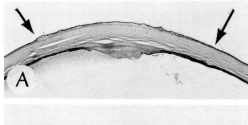
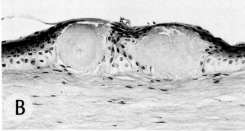
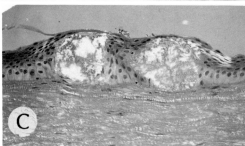

FIG. 8–39. Amyloid. **A.** Ring (*arrows*) of intraepithelial deposits in case of chronic glaucoma secondary to retrolental fibroplasia. **B.** Higher power of intraepithelial deposits. **C.** Birefringence is easily elicited with polarized light. All other criteria for amyloid are present, viz., metachromasia, Congo red positivity, fluorescence with thioflavine-T and ultraviolet light, dichroism and filamentary composition by electron microscopy. **A,** H&E, ×9; **B,** H&E, ×145; **C,** H&E, polarized, ×145.

1. The condition is inherited as an autosomal dominant and appears in the first or second year of life.
2. Myriads of tiny, fine, punctate vacuoles are present within the corneal epithelium. These rarely give visual problems until later in life, and then only on rare occasions.
3. The involved corneas are prone to recurrent irritations.
4. Histologically, increased amounts of epithelial basement membrane may be variably present between the epithelium and Bowman's membrane, and may protrude irregularly into the epithelium. By electron microscopy abnormal epithelial cells are seen and are recognizable by their content of a "peculiar substance," which appears to account for the diastase-resistant PAS positivity of the abnormal cells.

The cells with peculiar substance degenerate forming the tiny epithelial vacuoles that appear relatively transparent on retroillumination by slit-lamp examination. The epithelial cells in general contain an increased amount of glycogen due presumably to a more rapid turnover of cells.

of corneal stromal dehydration and corneal thinning due to a break in the continuity of the tear film layer secondary to elevation of surrounding structures, e.g., with pterygium, filtering bleb, suture granuloma or limbal tumor.
B. The histology is presumably a shrinkage or collapse of the stromal tissues due to dehydration.

DYSTROPHIES

These are primary, usually inherited bilateral disorders with fairly equal involvement of the corneas.

EPITHELIAL

I. Heredofamilial—primary in cornea.
  A. Meesmann's (Figs. 8–40 and 8–41) and Stocker Holt are probably the same dystrophy.
  B. Dot, fingerprint and geographic patterns (microcystic dystrophy) (Figs. 8–42 through 8–44)
    1. The condition occurs mainly in otherwise healthy persons.
    2. Clinically at least three pathologic configurations may be found, or any combinations thereof:

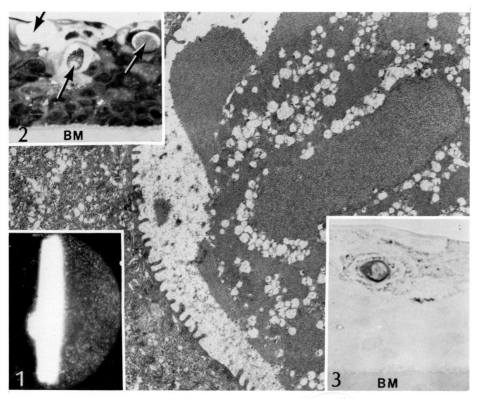

FIG. 8–40. Meesmann's dystrophy. **Inset 1** shows clinical appearances of dystrophy by retroillumination. **Inset 2** shows intra-epithelial cyst with content (right *arrow*), cyst containing cell with granular material (central *arrow*) and cyst opening onto epithelial surface (left *arrow*). Electron micrograph shows edge of single cyst. Cyst content is composed of masses of "peculiar substance" containing myriad tiny vacuoles. As seen in **inset 3,** cyst content is PAS-positive, diastase-resistant, as are many intracytoplasmic granules in adjacent cells. *BM,* Bowman's membrane. **Main figure,** ×7,200; **inset 1,** clinical; **inset 2,** 1.5 μ section, toluidine blue, ×395; **inset 3,** PAS, ×675.

FIG. 8–41. Meesmann's dystrophy. **A.** Cell containing characteristic "peculiar sub-stance" (*PS*) has reached most superficial layer of epithelium without completely degenerating into cystoid space. **B.** Cystoid space may reach surface and open, dis-charging its contents, thus forming short-lived pit. Such pits would account for some superficial punctate staining with fluorescein that is present clinically. **C.** Cell filled with peculiar substance (*PS*) attached normally by desmosomes (*arrows*) to adjacent, relatively normal cell on left. Note continuity of tono-filaments of desmosome with filamentary peculiar substance suggesting primary degeneration involving cytoplasmic fila-ments or "cytoskeleton" of epithelial cell. Involvement of desmosomes would then release degenerating cell to form microcyst. Although peculiar substance has been seen in basal cells, it becomes prominent in more superficial layers. **A,** ×22,500; **B,** ×7,200; **C,** ×42,000.

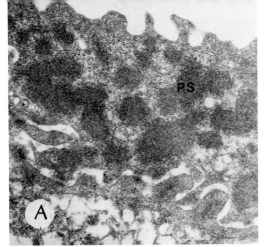

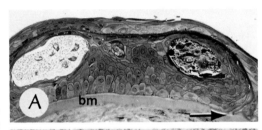

FIG. 8–42. Dot pattern. **A.** Two large intra-epithelial cysts and portion of third contain debris. They are surrounded by anomalous basement membrane continuous with normally positioned epithelial basement membrane (*arrow*). *bm*, Bowman's membrane. **B.** Electron micrograph shows cyst contents to consist of otherwise normal, desquamating surface epithelial cells (*EP*). *N*, nucleus of flattened epithelial cell near inverted surface. **A,** 1.5 μ section, PD, ×165; **B,** ×6,500.

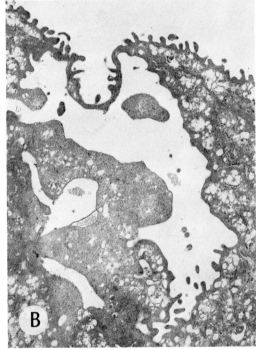

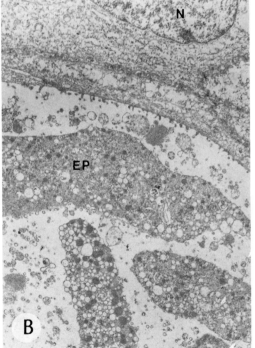

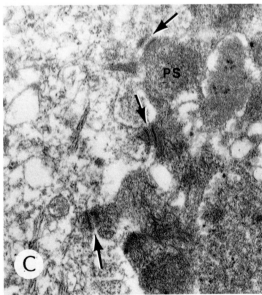

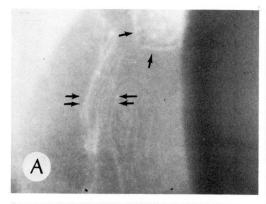

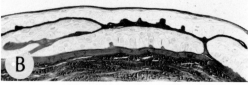

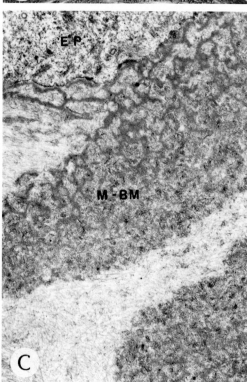

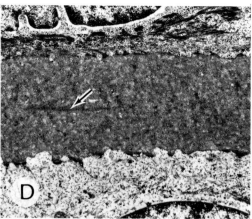

FIG. 8–43. Fingerprint pattern. **A.** Slit lamp photograph of fingerprint pattern (double *arrows*) as seen clinically. Single *arrows* indicate site of biopsy. **B.** Photomicrograph shows extensive intraepithelial pattern produced by aberrant production of basement membrane materials. **C.** Basement membrane consists of two separate multilaminar basement membranes (*M-BM*) produced by aberrant basal cells (*EP*). Collagenous fibrils separate two basement membranes as well as occasional foci of epithelial cells from their own multilaminar basement membrane. **D.** Apposition of adjacent multilaminar basement membranes obliterates intervening space. Separation continues to be identified by linear densities (*arrow*). **A,** clinical; **B,** 1.5 μ section, PD, ×145; **C,** ×16,500; **D,** ×12,000.

(inverted basal cells)

FIG. 8–44. Map pattern. **A.** Map or geographic patterns consist of mixture of accumulating subepithelial basement membrane (*arrows*) and collagenous tissue; the latter resembles subepithelial fibrous plaque. **B.** By electron microscopy multilaminar nature of irregular whorls of basement membrane are seen (*M-BM*). Collagenous fibrils (*C*) are interspersed between epithelial cells and basement membrane as well as throughout whorls of basement membrane. *EP,* basal cells of epithelium. **A,** 1.5 μ section, PD, ×350; **B,** ×7,500.

a. Groups of tiny, round or comma-shaped, grayish white, superficial epithelial opacities seen in the pupillary zones of both eyes.

b. A fingerprint pattern of sinuous, translucent lines, best seen with retroillumination.

c. A geographic or maplike disturbance, best seen on oblique illumination.

3. The hereditary pattern is uncertain.

4. Histologically three corresponding patterns can be observed:

a. The grayish dots represent small cystoid spaces in the epithelium

desquamated epithelial cells

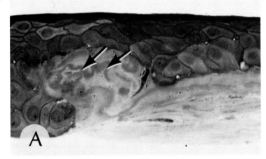

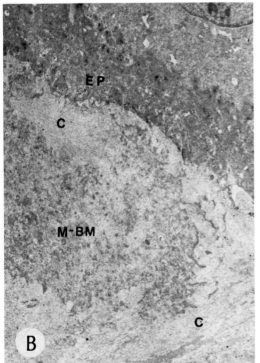

into which otherwise normal, superficial corneal epithelial cells desquamate.

Microcystic dystrophy is differentiated easily from Meesmann's dystrophy in that in the former the epithelial cells are not morphologically abnormal and contain a normal amount of glycogen.

b.m.

b. The fingerprint pattern is formed by production of abnormally large quantities of multilaminar basement membrane both by normally positioned and by inverted basal epithelial cells. The latter cells have migrated into the more superficial layers of the epithelium.

b.m. coll.

c. The map pattern is produced beneath the epithelium by elaboration of both multilaminar basement membrane and collagenous material by the basal epithelial cells and by keratocytes that have migrated from the superficial stroma.

II. Heredofamilial—secondary to systemic disease

A. Fabry's disease (angiokeratoma corporis diffusum) (Fig. 8–45)—see Table 11–2, p. 445 in Chapter 11.

sphingo-lipid

1. The typical macular-papular skin eruptions (angiokeratoma corporis diffusum), which are seen in a girdle distribution, start in male adolescence or in early manhood.

2. Whorllike (vortexlike) basal epithelial and subepithelial corneal opacities are seen. Clinically, tortuous retinal vessels with visible mural deposits may be seen. The deposits may be so pronounced as to partially obstruct the lumen resulting in sausage-shaped vessels; the blood in the arterioles becomes much darker than normal due to the stasis so produced.

Cornea verticillata (Fleischer-Gruber), the corneal manifestation of Fabry's disease, is the term found in the old literature.

FIG. 8–45. Fabry's disease. **A.** Laminated material accumulating mostly within basal epithelial cells in region of limbus (see **inset 1**). **Inset 2** shows fine laminations of lipoidal material at higher magnification. Material produces clinically observed corneal epithelial lines (cornea verticillata). **B. Inset 1** shows lipoidal materials accumulating within endothelial and periendothelial cells of limbal vessel. **Main figure** shows massive accumulation of lipoidal substances within endothelial cells (*EN*) of another limbal vessel. Note constrictions of lumen (*LU*) at single arrow and lumenal cleft at double arrow. **Inset 2** shows similar accumulations in small choroidal artery with characteristic accumulation in smooth muscle cells of vessel wall. **A.** ×13,500; **inset 1**, PD, ×275; **inset 2**, ×80,000. **B.** ×17,500; **inset 1**, PD, ×575; **inset 2**, PD, ×440.

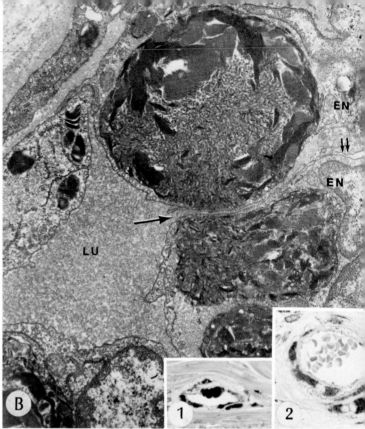

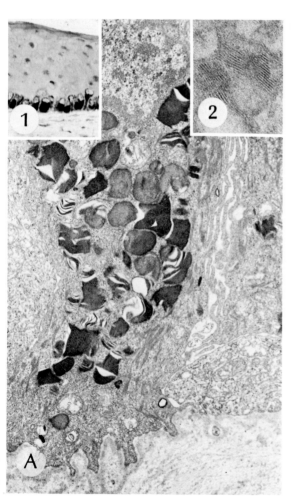

Color Plate II. **A, B,** and **C.** Granular ▶ dystrophy. **A.** Masses of eosinophilic, sharp-edged granules are present in stroma, replacing portions of Bowman's membrane, and are present in subepithelial regions. **B.** Higher magnification of region in **A** to show "granular" nature of deposits. **C.** Granular deposits stain brilliant red with Masson trichrome stain. Collagen (i.e., Bowman's membrane and corneal stroma) stains blue normally. **D.** and **E.** Macular dystrophy. In **D.** Keratocytes appear finely granular blue with colloidal iron stain for acid mucopolysaccharides. Small patches of blue can also be observed diffusely within stromal lamellas. **E.** Corneal endothelial cells like keratocytes contain granules of blue when stained with colloidal iron. **F, G,** and **H.** Lattice dystrophy. Characteristic ovoid or spindle-shaped "hyaline" lesions of lattice dystrophy, which are eosinophilic on H&E (**F**), show remarkable increased birefringence when examined by polarized light (**G**). **H.** Lesions of lattice dystrophy are positive for "amyloid" when stained with Congo red. **A,** H&E, ×145; **B,** H&E, ×395; **C,** trichrome, ×395; **D,** AMP, ×350; **E,** AMP, ×350; **F,** H&E, ×115; **G,** polarized H&E, ×115; **H,** Congo red, ×115.

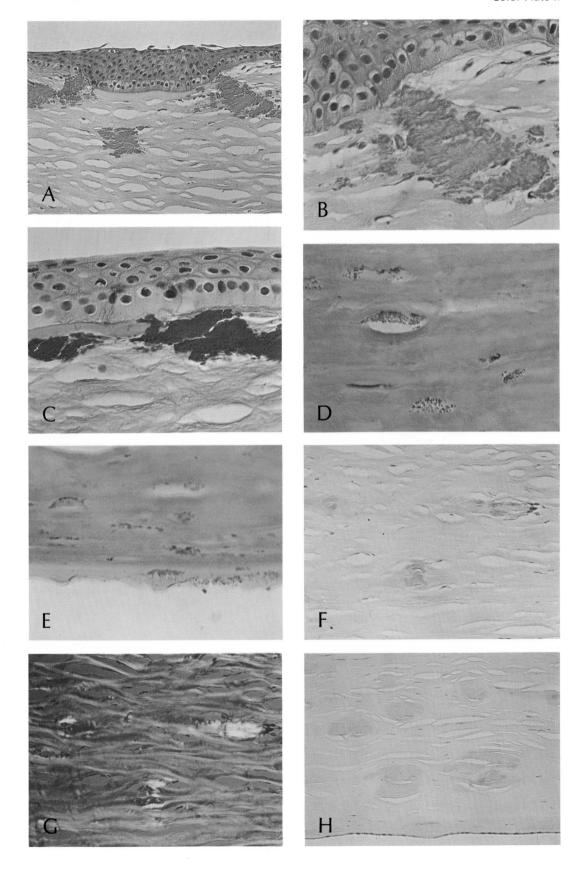

3. Fabry's disease is caused by a generalized inborn error of sphingolipid metabolism (see p. 445 in Chap. 11) wherein α-galactosidase deficiency results in an intracellular storage of ceramide trihexoside.

4. It has a sex-linked recessive inheritance pattern.

   Amniotic fluid can be analyzed at the 17th week of gestation for levels of α-galactosidase. In this way an affected child can be detected during the early part of the second trimester of pregnancy.

5. Histologically, lipid-containing inclusions are present in corneal epithelium, in lens epithelium, in endothelial cells in all organs, in liver cells, in fibrocytes of skin, in lymphocytes, in smooth muscle cells of arterioles, in capillary pericytes and in vascular endothelial cells in all organs.

BOWMAN'S MEMBRANE (Anterior Limiting Membrane or Layer)

Ringlike Dystrophy of Reis and Bücklers (Fig. 8–46)

A. Acute attacks of red, painful eyes due to recurrent erosions commence in early childhood. Usually by the fifth decade there is marked opacification of the corneas. Multiple, minute, discrete opacities are seen just beneath the epithelium.

B. The dystrophy is inherited as an autosomal dominant.

C. Histologically the corneal changes are limited to the plane of Bowman's membrane. The membrane or layer is replaced slowly by a scarring or increased layering of collagenous tissue that extends beneath the epithelium. Loss of hemidesmosomes and associated basement membrane appears to lead to the recurrent desquamations or erosions with consequent additional trauma to Bowman's membrane.

STROMAL

I. Heredofamilial—primary in cornea

A. Granular* (Groenouw I; Bücklers I; hyaline) (Color Plate II, Figs. 8–47 and 8–48)

1. Sharply defined, variably sized, white opacities or granules are seen in the axial region of the superficial corneal stroma. The stroma between the opacities is clear.

2. The dystrophy has a slow and insidious progression after initially appearing in the first or early second decade of life.

   The possibility that an inherited dystrophy may recur in otherwise normal donor material following a corneal graft has been demonstrated histologically in the case of granular dystrophy. The recurrence is exceedingly slow and is believed to be caused by the host keratocytes slowly replacing those of the donor.

3. The condition is inherited as an autosomal dominant.

4. Histologically, granular, eosinophilic deposits are scattered throughout the stroma but often are confined to the superficial layers.

B. Macular* (Groenouw II; Bücklers II; primary corneal acid mucopolysaccharidosis) (Color Plate II, Fig. 8–49)

1. Diffuse cloudiness of superficial stroma with aggregates of gray-white opacities in the axial region is seen. The stroma between the opacities is diffusely cloudy.

2. It usually develops rapidly so that vision in most patients is seriously impaired by 30 years of age.

3. The condition is inherited as an autosomal recessive.

4. Histologically basophilic deposits, which stain positively for acid mucopolysaccharides, are present in keratocytes, endothelial cells and in small pools lying extracellularly within or between stromal lamellas.

* See Table 8–1.

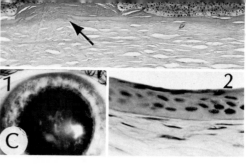

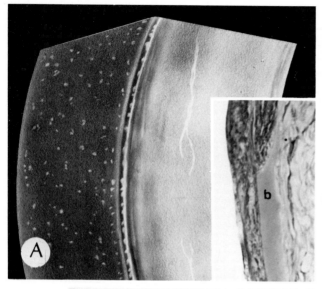

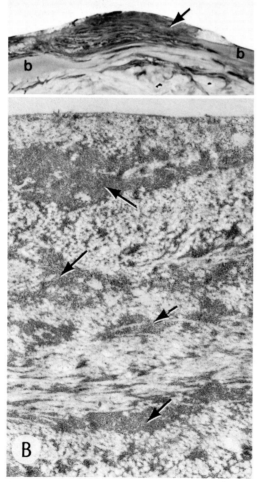

FIG. 8–46. Reis-Bücklers' dystrophy. **A.**
Clinically, myriad small white dots can be
seen, which appear in continuity with band
of relucency representing Bowman's
membrane. **Inset** is from biopsy of early
change oriented to correspond to drawing.
Destruction of Bowman's membrane is
primary disturbance. Exaggeration into focal
pannus formation produces overlying mound
of tissue. *b,* intact region of Bowman's
membrane. **B. Inset** shows focus of destruction of Bowman's membrane (*b*) in early
Reis-Bücklers' dystrophy. Corneal epithelium
has desquamated from area. *Arrow* indicates
accumulating pannus overlying plane of
Bowman's membrane. Electron micrograph
shows early changes within Bowman's layer
to consist of appearance of irregular masses
of dense, delicate filaments (*arrows*) and
aggregates of normal-diameter collagen
fibrils into lamellas. Epithelium is missing in
section. **C.** Late Reis-Bücklers' dystrophy
(**main figure** and **inset 1**). Note loss of
Bowman's membrane (*arrow*) and heavy
subepithelial pannus formation. Remainder
of stroma appears normal. Compare with
inset 2 of earlier changes in which Bowman's
membrane is lost but defect is filled with
cellular tissue. **A,** drawing; **inset,** 1.5 μ
section, PD, ×400. **B,** ×19,000; **inset,** 1.5 μ
section, PD, ×400. **C,** H&E, ×80; **inset 1,**
clinical; **inset 2,** H&E, ×395.

FIG. 8–48. Granular dystrophy. **A.** shows ▶
granular deposits in H&E stain, and **B** shows
granular deposits with trichrome stain. **C.**
"Granules" of granular dystrophy as seen
by light microscopy (**inset**) are seen to
consist of dense granules when observed by
electron microscopy. Many granules are
"apertured." **D.** By electron microscopy
close relationship of both dense and
apertured granules to packed, "folded"
macromolecules ("filaments") can be seen.
Latter are believed to be precursors of
granule formation. **A,** H&E, ×85; **B,** trichrome, ×85; **C,** ×4,500; **inset,** H&E, ×395;
D, ×16,500.

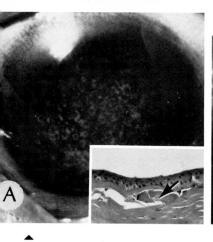

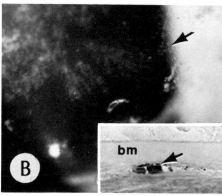

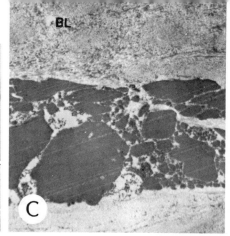

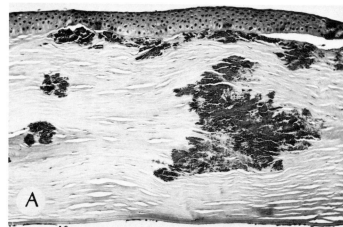

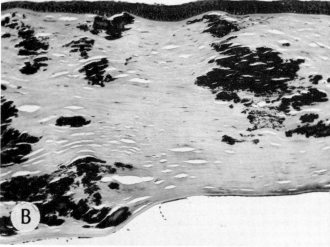

FIG. 8–47. Granular dystrophy. **A.** Clinical photo of granular dystrophy. **Inset** of biopsy shows presence of typical stromal granule (*arrow*). **B.** Clinical photo of recurrence of granular dystrophy in full thickness graft several years later. Note granules as seen by side illumination (*arrow*). **Inset** is from biopsy of new lesions within graft. Typical collection of granular material (*arrow*) lies within stroma beneath Bowman's membrane (*bm*). **C.** By electron microscopy granules from biopsy are typical of granular dystrophy. *BL,* Bowman's layer. **A,** clinical; **inset,** H&E, ×135. **B,** clinical; **inset,** 1.5 μ section, PD, ×485. **C,** ×12,000.

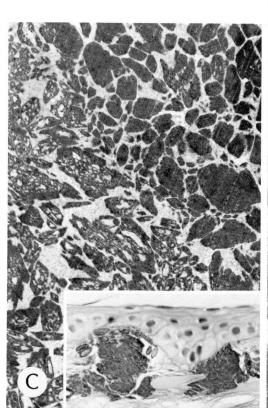

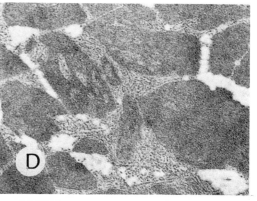

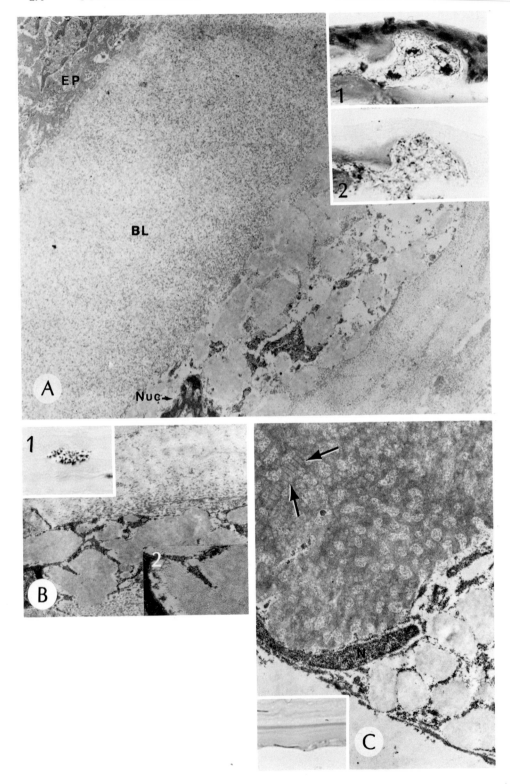

FIG. 8–49. Macular dystrophy. **A.** Cluster of vacuolated cells (**inset 1**) beneath epithelium. Vacuoles are filled with acid mucopolysaccharides (AMP) when stained with special stain (**inset 2**). Electron micrograph shows keratocyte beneath Bowman's layer (*BL*) filled with vesicles containing presumably AMP-positive substance. *EP*, epithelium; *Nuc*, nucleus of keratocyte. **B.** AMP-positive granules (**inset 1**) are due to presence of many intracytoplasmic vesicles when examined by electron microscopy. At higher magnification (**inset 2**) the vesicular content appears fibrillar. **C.** Vacuolated endothelium, which also may frequently produce excrescences on Descemet's membrane (**inset**), is seen by electron microscopy to be filled with cytoplasmic vesicles presumably containing AMP. Descemet's "wart" contains areas of banding or periodicity (*arrows*; as seen in cornea guttata) and myriad areas of rarefaction (type of thick multilaminar basement membrane formation) unlike cornea guttata. *N*, nucleus of endothelial cell. **A,** ×8,000; **inset 1,** trichrome, ×350; **inset 2,** colloidal iron, ×350. **B,** ×18,000; **inset 1,** colloidal iron, ×350; **inset 2,** ×36,000. **C,** ×16,500; **inset,** 1.5 μ section, ◀ PD, ×350.

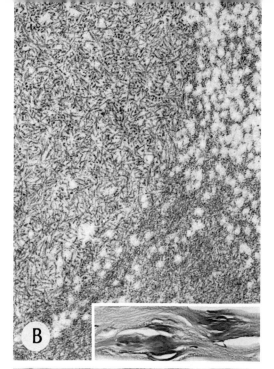

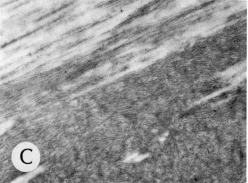

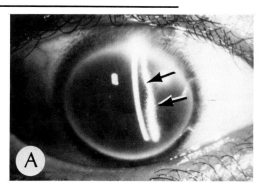

FIG. 8–50. Lattice dystrophy. **A.** Translucent branching lines of lattice dystrophy are seen best by retroillumination (*arrows*). **B.** "Hyaline" lesion of light microscopy (**inset**) is composed of myriad individual filaments either in disarray (as in **B**), and therefore nonbirefringent, or highly aligned (as in **C**), and therefore with birefringence exaggerated. **D.** Alterations in overlying epithelium are nonspecific. Here there is loss of basal cell hemidesmosomes, accumulation of abnormal quantity of thick homogeneous basement membrane (*bm*), and apparently similar material between adjacent basal cells (*arrows*). *d*, desmosomes; *ne*, intraepithelial neurite. **A,** clinical; **B,** ×36,000; **inset,** H&E, ×300; **C,** ×27,500; **D,** ×19,000.

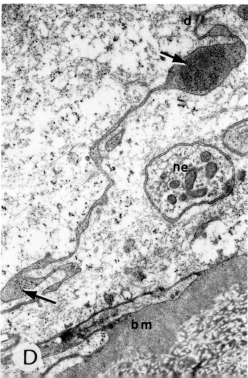

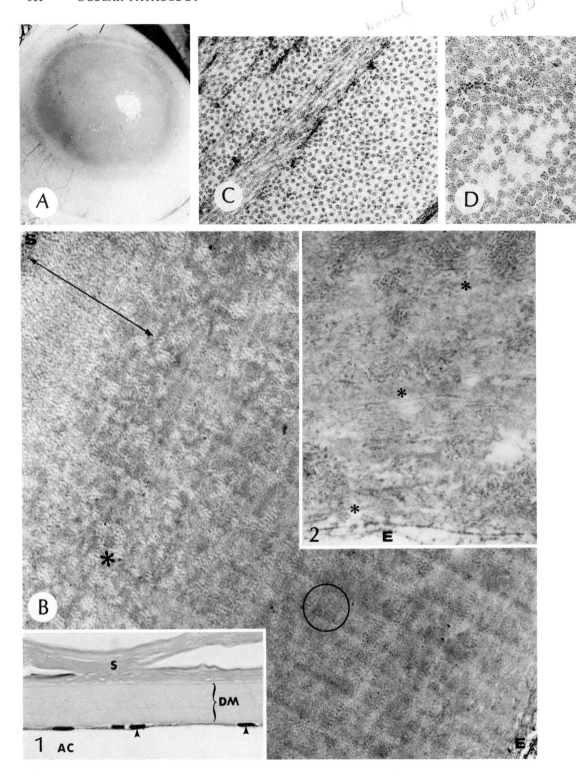

S

Namel

CHED

A

C

D

B

*

1 AC

S

DM

2   E

E

FIG. 8–51. Congenital hereditary endothelial dystrophy (CHED). **A.** Clinical appearance of cornea. **B.** Light micrograph (**inset 1**) shows markedly thickened (~ 23 μ) Descemet's membrane (*DM*) and attenuated endothelial layer (*arrowheads*). *S*, stroma; *AC*, anterior chamber. **Main figure** with banded (*arrow*) Descemet's membrane near stroma (*S*) and thickened posterior layer interspersed with fibrous basement membrane (*asterisk*) and patches of basement membrane (*circle*) of banded type. **E**, endothelium. **Inset 2** is higher magnification showing multilaminar patches (*asterisks*) of homogeneous basement membrane interspersed with multi-laminar sheets of fibrous basement membrane. *E*, endothelium. **C**, Collagen fibrils in normal corneal stroma measure approximately 240 A in diameter. **D.** Stromal collagen fibrils in CHED often measure approximately 480 A with some reaching diameters of up to 720 A. **A**, clinical; **B**, ×9,200; **inset 1**, H&E, ×600; **inset 2**, ◀×41,600; **C**, ×45,000; **D**, ×45,000.

Some cases show excrescences on Descemet's membrane.

C. Lattice* (Bücklers III; Biber-Haab-Dimmer; primary corneal amyloidosis) (Color Plate II, Fig. 8–50)—see p. 248 in Chapter 7.
   1. Lines forming a lattice configuration are present centrally in the anterior stroma leaving the peripheral cornea clear.

   Some authors feel that the lattice may represent nerves or nerve degeneration. Proof for this hypothesis is lacking.

   2. The dystrophy can progress to involve deeper stromal layers.
   3. Epithelial abnormalities also are present:
      a. Recurrent erosion.
      b. Loss of surface luster, which may be due to epithelial basement membrane abnormalities.

* See Table 8–1.

4. The condition begins in the first decade or early second decade and may progress fairly rapidly; many affected individuals develop marked visual impairment by 40 years of age.
5. The condition is inherited as an autosomal dominant.
6. Histologically an eosinophilic, metachromatic, PAS and Congo red positive, birefringent and dichroic deposit is present in the stroma, mainly superficially. The epithelium is abnormal with areas of hypertrophy and atrophy and with excessive basement membrane production.

The stromal lesions are characteristic of amyloid in all respects. Amyloidosis may be classified into two basic groups: systemic (primary and secondary) and localized (primary and secondary). Secondary systemic amyloidosis, the most frequently encountered type, rarely involves the eyes and is not an important ophthalmologic entity. Lattice dystrophy of the cornea is now considered by many to be a hereditary form of primary localized amyloidosis. The epithelial basement membrane abnormalities are responsible for secondary epithelial erosions and are partially responsible for the visual impairment.

D. Congenital hereditary endothelial dystrophy (Fig. 8–51)
   1. Clinically a diffuse bluish white opacity (ground glass) involves the total corneal thickness. It tends to be bilateral and stationary.
   2. Histologically, increased diameter of the stromal collagen fibrils may produce a thick cornea. There is fibrous thickening of Descemet's membrane (similar, if not identical, to cornea guttata), which implies an endothelial abnormality.
E. Hereditary corneal edema
   1. Corneal clouding with a thickened, edematous cornea develops within the first few years of life.
   2. The cornea may show incomplete clearing as children become older.

TABLE 8–1
Histopathologic Differentiation of Granular, Macular and Lattice Dystrophies

Dystrophy	Trichrome	AMP*	PAS	Amyloid†	Birefringence‡	Heredity
Granular	+	−	−	− or +§	−	Dominant
Macular	−	+	−	−	−	Recessive
Lattice	+	−	+	+	+	Dominant

* Stains for acid mucopolysaccharides, e.g., alcian blue and colloidal iron.
† Stains for amyloid, e.g., Congo red and crystal violet.
‡ To polarized light.
§ Periphery of granular lesion (and occasionally within the lesion) stains positively for amyloid.

3. Histology:
   a. There is corneal edema with the middle or posterior stroma swollen.
   b. The collagen fibrils have variable diameters from one-half to one and one-half times normal diameter, and areas free of fibrils ("lakes") are present.
   c. Degenerative changes are found in the keratocytes.
   d. Descemet's membrane is undulated, thinned and contains banded material.
   e. The corneal endothelium is replaced by fibroblastlike cells.
F. Hereditary fleck dystrophy (hérédo-dystrophie mouchetée)
   1. Clinically the condition is characterized by small opacities, which vary in size, shape and depth in the corneal stroma and are ring or wreathlike with clear centers and distinct margins.
   2. The condition tends to be bilateral, nonprogressive and congenital with little or no interference with vision.
   3. The condition has an autosomal dominant inheritance pattern.

   In one of the pedigrees studied by Francois and Neetens (1956) a case of central cloudy dystrophy occurred.

   4. No pathology is available.
G. Central stromal crystalline corneal dystrophy (hereditary dystrophy of Schnyder)

1. Clinically five morphologic phenotypes have been described:
   a. A disc-shaped central opacity lacking crystals.
   b. A central crystalline disc-shaped opacity with an ill-defined edge.
   c. A crystalline discoid opacity with a garlandlike margin of sinuous contour.
   d. A ring opacity that exhibits local crystal agglomerations with a clear center.
   e. A crystalline ring opacity with a clear center.
2. The bilateral, symmetrical, relatively nonprogressive condition probably is not related to blood lipoprotein abnormalities but may occasionally coexist with a hyperlipoproteinemia.
3. An autosomal dominant inheritance pattern is seen.
4. Histologically cholesterol and neutral fats are seen in corneal stroma. The dystrophy appears to be related to primary lipoidal degeneration of the cornea (Fig. 8–38).
II. Heredofamilial—secondary to systemic disease
   A. *Mucopolysaccharidoses* (Fig. 8–52) can be divided into seven major classes (Table 8–2). They all have mucopolysacchariduria, and all but MPS IV have an impairment in degradation of acid mucopolysaccharides. These genetic mucopolysaccharidoses may be considered as lysosomal diseases with deficiencies of lysosomal enzymes. Histologically, vacuolated cells

TABLE 8–2
Types of Mucopolysaccharidoses*

	Designation	Clinical Features	Genetics	Excessive Urinary MPS	Deficient Substance
MPS I H	Hurler syndrome	Early clouding of cornea, grave manifestations, death usually before age ten	Homozygous for MPS I H gene	Dermatan sulfate Heparan sulfate	α-L-Iduronidase (formerly called Hurler corrective factor)
MPS I S	Scheie syndrome	Stiff joints, cloudy cornea, aortic regurgitation, normal intelligence, ?normal life-span	Homozygous for MPS I S gene	Dermatan sulfate Heparan sulfate	α-L-Iduronidase
MPS I H/S	Hurler-Scheie compound	Phenotype intermediate between Hurler and Scheie	Genetic compound of MPS I H and I S genes	Dermatan sulfate Heparan sulfate	α-L-Iduronidase
MPS II A	Hunter syndrome, severe	No clouding of cornea, milder course than in MPS I H but death usually before age 15	Hemizygous for X-linked gene	Dermatan sulfate Heparan sulfate	Hunter corrective factor
MPS II B	Hunter syndrome, mild	Survival to 30s to 50s, fair intelligence	Hemizygous for X-linked allele for mild form	Dermatan sulfate Heparan sulfate	Hunter corrective factor
MPS III A	Sanfilippo syndrome A	Mild somatic, severe central nervous system effects (identical phenotype)	Homozygous for Sanfilippo A gene	Heparan sulfate	Heparan sulfate sulfatase
MPS III B	Sanfilippo syndrome B		Homozygous for Sanfilippo B gene (at different locus)	Heparan sulfate	N-Acetyl-α-D-glucosaminidase
MPS IV	Morquio syndrome (probably more than one allelic form)	Severe bone changes of distinctive type, cloudy cornea, aortic regurgitation	Homozygous for Morquio gene	Keratan sulfate	Unknown
MPS V	Vacant				
MPS VI A	Maroteaux-Lamy syndrome, classic form	Severe osseous and corneal change, normal intellect	Homozygous for Maroteaux-Lamy gene	Dermatan sulfate	Maroteaux-Lamy corrective factor
MPS VI B	Maroteaux-Lamy syndrome, mild form	Severe osseous and corneal change, normal intellect	Homozygous for allele at Maroteaux-Lamy locus	Dermatan sulfate	Maroteaux-Lamy corrective factor
MPS VII	β-glucuronidase deficiency (more than one allelic form?)	Hepatosplenomegaly, dysostosis multiplex, white cell inclusions, mental retardation	Homozygous for mutant gene at β-glucuronidase locus	Dermatan sulfate	β-Glucuronidase
—	Macular corneal dystrophy	Corneal clouding	Autosomal recessive	—	—

* Modified from Table 11-2 in McKusick VA: Heritable Disorders of Connective Tissue, 4th ed. St. Louis, Mosby, 1972, p 525

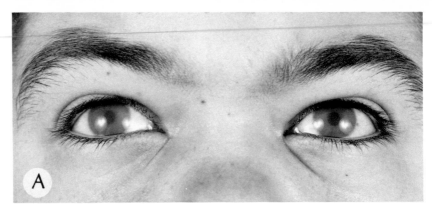

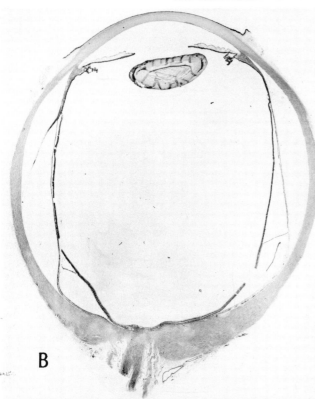

FIG. 8–52. Mucopolysaccharidoses type VI, Maroteaux-Lamy syndrome. **A.** Patient at 10 years of age. Note diffuse corneal clouding, saddle nose and prominent eyebrows. **B.** Section through whole eye shows moderate corneal thickening and marked thickening of posterior sclera. **C.** Cytoplasmic vacuolation most prominent in basal layer of corneal epithelium. Foamy histiocytes present in region of Bowman's membrane. **D.** Keratocytes are swollen by foamy-appearing cytoplasm. **E.** Intracytoplasmic vacuoles (*V*) in basal cells of corneal epithelium. Within Bowman's membrane (*BM*) abnormal extracellular material (*asterisk*) and vacuolated histiocyte (*H*) are seen. *N*, nucleus. **Inset** shows vacuoles bounded by single-unit membrane and containing clear to fibrillogranular material or occasional electron-dense inclusions. **F.** Keratocyte contains predominantly membranous lamellar vacuoles (*arrows*) and electron-dense inclusions. Granular material is interspersed among stromal collagen fibrils (circled). **A,** clinical; **B,** H&E, ×3; **C,** 1.5 μ section, PD, phase contrast, ×1,050; **D,** 1.5 μ section, PD, phase contrast, ×1,050; **E,** ×7,100; **inset,** ×17,000; **F,** ×31,000.

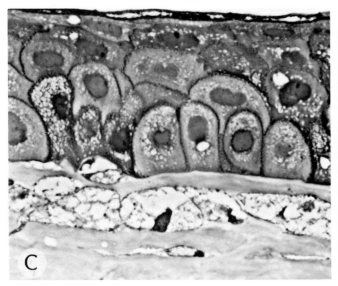

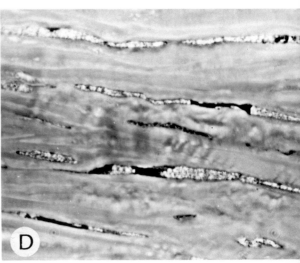

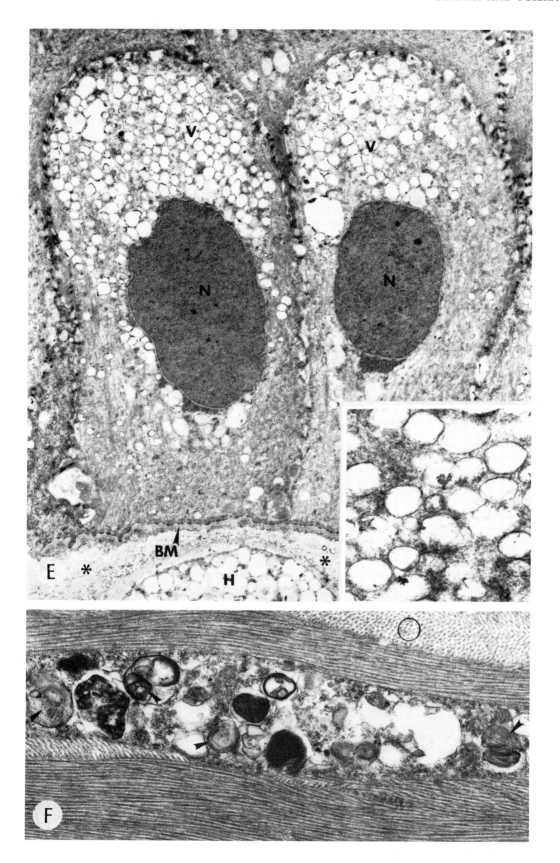

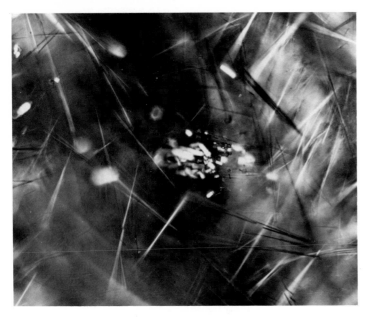

FIG. 8–53. Cystinosis. A mixture of typical, birefringent, rectangular, cystine crystallites and fusiform bodies observed near limbus. Polarized light, ×420.

(histiocytes, corneal epithelium and endothelium, keratocytes and iris and ciliary body epithelia) contain acid mucopolysaccharides within the vacuoles. The different classes show varying pathologic findings, fairly consistent within each class.

B. Mucolipidosis—see p. 440 in Chapter 11.

C. Sphingolipidosis—see p. 440 in Chapter 11.

D. Ochronosis—see p. 315 in this chapter.

E. Cystinosis (Lignac's disease) (Fig. 8–53)

  1. The disease, which is inherited as an autosomal recessive, is characterized by dwarfism and progressive renal dysfunction resulting in acidosis, hypophosphatemia, renal glycosuria and rickets.

  2. Patients with infantile or juvenile cystinosis may show a peripheral retinopathy that does not seem to cause any modification in retinal function.

Although cystine crystals are stored in the liver, spleen, lymph nodes, bone marrow, eyes and kidneys (and probably other organs), they seem to be relatively innocuous. Progressive renal failure starts in the first decade of life with proximal tubular involvement (*Toni-Febré-Fanconi syndrome*), but it does not seem to be related directly with renal cystine storage. The underlying enzyme defect is not yet known.

  3. Histologically cystine crystals are deposited in many tissues including the conjunctiva and cornea.

The cystine crystals can be seen clinically with a slit lamp as tiny, multicolored crystals.

III. Nonheredofamilial

A. Keratoconus (Color Plate I, Fig. 8–54)

  1. Ectasia of the central cornea usually becomes manifest in youth or adolescence, progresses for 5 to 6 years and then tends to arrest.

  2. Majority (~70 percent) of cases occurs in girls.

  3. The apex of the cone is slightly inferior and nasal to the anterior pole of the cornea.

  4. Munson's sign occurs when the lower lid bulges on down gaze.

  5. Vogt's vertical lines are present in the stroma.

  6. *Fleischer's ring* is due to iron deposition in the epithelium around the base of the cone, best seen with

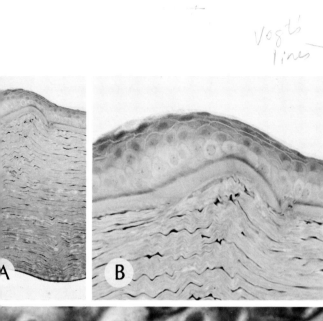

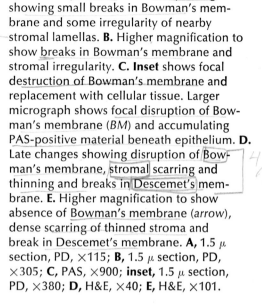

FIG. 8–54. Keratoconus. **A.** Early changes showing small breaks in Bowman's membrane and some irregularity of nearby stromal lamellas. **B.** Higher magnification to show breaks in Bowman's membrane and stromal irregularity. **C. Inset** shows focal destruction of Bowman's membrane and replacement with cellular tissue. Larger micrograph shows focal disruption of Bowman's membrane (*BM*) and accumulating PAS-positive material beneath epithelium. **D.** Late changes showing disruption of Bowman's membrane, stromal scarring and thinning and breaks in Descemet's membrane. **E.** Higher magnification to show absence of Bowman's membrane (*arrow*), dense scarring of thinned stroma and break in Descemet's membrane. **A,** 1.5 μ section, PD, ×115; **B,** 1.5 μ section, PD, ×305; **C,** PAS, ×900; **inset,** 1.5 μ section, PD, ×380; **D,** H&E, ×40; **E,** H&E, ×101.

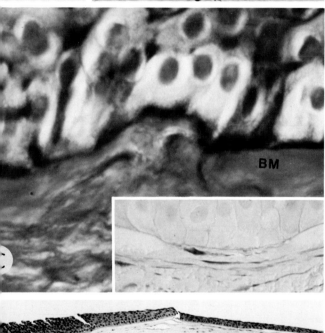

BM

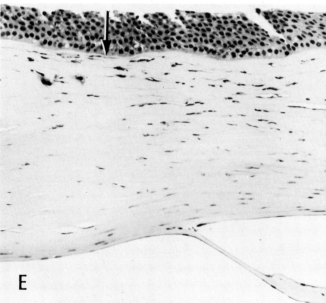

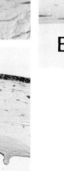

E

the light of the slit lamp through a cobalt blue filter.

7. Ruptures in Bowman's (early) and Descemet's (late) membranes and increased visibility of corneal nerves are common findings.

8. Most cases are not inherited, but a recessive or dominant inheritance pattern may occur.

9. Histologically the central cornea is thinned with the central portion of Bowman's membrane destroyed, the central stroma scarred and the central portion of Descemet's membrane frequently showing ruptures. Iron is found in epithelial cells at all levels in the peripheral region of the thinned central cornea.

ENDOTHELIAL

I. Cornea guttata (Fuchs's combined dystrophy) (Figs. 8–55 and 8–56)

A. Fuchs described the epithelial component, which is really a degeneration, secondary to the primary endothelial dystrophy (cornea guttata).

B. It occurs predominantly in elderly women and is bilateral.

C. There are four stages as seen clinically and histologically:

1. With cornea guttata there are excrescences that resemble Hassall-Henle warts except that they are present centrally. Electron microscopic studies of cornea guttata demonstrate regions of diffuse thickening and abnormal collagenous posterior layers of Descemet's membrane.

2. An early change in the epithelial area is a subepithelial ingrowth of a layer of cells from the superficial stroma through Bowman's membrane which leads to production of a subepithelial fibrous pannus of variable thickness.

3. Edema of stroma and epithelium with epithelial bullae develops later.

4. Late complications include glaucoma, ruptured bullae and infection.

II. Hereditary deep dystrophy (posterior polymorphous dystrophy)

A. Irregular, polymorphous opacities and vesicles with central pigmentation and surrounding opacification are seen in the central cornea at the level of endothelium, Descemet's membrane and deep stroma.

B. Ruptures in Descemet's membrane and glaucoma may be associated.

C. The condition is inherited as an autosomal dominant or recessive.

D. Histologically the deep corneal stroma shows nodules that contain crystals of calcium. Stromal folding is present in the deep corneal tissue. Descemet's membrane may be thickened focally or diffusely and the endothelial cells may take on the appearance of epithelial cells (i.e., multilayering, intracytoplasmic filaments and desmosomes).

FIG. 8–55. Cornea guttata. **A.** Posterior or abnormal layers cause marked thickening of Descemet's membrane by addition of alternating layers of collageous fibrils, filaments and basement membrane. Focal aggregations are called "warts" or cornea guttata clinically. Endothelium is generally attenuated, especially where present over wart. **Inset 1** shows additional fibrous thickening of the membrane superimposed on the warts. By TEM the warts characteristically include numerous patches of banded material (basement membrane) in disarray (**inset 2,** longitudinal; **inset 3,** transverse), reminiscent of the orderly pattern of the normal anteriormost part of Descemet's membrane. **B.** Posteriorly, early stromal changes occur anterior to Descemet's membrane (*DE*) as accumulating "lakes" or pools of fluid (X) separating collagenous lamellas or fibrils within a lamella. **C.** Early changes anteriorly consist of migration of cells from superficial stroma into subepithelial plane (*arrows*), presumably initially through normal nerve apertures present in Bowman's membrane. **D.** Accumulation of subepithelial cells with filamentous cytoplasm produces early pannus (*arrow*). Overlying epithelial cells assume bizarre shapes and in later stages become edematous. *BM,* Bowman's membrane. **E.** By electron microscopy filamentous cells (fibroblasts, i.e., presumably altered keratocytes) lie along plane of Bowman's layer (*BL*) and are separated from epithelium by band of collagenous material and normal, thin basement membrane (*arrows*). *N,* nucleus of filamentous cell; *EP,* basal epithelial cell. **A,** ×21,000; **inset 1,** TB, ×300; **inset 2,** ×22,000; **inset 3,** ×22,000; **B,** ×20,000; **C,** 1.5 μ section, PD, ×395; **D,** 1.5 μ section, PD, ×440; **E,** ×16,000.

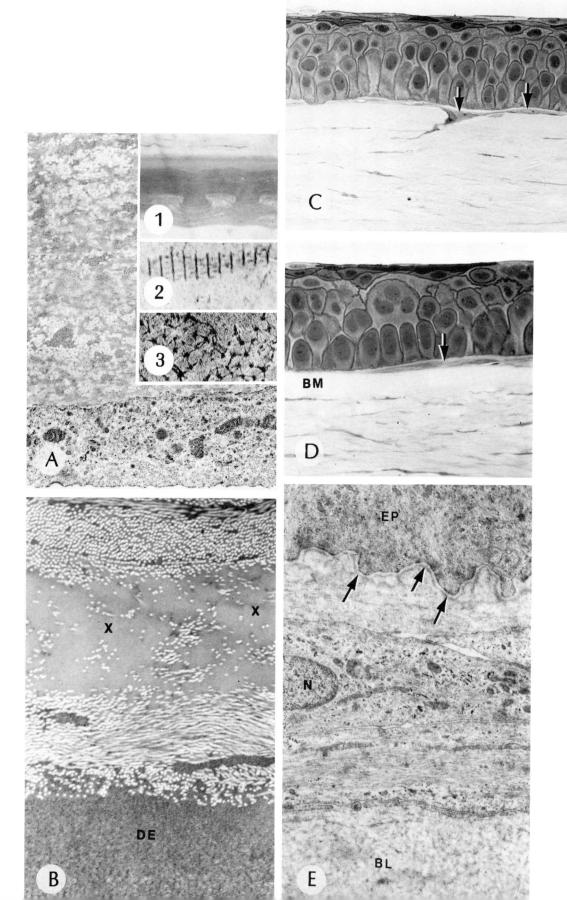

PIGMENTATIONS

MELANIN

I. Pigmentation of the basal layer of epithelium, especially in the peripheral cornea, is found normally in dark races (Fig. 8–57).

II. A posterior corneal membrane. This may be due to a proliferation of uveal melanocytes or pigment epithelial cells onto the posterior cornea following an injury.

III. Krukenberg spindle (see p. 610 in Chap. 16 and Fig. 16–20)

   A. Melanin pigment is present on the posterior corneal surface, phagocytosed by endothelial cells.

   B. The condition is most common in young myopes.

   C. In the vast majority the condition is bilateral and may be associated with the pigment dispersion syndrome as well as with glaucoma.

     When a Krukenberg spindle is present unilaterally, ocular trauma is the usual cause. When bilateral and the patient also has elevated ocular pressure, the condition of "pigmentary glaucoma" may be present (see p. 606 in Chap. 16).

BLOOD (Color Plate I, Fig. 8–58)

I. Staining of the cornea occurs in the presence of a hyphema in which there is at least 48 hours of increased intraocular pressure.

     Staining may occur earlier or even without glaucoma if the endothelium is diseased.

II. Staining of the cornea is due to hemoglobin and other breakdown products of erythrocytes with very little hemosiderin present and that usually within keratocytes.

III. The cornea clears first peripherally and may take several years to clear completely.

IV. Histologically, amorphous globules and tiny round spheres and rods (all orange in color in H&E-stained sections) are seen mainly between corneal lamellas but also in keratocytes and in Bowman's membrane.

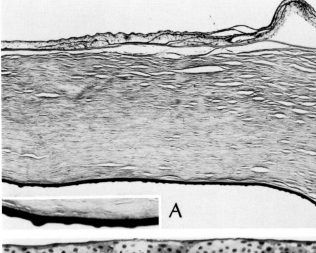

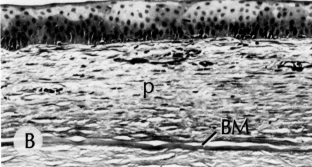

FIG. 8–56. Cornea guttata (Fuchs's combined dystrophy). **A.** Epithelium edematous with abnormal basement membrane secretion and formation of bulla. **Inset** shows higher magnification of Descemet's membrane to show guttate lesions. **B.** Advanced changes are present with epithelial edema and thick pannus (p). BM, Bowman's membrane. **A,** PAS, ×40; **inset,** PAS, ×101; **B,** trichrome, ×101.

IRON LINES

I. Fleischer ring (Color Plate I, Fig. 8–59) (see section Dystrophies, subsection Stroma above).

II. Hudson-Stahli line (Color Plate I, Fig. 8–60). This is due to a deposition of iron in the epithelium in a horizontal line just inferior to the center of the interpalpebral fissure.

FIG. 8–57. Melanin pigment may extend into *sub-* epithelium of cornea as depicted in diagram.

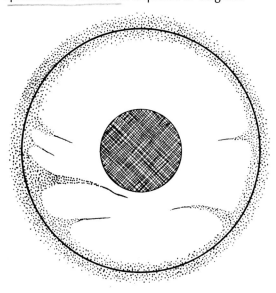

FIG. 8–58. Blood staining of cornea present. Compare small size of hemoglobin particles in corneal stroma to large erythrocytes in anterior chamber. *d*, Descemet's membrane. H&E, ×680.

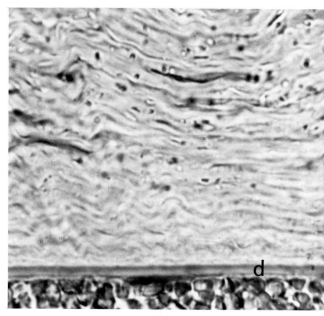

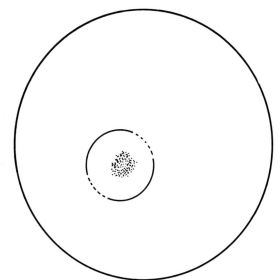

FIG. 8–59. Fleischer ring of keratoconus drawn as it would appear in left eye, i.e., slightly nasal and inferior to center of cornea.

FIG. 8–60. Ferry line depicted at top in front ▶ (i.e., below) filtering bleb; Stocker line depicted on right in front (to left) of advancing edge of pterygium; and Hudson-Stahli line across (horizontal) cornea just below center of cornea. All three lines due to presence of iron within epithelial cells.

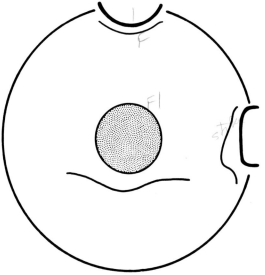

III. Stocker line (Fig. 8–60). This line results from a deposition of iron in the epithelium at the advancing edge of a pterygium.

IV. Ferry line (Fig. 8–60). This is due to a deposition of iron in the epithelium at the corneal margin of a filtering bleb.

KAYSER-FLEISCHER RING (Fig. 8–61)

I. The Kayser-Fleischer ring is associated with *hepatolenticular degeneration* (*Wilson's disease*):
   A. Increased absorption of copper from gut.
   B. Decrease in serum ceruloplasmin.
   C. Usually a recessive but may have a dominant type of autosomal inheritance pattern.

II. The Kayser-Fleischer ring, i.e., copper in Descemet's membrane, generally is apparent by late childhood or early adolescence and may be accompanied by a *"sunflower"* cataract.

The Kayser-Fleischer ring can be simulated exactly as a result of a retained intraocular copper foreign body. In this event, however, the ring is present only in the eye containing the foreign body.

III. Histologically the copper is deposited in the posterior half of the peripheral portion of Descemet's membrane and in the deeper layers of the anterior lens capsule.

TATTOO (Fig. 8–62)

I. Generally corneal tattooing is done to disguise unsightly leukomas.

II. The tattoo is performed by chemical reduction of metallic salts, e.g., gold chloride or platinum black.

III. Histologically the foreign material is seen in the corneal stroma.

DRUG INDUCED

I. Oxidized epinephrine (Figs. 7–16 and 8–63)
   A. Conjunctiva or corneal deposition can follow chronic use of epinephrine for treatment of glaucoma.
   B. Epinephrine may deposit under a corneal epithelial bleb where it becomes

FIG. 8–61. Kayser-Fleischer ring. **A.** Clinical photo showing peripheral corneal Kayser-Fleischer ring and "sunflower" or disciform cataract present in lens of patient with Wilson's disease. **B.** Line of copper is present within periphery of Descemet's membrane (*arrows*). Copper line accounts for color of Kayser-Fleischer ring observed clinically. **C.** Similar line of copper (*arrow*) is present deep within anterior lens capsule accounting for clinically observed cataract. (Stains for copper, including ruthenium red, were all positive but are not considered as entirely specific.) **A,** clinical; **B,** H&E, ×395; **C,** H&E, ×395.

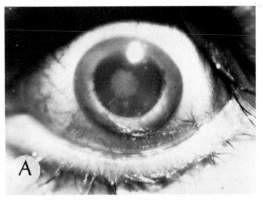

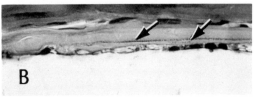

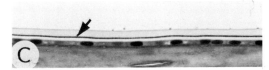

oxidized to a compound with properties similar to melanin.

On occasion the black corneal deposit has been mistaken for malignant melanoma of the cornea.

C. Histologically an amorphous pink material that stains black with silver stains and bleaches with hydrogen

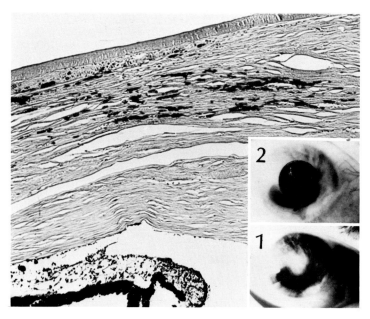

FIG. 8–62. Tattoo of cornea is noted histologically as dark, black deposits of platinum in upper corneal stroma. **Inset 1** shows corneal scar before tattooing and **inset 2** after tattooing. **Main figure,** H&E, ×40; **inset 1,** clinical; **inset 2,** clinical.

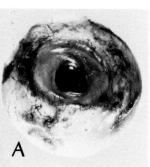
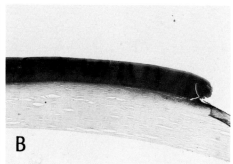

FIG. 8–63. Oxidized epinephrine. **A.** Well-circumscribed black mass present on cornea of enucleated eye. **B.** Black mass consists of oxidized epinephrine lying between epithelium and Bowman's membrane. Patient, who had been treated with epinephrine bitartrate for control of glaucoma, had his eye enucleated because of possible malignant melanoma of cornea. **A,** macroscopic; **B,** H&E, ×21.

peroxide is found between corneal epithelium and Bowman's membrane.

II. Cloroquine
   A. Chronic chloroquine use systemically causes a decreased corneal sensitivity.
   B. The corneal epithelial deposits vary from diffuse, fine, punctate opacities to focal aggregations arranged in radial, whorling lines, which diverge from just below the center of the cornea. These deposits tend to disappear when chloroquine usage is stopped.
III. Chlorpromazine
   A. The pigmentation (melaninlike) is present immediately under the anterior capsule of the lens in the central

(axial) area and in the conjunctival substantia propria in the interpalpebral fissure area.
   B. The corneal pigmentation appears as epithelial curvilinear and linear opacifications in the area of the interpalpebral fissure, as diffuse, granular yellow pigmentations in the corneal stroma and as fine deposits in the corneal endothelium.
IV. Indomethacin
   Indomethacin keratopathy may resemble chloroquine keratopathy both in its whorling distribution and reversibility, or it may appear only as fine, stromal, speckled opacities.

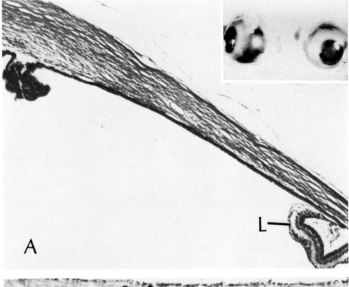

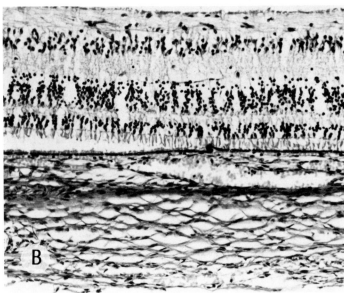

FIG. 8–64. Osteogenesis imperfecta. **A. Inset** shows enucleated eyes from baby who died from osteogenesis imperfecta. Histologic section shows thinned sclera over elongated pars plana of ciliary body. Note Lange's fold (*L*). **B.** Posterior sclera is thinned, even thinner than normal-appearing retina. **A,** trichrome, ×28; **inset,** macroscopic; **B,** H&E, ×101.

SCLERA

CONGENITAL ANOMALIES

BLUE SCLERA

I. Blue sclera may occur alone or with *brittle bones* and deafness.

II. There are three types of brittle bones:

    A. Osteogenesis imperfecta (Fig. 8–64)— usually apparent at birth.

    B. Osteopsathyrosis—a variant of brittle bones without blue sclera.

    C. Osteogenesis imperfecta tarda—delayed onset with levis and gravis forms.

III. The sclera retains its normal fetal transparency so that the blue uvea shows through.

IV. In the majority of cases the disease is inherited as an autosomal dominant, but autosomal recessive inheritance may occur.

V. Histologically the sclera is usually thinner than normal but may be thicker and more cellular than normal.

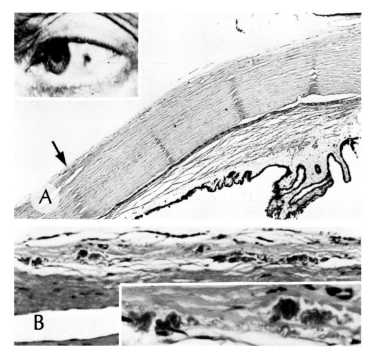

FIG. 8–65. Ochronosis. **A. Inset** shows pigmented spot of homogentisic acid deposition. Histologic section of same eye shows location of deposit (*arrow*). **B.** Higher magnification to show typical "curlicues" within superficial sclera and episclera (highest magnification in **inset**). **A,** H&E, ×16; **inset,** clinical; **B,** H&E, ×101; **inset,** H&E, ×252.

FIG. 8–66. Episcleritis. Episclera contains marked chronic inflammatory infiltrate in eye removed from child with Still's disease. **Inset** shows adult with episcleritis of right eye. **Main figure,** H&E, ×40; **inset,** clinical.

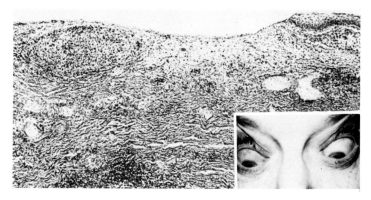

OCHRONOSIS (Alkaptonuria) (Fig. 8–65)

I. Because the enzyme homogentisic oxidase is lacking, homogentisic acid deposits in tissues (especially cartilage, elastic and collagen, e.g., sclera) and forms a melanin-like substance. The condition is inherited as an autosomal recessive.

II. Histologically, amorphous strands and curlicues are seen within the sclera and overlying substantia propria of the conjunctiva.

INFLAMMATIONS

EPISCLERITIS (Fig. 8–66)

I. Episcleritis may be associated with collagen diseases, but the majority are not.

II. Typically it occurs as a localized, painful, inflammatory, episcleral nodule in middle or old age.

III. Generally it is self-limiting and regresses over a period of 1 to 3 months.

IV. Histologically, usually a chronic, non-

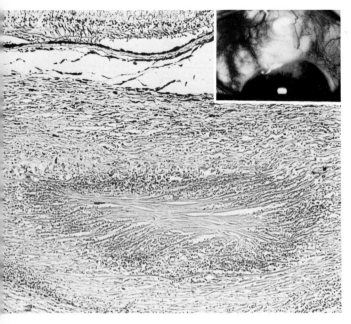

FIG. 8–67. Scleral nodule in patient with rheumatoid arthritis. Granulomatous inflammatory reaction surrounds necrotic scleral collagen. **Inset** shows clinical picture of necrotizing nodular scleritis. **Main figure,** H&E, ×54; **inset,** clinical.

fibrin

FIG. 8–68. Brawny scleritis. Chronic nongranulomatous (uvea) and granulomatous (sclera) inflammation involves and thickens sclera, anterior uveal tract and retina. H&E, ×8.

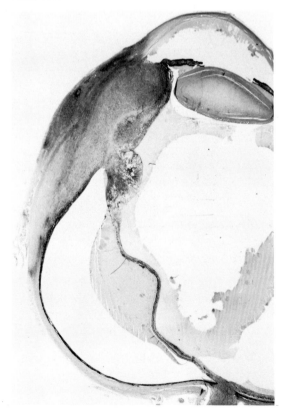

non- granulomatous infiltrate of lymphocytes and plasma cells is found in the episcleral tissue. Rarely, a granulomatous inflammatory infiltrate may be seen.

as in H. Zoster

SCLERITIS

I. Scleritis has a spectrum of involvement:

   A. Necrotizing nodular scleritis (Fig. 8–67)

     1. Necrotizing nodular scleritis is similar to episcleritis clinically, but it has more extensive and deeper involvement.

     2. There are repeated acute attacks with raised, painful, necrotic lesions. The lesions heal with sloughing of tissue, thereby exposing the underlying uvea.

     3. Histologically it resembles a rheumatoid subcutaneous nodule with a granulomatous inflammatory reaction surrounding degenerating collagen (see p. 101 in Chap. 4).

   B. Anterior scleritis

     1. Anterior scleritis is similar to necrotizing nodular scleritis but more extensive; it may develop into an *annular scleritis* by coalescence of many lesions.

2. The condition is found most frequently in young women and has a bilateral tendency.
C. Brawny scleritis (Fig. 8–68)
   1. Brawny scleritis is more serious than anterior scleritis.
   2. It tends to be a bilateral annular scleritis in elderly people with the addition of corneal involvement, i.e., *sclerosing keratitis.*
   3. Loss of an eye due to the corneal involvement is not uncommon.
D. Sclerokeratitis (Figs. 8–69 and 8–70) Sclerokeratitis is the most virulent type and combines a severe annular scleritis with a marked sclerosing keratitis.
E. Scleromalacia perforans
   1. Scleromalacia perforans uncommonly may result from any of the previous four entities.
   2. Most commonly, however, a painless necrotic nodule starts de novo between the limbus and equator with eventual sloughing after 6 months or longer.
   3. The nodules may be multiple or may occur at different times in different areas.
   4. Mainly middle-aged and elderly women are affected.

   Scleromalacia perforans may be seen in rheumatoid arthritis (most commonly), systemic lupus erythematosus, periarteritis nodosa and Wegener's granulomatosis. Rarely, it may be noted in porphyria, Herpes zoster and Crohn's disease.

II. Scleritis is associated with rheumatoid arthritis or other collagen disease in less than 25 percent of cases.
III. Rarely does the sclera actually perforate unless a subconjunctival steroid injection is given.
IV. Histologically a granulomatous lesion is present (see p. 101 in Chap. 4).

INJURIES

See section Normal Wound Healing in Chapter 5.

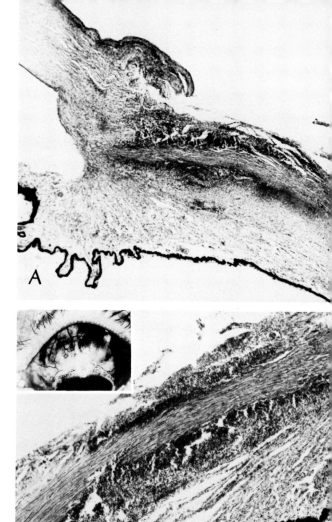

FIG. 8–69. Sclerokeratitis in adult with Wegener's granulomatosis. **A.** Necrotizing granulomatous reaction surrounds necrotic scleral collagen and extends to limbal cornea. **B.** Sclera thinned, necrotic and surrounded by granulomatous reaction. **Inset** shows clinical picture of healed scleral necrosis, i.e., scleromalacia perforans. **A,** H&E, ×21; **B,** H&E, ×28; **inset,** clinical.

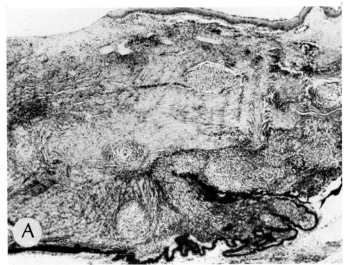

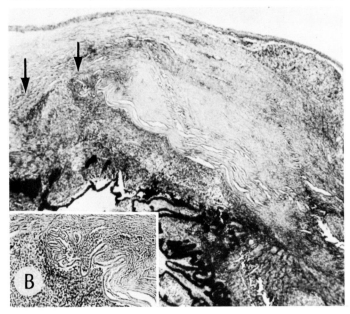

FIG. 8–70. Sclerokeratitis in child with Still's disease. **A.** Granulomatous inflammatory reaction involving cornea, sclera, iris and ciliary body. **B.** Iridocorneal granulomas have ruptured through Descemet's membrane (*arrows*), which is coiled up (see **inset**). A, H&E, ×21; **B,** H&E, ×21; **inset,** H&E, ×40.

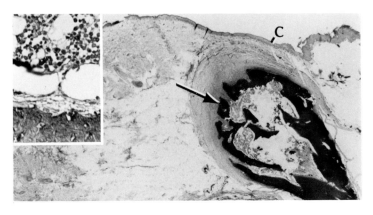

FIG. 8–71. Episcleral osseous choristoma (*arrow*) is episcleral tumor composed of bone; c, conjunctival epithelium. **Inset** shows higher magnification of bone, which contains hematopoietic tissue in marrow. **Main figure,** H&E, ×16; **inset,** H&E, ×170.

TUMORS

FIBROMAS

See section Mesenchymal Tumors in Chapter 14.

NODULAR FASCIITIS

See section Mesenchymal Tumors in Chapter 14.

HEMANGIOMAS

See section Mesenchymal Tumors in Chapter 14.

NEUROFIBROMAS

See section Mesenchymal Tumors in Chapter 14.

CONTIGUOUS TUMORS

- I. Conjunctiva.
- II. Malignant melanoma.

EPISCLERAL OSSEOUS CHORISTOMA (Fig. 8–71)

I. The tumor is present typically between the lateral and upper recti.
II. It is symptomless, is present at birth and characteristically contains bone.
III. Histologically, normal appearing bone is seen in the abnormal episcleral location.

ECTOPIC LACRIMAL GLAND

See p. 526 in Chapter 14.

BIBLIOGRAPHY

CORNEA

Congenital Defects

Alkemade PPH: Dysgenesis Mesodermalis of the Iris and the Cornea. Springfield, Thomas, 1969

Axenfeld T: Embryotoxon corneae posterius. Ber Dtsch Ophthalmol Ges 42:301, 1920

De Hauwere RC, Leroy JG, Adriaenssens K, van Heule R: Iris dysplasia, orbital hypertelorism, and psychomotor retardation: a dominantly inherited developmental syndrome. J Pediatr 82:679, 1973

Fernandez I, Arrivillaga R: Megalocornea. Rev Oftalmol Venez 17:204, 1968

Fischer F: Abnorme ciliarkörperanlage in einem Mikrophthalmus. Graefe's Arch Ophthalmol 132:71, 1934

Henkind P, Friedman AH: Iridogoniodysgenesis with cataract. Am J Ophthalmol 72:949, 1971

Henkind P, Marinoff G, Manas A, Friedman A: Bilateral corneal dermoids. Am J Ophthalmol 76:972, 1973

Henkind P, Siegel IM, Carr RE: Mesodermal dysgenesis of the anterior segment: Rieger's anomaly. Arch Ophthalmol 73:810, 1965

Hyams SW, Neumann E: Congenital microcornea and combined mechanism glaucoma. Am J Ophthalmol 68:326, 1969

Jacobs HB: Posterior conical cornea. Br J Ophthalmol 41:31, 1957

Jensen OA: Arcus corneae chez les jeunes. Arch Ophtalmol (Paris) 20:154, 1960

Kanai A, Wood TC, Polack FM, Kaufman HE: The fine structure of sclerocornea. Invest Ophthalmol 10:687, 1971

Kolker AE, Hetherington J: Becker-Shaffer's Diagnosis and Therapy of the Glaucomas, 3rd ed, Saint Louis: C. V. Mosby, 1970, p 284

Larson V, Eriksen A: Cornea plana. Acta Ophthalmol 27:275, 1949

Mandelcorn MS, Merin S, Cardarelli J: Goldenhar's syndrome and phocomelia. Case report and etiologic considerations. Am J Ophthalmol 72:618, 1971

March WF, Chalkley THF: Sclerocornea associated with Dandy-Walker cyst. Am J Ophthalmol 78:54, 1974

Nakanishi I, Brown SE: The histopathology and ultrastructure of congenital, central corneal opacity (Peters' anomaly). Am J Ophthalmol 72:801, 1971

O'Grady RB, Kirk HQ: Corneal keloids. Am J Ophthalmol 73:206, 1972

Peters A: Ueber angeborene Defektbildungen der Descemetschen Membran. Klin Monatsbl Augenheilkd 44:27, 1906

Reese AB, Ellsworth RM: The anterior chamber cleavage syndrome. Arch Ophthalmol 75:307, 1966

Rieger H: Beiträge zur Kenntnis seltener Missbildungen der Iris: I. Membrana iridopupillaris persistens. Graefe's Arch Ophthalmol 131:523, 1934

Rieger H: Beiträge zur Kenntnis seltener Missbildungen der Iris: II. Ueber Hypoplasie des Irisvorderblattes mit Verlagerung und Entrundung der Pupille. Graefe's Arch Ophthalmol 133:602, 1935

Rieger H: Demonstrationen (Gesellschaftsberichte). Z Augenheilkd 84:98, 1934

Rieger H: Erbfragen in der Augenheilkunde. Graefe's Arch Ophthalmol 143:227, 1941

Rodrigues MM, Calhoun J, Weinreb S: Sclerocornea with an unbalanced translocation. Am J Ophthalmol 78:49, 1974

Rogers GL, Polomeno RC: Autosomal-dominant inheritance of megalocornea associated with Down's syndrome. Am J Ophthalmol 78:526, 1974

Scheie HG, Yanoff M: Peter's anomaly and total posterior coloboma of retinal pigment epithelium and choroid. Arch Ophthalmol 87:525, 1972

Sugar HS: The oculoauriculo-vertebral syndrome of Goldenhar. Am J Ophthalmol 62:678, 1966

Townsend WM: Congenital corneal leukomas. 1.

Central defect in Descemet's membrane. Am J Ophthalmol 77:80, 1974

Townsend WM, Font RL, Zimmerman LE: Congenital corneal leukomas. 2. Histopathologic findings in 19 eyes with central defect in Descemet's membrane. Am J Ophthalmol 77:192, 1974

Townsend WM, Font RL, Zimmerman LE: Congenital corneal leukomas. 3. Histopathologic findings in 13 eyes with noncentral defect in Descemet's membrane. Am J Ophthalmol 77:400, 1974

Vail DT: Adult hereditary anterior megalophthalmus sine glaucoma: A definite disease entity. Arch Ophthalmol 6:39, 1931

Inflammations: Nonulcerative

Cairns JE: Cutaneous leishmaniasis (oriental sore): case with corneal involvement. Br J Ophthalmol 52:481, 1968

Cordero-Moreno R: Etiologic factors in tropical eye diseases. Am J Ophthalmol 75:349, 1973

Dawson CR, Hanna L, Togni B: Adenovirus type 8 infections in the United States. IV. Observations on the pathogenisis of lesions in severe eye disease. Arch Ophthalmol 87:258, 1972

Gilbert WS, Talbot FJ: Cogan's syndrome: signs of periarteritis nodosa and cerebral venous sinus thrombosis. Arch Ophthalmol 82:633, 1969

Hunter GW III, Frye WW, Swartzwelder JC: A Manual of Tropical Medicine, 4th ed. Philadelphia, Saunders, 1966, pp 372–414

Laibson PR, Dhiri S, Oconer J, Ortolan G: Corneal infiltrates in epidemic keratoconjunctivitis. Arch Ophthalmol 84:36, 1970

Lemp MA, Chambers RW, Lundy J: Viral isolate in superficial punctate keratitis. Arch Ophthalmol 91:8, 1974

Montenegro ENR, Israel CW, Nicol WG, Smith JL: Histopathologic demonstration of spirochetes in the human eye. Am J Ophthalmol 67:335, 1969

Naumann G, Gass JDM, Font RL: Histopathology of Herpes zoster ophthalmicus. Am J Ophthalmol 65:533, 1968

Naumann G, Gunders AE: Pathogenesis of the posterior segment lesion of ocular onchocerciasis. Am J Ophthalmol 75:82, 1973

Remky H: Augensymptome bei Protozoonosen (unter besonderer Berücksichtigung der Uveitis), in XX Concilium Ophthalmologicum Germania 1966, Acta, Pars II. Edited by E Weigelin. Amsterdam, Excerpta Medica Foundation, 1967, p 713

Scheie HG, Shannon RE, Yanoff M: Onchocerciasis (ocular). Ann Ophthalmol 3:697, 1971

Thygeson P: Superficial punctate keratitis. J Am Med Assoc 144:1544, 1950

Tripathi RC, Bron AJ: Ultrastructural study of nontraumatic recurrent corneal erosion. Br J Ophthalmol 56:73, 1972

Whitfield R, Wirostko E: Uveitis and intraocular treponemes. Arch Ophthalmol 84:12, 1970

Inflammations: Ulcerative

Allen HG: Current status of prevention, diagnosis and management of bacterial corneal ulcers. Ann Ophthalmol 3:235, 1971

Aronson SB, Elliott JH, Moore TE, O'Day D: Pathogenetic approach to therapy of peripheral corneal inflammatory disease. Am J Ophthalmol 70:65, 1970

Brown DC: Ocular herpes simplex. Invest Ophthalmol 10:210, 1971

Coskey RJ, Bryan HG: Vaccinia of the ocular region. J Pediatr Ophthalmol 5:157, 1968

Ferry AP, Leopold IH: Marginal (ring) corneal ulcer as presenting manifestation of Wegener's granuloma: clinicopathologic study. Trans Am Acad Ophthalmol Otolaryngol 74:1276, 1970

Fine BS: Mycotic Keratitis, in The Cornea World Congress. Edited by JH King, JW McTigue. Washington, DC, Butterworths, 1965, p. 207

Font RL: Chronic ulcerative keratitis caused by Herpes simplex virus. Arch Ophthalmol 90:382, 1973

Frayer WC: The histopathology of perilimbal ulceration in Wegener's granulomatosis. Arch Ophthalmol 64:58, 1960

Ginsberg HS: Adenoviruses. Am J Clin Pathol 57:771, 1972

Kaplan AS: Recent studies of the herpes viruses. Am J Clin Pathol 57:783, 1972

MacKeen D, Fine S, Aaron A, Fine BS: Preventable hazards at UV wavelengths, in Laser Focus Magazine. April 1971, p 29

Matas BR, Spencer WH, Hayes TL, Dawson CR: Morphology of experimental vaccinial superficial punctate keratitis—a scanning and transmission electron microscopic study. Invest Ophthalmol 10:348, 1971

Nahmias AJ, Hagler WS: Ocular manifestations of herpes simplex in the newborn (neonatal ocular herpes). Int Ophthalmol Clin 12:191, 1972

Naumann G, Green WR, Zimmerman LE: Mycotic keratitis. Am J Ophthalmol 64:668, 1967

Pavan-Langston D, McCulley JP: Herpes zoster dendritic keratitis. Arch Ophthalmol 89:25, 1973

Prebenga LW, Laibson PR: Dendritic lesions in herpes zoster ophthalmicus. Arch Ophthalmol 90:268, 1973

Spencer WH, Hayes TL: Scanning and transmission electron microscopic observations of the topographic anatomy of dendritic lesions in the rabbit cornea. Invest Ophthalmol 9:183, 1970

Verhoeff FM, Bell L: The pathological effects of radiant energy on the eye. Proc Am Acad Arts Sci 51:630, 1916

Wood WJ, Nicholson DH: Corneal ring ulcer as the presenting manifestation of acute monocytic leukemia. Am J Ophthalmol 76:69, 1973

Zimmerman LE: Keratomycosis, Survey Ophthalmol 8:1, 1963

Degenerations: Epithelial

Dodds HT, Laibson PR: Filamentary keratitis following cataract extraction. Arch Ophthalmol 88:609, 1972

Fells P, Bors F: Ocular complications of self-induced vitamin A deficiency. Trans Ophthalmol Soc UK 89:221, 1969

Font RL, Yanoff M, Zimmerman LE: Godwin's benign lymphoepithelial lesion of the lacrimal gland and its relationship to Sjögren's syndrome. Am J Clin Pathol 48:365, 1967

Gudas PP, Altman B, Nicholson DH, Green WR: Corneal perforation in Sjögren syndrome. Arch Ophthalmol 90:470, 1973

Levine RA, Rabb MF: Bitot's spot overlying a pinguecula. Arch Ophthalmol 86:525, 1971

Sood NN: Ocular manifestations in malnourished children. J Ped Ophthalmol 7:106, 1970

Sullivan WR, McCulley JP, Dohlman CH: Return of goblet cells after vitamin A therapy in xerosis of conjunctiva. Am J Ophthalmol 75:720, 1973

Zauberman H, Shapira Y, Gailer M: Sporadic keratomalacia. J Pediatr Ophthalmol 7:229, 1970

Degenerations: Stromal

Ansari MW, Rahi AHS, Shukla BR: Pseudoelastic nature of pterygium. Br J Ophthalmol 54:473, 1970

Aronson SB, Elliott JH, Moore TE, O'Day D: Pathogenetic approach to therapy of peripheral corneal inflammatory disease. Am J Ophthalmol 70:65, 1970

Berkow JW, Fine BS, Zimmerman LE: Unusual ocular calcification in hyperparathyroidism. Am J Ophthalmol 66:812, 1968

Brown SI, Grayson M: Marginal furrows: characteristic corneal lesion of rheumatoid arthritis. Arch Ophthalmol 79:563, 1968

Brownstein S, Rodrigues MM, Fine BS, Albert EN: The elastotic nature of hyaline corneal deposits. A histochemical, fluorescent, and electron microscopic examination. Am J Ophthalmol 75:799, 1973

Christensen GR: Proteinaceous corneal degeneration. A histochemical study. Arch Ophthalmol 89:30, 1973

Cogan DG, Albright F, Bartter FC: Hypercalcemia and band keratopathy: report of nineteen cases. Arch Ophthalmol 40:624, 1948

Cogan DG, Kuwabara T: Arcus senilis. Its pathology and histochemistry. Arch Ophthalmol 61:353, 1959

Fine BS, Berkow JW, Fine S: Corneal calcification. Science 162:129, 1968

Fine BS, Townsend WH, Zimmerman LE, Lashkari MH: Primary lipoidal degeneration of the cornea. Am J Ophthalmol 78:12, 1974

Francois J, Hanssens M, Stockmans L: Dégénerescence marginale pellucide de la cornée. Ophthalmologica 155:337, 1968

Fraunfelder FT, Hanna C: Spheroidal degeneration of cornea and conjunctiva. 3. Incidences, classification, and etiology. Am J Ophthalmol 76:41, 1973

Garner A, Morgan G, Tripathi RC: Climatic droplet keratopathy. II. Pathologic findings. Arch Ophthalmol 89:198, 1973

Houber JP: Bilateral recurrence of Salzmann's dys-

trophy after perforating keratoplasty. Ophthalmologica 161:90, 1970

Iwamoto T, DeVoe AG, Farris RL: Electron microscopy in cases of marginal degeneration of the cornea. Invest Ophthalmol 11:241, 1972

Jack RL, Luse SA: Lipid keratopathy. An electron microscopic study. Arch Ophthalmol 83:678, 1970

Klintworth GK: Chronic actinic keratopathy—a condition associated with conjunctival elastosis (pingueculae) and typified by characteristic extracellular concretions. Am J Pathol 67:327, 1972

O'Connor GR: Calcific band keratopathy. Trans Am Ophthalmol Soc 70:58, 1972

Porter R, Crombie AL: Corneal and conjunctival calcification in chronic renal failure. Br J Ophthalmol 57:339, 1973

Porter R, Crombie AL: Corneal calcification as a presenting and diagnostic sign in hyperparathyroidism. Br J Ophthalmol 57:665, 1973

Ramsey MS, Fine BS, Cohen SW: Localized corneal amyloidosis. Case report with electron microscopic observations. Am J Ophthalmol 73:560, 1972

Stafford WR, Fine BS: Amyloidosis of the cornea: report of a case without conjunctival involvement. Arch Ophthalmol 75:53, 1966

Süveges I, Levai G, Alberth B: Pathology of Terrien's disease. Histochemical and electron microscopic study. Am J Ophthalmol 74:1191, 1972

Terrien F: Dystrophie marginale symétrique des deux cornées avec astigmatisme régulier consécutif et guérison par la cautérisation ignée. Arch Ophtalmol (Paris) 20:12, 1900

Tragakis MP, Brown SI: The tear film alteration associated with dellen. Ann Ophthalmol 6:757, 1974

Wood TO, Kaufman HE: Mooren's ulcer. Am J Ophthalmol 71:417, 1971

Dystrophies: Epithelial

Akiya S, Brown SL: The ultrastructure of Reis-Bücklers' dystrophy. Am J Ophthalmol 72:549, 1971

Brady RO, Uhlendorf BW, Jacobson CB: Fabry's disease: antenatal detection. Science 172:174, 1971

Bron AJ, Tripathi RC: Cystic disorders of the corneal epithelium. I. Clinical aspects. Br J Ophthalmol 57:361, 1973

Burns R: Meesmann's corneal dystrophy. Trans Am Ophthalmol Soc 66:530, 1968

Font RL, Fine BS: Ocular pathology in Fabry's disease. Histochemical and electron microscopic observations. Am J Ophthalmol 73:419, 1972

Griffith DG, Fine BS: Light and electron microscopic observations in a superficial corneal dystrophy. Probably early Reis Bücklers' type. Am J Ophthalmol 63:1659, 1967

Guerry D: Observations on Cogan's microcystic dystrophy of the corneal epithelium. Trans Am Ophthalmol Soc 63:320, 1965

Jones ST, Stauffer LK: Reis-Bücklers' corneal dystrophy. A clinicopathologic study. Trans Am Acad Ophthalmol Otolaryngol 74:417, 1970

Kanai A, Kaufman HE, Polack FM: Electron microscopic study of Reis-Bücklers' dystrophy. Ann Ophthalmol 5:953, 1973

King RG Jr, Geeraets R: Cogan-Guerry microcystic corneal epithelial dystrophy. A clinical and electron microscopic study. Med Col Va Q 8:241, 1972

Kuwabara T, Ciccarelli EC: Meesmann's corneal dystrophy: a pathologic study. Arch Ophthalmol 71:676, 1964

Levitt JM: Microcystic dystrophy of the corneal epithelium. Am J Ophthalmol 72:381, 1971

Meesmann A, Wilke F: Klinische und anatomische Untersuchungen über eine bisher unbekannte, dominant vererbte Epitheldystrophie der Hornhaut. Klin Monatsbl Augenheilkd 103:361, 1939

Rice NSC, Ashton N, Jay B, Black RK: Reis-Bücklers' dystrophy. Clinico-Pathological Study. Br J Ophthalmol 52:577, 1968

Rodrigues MM, Fine BS, Laibson PR, Zimmerman LE: Disorders of the corneal epithelium—a clinicopathologic study of dot, geographic and fingerprint patterns. Arch Ophthalmol 92:475, 1974

Stocker W, Holt LB: Rare form of hereditary epithelial dystrophy. Arch Ophthalmol 53:536, 1955

Tripathi RC, Bron AJ: Cystic disorders of the corneal epithelium. II. Pathogenesis. Br J Ophthalmol 57:376, 1973

Trobe JD, Laibson PR: Dystrophic changes in the anterior cornea. Arch Ophthalmol 87:378, 1972

Dystrophies: Stromal—Heredofamilial

Akiya S, Brown SI: Granular dystrophy of the cornea. Arch Ophthalmol 84:179, 1970

Birndorf LA, Ginsberg SP: Hereditary fleck dystrophy associated with decreased corneal sensitivity. Am J Ophthalmol 73:670, 1972

Bron AJ, Williams HP, Corruthers ME: Hereditary crystalline stromal dystrophy of Schnyder. I. Clinical features of a family with hyperlipoproteinemia. Br J Ophthalmol 56:383, 1972

Brownstein S, Fine BS, Sherman ME, Zimmerman LE: Granular dystrophy of the cornea—light and electron microscopic confirmation of recurrence in a graft. Am J Ophthalmol 77:701, 1974

Fine BS, Townsend WM, Zimmerman LE, Lashkari MH: Primary lipoidal degeneration of the cornea. Am J Ophthalmol 78:12, 1974

Francois J, Neetens A: Nouvelle dystrophie hérédo-familiale du parenchyme corneen (Hérédo-dystrophie Mouchetée). Bull Soc Belge Ophthalmol 114:641, 1956

Garner A: Histochemistry of corneal macular dystrophy. Invest Ophthalmol 8:475, 1969

Garner A, Tripathi RC: Hereditary crystalline stromal dystrophy of Schnyder. II. Histopathology and ultrastructure. Br J Ophthalmol 56:400, 1972

Harboyen G, Mamo J, Kaloustian VD, Karam F: Congenital corneal dystrophy: progressive sensorineural deafness in a family. Arch Ophthalmol 85:27, 1971

Jones ST, Zimmerman LE: Macular dystrophy of the cornea (Groenouw type II). Am J Ophthalmol 47:1, 1959

Jones ST, Zimmerman LE: Histopathologic differentiation of granular, macular and lattice dystrophies of the cornea. Am J Ophthalmol 51:394, 1961

Kanai A, Kaufman HE: Further electron microscopic study of hereditary corneal edema. Invest Ophthalmol 10:545, 1971

Kenyon KR, Antine B: The pathogenesis of congenital hereditary endothelial dystrophy of the cornea. Am J Ophthalmol 72:787, 1971

Kenyon KR, Maumenee AE: The histological and ultrastructural pathology of congenital hereditary corneal dystrophy. Case report. Invest Ophthalmol 7:475, 1968

Kenyon KR, Maumenee AE: Further studies of congenital hereditary endothelial dystrophy of the cornea. Am J Ophthalmol 76:419, 1973

Klintworth GK: Lattice corneal dystrophy, an inherited variety of amyloidosis restricted to the cornea. Am J Pathol 50:371, 1967

Maumenee AE: Congenital hereditary corneal dystrophy. Am J Ophthalmol 50:114, 1960

McTigue JW, Fine BS: The stromal lesion in lattice dystrophy of the cornea: A light and electron microscopic study. Invest Ophthalmol 3:355, 1964

Rabb MF, Blodi F, Boniuk M: Unilateral lattice dystrophy of the cornea. Am J Ophthalmol 78:440, 1974

Ramsey MS, Fine BS, Cohen SW: Localized corneal amyloidosis. Case report with electron microscopic observations. Am J Ophthalmol 73:560, 1972

Smith ME, Zimmerman LE: Amyloid in corneal dystrophies: differentiation of lattice from granular and macular dystrophies. Arch Ophthalmol 79:407, 1968

Teng CC: Macular dystrophy of the cornea. A histochemical and electron microscopic study. Am J Ophthalmol 62:436, 1966

Dystrophies: Stromal—Heredofamilial: Secondary to Systemic Disease

Boniuk M, Hill LL: Ocular Manifestations of de Toni-Fanconi syndrome with cystine storage disease. South Med J 59:33, 1966

Brownstein MH, Elliott R, Helwig EB: Ophthalmologic aspects of amyloidosis. Am J Ophthalmol 69:423, 1970

Cogan DC, Kuwabara T: Ocular pathology of cystinosis with particular reference to the elusiveness of the corneal crystals. Arch Ophthalmol 63:51, 1960

Cogan DC, Kuwabara T, Moser H: Metachromatic leukodystrophy. Ophthalmologica 160:2, 1970

Davis P, Toussaint D: Histologic retinal changes in Hunter-type mucopolysaccharidosis (in French). Bull Soc Belge Ophtalmol 157:365, 1971

Emery JM, Green WR, Wyllie RG, Howell RR: G_{M1}-Gangliosidosis: ocular and pathological manifestations. Arch Ophthalmol 85:177, 1971

Francois J, Hanssens M, Coppieters R, Evans L: Cystinosis: clinical and histopathologic study. Am J Ophthalmol 73:643, 1972

Goldberg MF, Maumenee AE, McKusick VA: Corneal

dystrophies associated with abnormalities of mucopolysaccharide metabolism. Arch Ophthalmol 74:516, 1965

Hambrick GW Jr, Scheie HG: Studies of the skin in Hurler's syndrome. Arch Dermatol 85:455, 1962

Jensen OA: Mucopolysaccharidosis type III (Sanfillipo's syndrome): histochemical examination of the eyes and brain with a survey of the literature. Acta Pathol Microbiol Scand [A]79:257, 1971

Kenyon KR, Quigley HA, Hussels IE, Wyllie RG: The systemic mucopolysaccharidoses: ultrastructural and histochemical studies of the conjunctiva and skin. Am J Ophthalmol 73:811, 1972

Kenyon KR, Sensenbrenner JA: Mucolipidosis II (I-cell disease): ultrastructural observations of conjunctiva and skin. Invest Ophthalmol 10:555, 1971

Kenyon KR, Sensenbrenner JA: Electron microscopy of cornea and conjunctiva in childhood cystinosis. Am J Ophthalmol 78:68, 1974

Kenyon KR, Topping RM, Green WR, Maumenee AE: Ocular pathology of the Maroteaux-Lamy syndrome (systemic mucopolysaccharidosis type VI): histologic and ultrastructural report of two cases. Am J Ophthalmol 73:718, 1972

Krause E, Lutz P: Ocular cystine deposits in an adult. Arch Ophthalmol 85:690, 1971

Kroll WA, Schneider JA: Decrease in free cystine content of cultured fibroblasts by ascorbic acid. Science 186:1040, 1974

McKusick VA: Heritable Disorders of Connective Tissue 4th ed. Mosby, 1972, pp 521–686

Quigley HA, Goldberg MF: Scheie syndrome and macular corneal dystrophy. An ultrastructural comparison of conjunctiva and skin. Arch Ophthalmol 85:553, 1971

Quigley HA, Goldberg MF: Conjunctival ultrastructure in mucolipidosis III (pseudo-Hurler polydystrophy). Invest Ophthalmol 10:568, 1971

Sanderson PO, Kuwabara T, Stark WJ, Wong VG, Collins EM: Cystinosis. A clinical, histopathologic and ultrastructural study. Arch Ophthalmol 91:270, 1974

Seringe P, Dhermy P, Aron J-J: Les manifestations oculaires de la gangliosidose généralisée à G_{M1} (Maladie de Norman-Landing). Arch Ophtalmol (Paris) 30:113, 1970

Snip RC, Kenyon KR, Green WR: Macular corneal dystrophy: ultrastructural pathology of corneal endothelium and Descemet's membrane. Invest Ophthalmol 12:88, 1973

Spaeth GL: Ocular manifestations of the lipidoses, in Retinal Diseases in Children. Edited by W Tasman. New York, Harper & Row, 1971, pp 127–206

Spranger JW, Wiedemann HR: The genetic mucolipidoses. Diagnosis and differential diagnosis. Humangenetik 9:113, 1970

Topping TM, Kenyon KR, Goldberg MF, Maumenee AE: Ultrastructural ocular pathology of Hunter's syndrome: systemic mucopolysaccharidosis type II. Arch Ophthalmol 86:164, 1971

Tso MOM, Fine BS, Thorpe HE: Kayser-Fleischer ring and associated cataract in Wilson's disease. Am J Ophthalmol, 79:479, 1975

Vogel MH, Müller K-M, Witting C: Ocular histopathology in mucopolysaccharidosis III (Sanfilippo). Ophthalmologica 169:311, 1974

Weingeist TA, Blodi FC: Fabry's disease: ocular findings in a female carrier. A light and electron microscopic study. Arch Ophthalmol 85:169, 1971

Zimmerman TJ, Hood I, Gasset AR: "Adolescent" cystinosis; a case presentation and review of the recent literature. Arch Ophthalmol 92:265, 1974

Dystrophies: Stromal—Nonheredofamilial

McTigue JW: The human cornea. A light and electron microscopic study of the normal cornea and its alterations in various dystrophies. Trans Am Ophthalmol Soc 65:591, 1967

Pataa C, Joyon L, Roucher F: Ultra-structure de kératocône. Arch Ophtalmol (Paris) 30:403, 1970

Dystrophies: Endothelial

Boruchoff SA, Kuwabara T: Electron microscopy of posterior polymorphous degeneration. Am J Ophthalmol 72:879, 1971

Cross HE, Maumenee AE, Cantolino SE: Inheritance of Fuchs' endothelial dystrophy. Arch Ophthalmol 85:268, 1971

Gasset AR, Zimmerman TJ: Posterior polymorphous dystrophy associated with keratoconus. Am J Ophthalmol 78:535, 1974

Hogan MJ, Bietti G: Hereditary deep dystrophy of the cornea (polymorphous). Am J Ophthalmol 68:777, 1969

Hogan MJ, Wood I, Fine M: Fuchs' endothelial dystrophy of the cornea. Am J Ophthalmol 78:363, 1974

Iwamoto T, DeVoe AG: Electron microscopic studies on Fuchs' combined dystrophy. I. Posterior portion of cornea. Invest Ophthalmol 10:9, 1971

Iwamoto T, DeVoe AG: Electron microscopic studies on Fuchs' combined dystrophy. II. Anterior portion of cornea. Invest Ophthalmol 10:29, 1971

Michels RG, Kenyon KR, Maumenee AE: Retrocorneal fibrous membrane. Invest Ophthalmol 11:822, 1972

Schroeder GT, Hanna C: Unusual epithelial changes in a case of combined corneal dystrophy of Fuchs. Am J Ophthalmol 72:542, 1971

Pigmentations

Burns CA: Indomethacin, reduced retinal sensitivity and corneal deposits. Am J Ophthalmol 66:825, 1968

Calkins LD: Corneal epithelial changes occurring during chloroquine (Aralen) therapy. Arch Ophthalmol 60:981, 1958

Ferry AP: A "new" iron line of the superficial cornea: occurrence in patients with filtering blebs. Arch Ophthalmol 79:142, 1968

Ferry AP, Zimmerman LE: Black cornea: a complication of topical use of epinephrine. Am J Ophthalmol 58:205, 1964

Gass JE: The iron lines of the superficial cornea. Arch Ophthalmol 71:348, 1964

Goldberg MF, Von Noorden GK: Ophthalmic findings in Wilson's hepatolenticular degeneration. Arch Ophthalmol 75:162, 1966

Johnson BL: Ultrastructure of the Kayser-Fleischer ring. Am J Ophthalmol 76:455, 1973

Kaufer G, Fine BS, Green WR, Zimmerman LE: Retrocorneal pigmentation with special reference to the formation of retrocorneal membranes by uveal melanocytes. Am J Ophthalmol 64:567, 1967

Madge GE, Geeraets WJ, Guerry DP: Black cornea secondary to topical epinephrine. Am J Ophthalmol 71:402, 1971

Pouliquen Y, Graf B, Bisson J, Feuvrier YM, Dellattre A: Ultrastructural study of corneal thickening in the course of chlorpromazine treatment (in French). Arch Ophtalmol (Paris) 30:769, 1970

Prien RF, Cole JO, deLong SL, Levine J: Ocular effects of long term chlorpromazine. Arch Gen Psychiatry 23:464, 1970

Reinecke RD, Kuwabara T: Corneal deposits secondary to topical epinephrine. Arch Ophthalmol 70:170, 1963

Rones B: Ochronosis oculi in alkaptonuria. Am J Ophthalmol 49:440, 1960

Tso MOM, Fine BS, Thorpe HE: Kayser-Fleischer ring and associated cataract in Wilson's disease. Am J Ophthalmol, 79:479, 1975

SCLERA

Congenital Anomalies

Daicker B, Riede UN: Histologische and ultrastrukturelle Befunde bei alkaptonurischer Ochronosis oculi. Ophthalmologica 169:377, 1974

McKusick VA: Heritable Disorders of Connective Tissue, 4th ed., St. Louis, Mosby, 1972, pp 390–474

O'Brien WM, LaDu BN, Bunim JJ: Biochemical, pathologic and chemical aspects of alcaptonuria, ochronosis and ochronotic arthropathy. Am J Med 34:813, 1963

Inflammations

Anderson B Sr: Ocular lesions in relapsing polychondritis and other rheumatoid syndromes. Trans Am Acad Ophthalmol Otolaryngol 71:227, 1971

Brubaker R, Font RL, Shepherd EM: Granulomatous sclerouveitis: regression of ocular lesions with cyclophosphamide and prednisone. Arch Ophthalmol 86:517, 1971

Evans PJ, Eustace P: Scleromalacia perforans associated with Crohn's disease treated with sodium versenate (EDTA). Br J Ophthalmol 57:330, 1973

Frayer WC: The histopathology of perilimbal ulceration in Wegener's granulomatosis. Arch Ophthalmol 64:58, 1960

Henkind P, Gold DH: Ocular Manifestations of rheumatic disorders. Rheumatology 4:13, 1973

Lyne AJ, Pikerthley DA: Episcleritis and scleritis. Arch Ophthalmol 80:171, 1968

Tumors

Ferry AP, Hein HF: Epibulbar osseous choristoma within an epibulbar dermoid. Am J Ophthalmol 70:764, 1970

CONGENITAL AND DEVELOPMENTAL DEFECTS

PERSISTENT PUPILLARY MEMBRANE (Fig. 9–1)

I. Persistence of a pupillary membrane, an extremely common finding, is due to incomplete atrophy (resorption) of the fetal vascular arcades and associated mesodermal tissue derived from the primitive annular vessel.

Incomplete persistence is the rule. Because the remnants represent fetal mesodermal tissue, they are nonpigmented except if they are attached to the anterior surface of the lens. The remnants may be attached to the iris alone (invariably to the collarette), or they may run from the collarette of the iris to attach onto the posterior surface of the cornea where occasionally there is an associated corneal opacity. Isolated nonpigmented or pigmented remnants may be found on the anterior lens capsule ("stars") or found drifting freely in the anterior chamber. Total persistence of the fetal pupillary membrane is extremely rare and usually associated with other ocular anomalies, especially microphthalmos.

II. Histologically, fine strands of mesodermal tissue occasionally with patent blood vessels are seen.

PERSISTENT TUNICA VASCULOSA LENTIS

I. Persistence of the tunica vasculosa lentis is due to incomplete atrophy (resorption) of the fetal tunica vasculosa lentis derived posteriorly from the primitive hyaloid vasculature and anteriorly from the primitive annular vessel posterior to the fetal pupillary membrane.

Persistence of the posterior part of the tunica vasculosa lentis generally is associated with persistence of a hyperplastic primary vitreous, the composite whole being known as persistent hyperplastic primary vitreous (PHPV; see p. 698 in Chap. 18), and may or may not be associated with persistence of the anterior part of the tunica vasculosa lentis. Persistence of the anterior part of the tunica vasculosa lentis alone probably does not occur. The entire tunica vasculosa lentis may persist without an associated primary vitreous, but this is extremely rare and usually is associated with other ocular anomalies, e.g., with the ocular anomalies of trisomy 13–15.

II. Histologically, fine strands of mesodermal tissue generally with patent blood vessels are seen closely applied to and surrounding the lens capsule. Persistence and hyperplasia of the primary vitreous may or may not be present.

HEMATOPOESIS (Fig. 9–2)

I. Hematopoesis within the choroid is a normal finding in premature infants and even in full-term infants for the first 3 to 6 months of life.

Hematopoetic tissue may occur as an acquired form associated with intraocular osseous metaplasia (the bone containing marrow spaces) generally in chronically inflamed eyes.

II. Histologically hematopoetic tissue containing blood cell precursors is seen in the uvea, especially in the choroid.

ECTOPIC INTRAOCULAR LACRIMAL GLAND TISSUE (Fig. 9–3)

I. Tissue appearing histologically similar to lacrimal gland tissue has been found in the iris, ciliary body, choroid, anterior chamber angle, sclera and limbus.

II. Histologically the tissue resembles normal lacrimal gland.

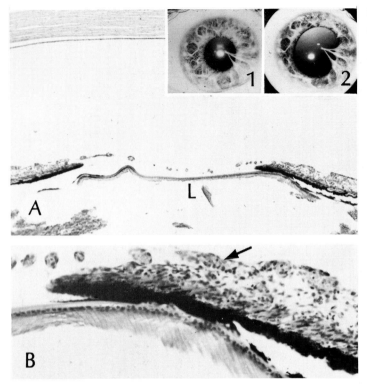

FIG. 9–1. Persistent pupillary membrane. A. Inset 1 shows persistent pupillary membrane extending from iris collarette (from 3 to 4 o'clock) to anterior surface of lens; **inset 2** same eye after dilatation. Photomicrograph shows vascular membrane extending across pupil in 3-day-old premature infant. *L*, lens. **B.** Higher magnification to show pupillary membrane (blood vessels) arising from iris collarette (*arrow*). **A,** H&E, ×21; **inset 1,** clinical; **inset 2,** clinical; **B,** H&E, ×101.

— up to 3–6 months

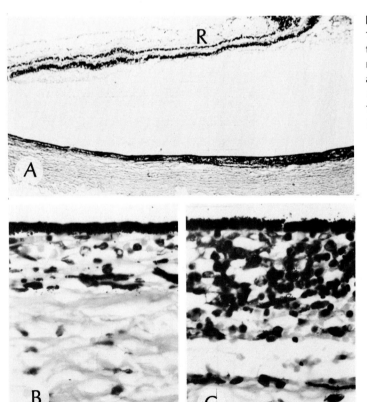

FIG. 9–2. Hematopoesis. Infant weighing 1,070 g died first day of life. **A.** Choroid thickened over most of right side of figure. *R*, retina. **B.** Higher magnification of normal area of choroid to compare with **C** (at same magnification), which shows choroid thickened by hematopoetic tissue. **A,** H&E, ×16; **B,** H&E, ×252; **C,** H&E, ×252.

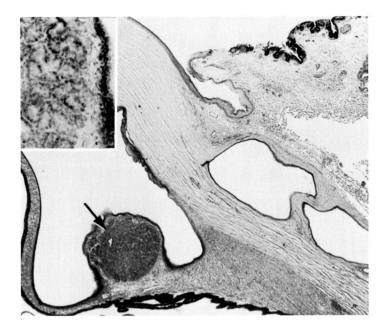

FIG. 9–3. Ectopic intraocular lacrimal gland tissue (*arrow* and shown with higher magnification in **inset**) present within iris in 2½-week-old child. Congenital epithelialization of anterior surface of iris (right side of **inset**), anterior chamber angle and posterior cornea is present. **Main figure,** H&E, ×16; **inset,** H&E, ×101.

Peters : ō Descemets
ō Endithelin
ō Bowmans !!

CONGENITAL AND DEVELOPMENTAL DEFECTS OF THE PIGMENT EPITHELIUM

See p. 638 in Chapter 17.

HYPOPLASIA OF THE IRIS (Fig. 9–4)

I. Although commonly called *aniridia*, complete absence of the iris is exceedingly rare. Gonioscopically a rudimentary iris can be seen in continuity with the ciliary body.

The rudimentary iris may be clinically invisible unless gonioscopy is used. The amount of iris tissue present varies in different quadrants. Generally the equator of the lens is seen easily when focal illumination is used. Photophobia, nystagmus and poor vision may be present but not invariably. Glaucoma frequently is associated with hypoplasia of the iris. Other ocular anomalies are found commonly.

II. The condition may be inherited as an autosomal dominant or less commonly as an autosomal recessive.

III. Histologically a rim of rudimentary iris tissue is found encircling the periphery. The iris musculature generally is underdeveloped or absent.

MESODERMAL DYSGENESIS OF THE CORNEA AND IRIS (*Riegers*) — *no ulcer*

See p. 268 in Chapter 8.

COLOBOMA (Figs. 9–4 through 9–7)

I. A coloboma, i.e., localized absence or defect, of the iris may occur alone or in association with a coloboma of the ciliary body and choroid.
   A. Typical colobomas occur in the region of the embryonic cleft, inferonasally, and may be complete, incomplete (e.g., iris stromal hypoplasia) or, in the region of the choroid, cystic.
   B. Atypical colobomas occur in regions other than in the inferonasal area.
   C. Typical colobomas are due to some interference with the normal closure of the embryonic cleft, producing defective ectoderm. The cause of atypical colobomas is poorly understood.

The anterior pigment epithelium seems primarily to be defective. Except in the rare iris bridge coloboma, no tissue spans the defect so that an area of complete absence results. Iridodiastasis is a coloboma of the iris periphery that resembles an iridodialysis. In the ciliary body fre-

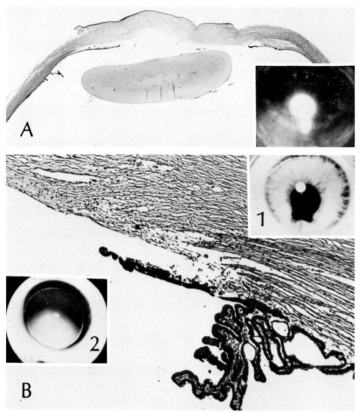

FIG. 9–4. Hypoplasia of iris. **A.** Hypoplasia is more marked on right iris leaf than left. Peculiar shape of lens ("blunting" on right side) due to "coloboma" of lens on right side (inferiorly) in area where zonules are absent (see Figures 8–13 and 10–1). **Inset** shows transillumination of same eye to demonstrate coloboma (hypoplasia) of iris inferiorly. **B.** Higher magnification of hypoplastic iris. **Insets** show range of iris hypoplasia from partial stromal coloboma (**1**) to "aniridia" or marked hypoplasia (**2**). **A,** H&E, ×6; **inset,** macroscopic; **B,** H&E, ×40; **inset 1,** clinical; **inset 2,** clinical.

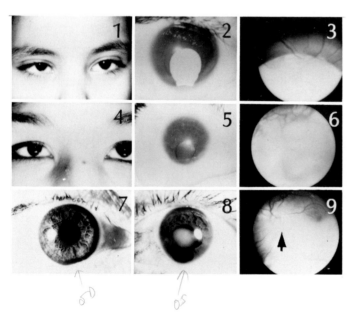

FIG. 9–5. Coloboma. **1, 2** and **3** from same patient show microcornea of right eye (OD), iris coloboma OD and choroidal coloboma OD with involvement of optic disc. **4, 5** and **6** from second patient show microcornea OD, iris coloboma OD and choroidal coloboma OD with involvement of optic disc and of area superior to disc. **7, 8** and **9** from third patient show heterochromia with lighter iris OD and darker iris (containing inferior nasal coloboma) of left eye. Left eye contains cataract, which induced acute attack of angle closure glaucoma. Following cataract extraction (**9**) coloboma of choroid, not involving optic disc, was observable (*arrow* points to inferior margin of disc). Case illustrates that iris colobomas are rarely complete and some peripheral iris had to be present to cause acute angle closure glaucoma. (**1,** clinical, both eyes; **2,** clinical, right eye; **3,** fundus; **4,** clinical, both eyes; **5,** clinical, right eye; **6,** fundus; **7,** clinical, right eye; **8,** clinical, left eye; **9,** fundus.

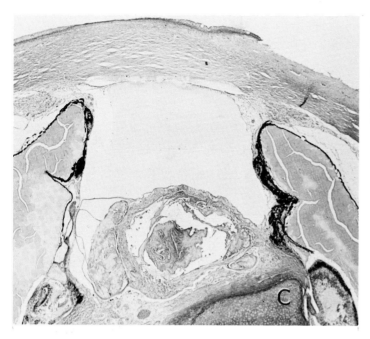

FIG. 9–6. Massive coloboma of iris and ciliary body in case of 13–15 trisomy. Note cartilage (C) behind cataractous lens. H&E, ×16.

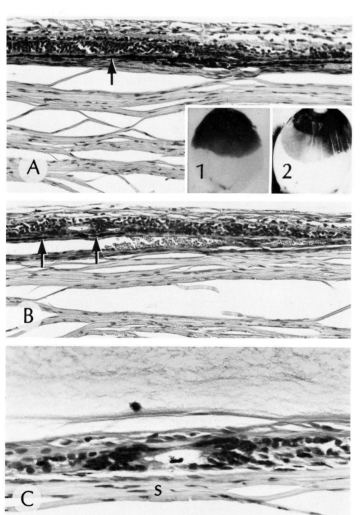

FIG. 9–7. Coloboma of retinal pigment epithelium and choroid. **A. Inset 1** shows transilluminated whole eye to demonstrate lack of pigment posteriorly, better shown in opened eye (**inset 2**). Photomicrograph shows anterior retina with pigment epithelium (*arrow*) intact. **B.** Transitional area in equatorial region shows discontinuous pigment epithelium (*arrows*); choroid is intact. **C.** Posterior area. Pigment epithelium and choroid are not present. Retina is dysplastic with rosette formation. *s*, sclera. **A,** H&E, ×130; **inset 1,** macroscopic (unopened eye); **inset 2,** macroscopic; **B,** H&E, ×130; **C,** H&E, ×365.

quently the tissue underlying the pigment epithelial defect consists of mesoderm and vascular tissue that fills the region of the coloboma, whereas there is hyperplasia of the ciliary processes on either side of the defect. The mesodermal tissue may contain cartilage in trisomy 13–15. Overlying the pigment epithelial defect, there may be an absence of zonules so that the lens becomes notched, producing the appearance of a *coloboma of the lens*. The retinal pigment epithelium is absent in the area of a choroidal coloboma, although it is usually hyperplastic at the edges; the sensory retina is atrophic and gliotic and may contain rosettes; the underlying choroid is absent (partially or completely); and the sclera may be thin or ectatic sometimes appearing as a large cyst often associated with a microphthalmic eye; see p. 516 in Chap. 14.

II. The extent of a coloboma of the choroid is variable. It may be complete from the optic nerve to the ora serrata inferonasally. It may be incomplete and consist of an *inferior crescent* at the inferonasal portion of the optic nerve, or it may consist of a linear area of pigmentation or retinal pigment epithelial and choroidal thinning in any part of the fetal fissure.

III. Colobomas may occur alone or in association with other ocular anomalies.

IV. The condition may be inherited as an irregular autosomal dominant.

V. Histology:

    A. The iris coloboma shows a complete absence of all tissue in the involved area; either a complete sector from pupil to periphery may be involved or only a part of the iris.

    B. The ciliary body coloboma shows a defect filled with mesoderm and vascular tissues (also cartilage in trisomy 13–15) with hyperplastic ciliary processes at the edges.

    C. The choroidal coloboma shows an absence of retinal pigment epithelium with atrophic and gliotic retina, sometimes containing rosettes, overlying the area and absent or atrophic choroid underlying it. The retinal pigment epithelium tends to be hyperplastic at the edge of the defect. The sclera in the region generally is thinned and may be

cystic; the cystic space often is filled with proliferated glial tissue.

The proliferated glial tissue may become so extensive (i.e., massive gliosis) so as to be confused with a glial neoplasm.

CYSTS OF THE IRIS AND ANTERIOR CILIARY BODY

I. Iris stroma cysts (Fig. 9–3) resemble implantation iris cysts following nonsurgical and surgical trauma.

    A. The cysts can become quite large and cause visual problems by impinging on the pupil; they may also occlude the angle and cause secondary angle closure glaucoma.

    B. The origin of the cysts is poorly understood, although evidence suggests a two-part derivation, a mesodermal component from cells of the iris stroma and an epithelial component from nonpigmented neuroepithelial cells.

    C. Histologically the cysts are lined by a multilayered epithelium resembling cornea or conjunctival epithelium, which may even have goblet cells. The cysts generally contain a clear fluid.

II. Iris or ciliary body epithelial cysts (Figs. 9–8 through 9–10) are associated with the nonpigmented epithelium of the ciliary body or the pigmented neuroepithelium on the posterior surface of the iris or at the pupillary margin.

    A. With the possible exception of the production of a secondary angle closure glaucoma or pupillary obstruction, the clinical course of the cysts usually is benign.

Multiple iris and ciliary body cysts may be found in congenital syphilis. These eyes frequently develop a secondary angle closure glaucoma.

    B. The cysts form as a proliferation of the posterior layer of iris pigment epithelium or of the inner layer of ciliary epithelium.

Occasionally a cyst may break off and float freely in the anterior chamber. The cysts then may implant in the anterior

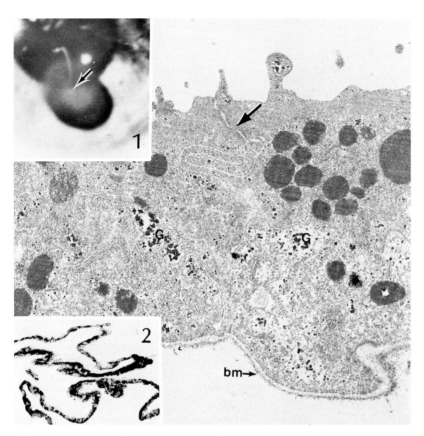

FIG. 9–8. Iris epithelial cyst. **Inset 1.** Clinical photograph of pigmented cyst floating freely in lower part of anterior chamber. Note that iris can be seen through translucency of the cyst (*arrow*). **Inset 2.** Wall of collapsed cyst appears to be composed of single layer of pigmented epithelium, confirmed on examination by electron microscopy. Thin basement membrane (*bm*), apical tight junction (*arrow*) and apical villi indicate polarization of cells in layer, like that of normal posterior iris pigment epithelium. Presence of glycogen (*G*) also is feature of normal iris pigment epithelium. **Main figure,** TSC, ×16,500; **inset 1,** clinical; **inset 2,** 1.5 μ section, PD, ×130.

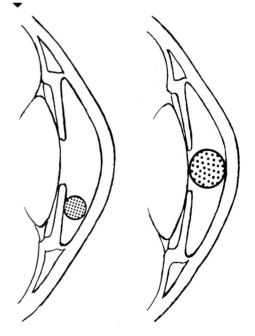

FIG. 9–9. Enlarging free cyst of necessity will occupy pupillary region of anterior chamber and must be removed for reasons of vision.

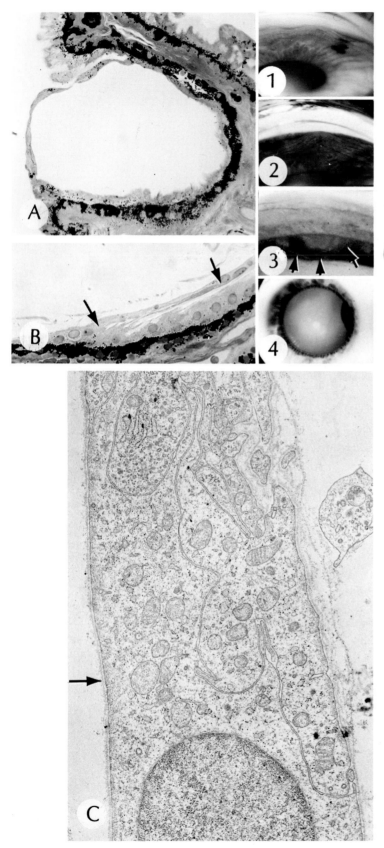

FIG. 9–10. Nonpigmented ciliary epithelial cysts are common in region of pars plicata. **A.** They generally are due to proliferations of nonpigmented epithelium and are frequently incidental findings on gross examination of enucleated postmortem eyes. **B.** Note (*arrows*) nonpigmented epithelial layer proliferating to form wall of cyst. **1** and **2** show tenting up of iris in region of pars plicata ciliary body cysts; **3** shows clear cyst (*arrows*) seen behind dilated pupil (note ciliary processes seen through transparent cyst); **4** shows pigmented cyst. **C.** Electron microscopy of wall of cyst shows proliferating nonpigmented epithelial cells. Note presence of thin basement membrane-like layer on one side (*arrow*) and poorly formed multilaminar basement membrane on other. **A,** 1.5 μ section, PD, $\times$220; **B,** 1.5 μ section, PD, $\times$300; **1,** clinical; **2,** clinical; **3,** clinical; **4,** clinical; **C,** $\times$8,800.

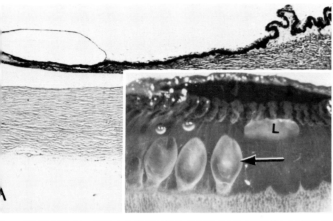

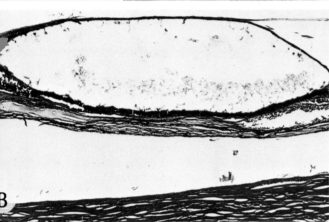

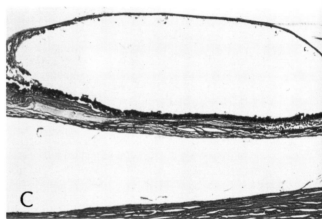

chamber angle where they have on occasion been mistaken for a malignant melanoma. Occasionally a cyst may float freely, enlarge and so obstruct the pupil that surgical removal of the cyst is necessary.

III. Histologically the pigmented cysts are lined by epithelial cells having all the characteristics of mature pigment epithelium. The lumen is filled with an as yet unidentified watery substance.

CYSTS OF THE POSTERIOR CILIARY BODY (PARS PLANA) (Figs. 9–11 through 9–13)

I. Most cysts of the pars plana of the ciliary body are acquired rather than congenital.

II. Pars plana cysts are intraepithelial cysts of the nonpigmented ciliary epithelium and are apparently analogous to the cysts of microcystoid degeneration of the retina (see p. 412 in Chap. 11).

Clinically the garden-variety pars plana cysts and those of multiple myeloma appear almost identical. With fixation, however, the multiple myeloma cysts turn white or milky, whereas the other cysts remain clear. The *multiple myeloma cysts* contain α-globulin (immunoglobulin). Cysts similar to the myeloma cysts but extending over the pars plicata have been seen in nonmyelomatous hypergammaglobulinemic conditions.

III. Histologically, large intraepithelial cysts are present within the nonpigmented ciliary epithelium of the pars plana. The cysts appear empty in routinely stained sections but contain a hyaluronidase-sensitive material, presumably hyaluronic acid, when stained with special stains to demonstrate acid mucopolysaccharides.

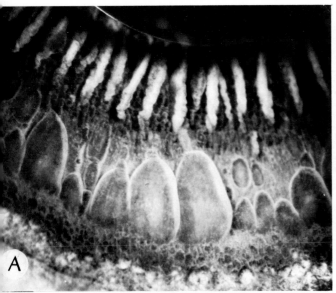

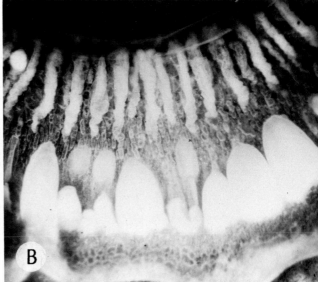

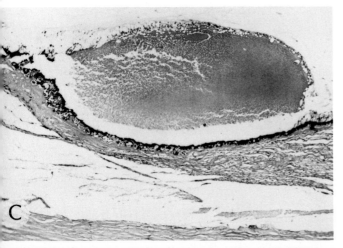

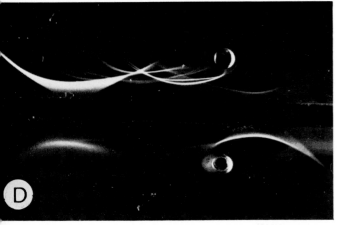

FIG. 9–12. Multiple myeloma. **A.** Ciliary body pars plana cysts are clear in normal or unfixed state, but in **B** are shown to become milky after 60 minutes' fixation in formaldehyde. **C.** Deeply staining proteinaceous material fills pars plana cyst. **D.** Immunoelectrophoretic pattern. Top well filled with patient's serum and bottom well with cyst material. Trough loaded with antisera directed against whole serum (anode is at left). **A,** macroscopic; **B,** macroscopic; **C,** H&E, ×40; **D,** immunoelectrophoretic pattern.

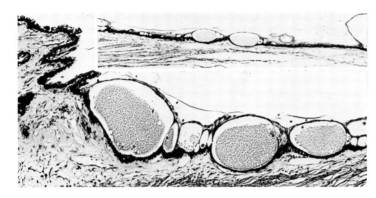

FIG. 9–13. Multiple myeloma. Cysts involve both pars plicata (left side of **main figure**) and pars plana (**inset**). **Main figure,** H&E, ×40; **inset,** H&E, ×16.

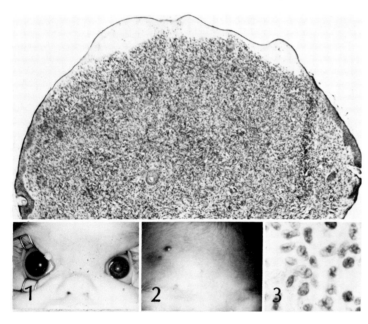

FIG. 9–14. Juvenile xanthogranuloma. **Inset 1** shows infant with bilateral spontaneous hyphema, buphthalmos of right eye and orange skin lesions on forehead (**inset 2**). Biopsy of skin lesion shows replacement of dermis by histiocytes (higher magnification in **inset 3**). **Main figure,** H&E, ×28; **inset 1,** clinical, both eyes; **inset 2,** clinical; **inset 3,** H&E, ×252.

INFLAMMATIONS

See Chapters 3 and 4.

INJURIES

See Chapter 5.

SYSTEMIC DISEASES

DIABETES MELLITUS

See sections Iris, Ciliary Body and Choroid in Chapter 15.

VASCULAR DISEASES

See section Vascular Disease in Chapter 11.

CYSTINOSIS

See p. 306 in Chapter 8.

HOMOCYSTINURIA

See p. 380 in Chapter 10.

AMYLOIDOSIS

See p. 248 in Chapter 7 and p. 480 in Chapter 12.

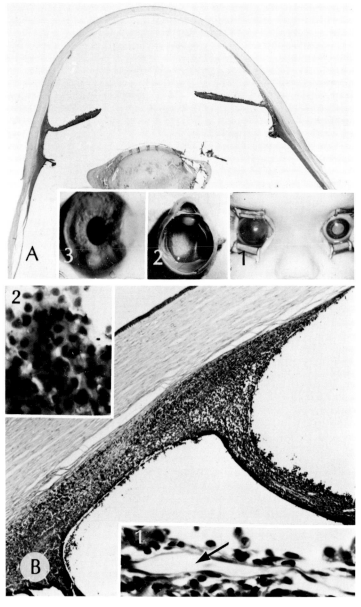

FIG. 9–15. Juvenile xanthogranuloma. **A.** Right eye (**inset 1**) enucleated (**inset 2**) because of glaucoma, opaque media and suspected retinoblastoma. Photomicrograph shows diffuse involvement of iris and ciliary body by histiocytes. **Inset 3** shows another patient with segmental involvement of iris temporally. **B.** Higher magnification to show diffuse histiocytic infiltrate. **Inset 1** shows thin-walled capillary (*arrow*) near surface of iris. **Inset 2** shows positive lipid staining of histiocytes. **A,** H&E, ×5; **inset 1,** clinical, both eyes; **inset 2,** macroscopic; **inset 3,** clinical, left eye; **B,** H&E, ×28; **inset 1,** H&E, ×252; **inset 2,** oil red-O, ×252.

JUVENILE XANTHOGRANULOMA
(Nevoxanthoendothelioma)
(Figs. 1–23, 9–14, 9–15 and figure H in Color Plate III)

I. Juvenile xanthogranuloma (JXG) is a benign cutaneous disorder observed in infants and young children. The typical raised orange skin lesions, which occur singly or in crops, tend to regress spontaneously.

II. Ocular findings include mainly iris involvement, diffusely or discretely, but also on occasion ciliary body and anterior choroid lesions, epibulbar involvement, corneal lesions, nodules on the lids and orbital granulomas may be seen.

A. Most ocular lesions occur in the very young, usually under 1 year of age.

B. The iris lesions are quite vascular and bleed easily. A spontaneous hyphema in an infant must be considered JXG until proven otherwise.

III. JXG probably should be included in the group of nonlipid reticuloendothelioses called histiocytosis X (eosinophilic granuloma, Letterer-Siwe disease and Schuller-Christian disease; see subsection Reticuloendothelioses in Chap. 14).

IV. Histologically there is a diffuse granulomatous inflammatory reaction with many histiocytes and often with Touton giant cells. Frequently the lesions are quite vascular.

HISTIOCYTOSIS X

See subsection Reticuloendotheliosis in Chapter 14.

COLLAGEN DISEASES

See section Collagen Diseases in Chapter 6.

MUCOPOLYSACCHARIDOSES

See p. 302 in Chapter 8.

ATROPHIES AND DEGENERATIONS

See sections Atrophy and Degeneration in Chapter 1.

RUBEOSIS IRIDIS (Figs. 9–16 and 9–17)

I. Many causes.
   A. Vascular hypoxia.
      1. Central retinal vein occlusion.
      2. Central retinal artery occlusion.
      3. Temporal arteritis.
      4. Aortic arch syndrome.
      5. Carotid artery disease.
      6. Retinal vascular disease.
   B. Neoplastic.
      1. Uveal malignant melanoma.
      2. Retinoblastoma.
      3. Metastatic carcinoma (uveal).
      4. Embryonal medulloepithelioma (dyktyoma).
   C. Inflammatory.
      1. Chronic uveitis, e.g., Fuchs's heterochromic iridocyclitis.
      2. Following retinal detachment surgery.

3. Following radiation therapy.
4. Fungus endophthalmitis.
5. Following trauma (surgical or nonsurgical).
   D. Retinal diseases.
      1. Diabetes mellitus (generally only when advanced diabetic retinopathy is present).
      2. Chronic retinal detachment.
      3. Coats's disease.
      4. Chronic glaucoma (almost never with primary chronic open angle glaucoma unless surgical trauma has occurred).
      5. Sickle cell retinopathy.
      6. Retrolental fibroplasia.
      7. Eales's disease.
      8. Persistent hyperplastic primary vitreous.
      9. Leber's miliary microaneurysms.
      10. Norrie's disease.

II. Rubeosis iridis may be induced by hypoxia, products of tissue breakdown or an as yet unidentified "specific rubeogenic factor."

III. The neovascularization generally starts concurrently on the pupillary margin and the trabecular meshwork area, but it can start in either place first; the midstromal portion rarely is involved early.

Early, rubeosis iridis in the angle does not cause synechias and angle closure but rather a secondary open angle glaucoma due to a mechanical obstruction of outflow by the fibrovascular membrane. Rapidly, however, synechias are induced and a chronic secondary angle closure glaucoma ensues. Rarely, as in *Fuchs's heterochromic iridocyclitis*, the rubeosis iridis involves the angle structures and anterior iris surface but does not cause synechias.

IV. The main complications of rubeosis iridis are hyphema and a secondary angle closure glaucoma called *neovascular glaucoma.*

Occasionally rubeosis iridis may be difficult to differentiate from normal iris vessels. The differentiation may be especially hard with ocular inflammation and secondarily dilated iris vessels. Even with such dilatation, however, the normal iris vessels are seen to course radially as against the random distribution found with rubeosis iridis.

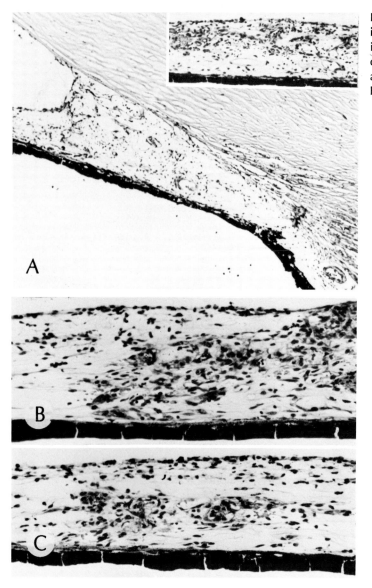

FIG. 9–16. Rubeosis iridis. **A** (including **inset**), **B** and **C** all from same eye to show intrairidal neovascularization, which grows out onto surface of iris to cause peripheral anterior synechia (**A**). **A,** H&E, ×54; **inset,** H&E, ×40; **B,** H&E, ×101; **C,** H&E, ×101.

FIG. 9–17. Rubeosis iridis. **A.** Case of polycythema vera with central retinal vein occlusion. **Inset** shows hemorrhagic necrosis of retina. **B.** Case of sickle cell trait with central retinal vein occlusion. Note marked ectropion uveae. **Inset 1** shows hemorrhagic necrosis of retina; **inset 2** shows sickled erythrocytes in vitreous. **C.** Case of familial interstitial nephritis with hypertensive retinopathy (severe) and retinal detachment in this eye. Note marked ectropion uveae. **D.** Case of Turner's syndrome and Coats's disease. **A,** H&E, ×101; **inset,** H&E, ×40; **B,** H&E, ×28; **inset 1,** H&E, ×40; **inset 2,** H&E, ×176; **C,** PAS, ×21; **D,** PAS, ×80.

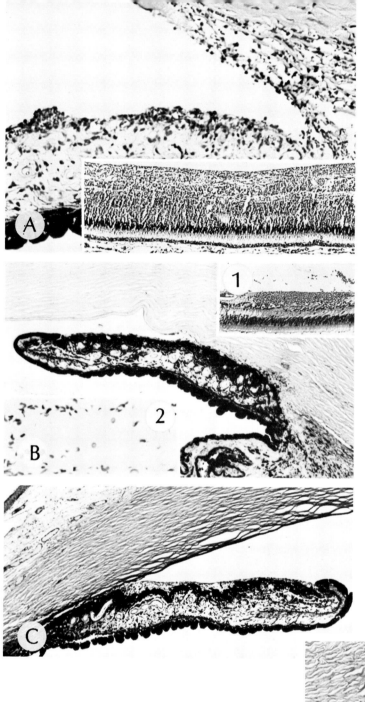
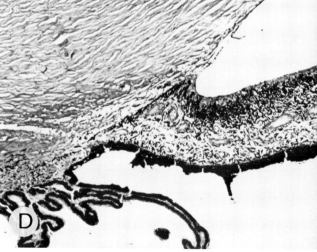

V. Histologically fibrovascular tissue is found almost exclusively on the anterior surface of the iris. The blood vessels, however, are derived initially from the ciliary body near the iris root or from iris stroma (most commonly toward the pupil). The abnormal tissue is also seen in the anterior chamber angle.

With contracture of the fibrovascular tissue, the pupillary border of the iris is turned anteriorly (*ectropion uveae**). Synechias generally are present only in the area of the anterior chamber angle peripheral to the end of Descemet's membrane, thereby differentiating these synechias from such broad-based synechias as may be caused by a persistent flat chamber, chronic angle closure glaucomas or an iris bombé.

MACULAR DEGENERATION

See p. 421 in Chapter 11.

DYSTROPHIES

ESSENTIAL IRIS ATROPHY

See p. 598 in Chapter 16.

CHANDLER'S SYNDROME

See p. 598 in Chapter 16.

IRIDOSCHISIS

See p. 598 in Chapter 16.

CHOROIDAL DYSTROPHIES

I. Regional choroidal dystrophies
   A. Choriocapillaris atrophy involving the posterior eyegrounds
      1. Involvement of the macula alone— also called *central areolar choroidal sclerosis,* central progressive areolar choroidal dystrophy and central

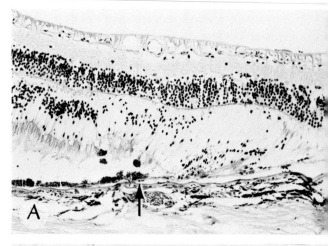

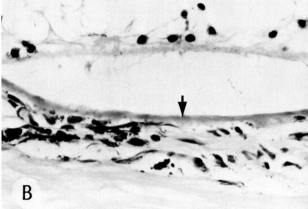

FIG. 9–18. Central areolar choroidal sclerosis. **A.** Temporal border of macular lesion. To left of arrow retinal pigment epithelium (RPE) and neural retina are relatively normal; to right is abrupt transition to area of chorioretinal abnormality involving outer retinal layers, RPE and choroid. Ganglion cell and nerve fiber layers are atrophic consequent to glaucoma. **B.** Center of lesion shows prominent Bruch's membrane (*arrow*) and loss of photoreceptors and RPE. Choriocapillaris is obliterated and no blood-containing vessels are seen in remainder of choroid. **A,** H&E, ×25; **B,** H&E, ×480.

---

* The old anatomic name (circa 1850) for the pigment epithelium of the iris was pigment epithelium uveae. Hence the name given to a turning out of the pigment seam of the pupil (composed of iris pigment epithelium) was ectropion uveae.

choroidal angiosclerosis (Fig. 9–18).

a. Choriocapillaris atrophy involving the macular area alone probably has an autosomal (recessive or dominant) inheritance pattern and is characterized by the onset of an exudative and edematous maculopathy in the third to the fifth decade.

In the early stage the macular lesion may resemble a macular degeneration or dystrophy.

b. With the typical slow progression of the lesion, it takes on a sharply demarcated, atrophic appearance involving only the posterior pole area and causes a central scotoma but no night blindness.

c. Histologically the area of involvement shows an incomplete or complete loss or degeneration of the choriocapillaris, the retinal pigment epithelium and the outer retinal layers.

2. Involvement of the peripapillary area—also termed peripapillary choroidal sclerosis.*

Angioid streaks may be associated with this form.

3. Involvement of the paramacular area—also called circinate choroidal sclerosis.*

B. Total choroidal vascular atrophy involving the posterior eyegrounds

1. Involvement of the macula alone or throughout most of the posterior eyegrounds—also termed choroidal vascular abiotrophy helicoid, serpiginous degeneration of the choroid and central gyrate atrophy.*

2. Involvement with nasal and temporal foci—also called progressive bifocal chorioretinal atrophy.*

3. Involvement of the disc—also called helicoid peripapillary chorioretinal atrophy, choroiditis areata, circumpapillary dysgenesis of the pigment

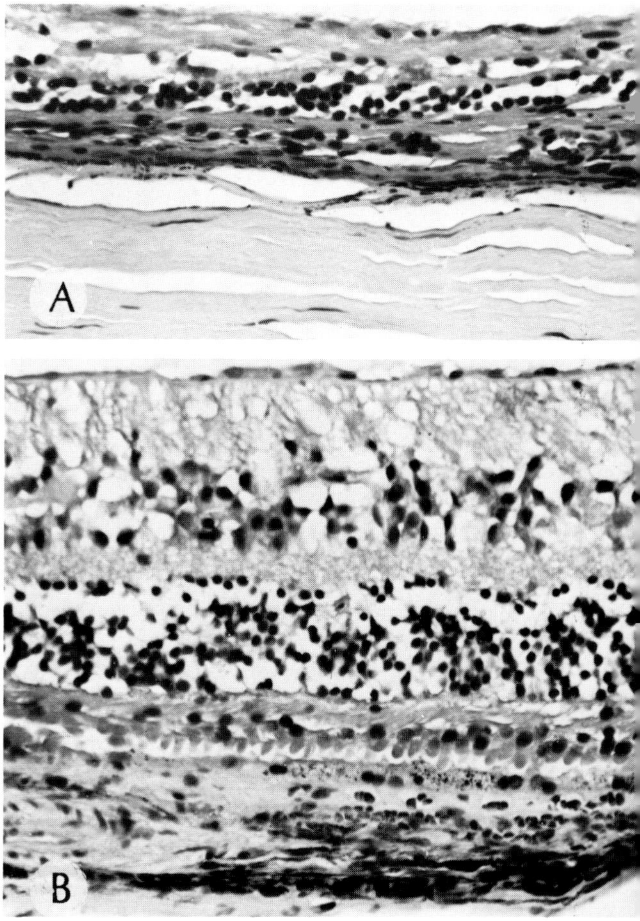

FIG. 9–19. Choroideremia. **A.** Peripheral area showing absence of choroid and retinal pigment epithelium and marked atrophy of retina. **B.** Macular area showing atrophy of choroid, retinal pigment epithelium and outer retinal layers. **A,** H&E, ×176; **B,** H&E, ×176.

---

* The histology of these entities is unknown or not worked out well.

epithelium and chorioretinitis striata.*

4. Malignant myopia (see p. 420 in Chapter 11).

II. Diffuse choroidal dystrophies

A. Diffuse choriocapillaris atrophy—also called generalized choroidal angiosclerosis, diffuse choroidal sclerosis and generalized choroidal sclerosis.

Histologically there is a complete loss or degeneration of the choriocapillaris, the retinal pigment epithelium and the outer retinal layers.

B. Diffuse total choroidal vascular atrophy

1. Autosomal recessive or irregular dominant inheritance—also called *gyrate atrophy* of the choroid.

a. Diffuse total choroidal vascular atrophy of the autosomal recessive (or irregular dominant) inherited type is a condition characterized by the development of atrophic chorioretinal patches in the periphery, which progress, move centrally and partially fuse. Patients have hyperornithinaemia probably due to defective activity of the enzyme ornithine ketoacid aminotransferase.

A peripapillary atrophy may develop simultaneously. In the final stage all of the fundus except the macula may be involved so that the condition may resemble the sex-linked type of diffuse total choroidal vascular atrophy.

b. The condition becomes manifest in the second or third decade of life and slowly progresses with decreasing vision and night blindness as prominent symptoms.

c. Other ocular findings include posterior subcapsular cataracts and myopia (and rarely retinopathia pigmentosa).

d. Histology is not available but

would probably resemble the sex-linked type of diffuse total choroidal vascular atrophy.

2. Sex-linked inheritance—also called *choroideremia*, progressive tapetochoroidal dystrophy and progressive chorioretinal degeneration (Fig. 9–19).

a. Diffuse total choroidal vascular atrophy of the sex-linked intermediate inherited type is a condition characterized by almost complete degeneration of the retina and choroid (except in the macula) in affected men. The condition becomes manifest in childhood and progresses slowly until complete at about age 50 years.

The fundus picture in carrier women resembles that seen in the early stages in affected men, namely, degeneration of the peripheral retinal pigment epithelium giving a salt-and-pepper appearance to the peripheral fundus.

b. It is unclear whether the earliest changes are in the choroid or the retinal pigment epithelium, but they probably are in the latter.

c. Histologically the choroid is absent or markedly atrophic, and the overlying retina is atrophic, especially in its outer layers.

III. All of the above choroidal entities, although usually called atrophies, should more properly be called dystrophies with secondary retinal changes; it is most likely that the primary dystrophic abnormality resides in the retinal pigment epithelium.

ANGIOID STREAKS

See p. 440 in Chapter 11.

TUMORS

EPITHELIAL

I. Hyperplasias (Fig. 9–20 and figures A, B, C, and D in Color Plate III)—see p. 22 in Chapter 1 and section Melanotic Tumors

---

* The histology of these entities is unknown or not worked out well.

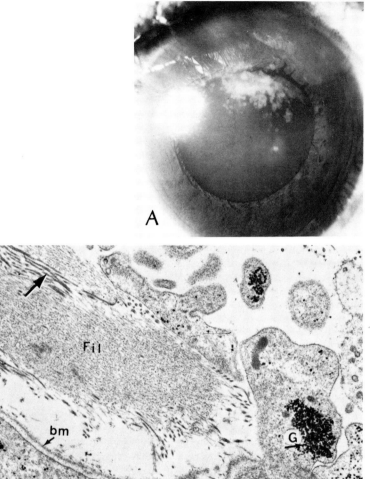

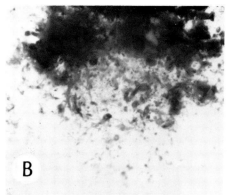

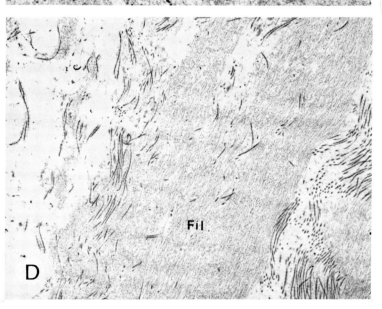

FIG. 9–20. Hyperplasia. **A.** Adenomatous proliferations of nonpigmented ciliary epithelium may, on rare occasions, proliferate so profusely as to appear in anterior chamber. Fronds and tiny vesicles of whitish proliferating cells lie suspended in primitive or infantile vitreouslike material that can be observed biomicroscopically. **B.** Macroscopic specimen of proliferation lying within anterior chamber. Cells are colored black by osmium tetroxide, whereas primitive vitreous in which they are suspended remains transparent. **C.** By electron microscopy cells contain glycogen (*G*) and possess thin basement membrane (*bm*), and extracellular materials consist of filaments (*Fil*) reminiscent of vitreous body or zonules, as well as fibrils of larger diameter (*arrow*). **D.** Another region of "primitive vitreous" to show masses of filaments (*Fil*) and associated larger fibrils. (Same case shown figures A, B, C and D in Color Plate III.) **A,** clinical; **B,** macroscopic; **C,** TSC, ×15,500; **D,** TSC, ×15,500.

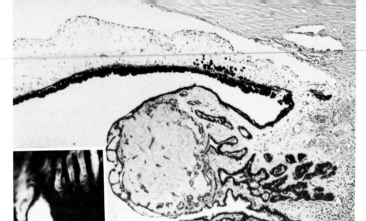

see p. 648

FIG. 9–21. Fuchs's adenoma consists of nonvascular, acid mucopolysaccharide and glycoprotein-containing proliferation of nonpigmented ciliary epithelium. **Inset** shows macroscopic appearance of same tumor. **Main figure,** H&E, ×28; **inset,** macroscopic.

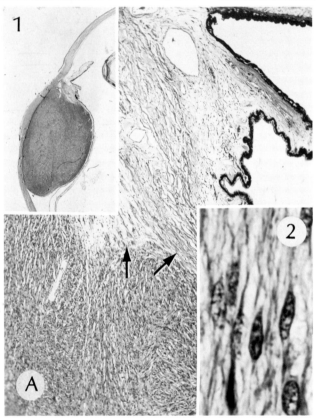

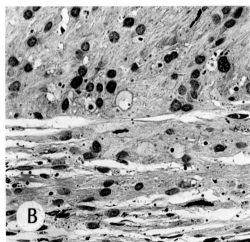

FIG. 9–22. A. Leiomyoma of ciliary body (**inset 1**) contains large spindle-shaped cells with "open" or light-staining nuclei and filamentous appearance of attenuated cytoplasm (**inset 2**). Blending of ciliary musculature (*arrows*) with mass of spindle-shaped cells is shown. **B.** Sample showing area of tumor above and relatively normal smooth muscle cells below. Such sample enables comparison between cell types under similar conditions of fixation. **C.** Electron microscopy of routinely fixed (i.e., formaldehyde) tissue clarifies differential diagnosis of leiomyoma from nonpigmented spindle cell malignant melanoma. All characteristics of smooth muscle cell are found, including presence of densities (*D*) among cytoplasmic filaments, plasmalemmal associated pinocytotic vesicles (*arrows* and enlarged in **inset**) and thin basement membranes, all of which are absent in well-fixed spindle melanomas. **A,** H&E, ×40; **inset 1,** H&E, ×3.5; **inset 2,** H&E, ×1,040; **B,** 1.5 μ section, PD, ×300; **C,** ×12,600; **inset,** ×18,000.

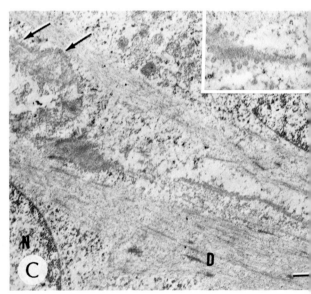

of Pigment Epithelium of Iris, Ciliary Body and Retina in Chapter 17.

Occasionally adenomatous hyperplasias may become extreme and produce masses that are noted clinically, either localized to the posterior chamber or, rarely, proliferated into the anterior chamber.

II. Benign epithelioma (adenoma) of Fuchs (Fig. 9–21).
A. The tumor is present in over 25 percent of older people, generally is located in the pars plicata of the ciliary body, is benign and usually is found incidentally when examining microscopically an enucleated globe.
B. It rarely may cause localized occlusion of the anterior chamber angle.
C. There is some question whether the tumor is neoplastic or proliferative, but it is probably the latter.
D. Histologically the tumor is a nonvascular proliferation of the nonpigmented ciliary epithelium and contains acid mucopolysaccharides (mainly hyaluronic acid) and glycoproteins.

III. Medulloepithelioma (embryonal and adult types)—see p. 642 in Chapter 17 and p. 702 in Chapter 18.

MUSCULAR (Fig. 9–22)

I. Leiomyomas rarely may occur in the anterior uvea.
A. It is difficult, if not impossible, to differentiate a leiomyoma from an amelanotic spindle cell melanoma without the use of electron microscopy.
B. The electron microscopic criteria for smooth muscle cells include an investing thin basement membrane, plasmalemmal vesicles, plasmalemmal associated densities and myriad longitudinally aligned intracytoplasmic filaments with scattered associated densities.
C. *Leiomyosarcoma* has been reported as a rare iris neoplasm.

II. A rhabdomyosarcoma is an extremely rare tumor of the iris and probably is atavistic in nature.

VASCULAR (Fig. 9–23)

I. True hemangiomas of the iris and ciliary body are extremely rare.

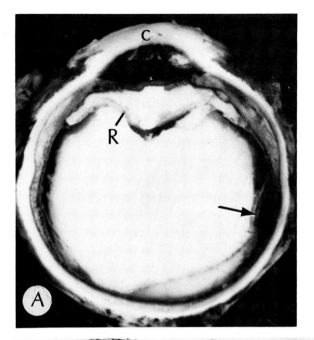

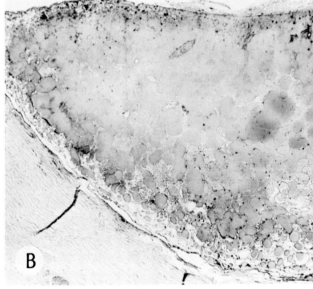

FIG. 9–23. Hemangioma of choroid. **A.** Hemangioma (*arrow*) is incidental finding in eye enucleated because of blindness and long-standing retinal detachment. *R*, retina; *c*, cornea. **B.** Photomicrograph of same hemangioma shows cavernous pattern. **A,** macroscopic; **B,** H&E, ×16.

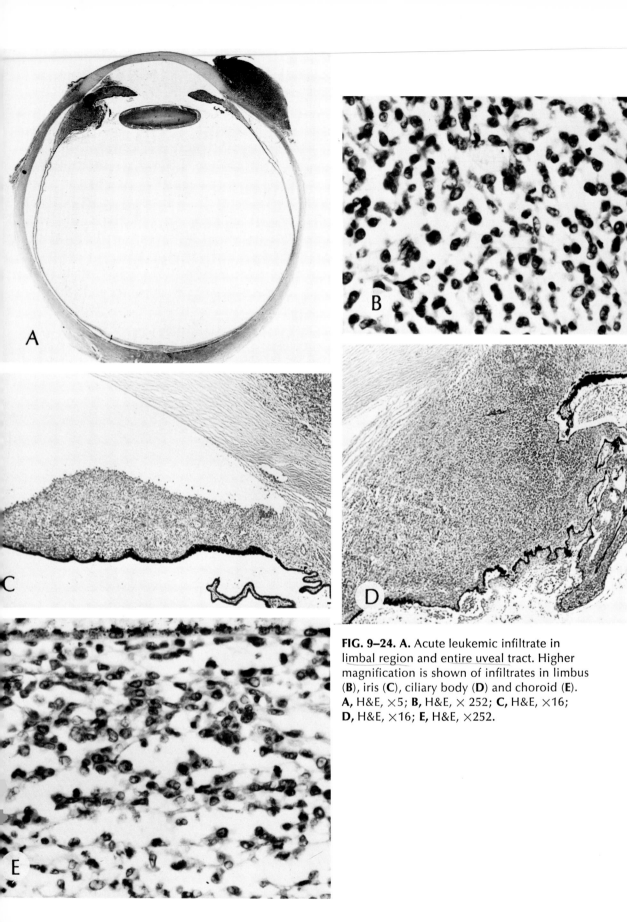

FIG. 9–24. A. Acute leukemic infiltrate in limbal region and entire uveal tract. Higher magnification is shown of infiltrates in limbus (**B**), iris (**C**), ciliary body (**D**) and choroid (**E**). **A,** H&E, ×5; **B,** H&E, × 252; **C,** H&E, ×16; **D,** H&E, ×16; **E,** H&E, ×252.

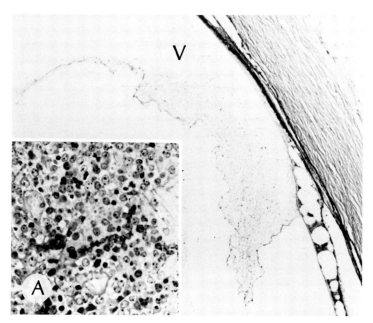

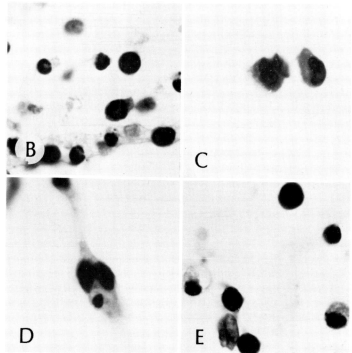

FIG. 9–25. Patient was treated for posterior uveitis OU for over a year before central nervous symptoms developed. **A.** Vitreous (*V*) is detached posteriorly and contains many cells. **Inset** shows section of brain infiltrated with reticulum cell sarcoma. **B, C, D** and **E** are higher magnifications to show sarcoma cells in vitreous. Reticulum cell sarcoma found only in brain and vitreous of both eyes; no other tissues involved. **A,** PAS, ×16; **inset,** 1.5 μ section, PD, ×176; **B,** H&E, ×630; **C,** H&E, ×630; **D,** H&E, ×630; **E,** H&E, ×630.

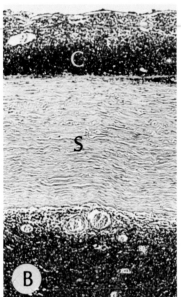

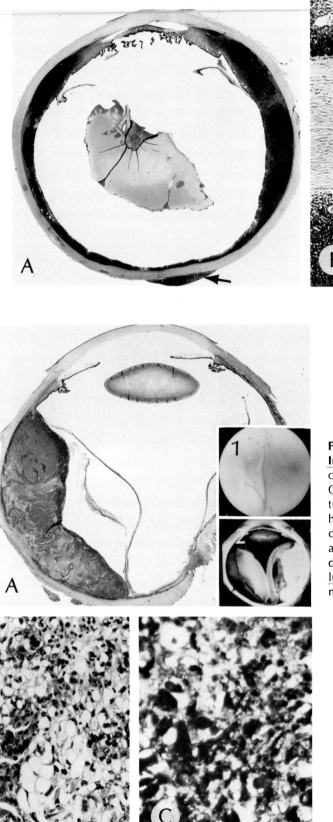

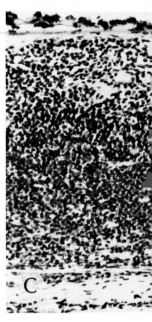

FIG. 9–26. Benign lymphoid infiltrate of uvea. **A.** Entire uveal tract and extraocular area (*arrow*) involved. **B.** Higher magnification of area at *arrow* in **A.** S, sclera; C, choroid. **C.** High magnification to show benign lymphoid choroidal infiltrate. **A,** H&E, ×5; **B,** H&E, ×40; **C,** H&E, ×136.

FIG. 9–27. Metastatic adenocarcinoma. **A. Inset 1** shows solid detachment thought clinically to be malignant melanoma. Opened enucleated eye with large choroidal tumor shown macroscopically (**inset 2**) and histologically. **B.** Photomicrograph shows carcinoma with vacuolated cells. **C.** Vacuoles are PAS-positive, diastase-resistant. Patient died from metastatic adenocarcinoma of lung. **A,** H&E, ×5; **inset 1,** fundus; **inset 2,** macroscopic; **B,** H&E, ×101; **C,** PAS, ×252.

II. Hemangioma of the choroid may occur as an isolated finding, but more often it is part of the Sturge-Weber syndrome (see p. 30 in Chap. 2).

MELANOMATOUS

See Chapter 17.

LEUKEMIC AND LYMPHOMATOUS

I. Acute granulocytic (myelogenous) and lymphocytic leukemias (Fig. 9–24) not infrequently have uveal, usually posterior choroidal, infiltrates as part of the generalized disease.
II. Malignant lymphomas rarely involve the uveal tract (Fig. 9–25).
   Reticulum cell sarcoma of the brain (histiocytic lymphoma; microgliomatosis) may be associated with a similar neoplastic infiltrate in the vitreous, presenting clinically as a uveitis. The retina and choroid also may be involved. The neoplasm probably arises in the brain and eye due to multicentric origin rather than to metastasis.
III. Occasionally benign lymphoid infiltrates containing lymphocytes, plasma cells and reticulum cells may be seen in the uveal tract (Fig. 9–26).
   A. The infiltrates generally are unilateral but may be bilateral.
   B. They resemble the inflammatory pseudotumors, especially benign reactive lymphoid hyperplasia (see p. 556 in Chap. 14) seen in the orbit.

NEURAL

I. *Neurofibromas* of the uvea occur as part of diffuse neurofibromatosis (see p. 32 in Chap. 2).
II. Neurilemmomas are exceedingly rare in the uveal tract (see p. 541 in Chap. 14).

SECONDARY NEOPLASMS

I. By direct extension:
   A. Basal cell carcinoma of conjunctiva.
   B. Malignant melanoma of conjunctiva.
   C. Retinoblastoma.
   D. Malignant melanoma of uvea (e.g., ciliary body melanoma extending into choroid or iris).

E. Embryonal and adult medulloepitheliomas.
F. Glioma of optic nerve.
G. Meningioma of optic nerve sheaths.

It is extremely rare for an orbital neoplasm to invade through the sclera into the uvea or through the meninges into the optic nerve.

II. Metastatic—second most common adult intraocular neoplasm (Figs. 9–27 through 9–29)

Although metastatic neoplasms are considered to be the second most common intraocular neoplasm (second to primary uveal malignant melanomas), if the true incidence were known, metastatic neoplasms might very well be the most common intraocular neoplasm.

   A. Lung—most common metastatic lesion in men (usually occurs early in the course of the disease and may be the initial finding).
   B. Breast—most common metastatic lesion in women (usually occurs late in the course of the disease and generally breast surgery has been performed).
   C. All other primary sites are relatively uncommon as a source of intraocular metastases.
   D. Metastatic intraocular neoplasms are more common in women and are bilateral in about 20 to 25 percent of cases.

UVEAL EDEMA (uveal detachment; uveal hydrops)

TYPES

I. Uveal effusion with choroidal and ciliary body detachment (spontaneous serous detachments)
   A. Uveal effusion is characterized by a slowly progressive, often bilateral, retinal detachment with shifting fluid found mainly in middle-aged men.
   B. Choroidal effusion presumably is the underlying cause. Signs of uveitis are minimal or absent.
   C. The retinal detachment may reattach after months or even years, although it may remain permanently detached.

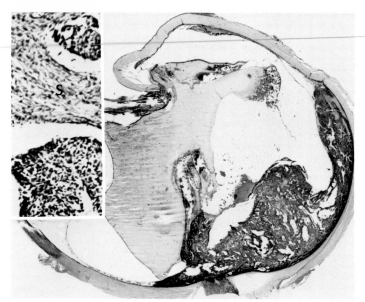

FIG. 9–28. Metastatic carcinoma discovered after cataract extraction. Note thick band of supporting stroma (s) between nests of carcinoma cells in **inset.** Melanomas do not have supporting stroma, but stroma is characteristic of carcinomas. **Main figure,** H&E, ×5; **inset,** H&E, ×69.

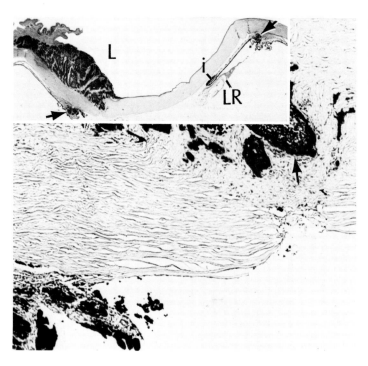

FIG. 9–29. Metastatic carcinoma (**inset**) involves limbus (L), iris root and anterior ciliary body (*arrows*) and surface of iris (*i*). *LR,* lens remnants. "Oat-cell" bronchogenic carcinoma is present in cataract scar (*arrow* in **main figure**). **Main figure,** H&E, ×40; **inset,** H&E, ×6.

II. Posttrauma—either surgical or nonsurgical trauma.
   A. Hypotony and vasodilation following penetration of the globe combine to produce transudation of fluid through uveal vessels, leading to uveal edema. Clinically this appears as a *combined detachment* of uveal tract and retina.
   B. Uveal hemorrhage may occur secondary to the trauma and result in uveal detachment.

III. Vascular—malignant hypertension, eclampsia, nephritis and other conditions that affect the ciliary vessels can lead to uveal edema.
IV. Inflammatory—any type of ocular inflammation (i.e., acute, nongranulomatous or granulomatous) can induce uveal edema.
V. Sequelae—in atrophic eyes with or without shrinkage, secondary to any cause, traction bands and organized scar tissue may induce uveal detachment.

BIBLIOGRAPHY

CONGENITAL AND DEVELOPMENTAL DEFECTS

Baker TR, Spencer WH: Ocular findings in multiple myeloma. A report of two cases. Arch Ophthalmol 91:110, 1974

Duke-Elder S: System of Ophthalmology, Vol III, Normal and Abnormal Development, Part 2, Congenital Deformities. St. Louis, Mosby, 1963, pp 456–472

Fine BS: Free-floating pigmented cyst in the anterior chamber. Am J Ophthalmol 67:493, 1969

Gärtner J: Fine structure of pars plana cysts. Am J Ophthalmol 73: 971, 1972

Hayreh SS, Cullen JF: Atypical minimal peripapillary choroidal colobomata. Br J Ophthalmol 56:86, 1972

Hoepner J, Yanoff M: Spectrum of ocular anomalies in trisomy 13–15: analysis of 13 eyes with two new findings. Am J Ophthalmol 74:729, 1972

Johnson BL, Storey JD: Proteinaceous cysts of the ciliary epithelium I. Their clear nature and immunoelectrophoretic analysis in a case of multiple myeloma. Arch Ophthalmol 84:166, 1970

Johnson BL: Proteinaceous cysts of the ciliary epithelium. II. Their occurrence in nonmyelomatous hypergammaglobulinemic conditions. Arch Ophthalmol 84:171, 1970

Karlsberg RC, Emery JM, Green WC, Valdes-Depena M, Coulombre AJ: Anomalies of iris and anterior-chamber angle. Arch Ophthalmol 86:287, 1971

Kozart DM, Scheie HG: Spontaneous cysts of the ciliary epithelium. Trans Am Acad Ophthalmol Otolaryngol 74:534, 1970

Merin S, Crawford JS, Cardarelli J: Hyperplastic persistent pupillary membrane. Am J Ophthalmol 72:717, 1971

Morgan G, Mushin A: Ectopic intraocular lacrimal gland. Br J Ophthalmol 56:690, 1972

Naumann G, Green WR: Spontaneous nonpigmented iris cysts. Arch Ophthalmol 78:496, 1967

Rosen E, Rosen RJ: Ciliary body cysts. Eye Ear Nose Throat Mon 50:288, 1971

Roy FH, Hanna C: Spontaneous congenital iris cyst. Am J Ophthalmol 72:97, 1971

Scheie HG, Yanoff M: Peters' anomaly and total posterior coloboma of retinal pigment epithelium and choroid. Arch Ophthalmol 87:525, 1972

Sugar HS, Blau RP: Free-floating cysts of the ocular media. Ann Ophthalmol 5:445, 1973

Yanoff M, Zimmerman LE: Pseudomelanoma of anterior chamber caused by implantation of iris pigment epithelium. Arch Ophthalmol 74:302, 1965

Zimmerman LE, Fine BS: Production of hyaluronic acid by cysts and tumors of the ciliary body. Arch Ophthalmol 72:365, 1964

SYSTEMIC DISEASES

Helwig EB, Hackney VC: Juvenile xanthogranuloma (nevoxanthoendothelioma). Am J Pathol 30:625, 1954

Lahav M, Albert DM: Unusual ocular involvement in acute disseminated histiocytosis X. Arch Ophthalmol 91:455, 1974

Mittleman D, Apple DJ, Goldberg MF: Ocular involvement in Letterer-Siwe disease. Am J Ophthalmol 75:261, 1973

Rupp RH, Holloman KR: Histiocytosis X affecting the uveal tract. Arch Ophthalmol 84:468, 1970

Schwartz LW, Rodrigues MM, Hallett JW: Juvenile xanthogranuloma diagnosed by paracentesis. Am J Ophthalmol 77:243, 1974

Zimmerman LE: Ocular lesions of juvenile xanthogranuloma. Nevoxanthoendothelioma. Trans Am Acad Ophthalmol Otolaryngol 69:412, 1965

ATROPHIES AND DEGENERATIONS

Anderson D, Morin D, Hunter W: Rubeosis iridis. Can J Ophthalmol 6:138, 1971

Cameron JD, Yanoff M, Frayer WC: Coats' disease and Turner's syndrome. Am J Ophthalmol 78:852, 1974

DYSTROPHIES

Ferry AP, Llovera I, Shafer DM: Central areolar choroidal dystrophy. Arch Ophthalmol 88:39, 1972

Krill AE, Archer D: Classification of the choroidal atrophies. Am J Ophthalmol 72:562, 1971

Rafuse EV, McCulloch C: Choroideremia. A pathologic report. Can J Ophthalmol 3:347, 1968

Sarks SH: Senile choroidal sclerosis. Br J Ophthalmol 57:98, 1973

Schatz H, Maumenee AE, Patz A: Geographic helicoid peripapillary choroidopathy: clinical presentation and fluorescein angiographic findings. Trans Am Acad Ophthalmol Otolaryngol 78:747, 1974

Takki K: Gyrate atrophy of the choroid and retina associated with hyperornithinaemia. Br J Ophthalmol 58:3, 1974

Takki K: Differential diagnosis between the primary total choroidal vascular atrophies. Br J Ophthalmol 58:24, 1974

TUMORS

Albert DM, Gaasterland DE, Caldwell JBH, Howard RO, Zimmerman LE: Bilateral metastatic choroidal melanoma, nevi, and cavernous degeneration. Involvement of the optic nervehead. Arch Ophthalmol 87:39, 1972

Dugmore WN: 11-year follow-up of a case of iris leiomyosarcoma. Br J Ophthalmol 56:366, 1972

Ferry AP: Hemangiomas of the iris and ciliary body: do they exist? A search for a histologically proved case. Int Ophthalmol Clin 12:225, 1972

Ferry AP: The biological behavior and pathological features of carcinoma metastatic to the eye and orbit. Trans Am Ophthalmol Soc 71:373, 1973

Fine BS, Yanoff M: Ocular Histology: A Text and Atlas. Hagerstown, Harper & Row, 1972, pp 208–211

Hillemann J, Naumann G: Beitrag zum benignen Epitheliom (Fuchs) des Ziliarkörpers. Ophthalmologica 164:321, 1972

Johnston SS, Ware CF: Iris involvement in leukaemia. Br J Ophthalmol 57:320, 1973

Klingele TG, Hogan MJ: Ocular reticulum cell sarcoma. Am J Ophthalmol 79:39, 1975

Meyer SL, Fine BS, Font RL, Zimmerman LE: Leiomyoma of the ciliary body. Electron microscopic verification. Am J Ophthalmol 66:1061, 1968

Naidoff MA, Kenyon KR, Green WR: Iris hemangioma and abnormal retinal vasculature in a case of diffuse congenital hemangiomatosis. Am J Ophthalmol 72:633, 1971

Naumann G, Font RL, Zimmerman LE: Electron microscopic verification of primary rhabdomyosarcoma of the iris. Am J Ophthalmol 74:110, 1972

Naumann G, Ruprecht KW: Xanthoma der Iris. Ein klinisch-pathologischer Befundbericht. Ophthalmologica 164:293, 1972

Neault RW, van Scoy RE, Okazaki H, MacCarty CS: Uveitis associated with isolated reticulum cell sarcoma of the brain. Am J Ophthalmol 73:431, 1972

Ryan SJ Jr, Frank RN, Green WR: Bilateral inflammatory pseudotumors of the ciliary body. Am J Ophthalmol 72:586, 1971

Ryan SJ Jr, Zimmerman LE, King FM: Reactive lymphoid hyperplasia: an unusual form of intraocular pseudotumor. Trans Am Acad Ophthalmol Otolaryngol 76:652, 1972

Vogel MH, Font RL, Zimmerman LE, Levine RA: Reticulum cell sarcoma of the retina and uvea. Report of six cases and review of the literature. Am J Ophthalmol 66:205, 1968

Woyke S, Chwirot R: Rhabdomyosarcoma of the iris. Report of the first recorded case. Br J Ophthalmol 56:60, 1972

Zimmerman LE: Verhoeff's "Terato-Neuroma": a critical reappraisal in light of new observations and current concepts of embryonic tumors. Am J Ophthalmol 72:1039, 1971

UVEAL EDEMA

Brockhurst RJ, Lam K-W: Uveal effusion. II. Report of a case with analysis of subretinal fluid. Arch Ophthalmol 90:399, 1973

Schepens CL, Brockhurst RJ: Uveal effusion. I. Clinical picture. Arch Ophthalmol 70:189, 1963

chapter 10

Lens

From birth on the lens may be considered as a sequestered colony of modified epithelial cells (modified epidermis), which have maintained their transparency.

Normally there are no blood vessels or nerves within, or attached to, the lens. The interior contains no connective tissue.

Because of the complete enclosure of the lens by the epithelial basement membrane (capsule of the lens), desquamation of aging cells is impossible. The older lens cells ("fibers") become compressed into the center of the lens. The cells are formed constantly throughout life and are laid down externally to the old cells.

CONGENITAL ANOMALIES

INTRODUCTION

I. Congenital anomalies of the lens usually are associated with other ocular anomalies.

II. Such entities as coloboma of the lens, spherophakia and congenital dislocation of lens may be related to problems of zonular rather than lenticular development.

A true coloboma of the lens probably does not exist. A coloboma of the zonules may result in a deformation of the equator of the lens simulating a coloboma of the lens (Fig. 10–1).

III. The histology of the anomaly depends to a large extent upon the underlying cause.

CONGENITAL AND NEONATAL LENS OPACITIES
MITTENDORF DOT

See p. 470 in Chapter 12.

CONGENITAL APHAKIA

I. Congenital aphakia is a rare anomaly and exists in two forms:

A. Primary congenital aphakia in which no lens "anlage" has developed.

B. Secondary congenital aphakia in which a lens has developed to some degree but has been resorbed or extruded through a corneal perforation before or during birth.

II. Histologically primary congenital aphakia is characterized by an absent lens and an aplasia of the anterior segment. The secondary form has findings dependent on the underlying cause.

FLECK CATARACT

I. Fleck cataract consists of multiple, stationary, tiny, white anterior subcapsular or anterior cortical flecks associated with adhesions of persistent pupillary membranes.

FIG. 10–1. "Coloboma" of lens actually is due to coloboma of zonules causing notch (*arrow*) in lens. Eye has coloboma of iris in same area and abnormal proliferation of ciliary epithelium (ce) on posterior surface of lens (see Figures 8–13 and 9–4). Macroscopic.

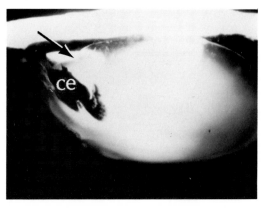

II. Frequently pigment cells are present on the anterior surface of the lens capsule in the pupillary area at the site of attachment of the pupillary membrane overlying the tiny opacity.

All degrees of changes can be seen (especially with the slit lamp). Sometimes only the white flecks, other times only the membrane adhesions, other times only the pigment cells, or any combination, can be seen.

III. More rarely the same type of fleck cataract can occur posteriorly associated with remnants of the hyaloid vessels or of the posterior tunica vasculosa lentis.

ANTERIOR POLAR CATARACT

I. An anterior polar cataract appears similar clinically and histologically to the acquired anterior subcapsular cataract.
II. The cataract is almost always stationary.
III. Most of the time the cause of the cataract is unknown, although occasionally it may be inherited as an autosomal dominant.

Rarely congenital anterior polar cataract may be secondary to intrauterine keratitis. The capsule of the lens may become adherent to the inflamed cornea causing lens traction during fetal development. The traction may distort the lens by drawing its axial area out to form an *anterior pyramidal cataract.*

POSTERIOR POLAR CATARACT (Fig. 10–2)

I. A posterior polar cataract, rarer than its anterior counterpart, appears similar clinically and histologically to the acquired posterior subcapsular cataract.

II. The cataract usually is stationary but may be progressive when associated with persistent hyperplastic primary vitreous (see p. 698 in Chap. 18) in which case there may be a dehiscence in the lens capsule posteriorly with fibrovascular tissue within the posterior lens substance.

ANTERIOR LENTICONUS (Lentiglobus)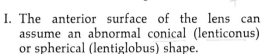

I. The anterior surface of the lens can assume an abnormal conical (lenticonus) or spherical (lentiglobus) shape.
II. Either condition predominates in males, usually is present as the only ocular anomaly and generally is bilateral.
III. Clinically an "oil globule" reflex is seen in the lens in the pupillary area.
IV. The cause is unknown, except rarely it may be inherited as an autosomal recessive.

Anterior lenticonus has been reported in *familial hemorrhagic nephritis (Alport's syndrome).* Spherophakia, anterior polar cataract and posterior cortical cataract have also been described in this syndrome.

V. Histologically thinning of the anterior lens capsule, decreasing number of lens epithelial cells and bulging of the anterior cortex are seen.

POSTERIOR LENTICONUS (Lentiglobus) (Fig. 10–3)

I. Posterior lenticonus, more properly called lentiglobus, consists of a spherical elevation or ridge on the posterior surface of the lens and is more common than its anterior counterpart.
II. The condition predominates in females,

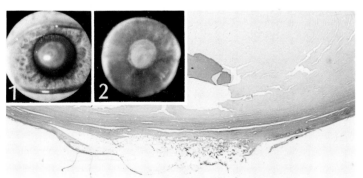

FIG. 10–2. Posterior congenital polar cataract (PCPC). Patient had bilateral PCPCs since birth. **Insets** show clinical (**1**) and macroscopic (**2**) appearance. Photomicrograph demonstrates posterior bulge, marked posterior subcapsular cortical degeneration and posterior migration of lens epithelial nuclei. Ruptures in lens capsule are artifacts. **Main figure,** H&E, ×16; **inset 1,** clinical; **inset 2,** macroscopic.

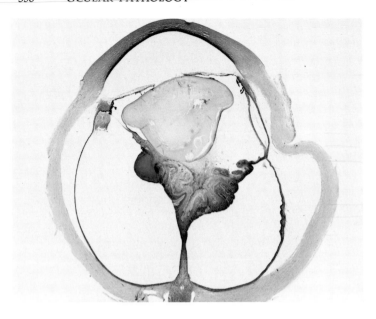

FIG. 10–3. Posterior lentiglobus and congenital nonattachment of retina present in eye enucleated from infant because of suspected retinoblastoma. PAS, ×6.

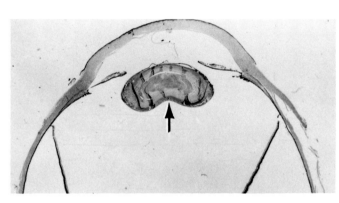

FIG. 10–4. Umbilication of lens posteriorly (*arrow*) commonly found as fixation artifact in infant eyes. H&E, ×6.

usually is present as the only ocular anomaly and generally is unilateral.

III. Clinically an "oil globule" reflex is seen in the pupillary area of the lens.

IV. The cause is unknown. The condition may occur in Lowe's syndrome.

V. Histologically the capsule is thinned posteriorly, the lens cortex bulges posteriorly and frequently abnormal nuclei, resembling either lens epithelium or pigmented and nonpigmented ciliary epithelium, can be seen in the area of the anomaly.

A bulging or umbilicated posterior polar lens abnormality is encountered frequently in enucleated infant eyes. The abnormality is due to a fixation artifact (Fig. 10-4).

OTHER CONGENITAL CATARACTS

I. Congenital cataracts such as *zonular, sutural, axial, membranous* and *filiform* have nonspecific changes histologically, changes quite similar to those described below under cortical and nuclear cataracts.

II. Cataracts secondary to intrauterine infection.

A. Anterior subcapsular cataract—see p. 366 in this chapter.

B. Posterior subcapsular cataract—see p. 368 in this chapter.

C. Rubella cataract—see pp. 48–50 in Chapter 2.

III. Galactosemia cataract—see p. 377 in this chapter.

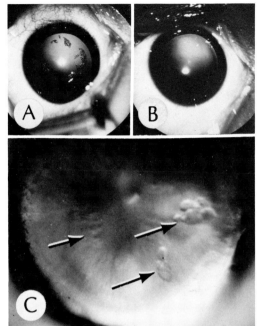

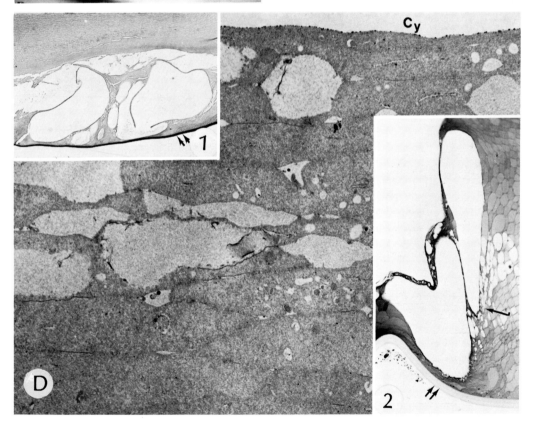

FIG. 10–5. Transient neonatal lens vacuoles. Vacuoles in posterior lens of infant (**A**) have disappeared three weeks later (**B**). **C.** Lens removed at autopsy from another child; lens viewed from behind by oblique illumination. *Arrows* point to more obvious clusters of vacuoles. **D. Inset 1** shows multiloculated subcapsular cysts. *Double arrows* indicate posterior lens capsule. **Inset 2** shows swollen lens cortical cells (*arrow*) adjacent to edge of cyst. *Double arrows* indicate posterior capsule. Electron micrograph shows edge of cyst (*Cy*) and adjacent cortical cells. Both inter- and intracellular enlargements are present. Latter are filled with watery material. Lowest cells in figure are relatively normal. **A,** clinical; **B,** clinical; **C,** macroscopic; **D,** ×8,700; **inset 1,** PAS, ×42; **inset 2,** 1.5 μ section, PD, ×195.

IV. Transient neonatal lens vacuoles (Fig. 10–5)

 A. Bilateral, symmetrical lens vacuoles situated predominantly in the posterior cortex near the Y sutures close to the lens capsule are seen.

 B. The vacuoles, seen mainly in premature infants, usually are not present at birth, generally appear between the eighth and fourteenth day and persist for about 2 weeks, but may remain up to 9 months before disappearing completely.

 C. Histologically swelling of lens cortical cells in several lamellas of both anterior and posterior cortex is seen. Large vacuoles with a nonstaining content (i.e., watery) are found in the posterior cortex. Lipoidal degenerative products also are seen in the involved areas.

 The vacuoles when exaggerated may be responsible for zonular types of cataracts if they do not disappear, and the lipoidal degenerative products may be responsible for clinically seen punctate opacities.

CAPSULE (EPITHELIAL BASEMENT MEMBRANE)

GENERAL REACTIONS

I. The lens capsule, which is the thickest basement membrane in the body, is resistant to the passage of particulate matter (e.g., bacteria and inflammatory cells) and is elastic and easily molded, thereby resisting rupture.

II. The lens capsule can undergo marked thinning, as in a mature cataract or anterior or posterior lenticonus (see pp. 357–358 in this chapter), or focal thickening as in Lowe's syndrome, Miller's syndrome and Down's syndrome (see pp. 43, 53 in Chap. 2).

 A. Oculocerebrorenal syndrome of Lowe (Fig. 10–6)

 1. Lowe's syndrome consists of systemic acidosis, organic aciduria, decreased ability to produce ammonia in the kidneys, renal rickets, generalized hypotonia and hydrophthalmos. The syndrome is transmitted as a sex-linked recessive.

 2. Ocular findings include congenital cataract and glaucoma.

 Most cases of genetic congenital cataract are not associated with glaucoma, and, conversely, most cases of genetic congenital glaucoma are not associated with cataract. The combination, therefore, of congenital cataract and glaucoma is highly suggestive of either Lowe's syndrome or congentital rubella.

 3. Histology

 a. The cataractous lens is small and discoid, frequently with a posterior lenticonus. Peculiar anterior and equatorial lens capsular excrescences, similar to those seen in trisomy 21 (i.e., Down's syndrome) and in Miller's syndrome may be found.

 b. The anterior chamber angle is similar to that seen in genetic congenital glaucoma (see pp. 588–590 in Chap. 16).

III. Rupture of the lens capsule (see pp. 148–150 in Chap. 5) may be healed over by the underlying lens epithelium (Fig. 10–7) or sealed by the overlying iris, if the rent is small enough.

 Most capsular ruptures result from trauma (Fig. 10–8). Rarely rupture may be spontaneous, e.g., in a hypermature cataract or in lenticonus, or even more rarely, rupture may be secondary to a purulent infection.

EXFOLIATION OF THE LENS CAPSULE
(Figs. 10–9 and 10–10)

I. True exfoliation of the lens capsule is a rare condition that results from prolonged ocular exposure to infrared radiation (a condition once common in glass and steel workers).

II. The anteriormost layers of the anterior lens capsule split off into one or more sheets that curl into the anterior chamber.

 The exfoliated lamellas frequently can be seen clinically as a "scroll" or "roll of parchment" on the anterior surface of the lens, waving in the aqueous. A senile or aging form of true exfoliation of the lens capsule that does not seem to be related to infrared heat

? fixation artifact
infant eyes (?! SHC)

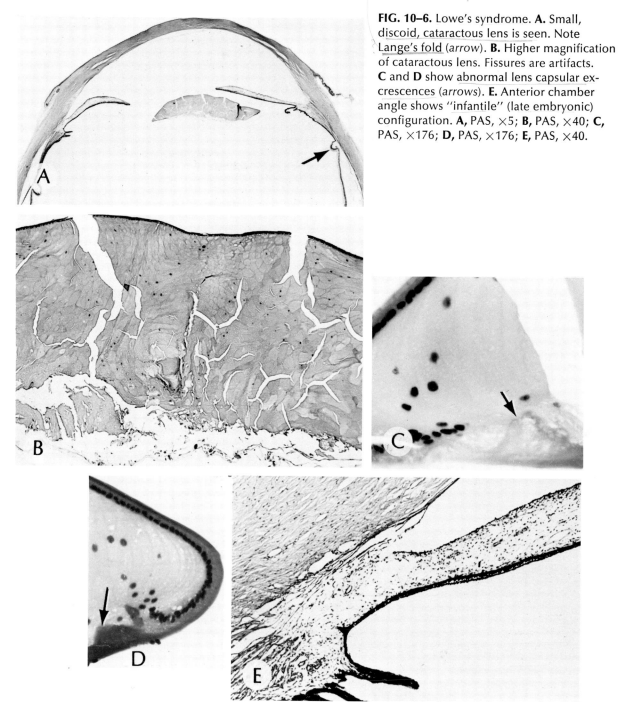

FIG. 10–6. Lowe's syndrome. **A.** Small, discoid, cataractous lens is seen. Note Lange's fold (*arrow*). **B.** Higher magnification of cataractous lens. Fissures are artifacts. **C** and **D** show abnormal lens capsular excrescences (*arrows*). **E.** Anterior chamber angle shows "infantile" (late embryonic) configuration. **A,** PAS, ×5; **B,** PAS, ×40; **C,** PAS, ×176; **D,** PAS, ×176; **E,** PAS, ×40.

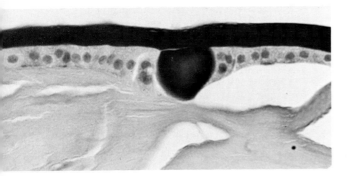

FIG. 10–7. Thickened, globular capsule marks site of healed capsular rent. PAS, ×500.

FIG. 10–8. Traumatically ruptured lens capsule has allowed lens cortical material to "spill out" into anterior chamber. PAS, ×80.

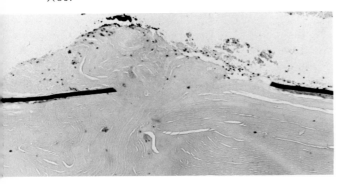

FIG. 10–9. Exfoliation of lens capsule. Anterior layers of anterior lens capsule split off and curl into anterior chamber.

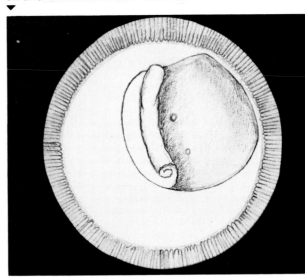

is currently the most common type of true exfoliation seen in the United States.

   III. Exfoliation of the lens does not affect the zonules and is not associated specifically with glaucoma.

PSEUDOEXFOLIATION OF THE LENS CAPSULE
(Fibrillopathia Epitheliocapsularis)
(Figs. 10–11 through 10–13)

   I. Pseudoexfoliation of the lens capsule has a worldwide distribution but seems to be most common in Scandinavian people (especially in Norway and Finland) and quite rare in black people. It is probably inherited, possibly as an autosomal dominant with incomplete penetrance and variable expressivity.

   II. The condition, which occurs mainly in people between 60 and 80 years of age, produces a deposition of a peculiar white, fluffy material of unknown origin on the lens capsule, the zonules, the ciliary epithelium, the iris pigment epithelium and the trabecular meshwork, i.e., limited to the anterior compartment of the eye.

Clinically the anterior surface of the lens shows a characteristic picture. There is a thin, homogeneous white deposit centrally, called the *central disc,* corresponding in extent to the smallest size of the pupil. Frequently the edge of the central disc is well defined by an inrolled edge. The central disc is surrounded by a relatively clear zone. On the outer third of

FIG. 10–10. True exfoliation of lens capsule (with exfoliated layer broken away). **Inset** shows cleavage (*arrow*) to lie within anterior half of lens capsule. e, epithelium. Electron micrograph reinforces bilaminar appearance of anterior capsule, having filamentous anterior part to this thick basement membrane and more homogeneous posterior portion. Separation clearly lies in middle of anteriormost (or filamentous) layer. **E,** lens epithelium. **Main figure,** ×10,000; **inset,** PD, ×300.

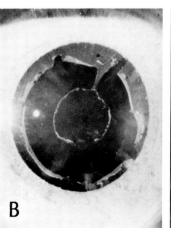

FIG. 10–11. Pseudoexfoliation of lens capsule. **A,** is drawing and **B** and **C** are clinical pictures to show central disc surrounded by relatively clear zone, surrounded in turn by peripheral granular area.

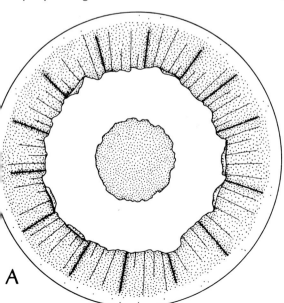

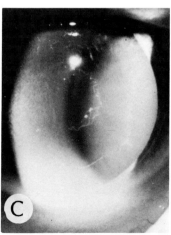

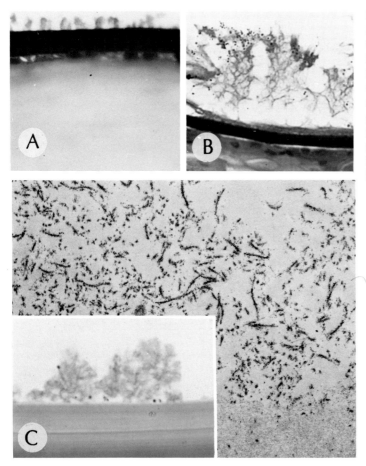

FIG. 10–12. Pseudoexfoliation of lens. **A.** Photomicrograph of central disc area of lens to show small, straight deposits resembling iron filings on magnet. **B.** Area of peripheral band shows dendritic appearance of material. **C. Inset** shows characteristic flocculent material on lens capsule. Electron micrograph shows same material as "crusted" filaments much larger in diameter than zonular filaments. Lens capsule is below. **A,** PAS, ×252; **B,** PAS, ×400; **C,** ×20,000; **inset,** 1.5 μ section, PD, ×615.

the anterior lens surface extending to the equator and usually not seen unless the iris is dilated is a *peripheral band* of a coarse, granular, "hoarfrost" material giving a frosted appearance to the lens surface. The band tends to have radial depressions, which correspond to the radial furrows on the posterior surface of the iris. Powdery, dandrufflike particles commonly are seen on the pupillary margin of the iris and occasionally attached to the corneal endothelium. The iris tends to be "leathery" and to dilate poorly, because of fusion and atrophy of groups of circumferential ridges on its posterior surface. Therefore, it is advisable to do a sector rather than a peripheral iridectomy prior to cataract extraction.

III. In slightly greater than 50 percent of people the condition is bilateral, and in about 70 percent glaucoma (*glaucoma capsulare*) is present.

There is often a degeneration of iris pigment epithelium with subsequent dense pigmentation of the anterior chamber angle resembling the picture seen in *pigmentary glaucoma*. *Sampaolesi's line* is a pigmented line lying on the corneal side of Schwalbe's line and is considered to be an early sign of the condition. The cause of the glaucoma is unknown, although it has been suggested that it is due to accumulations of the peculiar pseudoexfoliated material or to pigment in the angle. Most likely, however, the glaucoma is caused by a separate gene on a locus close to the gene that causes the other changes, or, conversely, the glaucoma may be caused by a single gene bearing three characteristics: (1) an abnormality of the aqueous drainage pathways causing glaucoma; (2) an abnormality causing the pseudoexfoliation material; and (3) an abnormality causing degeneration of the iris pigment epithelium. Variations of expressivity of this single gene would explain why the three events usually are found

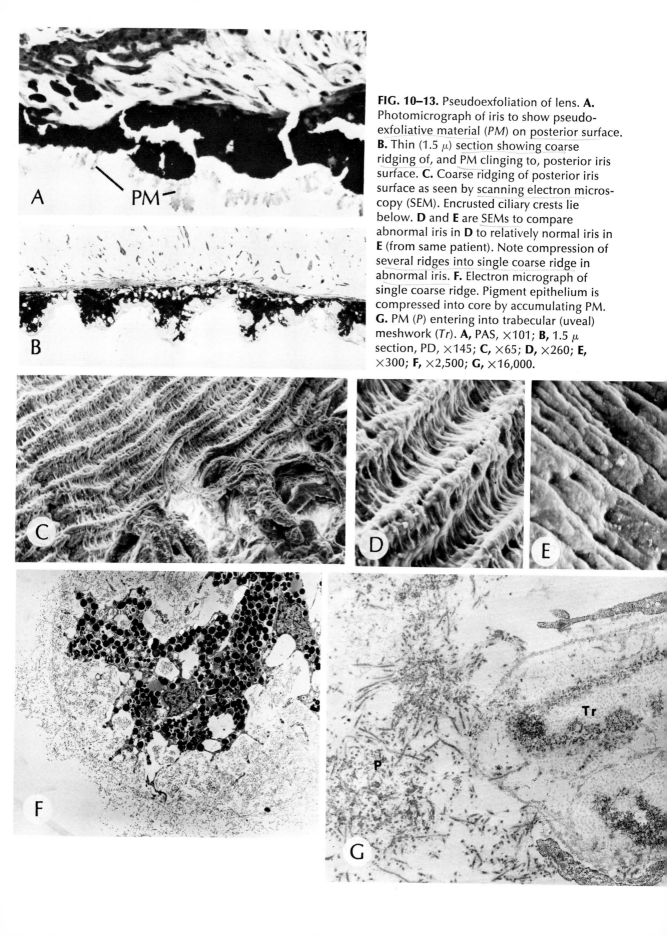

FIG. 10–13. Pseudoexfoliation of lens. **A.** Photomicrograph of iris to show pseudo-exfoliative material (*PM*) on posterior surface. **B.** Thin (1.5 μ) section showing coarse ridging of, and PM clinging to, posterior iris surface. **C.** Coarse ridging of posterior iris surface as seen by scanning electron microscopy (SEM). Encrusted ciliary crests lie below. **D** and **E** are SEMs to compare abnormal iris in **D** to relatively normal iris in **E** (from same patient). Note compression of several ridges into single coarse ridge in abnormal iris. **F.** Electron micrograph of single coarse ridge. Pigment epithelium is compressed into core by accumulating PM. **G.** PM (*P*) entering into trabecular (uveal) meshwork (*Tr*). **A**, PAS, ×101; **B**, 1.5 μ section, PD, ×145; **C**, ×65; **D**, ×260; **E**, ×300; **F**, ×2,500; **G**, ×16,000.

together but why sometimes only two or one is present.

IV. Histologically eosinophilic material is found on the anterior surface of the lens, on the zonular fibers, on and within both surfaces of the iris and ciliary body, in the anterior chamber, in the trabecular meshwork and around conjunctival blood vessels.

A. In the central disc area of the lens the small, straight, thin, eosinophilic deposits line up parallel to each other but perpendicular to the lens, looking much like iron filings lining up on a magnet.

B. In the area of the peripheral band and on the other ocular structures in the anterior segment of the eye, the deposits tend to have a dendritic appearance usually at right angles to the surface to which they are attached. They are prominent over the free surface of the iris pigment epithelium, which characteristically is aggregated into atrophic clusters of circumferential ridges.

FIG. 10–14. Anterior subcapsular cataract. **A** through **D** show change from normal lens epithelium through proliferating epithelial cells to final subcapsular fibrous plaque and formation of new continuous basement membrane or lens capsule.

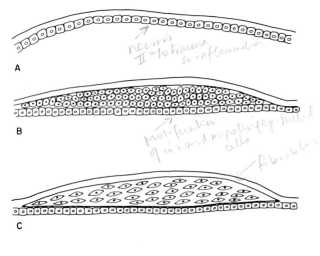

C. Electron microscopically a fibrogranular material is found within the deep (posterior) part of the anterior lens capsule most marked toward the equator and in the region of the zonular attachments. The abnormal material also seems to be present near the underlying lens epithelium.

D. The material's chemical nature and origin are unknown, but by electron microscopy it is seen to be made up of bundles of exceedingly fine filaments irregularly encrusted or banded together.

Currently the most appealing hypothesis is that the material consists of abnormal basement membrane. Preliminary chemical analysis indicates that the material is a protein, lacking in hydroxyproline. A relationship to the noncollagenous protein of basement membranes is possible.

EPITHELIUM

PROLIFERATION AND MIGRATION OF EPITHELIUM

Anterior subcapsular cataract (Figs 10–14 through 10–16)

I. After an injury (usually traumatic or noxious such as iritis or keratitis) to the anterior lens surface, the following sequence of events may take place resulting in an anterior subcapsular cataract:

A. The lens epithelial cells in the region of the anterior pole of the lens become necrotic.

B. Adjacent lens epithelial cells migrate into the area and proliferate under the capsule forming an epithelial plaque.

C. The epithelial cells, except the most posterior layer, then undergo fibrous metaplasia to become fibroblasts, which lay down a connective tissue plaque or scar containing collagen.

D. With time the fibroblasts largely disappear and the scar tissue shrinks, wrinkling the overlying lens capsule.

E. At the same time the remaining epithelial cells, which now line the posterior edge of the fibrous plaque, lay down a new lens capsule. The final

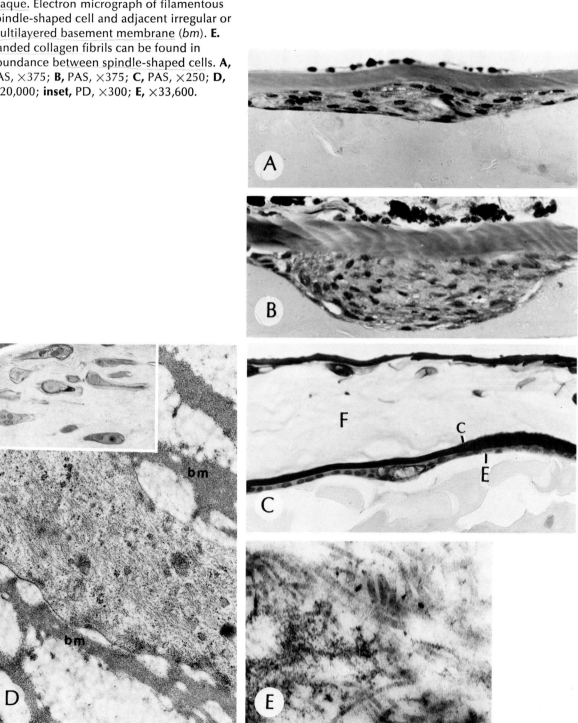

FIG. 10–15. Anterior subcapsular cataract. **A.** Early change with proliferation of subcapsular epithelium. **B.** More proliferation with start of fibrous metaplasia. **C.** Late phase with well-formed fibrous plaque (*F*), new capsule (*c*) and new epithelium (*E*). **D. Inset** shows proliferated spindle-shaped cells in fibrous plaque. Electron micrograph of filamentous spindle-shaped cell and adjacent irregular or multilayered basement membrane (*bm*). **E.** Banded collagen fibrils can be found in abundance between spindle-shaped cells. **A,** PAS, ×375; **B,** PAS, ×375; **C,** PAS, ×250; **D,** ×20,000; **inset,** PD, ×300; **E,** ×33,600.

result is a fibrous plaque at the anterior pole of the lens between a duplicated lens capsule. When the above process occurs to a marked degree resulting in a clinically evident opacity, an anterior subcapsular cataract is present.

An anterior subcapsular cataract of this type is seen infrequently clinically in its pure form because an occluded pupil is almost invariably superimposed.

II. Frequently the same injury that initially caused the damage to the epithelial cells, leading to the above described anterior subcapsular cataract (the end-stage fibrous plaque between a duplicated capsule), also causes an anterior cortical cataract. The combination of an anterior subcapsular cataract plus an anterior cortical cataract is called a *duplication cataract* (Fig. 10–17).

Posterior subcapsular cataract (Fig. 10–18)

I. Either idiopathically (the majority) or after an injury (usually a noxious injury, e.g., with choroiditis, retinopathia pigmentosa or anterior segment necrosis following retinal detachment surgery) to the posterior or equatorial area of the lens, the following sequence of events may take place resulting in a posterior subcapsular cataract:
   A. Early, in all probability, the subcapsular posterior cortical cells degenerate.
   B. Later the lens epithelial cells proliferate and migrate posteriorly, frequently reaching the posterior pole of the lens.

Any lens epithelial cells present between lens capsule and lens cortex posterior to the equator are always in an abnormal location and represent a pathologic change. The abnormal proliferation of epithelial cells may proceed so that the entire lens capsule appears lined by a continuous uninterrupted layer of cells.

   C. The abnormally positioned epithelial cells enlarge in a grossly abnormal manner producing large, bizarrely-shaped cells with abundant, pale-staining, vesicular cytoplasm and small nuclei, i.e., a *bladder cell* (of Wedl).

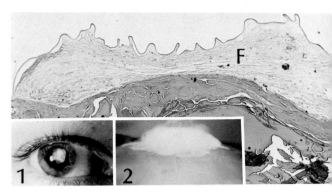

FIG. 10–16. Anterior subcapsular cataract (ASC) with thick fibrous plaque (F) and wrinkled capsule. **Insets** show clinical (**1**) and macroscopic (**2**) appearance of ASC. **Main figure,** H&E, ×30; **inset 1,** clinical; **inset 2,** macroscopic.

FIG. 10–17. Duplication cataract is due to combination of anterior subcapsular cataract (F) and anterior cortical cataract (arrows). H&E, ×60.

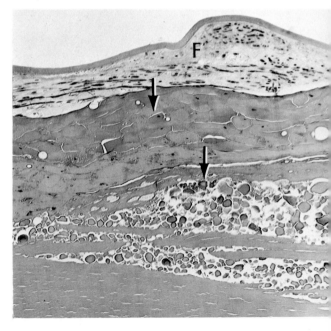

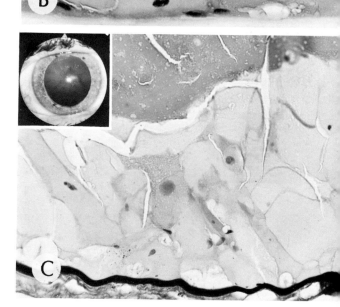

When the changes, mainly bladder cell formation, become significant enough to be seen clinically, a posterior subcapsular cataract is present.

II. The proliferating epithelial cells, including the aberrant forms (bladder cells), may move anteriorly into the posterior cortex resulting in a posterior cortical cataract in addition to the posterior subcapsular cataract.

Elschnig's pearls (Fig. 10–19)

See pp. 129, 150 in Chapter 5.

DEGENERATION AND ATROPHY OF THE EPITHELIUM (Fig. 10–20)

Degeneration and atrophy of the lens epithelium may occur as the result of aging or secondary to acute or chronic glaucoma, to iritis or iridocyclitis, to hypopyon, to hyphema, to chemical injury (especially alkali burn), to noxious products in the aqueous (e.g., with a uveal malignant melanoma or anterior segment necrosis) or to stagnation of the aqueous (e.g., with posterior synechias and iris bombé).

The epithelial damage may be minimal, resulting in no clinically detectable opacity. The damage may be extensive, resulting in widespread cortical degeneration and opacification. Between the two extremes a wide range of abnormalities may occur. Neighboring epithelial cells may proliferate to heal a small epithelial defect, sometimes forming irregular tufts dipping into the lens substance, or they may overproliferate forming anterior or posterior subcapsular cataracts. Localized, focal areas of epithelial necrosis as occurs frequently after an acute attack of glaucoma may result in multiple, discrete, stationary, permanent subcapsular opacities often called *glaukomflecken* (*cataracta disseminata subcapsularis glaucomatosa*). Undoubtedly stagnation of aqueous secondary to aqueous outflow blockage along with a buildup of noxious materials in the aqueous, especially from iris necrosis, play a role in the development of glaukomflecken.

FIG. 10–18. Posterior subcapsular cataract (PSC). **A.** Early PSC (*arrow*) shown macroscopically in **inset** next to ciliary body malignant melanoma (*m*). Photomicrograph of same case shows posterior migration of lens epithelial cells and minimal posterior subcapsular cortical degeneration. **B.** Moderate PSC changes in lens from patient with primary retinopathia pigmentosa (see Figure 11–49). **C.** Marked PSC changes with posterior cortical bladder cell formation. **Inset** shows clinical appearance of PSC. **A,** H&E, ×250; **inset,** macroscopic; **B,** H&E, ×250; **C,** PAS, ×250; **inset,** clinical.

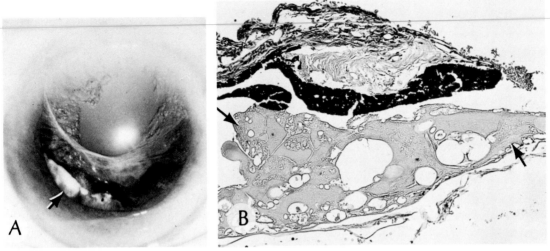

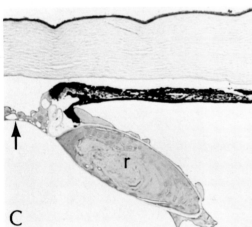

FIG. 10–19. Elschnig's pearls. **A.** Pearls look like fish eggs in periphery of pupillary space. Cortical material (*arrow*) seen partially covered by pupillary iris. **B** and **C** show aberrant proliferation (*arrows*) of lens epithelial cells. Note part of Soemmerring's ring (*r*) in **C. A,** clinical; **B,** H&E, ×100; **C,** H&E, ×16.

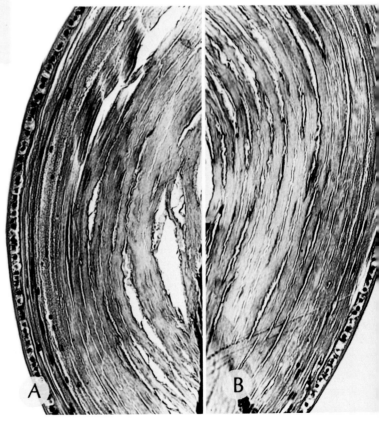

FIG. 10–20. Equatorial epithelial cells nasally (**A**) are relatively normal, whereas cells temporally (**B**), on side of anterior segment necrosis, show vacuolization of cytoplasm and pyknosis of nuclei. **A,** H&E, ×150; **B,** H&E, ×150.

CORTEX AND NUCLEUS (LENS CELLS OR "FIBERS")

CORTEX ("Soft Cataract") (Figs. 10–21 through 10–27)

I. Biochemical changes in the lens cortex due to any cause (congenital, inflammatory, traumatic) may result in clinically detectable opacities, i.e., cortical cataracts.

II. Many clinical types of cataracts are recognized (e.g., cuneiform, coronal, spokelike), but they do not as yet have well-characterized pathologic counterparts in specific histologic findings.

III. Histologically the following pathologic changes may be found in cortical cataracts:

A. *Clefts* seen clinically and histologically are made up of diffuse watery or eosinophilic material, probably representing altered or denatured cell proteins.

B. *Cell fragments* represent pieces of broken up lens cortical cells. They are distinguished from artifactitious fragments by the rounding off of their fractured ends due to retraction of the tenacious cytoplasm of the cell. Cortical fragmentation and rounding, or liquefaction, of their cytoplasm results in the production of morgagnian globules.

C. *Morgagnian globules* represent small or large fragments of cortical cells, which appear rounded due to the increased liquidity of the cytoplasm. They may be present within small or large clefts in otherwise normal-appearing cortex, or they may completely dominate the picture so that no normal-appearing cortex may be seen.

As more and more morgagnian globules together with altered or denatured protein replace the normal lens cortex, the lens becomes hyperosmolar and absorbs fluid. A swollen (mainly in the anterior–posterior diameter) or *intumescent* cataract* results. The globules or abnormal protein may replace the entire cortex resulting in a *mature (liquefied or morgagnian) cataract* in which case the nucleus (generally small and shrunken) sinks by gravity inferiorly. The whole lens looks clinically like a milk-filled sac (the free-floating nucleus usually cannot be seen clearly through an opacified liquid cortex). During the above process of cortical liquefaction, fluid, if of sufficiently small molecular size, may escape through the intact capsule, resulting in a smaller than normal lens with a wrinkled capsule, called a *hypermature cataract*. Rarely the capsule of a mature cataract may rupture spontaneously spilling its contents into the aqueous fluid. In both a mature and a hypermature cataract the capsule fre-

FIG. 10–21. Types of changes that lens "fibers" can undergo.

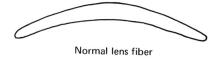

Normal lens fiber

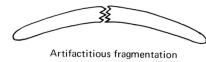

Artifactitious fragmentation

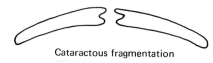

Cataractous fragmentation

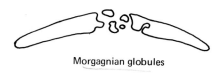

Morgagnian globules

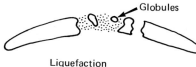

Globules

Liquefaction (hypermature material)

* Clinically the term mature cataract refers to the appearance of a swollen (intumescent) lens as well as to the fact that no clear cortex is detectable beneath the anterior capsule. An immature cataract clinically has some clear cortex between the anterior cortical opacity and the lens capsule, and the lens may be normal in size or swollen. If it is swollen, it is an intumescent cataract. Clinically a hypermature cataract is smaller than normal with a wrinkled capsule and a dense nucleus, usually out of its normal position (the nucleus tends to sink inferiorly as a result of gravity). If cortical clefts filled with morgagnian globules are present histologically but are not seen clinically, they represent the histologic counterpart of an incipient cataract.

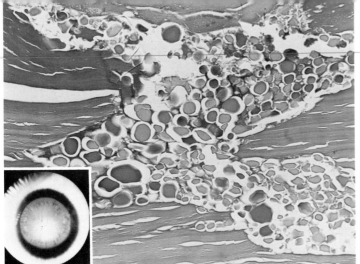

FIG. 10–22. Morgagnian globules between fragmented lens fibers. **Inset** shows peripheral cataractous clefts presumably due to similar type of process. **Main figure,** PAS, ×200; **inset,** clinical.

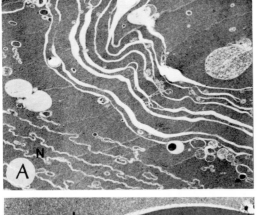

FIG. 10–23. Cortical fragmentation and globule formation. H&E, ×69.

FIG. 10–24. Cortical changes by electron microscopy. **A.** Gross irregularities of cortical cells above with few globules. Normal (*N*) cells are present below. **B.** Cell fragmentation and morgagnian globule (*G*) formation are present. **C.** Dense (*D*) and lucent (*L*) globules are present. The lucent globule appears more watery or liquid. **D.** Watery cell or possibly "hypermature" cell protein (*H*). **A,** ×7,000; **B,** ×7,000; **C,** ×7,000; **D,** ×7,000.

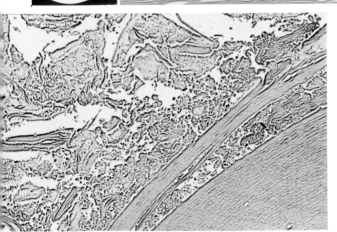

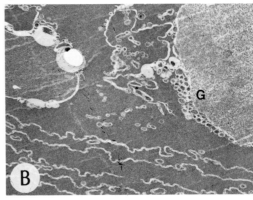

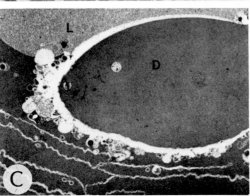

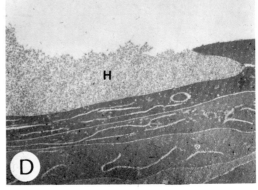

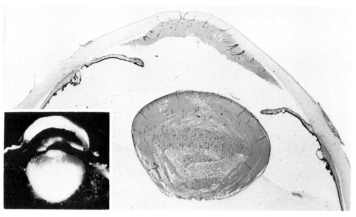

FIG. 10–25. Intumescent or swollen cataract with marked cortical morgagnian degeneration. Note peripheral anterior synechias and chronic secondary angle closure glaucoma. **Inset** shows intumescent lens with "milky" cortex and anterior subcapsular cataract. **Main figure,** H&E, ×8; **inset,** macroscopic.

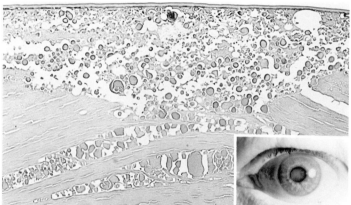

FIG. 10–26. Mature cataract shown in **inset.** Photomicrograph shows morgagnian cortical degeneration coming right up to anterior capsule so that no clear cortex would be seen clinically with slit lamp (i.e., mature cataract). **Main figure,** H&E, ×40; **inset,** clinical.

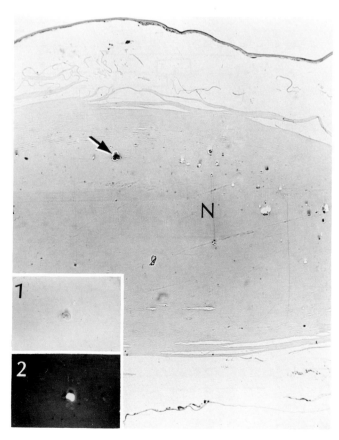

FIG. 10–27. Hypermature cataract characterized by wrinkled capsule. No cortex present (liquefied and "leaked" out), only nucleus (*N*). Calcium oxalate crystal (*arrow*) present in nucleus, seen with higher magnification in **insets** before polarization (**1**) and after polarization (**2**); crystal is birefringent to polarized light. **Main figure,** H&E, ×25; **inset 1,** H&E, ×101; **inset 2,** polarized, H&E, ×101.

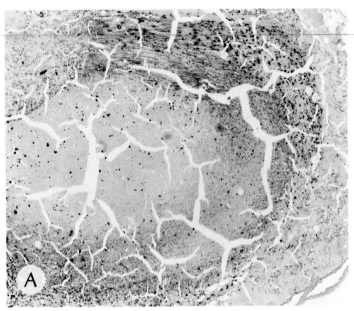

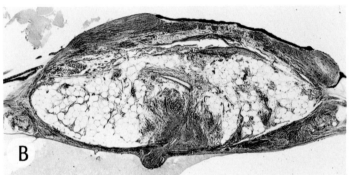

FIG. 10–28. Calcium salts (black dots in nuclear and cortical cataract in **A**) and adipose tissue (**B**) may form in cataractous lens. **A**, von Kossa, ×40; **B**, H&E, ×28.

FIG. 10–29. Soemmerring's ring cataracts shown in **A** and **B**. Note also postcontusion deformity of anterior chamber angle in both eyes. **A**, H&E, ×5; **B**, H&E, ×16.

▼

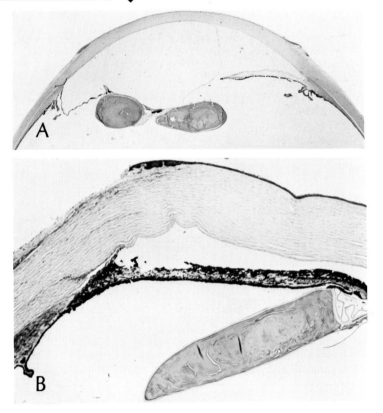

quently is thinned, and the epithelial cells often are degenerated. Because of complications or of surgical intervention, it is quite rare to see a hypermature lens in which all of the lens substance has been resorbed leaving only a clear capsule.

D. Numerous crystals such as calcium oxalate (Fig. 10–27), cholesterol and relatively insoluble amino acids may become deposited in long-standing cataracts.
E. *Calcium salts* may impregnate long-standing cataracts (cataracta calcarea). The abnormal calcification of the lens is an example of *dystrophic calcification* (Fig. 10–28A).
F. With a break in the lens capsule or on a congenital basis, mesenchymal tissue may grow into the cataract leading to bone formation (*cataracta ossea*) or the formation of adipose tissue (*cataracta adiposa* or *xanthomatosis lentis*) (Fig. 10–28B). A break in the anterior capsule may result in cortical material becoming trapped in the equatorial region of the lens, i.e., a *Soemmerring's ring* cataract (Fig. 10–29) (see p. 150 in Chapter 5).

NUCLEUS ("Hard Cataract") (Figs. 10–30 and 10–31)

I. The increasing pressure of cell on cell, the breakdown of intercellular membranes within the lens nucleus, the slow conversion of soluble to insoluble protein and the dehydration and accumulation of pigment (urochrome) all lead to optical and histologic densification of the nucleus and a nuclear cataract.

With more and more accumulation of pigment in the nucleus, the nuclear color changes from clear to yellow to brown (*cataracta brunescens*) to black (*cataracta nigra*). Both the change in color and the increase in refractive index of the nucleus impede the light entering the eye causing a decrease in visual acuity. The increase in index of refraction also causes greater bending of the entering light resulting in a lens-induced myopia.

II. Histologically the changes generally are subtle and are seen as a disappearance of the usual artifactitious nuclear clefts so that the nucleus appears more and more as an amorphous, homogeneous, eosinophilic mass, generally with increased eosinophilia. As seen by electron microscopy the cells become exceedingly folded, tightly packed with obliteration of the intercellular spaces and very electron dense.

SENILE CATARACTS

I. Senile cataracts consist of any cataracts that develop in elderly people (generally over 60 years of age) for which no other cause can be found.
A. Clinically senile cortical cataracts can be divided into three main types: (1) cuneiform (in the peripheral cortex); (2) punctate perinuclear (in the cortex next to the nucleus); and (3) cupuliform (in the posterior cortex).
B. A nuclear cataract is merely the acceleration of the normal densification process of the innermost lens "fibers," which occurs with aging.
II. Senile cataracts may subluxate or dislocate spontaneously. The histology of cortical and nuclear cataracts has been described above (Fig. 10–32).

SECONDARY CATARACTS

INTRAOCULAR DISEASE

I. Uveitis, malignant intraocular tumors (Fig. 10–18), glaucoma (Figs. 10–25 and 10–31), retinopathia pigmentosa (Fig. 10–18) and retinal detachment can all cause secondary cataracts.

The cataract secondary to intraocular disease has been termed a complicating cataract (*cataracta complicata*). Diseases in the anterior part of the eye tend to cause anterior cataract (anterior subcapsular or anterior cortical or both), whereas diseases in the posterior part of the eye tend to cause posterior cataract (posterior subcapsular or posterior cortical or both).

II. Histologically the lens changes are non-specific and are the same as those described above.

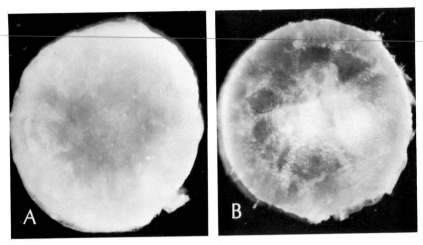

FIG. 10–30. Macroscopic appearance of cataracta brunescens (**A**) and cataracta nigra (**B**).

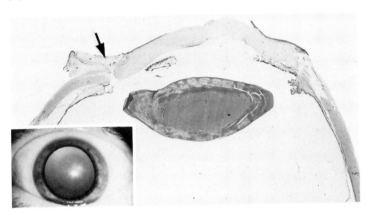

FIG. 10–31. Nuclear cataract (**inset**) is recognized histologically by relative homogeneity of nucleus. Note (*arrow*) area of peripheral iridectomy, scleral cautery and filtering bleb. **Main figure,** H&E, ×5; **inset,** clinical.

FIG. 10–32. Schematic comparison of histologic features in normal and abnormal lenses. ▼

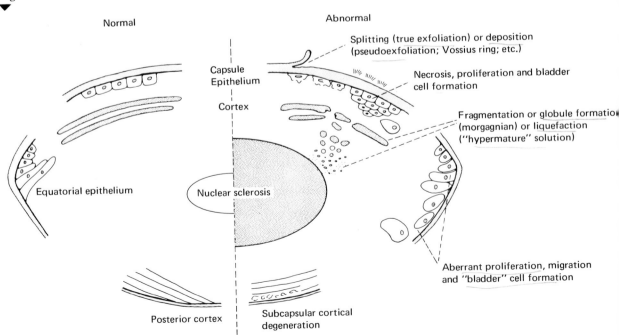

Normal   Abnormal

Splitting (true exfoliation) or deposition (pseudoexfoliation; Vossius ring; etc.)

Capsule
Epithelium

Necrosis, proliferation and bladder cell formation

Cortex

Fragmentation or globule formation (morgagnian) or liquefaction ("hypermature" solution)

Equatorial epithelium

Nuclear sclerosis

Aberrant proliferation, migration and "bladder" cell formation

Posterior cortex   Subcapsular cortical degeneration

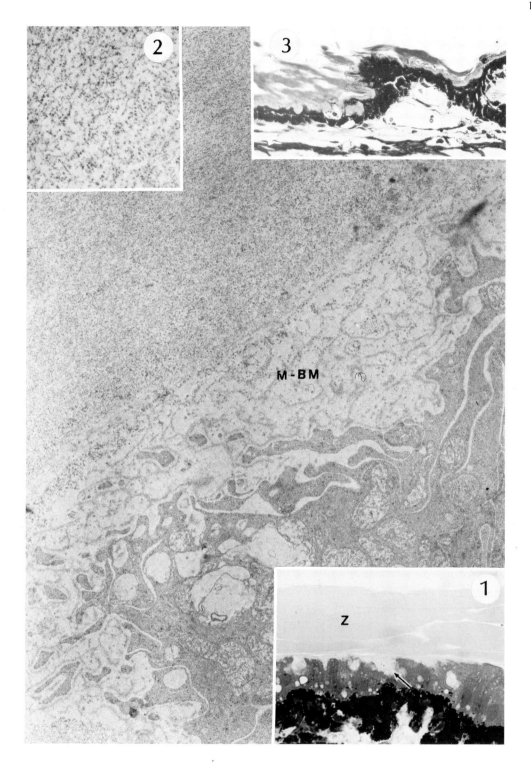

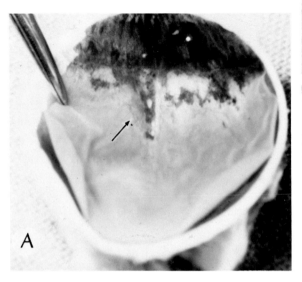

A

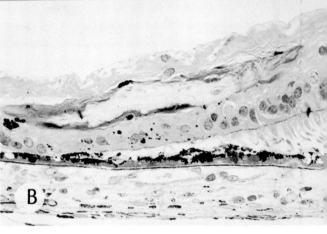

B

FIG. 10–37. Homocystinuria. **A.** Calotte showing extensive peripheral retinal degeneration and secondary pigmentary changes sharply demarcated (*arrow*) from normal retina. **B.** Abrupt transition is shown between normal retina on right and degenerate retina on left. **A,** macroscopic; **B,** 1.5 μ section, PD, ×350.

figuration, but this is variable and nonspecific.

2. The iris shows segmental hypopigmentation or absence of pigment from the posterior layer of the pigment epithelium, especially toward the periphery, with accompanying hypoplasia of the overlying iris dilator muscle.

The hypopigmentation of the posterior iris pigment epithelial layer is highly characteristic and explains the clinical observation of increased positive retro-illumination of the iris diaphragm where stromal pigmentation is not too dense.

3. The ciliary body processes or crests extend sporadically onto the back of the iris and are maldeveloped.
4. The lens is subluxated in the posterior chamber or dislocated into the anterior chamber or vitreous compartment.

IV. Weill-Marchesani Syndrome (Fig. 10–40)

A. Weill-Marchesani syndrome is a generalized disorder of connective tissues characterized by spherophakia, ectopia lentis, brachymorphism and joint stiffness.

B. The spherophakic lens subluxates frequently and usually in a down-and-in direction. High myopia often is present.

Spherophakia may be part of the Weill-Marchesani syndrome, may occur independently or, rarely, may occur in Marfan's syndrome. The small lens can cause a pupillary block glaucoma. Such a glaucoma is worsened by miotics but ameliorated by mydriatics. Peripheral anterior synechias may form secondarily to the pupillary block. The small lens dislocates frequently into the anterior chamber.

C. The condition is inherited as an autosomal recessive.
D. Histologically there is a filamentary degeneration of zonular fibers producing a thick periodic acid-Schiff positive layer overlying the ciliary epithelium. The picture is almost identical to that seen in homocystinuria.

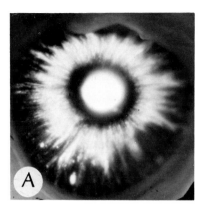

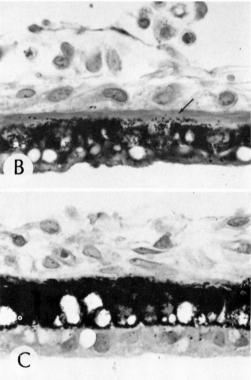

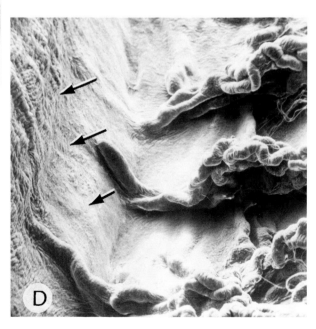

FIG. 10–38. Marfan's syndrome. **A.** Transillumination of enucleated eye shows widespread lucency of most of iris leaf. **B.** Posterior epithelium is pigmented slightly and thin dilator muscle is present (*arrow*). **C.** Posterior epithelium is amelanotic and dilator muscle appears absent. **D.** Scanning electron micrograph of posterior iris near its root. Ciliary crests on right are fetal in configuration and extend onto peripheral iris. Circumferential ridges and furrows of iris gradually disappear (*arrows*) as posterior iris surface becomes smooth in its periphery. Fragments lying within interciliary valleys are remnants of dissected zonules. **A,** macroscopic, transilluminated; **B,** 1.5 μ section, PD, $\times$575; **C,** 1.5 μ section, PD, $\times$575; **D,** $\times$65.

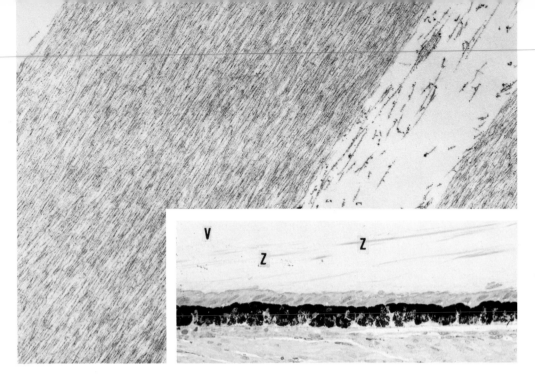

FIG. 10–39. Marfan's syndrome. **Inset** shows
sample region of pars plana. Epithelial
layers, nearby anterior vitreous body (*V*)
and zonular segments (*Z*) appear normal.
Electron micrograph shows normal arrangement of myriad filaments, highly aligned,
that make up fragment of zonular fiber.
Main figure, ×20,000; **inset** 1.5 μ section,
PD, ×265.

FIG. 10–40. Weill-Marchesani syndrome.
Inset shows heavy deposit of PAS-positive
material (*arrows*) over nonpigmented epithelium of ciliary body. Electron micrograph
shows that material is composed of dis-
integrated zonular filaments. Note deficiency
of multilaminar basement membrane
(*arrows*). **Main figure,** ×8,000; **inset,** PAS,
×50.

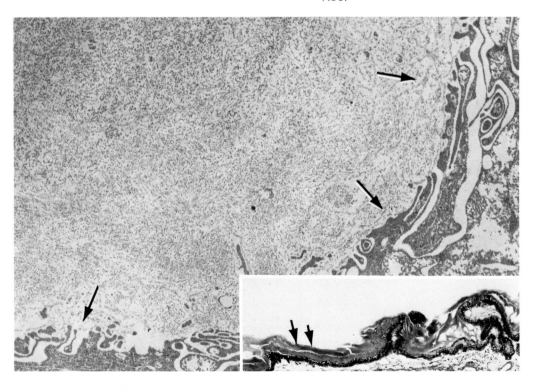

BIBLIOGRAPHY

GENERAL INFORMATION

Fine BS, Yanoff M: Ocular Histology: A Text and Atlas. New York, Harper & Row, 1972, pp. 129–139

CONGENITAL ANOMALIES

Brownell RD, Wolter JR: Anterior lenticonus in familial hemorrhagic nephritis. Arch Ophthalmol 71:481, 1964

Chavis RM, Groshong T: Corneal arcus in Alport's syndrome. Am J Ophthalmol 75:793, 1973

Duke-Elder S: System of Ophthalmology, Vol III, Normal and Abnormal Development, Part 2, Congenital Deformities. St. Louis, Mosby, 1963, pp 688–761

Henkind P, Prose P: Anterior polar cataract: electron microscopic evidence of collagen. Am J Ophthalmol 63:768, 1967

Hoepner J, Yanoff M: Craniosynostosis and syndactylism (Apert's syndrome) associated with a trisomy 21 mosaic. J Pediatr Ophthalmol 8:107, 1971

Manschot WA: Primary congenital aphakia. Arch Ophthalmol 69:571, 1963

Schatz H: Alport's syndrome in a negro kindred. Am J Ophthalmol 71:1236, 1971

Stevens PS: Anterior lenticonus and the Waardenburg syndrome. Br J Ophthalmol 54:621, 1970

Yanoff M, Fine BS, Schaffer DB: Histopathology of transient neonatal lens vacuoles: a light and electron microscopic study. Am J Ophthalmol 76:363, 1973

CAPSULE

Aasved H: Mass screening for fibrillopathia epitheliocapsularis. Acta Ophthalmol (Kbh) 49:334, 1971

Aasved H: The frequency of optic nerve damage and surgical treatment in chronic simple glaucoma and capsular glaucoma. Acta Ophthalmol (Kbh) 49:589, 1971

Aasved H: Intraocular pressure in eyes with and without fibrillopathia epitheliocapsularis. Acta Ophthalmol (Kbh) 49:601, 1971

Ashton N, Shakib M, Collyer R, Blach R: Electron microscopic study of pseudoexfoliation of the lens capsule. I. Lens capsule and zonular fibers. II. Iris and ciliary body. Invest Ophthalmol 4:141, 154, 1965

Bertelsen TI: Fibrillopathia epithelio-capsularis. The so-called senile exfoliation or pseudo-exfoliation of the anterior lens capsule. Acta Ophthalmol (Kbh) 44:737, 1966

Bertelsen TI, Drablös PA, Flood PR: The so-called senile exfoliation (pseudo-exfoliation) of the anterior lens capsule, a product of the lens epithelium. Fibrillopathia epithelio-capsularis. Acta Ophthalmol (Kbh) 42:1096, 1964

Blackstad TW, Sunde OA, Traetteborg J: On the ultrastructure of the deposits of Busacca in eyes with glaucoma simplex and so-called senile exfoliation of the anterior lens capsule. Acta Ophthalmol (Kbh) 38:587, 1960

Burde RM, Bresnick G, Uhrhammer J: True exfoliation of the lens capsule—an electron microscopic study. Arch Ophthalmol 82:651, 1969

Callahan A, Klein BA: Thermal detachment of the anterior lamella of the anterior lens capsule. A clinical and histologic study. Arch Ophthalmol 59:73, 1958

Ghosh M, Speakman JS: Inclusions in the human lens capsule and their relationship to senile exfoliation. Can J Ophthalmol 7:413, 1972

Ghosh M, Speakman JS: The ciliary body in senile exfoliation of the lens. Can J Ophthalmol 8:394, 1973

Gillies WE: Effect of lens extraction in pseudo-exfoliation of lens capsule. Br J Ophthalmol 57:46, 1973

Luntz MH: Prevalence of pseudo-exfoliation syndrome in an urban South African clinic population. Am J Ophthalmol 74:581, 1972

Pallisgaard G, Goldschmidt E: Oculo-cerebro-renal syndrome of Lowe in 4 generations of one family. Acta Paediatr Scand 60:146, 1971

Pohjanpelto PEJ: The fellow eye in unilateral hypertensive pseudoexfoliation. Am J Ophthamol 75:216, 1973

Ringvold A: Ultrastructure of exfoliation material (Busacca deposits). Virchows Arch [Pathol Anat] 350:95, 1970

Ringvold A: Electron microscopy of the limbal conjunctiva in eyes with pseudoexfoliation syndrome (PE syndrome). Virchows Arch [Pathol Anat] 355:275, 1972

Ringvold A: A preliminary report on the amino acid composition of the pseudoexfoliation material (PE material). Exp Eye Res 15:37, 1973

Ringvold A: On the occurrence of pseudo-exfoliation material in extrabulbar tissue from patients with pseudo-exfoliation syndrome of the eye. Acta Ophthalmol (Kbh) 51:411, 1973

Tarkkanen A: Pseudoexfoliation of the lens capsule. Acta Ophthalmol (Kbh) 40 [Suppl 71], 1962

Tarkkanen A: Treatment of chronic open-angle glaucoma associated with pseudoexfoliation. Acta Ophthalmol 43:514, 1965

Zimmerman LE, Font RL: Congenital malformations of the eye. J Am Med Assoc 196:684, 1966

EPITHELIUM

Eagle RC Jr, Yanoff M, Morse PH: Anterior segment necrosis following scleral buckling in hemoglobin SC disease. Am J Ophthalmol 75:426, 1973

Font RL, Brownstein S: A light and electron microscopic study of anterior subcapsular cataracts. Am J Ophthalmol 78:972, 1974

Henkind P, Prose P: Anterior polar cataract: electron microscopic evidence of collagen. Am J Ophthalmol 63:768, 1967

Wedl C: Atlas der pathologischen Histologie des Auges. Leipzig, Wigand, 1860–1861, LV IV, 44 and 55

Winstanley J: Iris atrophy in primary glaucoma. Trans Ophthalmol Soc UK 81:23, 1961

CORTEX AND NUCLEUS

Babel J: Recherches histochimiques sur le cristallin normal et cataracte. Bull Soc Ophtalmol Fr 78:413, 1965

Blodi FC: Developmental anomalies of the skull affecting the eye. Arch Ophthalmol 57:593, 1957

Brini A, Porte A, Stoeckel ME: Modifications ultrastructurales du cristallin dans certaines cataractes expérimentales et humaines. Bull Soc Ophtalmol Fr 76:193, 1963

Cowan TH: Pigmentation and coloration of the lens. Survey Ophthalmol 6:630, 1961

Meyer-Arendt J, Meyer-Arendt EA: Spectrophotometric studies on human lenses with cataracta brunescens (letter to ed). J Histochem Cytochem 8:75, 1960

SECONDARY CATARACTS

Becker B: The side effects of corticosteroids. Invest Ophthalmol 3:492, 1964

Leopold IH: Trends in ocular therapy. Am J Ophthalmol 65:297, 1968

Monteleone JA, Beutler E, Monteleone PL, Utz CL, Casey EC: Cataracts, galactosuria and hypergalactosemia due to galactokinase deficiency in a child. Am J Med 50:403, 1971

COMPLICATIONS OF CATARACTS

Flocks M, Littwin CS, Zimmerman LE: Phacolytic glaucoma. Arch Ophthalmol 54:37, 1955

Yanoff M, Scheie HG: Cytology of human lens aspirate. Its relationship to phacolytic glaucoma and phacoanaphylactic endophthalmitis. Arch Ophthalmol 80:166, 1968

ECTOPIC LENS

Cross HE, Jensen AD: Ocular manifestations in the Marfan syndrome and homocystinuria. Am J Ophthalmol 75:405, 1973

Gaull GE: Clinical importance of enzymatic diagnosis: the homocystinurias. J Pediatr Ophthalmol 10:247, 1973

Jensen AD, Cross HE: Ocular complications in the Weil-Marchesani syndrome. Am J Ophthalmol 77:261, 1974

McGavic JS: Weil-Marchesani syndrome—brachymorphism and ectopia lentis. Am J Ophthalmol 62:820, 1966

Ramsey MS, Fine BS, Shields JA, Yanoff M: The Marfan syndrome. A histopathologic study of ocular findings. Am J Ophthalmol 76:102, 1973

Ramsey MS, Fine BS, Yanoff M: The ocular histopathology of homocystinuria. A light and electron microscopic study. Am J Ophthalmol 74:377, 1972

Willi M, Kut L, Cotlier E: Pupillary-block galucoma in the Marchesani syndrome. Arch Ophthalmol 90:504, 1973

chapter 11

Retina

Handwritten margin notes: *p. 461* (top), *3/4/76* (left margin)

CONGENITAL ANOMALIES

ALBINISM

I. Systemically albinism generally is complete resulting in white, silky skin and fine, white or straw-colored hair, brow and lashes.

II. Incomplete (rather than complete) albinism usually occurs in ocular tissues with a deficiency, but rarely a complete lack, of melanin in pigment epithelium and in uveal melanocytes.

Pink or red eyes result from the decreased amount of melanin in the stromal and pigment epithelial cells of the iris with resultant translucency of the irises. Poor vision is due to hypoplasia of the foveomacular area of the retina. Near vision frequently is better than distant vision. Nystagmus and photophobia commonly accompany the defective vision.

III. The condition usually is inherited as an autosomal recessive but rarely may be sex-linked recessive or autosomal dominant.

IV. Chediak-Higashi syndrome. This syndrome is an autosomal recessive disease characterized by oculocutaneous albinism, photophobia, a distinctive granular anomaly of myeloid cells, inclusion bodies in lymphocytes and monocytes, granulocytopenia, abnormalities of lipid metabolism, neurologic defects and death by about 8 to 10 years of age from infection or hemorrhage.
Histologically chronic granulomatous choroiditis and nongranulomatous optic neuritis may be observed.

GROUPED PIGMENTATION (Bear Tracks) (Fig. 11–1)

I. Grouped pigmentation is seen clinically as discrete pigmented areas resembling the footprints of a bear.

II. The condition usually is unilateral and nonprogressive affecting a sector-shaped retinal area with the apex of the sector at the optic disc.

III. Histologically hypertrophy of the retinal pigment epithelium, sometimes accompanied by degeneration of the overlying receptors, is seen.

A familial case of grouped pigmentation of the macula has been described in two sisters. This may represent an autosomal recessive inheritance pattern in these two cases.

COLOBOMA

I. The typical coloboma involves the region of the embryonic cleft (fetal fissure) (i.e., inferonasally) and is bilateral in 60 percent of cases.

The coloboma may involve the total extent of the embryonic cleft, a large part of the region or one or more small isolated parts.

II. Histologically the retinal pigment epithelium is missing primarily with a secondary hypoplasia and dysplasia of the overlying sensory retina and the underlying choroid (see p. 332 in Chap. 9).

The sclera may be thinned or even absent in the area of the coloboma, and the retina may herniate through in the form of a cyst and/or undergo massive glial proliferation (*massive gliosis*). See pp. 516–517 in Chapter 14.

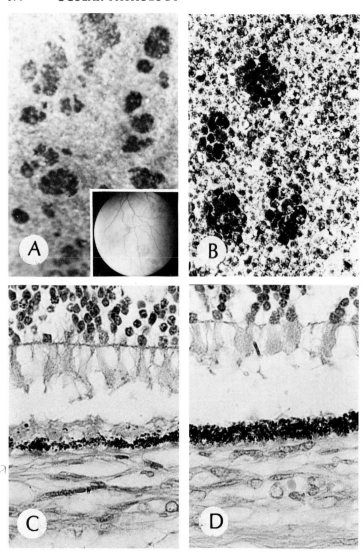

FIG. 11–1. Grouped pigmentation. **A.** Macroscopic appearance of pigmented plaques. Fundus (**inset**) shows typical grouped pigmentation. **B.** Flat preparation of RPE showing greater concentration of pigment granules in cells corresponding to grouped pigmentation. **C.** RPE in normal area adjacent to plaque. **D.** RPE in area of plaque shows greater concentration of pigment granules. Overlying retina detached artifactitiously. **A,** macroscopic; **inset,** fundus; **B,** flat preparation, H&E, ×256; **C,** H&E, ×640; **D,** H&E, ×640.

RETINAL DYSPLASIA (Fig. 11–2)

See p. 698 in Chapter 18.

LANGE'S FOLD (Fig. 11–3)

I. Lange's fold consists of an inward fold of retina at the ora serrata seen only in infants' and children's eyes.
II. The fold is not present in vivo or in the enucleated, nonfixed eye and is an artifact of fixation.

    Lange's fold can be considered a useful artifact because it helps to identify an eye in tissue section as that of a child.

CONGENITAL NONATTACHMENT OF THE RETINA* (see Fig. 10–3)

I. Nonattachment of the retina is the normal situation in the embryonic eye; persistence of the situation after birth is abnormal.
II. The condition frequently is associated with other ocular abnormalities such as microphthalmos, persistent hyperplastic primary vitreous, colobomas and others.

    * In this chapter the terms retina, neural retina and sensory retina are used synonymously. The terms refer to all the layers of the retina exclusive of its pigment epithelium.

III. Histologically the neural (sensory) retina and nonpigmented epithelium of the ciliary body are separated from the pigment epithelium of the retina and ciliary body. The retina may be normal, completely dysplastic or anything in between.

The space between the neural retina and its pigment epithelium normally closes progressively during fetal life. If something should happen shortly before birth to reverse this trend and rapidly separate the two layers, a *congenital retinal detachment,* secondary in nature, would result. A retinal *dialysis (disinsertion),* usually located nasally, may develop in utero and lead to a secondary congenital or developmental retinal detachment.

RETINAL CYSTS (Fig. 11–4)

I. A cyst of the (neural) retina is defined arbitrarily as an intraretinal space in which the internal–external diameter is greater than the thickness of the surrounding retina and of approximately equal dimension in any direction; retinoschisis, on the other hand, is an intraretinal space that has a smaller internal–external diameter than the thickness of the surrounding retina and much smaller than the width of the space lying parallel to the retina.

"Cyst" is a poor term because a cyst, by definition, is an epithelial-lined space. In ocular pathology, however, the term cyst (intraretinal, intracorneal, intrascleral, etc.) is used frequently to describe an intratissue space not necessarily lined by epithelium.

II. Congenital retinal cysts have been reported in the periphery, generally inferior temporal region, and in the macula.

It is not clear whether or not so-called congenital cysts are not in fact a manifestation of juvenile retinoschisis (see pp. 432, 434 in this chapter). *Secondary retinal cysts* may occur in congenital nonattachment of the retina and in secondary congenital or acquired retinal detachments.

III. Histologically the cysts usually are lined by gliotic retina and are filled with a periodic acid-Schiff positive material that is negative for stains that demonstrate acid mucopolysaccharides.

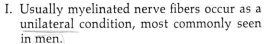

MYELINATED (MEDULLATED) NERVE FIBERS (Fig. 11–5)

I. Usually myelinated nerve fibers occur as a unilateral condition, most commonly seen in men.
II. Clinically they appear as an opaque white patch or arcuate band with "feathery" edges.

The area of myelination may be continuous with the optic disc or may be separated from it by an area of nonmyelinated retina. It may occur in any part of the retina. Rarely the condition may be inherited. The patch of myelination may become involved in multiple sclerosis.

III. Histologically myelin (and possibly oligodendrocytes) is present in the retinal nerve fiber layer, but the region of the lamina cribrosa is free of myelination.

OGUCHI'S DISEASE

I. Oguchi's disease, inherited as an autosomal recessive, is a stationary form of congenital night blindness.
II. The color of the fundus is unusual, varying from shades of gray to yellow; the retina may be involved totally or segmentally.
III. Mizuo's phenomenon, i.e., a more normal appearing fundus in the dark-adapted state, is present.
IV. Histologically the cones are more numerous than usual, and there are practically no rods, especially in the temporal area. There is a nondescript, amorphous material containing pigment granules between the cones and the retinal pigment epithelium.

FOVEOMACULAR ABNORMALITIES*

I. Hypoplasia
   A. Hypoplasia is characterized by a total or nearly total absence of the clinically

---

* There has been much confusion in recent years regarding the proper use of the terms fovea, macula and posterior pole by clinicians. The anatomic fovea is a

(continued)

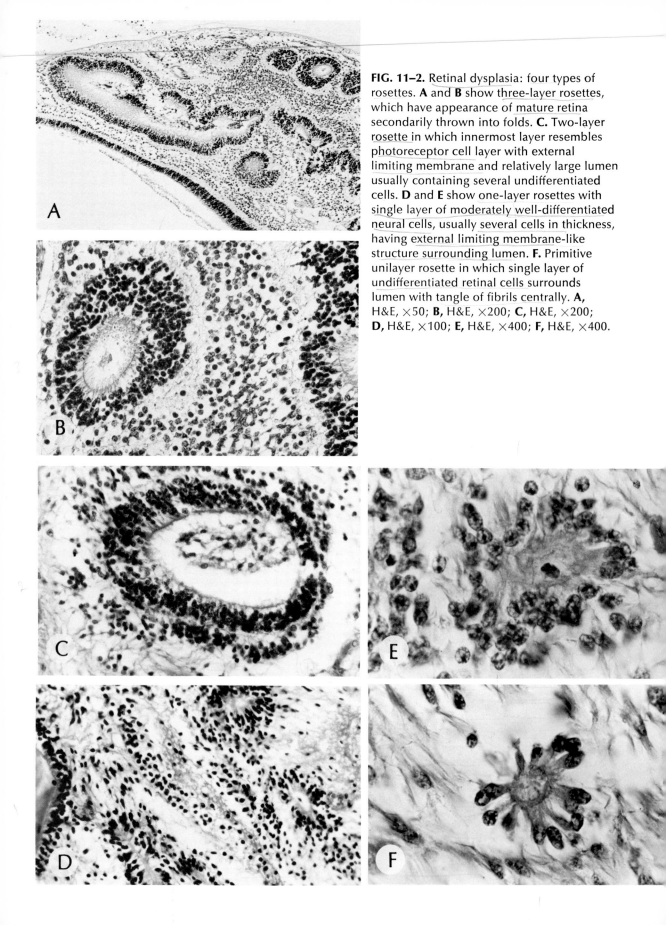

FIG. 11–2. Retinal dysplasia: four types of rosettes. **A** and **B** show three-layer rosettes, which have appearance of mature retina secondarily thrown into folds. **C.** Two-layer rosette in which innermost layer resembles photoreceptor cell layer with external limiting membrane and relatively large lumen usually containing several undifferentiated cells. **D** and **E** show one-layer rosettes with single layer of moderately well-differentiated neural cells, usually several cells in thickness, having external limiting membrane-like structure surrounding lumen. **F.** Primitive unilayer rosette in which single layer of undifferentiated retinal cells surrounds lumen with tangle of fibrils centrally. **A,** H&E, ×50; **B,** H&E, ×200; **C,** H&E, ×200; **D,** H&E, ×100; **E,** H&E, ×400; **F,** H&E, ×400.

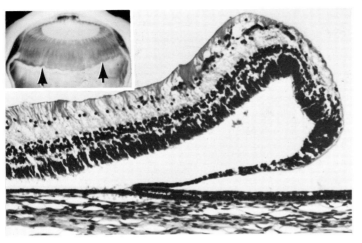

FIG. 11–3. Lange's fold (see in **inset** at *arrows*) consists of artifactitious, inward fold of retina at ora serrata. **Main figure,** H&E, ×101; **inset,** macroscopic.

fixation artefact in infants.

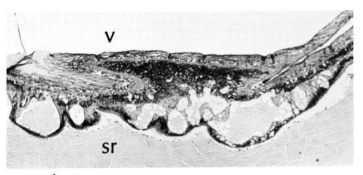

FIG. 11–4. Retinal cysts are present in detached retina. *v,* vitreous; *sr,* subretinal space containing eosinophilic coagulum. H&E, ×16.

FIG. 11–5. Myelinated nerve fibers. **A. Inset** is macroscopic photograph of patch of myelinated nerve fibers fanning out upper temporally from vicinity of optic disc (*d*). Note "feathered" edge (*arrows*) to heavily myelinated patch. Micrograph shows myelination of entire nerve fiber layer in this part of peripheral macula. **B.** Higher magnification shows myelination of all nerve fibers (ganglion cell axons) in this region. Fibers, or axons, are extremely variable in size. *ipl,* inner plexiform layer; *inl,* inner nuclear layer. **C.** Fundus appearance of myelinated nerve fibers. **Right,** child was referred by pediatrician because of suspected retinoblastoma. **A.** 1.5 µ section, PD, ×80; **inset,** macroscopic; **B.** 1.5 µ section, PD, ×300; **C,** right and left, fundus.

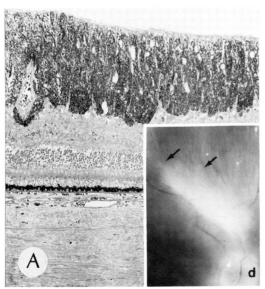

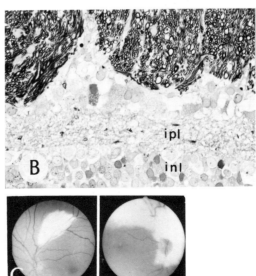

seen macular yellow, an absence or irregularity of the foveal and perifoveal reflexes and an irregular distribution of perifoveal capillaries.

B. Frequently it is associated with hereditary anomalies such as aniridia, achromatopsia, sex-linked hemeralopia, ocular and systemic complete and incomplete albinism and microphthalmos.

II. Dysplasia (Coloboma of Macula)

A. Many, if not most, of the foveomacular dysplasias or colobomas are secondary to congenital toxoplasmosis (see p. 94 in Chap. 4).

B. Hereditary forms have been described with both a dominant and recessive autosomal pattern.

VASCULAR DISEASE

DEFINITIONS

I. The retinal circulation is predominantly arteriolar, because very shortly after the central retinal artery enters the retina it loses its internal elastic lamina and continuous muscular coat and therefore becomes an arteriole (generally it becomes an arteriole by the first intraretinal bifurcation).

II. Similarly the central retinal vein loses its thick wall and becomes a venule usually by its first intraretinal bifurcation.

(continued)
depression or pit in the retina, which is approximately the same size, especially in horizontal measure, as the corresponding optic disc, i.e., 1.5 mm. The anatomic foveola is a small (~ 350 μ diameter) reddish disc comprising the floor of the fovea. It is a major portion of the avascular zone of the fovea (i.e. ~ 500 μ diameter). The anatomic macula (derived from the term macula lutea) is an area larger than the anatomic fovea and is frequently equated with the histologic appearance of more than a single layer of ganglion cells, i.e., area centralis.

For convenience and practical reasons the three clinical terms fovea, macula and posterior pole correspond best to the three anatomic terms foveola, fovea and macula (area centralis). With this simple equation in mind, the reader may easily convert clinical terminology to anatomic as well as the reverse. The widespread clinical use of the term macula for the general area encompassed by the anatomic fovea cannot in all likelihood be altered significantly.

III. The inner half of the retina (approximately) is supplied by the retinal circulation (retinal capillaries) and the outer half by the choroidal circulation (choriocapillaris).

Clinically, however, the largest retinal vessels are by common usage known as arteries and veins. These terms are carried over into ophthalmic pathology.

RETINAL ISCHEMIA

I. Causes

A. Choroidal vascular insufficiency

1. Choroidal tumors such as nevus, malignant melanoma, hemangioma and metastatic carcinoma may "compete" with the outer layers of the retina for nourishment from the choriocapillaris.

2. *Choroidal thrombosis* due to idiopathic thrombotic thrombocytopenic purpura, malignant hypertension, collagen diseases or *emboli* (Fig. 11–6) may occlude the choriocapillaris primarily or secondarily via effects on the choroidal arterioles.

Rarely large areas of choriocapillaris may be occluded chronically by such materials as accumulating amyloid with surprisingly good preservation of the overlying retina.

B. Retinal vascular insufficiency

1. Large artery disease anywhere from aortic arch to central retinal artery

a. Atherosclerosis (Fig. 11–7) has a patchy distribution, shows subendothelial lipid deposits and erosion of media.

b. *Takayasu's disease* occurs usually in young women, frequently Japanese, shows an adventitial giant cell reaction, also involves the media and produces intimal proliferation with obliteration of the lumen.

Takayasu's syndrome or aortic arch syndrome (Fig. 11–8) occurs in older patients of either sex and differs from the "usual" type of

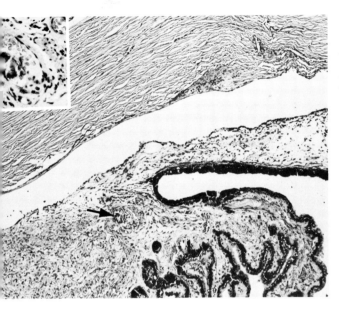

FIG. 11–6. Calcific embolus present in greater circle of iris (*arrow*). **Inset** shows embolus (*arrow*) at higher magnification. Note cyclodialysis with overgrowth of endothelial-produced Descemet's membrane, due to nonsurgical trauma 16 years previously. **Main figure,** H&E, ×40; **inset,** H&E, ×101.

FIG. 11–7. Atherosclerosis. **A.** Gross appearance of fundus of eye removed postmortem. *Arrow* indicates plaque in inferonasal arteriole, which is seen microscopically in **B. B.** Frozen section stained with oil red-O shows lipid deposits (*arrow*) in atheromatous plaque. Note fatty infiltration in muscular wall at edge of artifactitious cleft (*double arrow*). **A,** macroscopic; **B,** oil red-O, ×200.

atherosclerosis only in its site of predilection of the aortic arch. Another cause of the syndrome is syphilitic aortitis.

c. Temporal (cranial) arteritis (Fig. 11–9)
1) Temporal arteritis is most commonly found in middle-aged or elderly women.
2) It frequently is associated with malaise, weight loss, fever, severe headaches, scalp pain and visual loss.
3) The superficial temporal artery may be red, tender, firm, enlarged and pulseless, or it may be normal. The erythrocyte sedimentation rate becomes elevated, often to a high degree.
4) The aorta and its larger branches may be involved.
5) Marked impairment of visual acuity often with involvement of the second eye within days or weeks of involvement of the first eye is the most frequent ocular problem, but ptosis and muscle palsies also may occur.

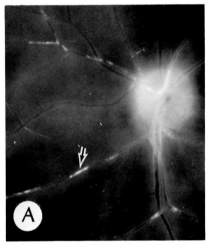

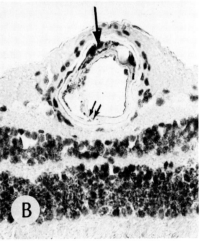

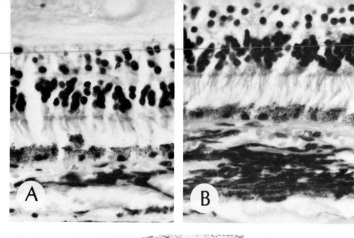

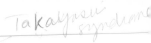

FIG. 11–8. Aortic arch syndrome in 69-year-old white man. **A** shows macular area and **B** peripheral area. Note acellularity of inner layers, lack of blood in vessel in **A** and degeneration of receptors. **A,** H&E, ×252; **B,** H&E, ×252. (Atherosclerotic)

FIG. 11–9. Temporal arteritis. **A.** Temporal artery shows vasculitis involving all coats. **B.** Special stain shows fragmentation of internal elastic lamina (*arrows*). **A,** H&E, ×40; **B,** elastica, ×40.

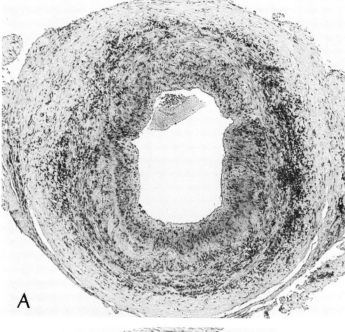

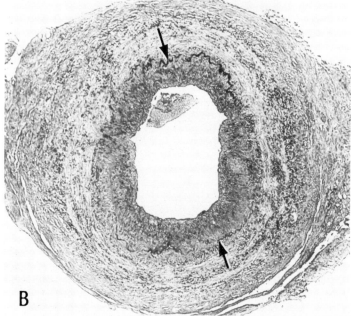

6) Histologically a granulomatous reaction centering about a fragmented internal elastic lamina and spreading into the media and adventitia of the temporal artery is characteristic.

Giant cells frequently are present but may be absent. Occasionally a chronic nongranulomatous reaction with lymphocytes and plasma cells without epithelioid or giant cells is seen. The inflammatory reaction tends to be spotty so that microscopic sections cut at many levels may have to be done; thus a positive finding is more significant than a negative one.

d. Central retinal artery occlusion
The many causes include atherosclerosis, emboli, temporal arteritis, collagen diseases, endarteritis and homocystinuria.
e. Collagen diseases, Wegener's granulomatosis, hypersensitivity angiitis, thromboangiitis obliterans (Buerger's disease) and midline lethal granuloma all may involve the larger retinal vessels and cause retinal ischemia.
2. Arteriolar and capillary disease of retinal vasculature
   a. *Arteriolarsclerosis* is invariably associated with hypertension and is characterized by a diffuse infiltration of the media of arterioles by lipids with late hyalinization.
   b. Branch retinal artery occlusion
The many causes include emboli (Fig. 11–10), arteriolarsclerosis, diabetes mellitus, arteritis, dysproteinemias, collagen diseases and malignant hypertension.
   c. Diabetes mellitus—see Chapter 15.
   d. Malignant hypertension (Fig. 11–11), toxemia of pregnancy, hemoglobinopathies, collagen diseases (Fig. 11–12), dysproteinemias, carbon monoxide

poisoning and blood dyscrasias of many kinds may involve the small retinal vessels and cause retinal ischemia.
II. Complications (Fig. 11–13)
   A. If localized, field defects may result.
   B. If massive, complete loss of vision may occur.
   C. Neovascular glaucoma may occur in 2 percent of eyes following central retinal artery occlusion; it is most rare after branch retinal artery occlusion.
III. Histology of retinal ischemia
   A. Early (Figs. 11–12, 11–14 and 11–15)
      1. The retina shows coagulative necrosis of its inner layers, which are supplied by the retinal arterioles. The neuronal cells rapidly become edematous during the first few hours after occlusion of the artery. The intracellular swelling accounts for the gray retinal opacity noted clinically.
      2. If the area of coagulative necrosis (see p. 24 in Chap. 1) is small and localized, it appears clinically as a *cotton-wool spot.*

The cotton-wool spot observed clinically is a result of a microinfarct of the nerve fiber layer of the retina. The cytoid body, which is observed microscopically, is a swollen, interrupted axon in the retinal nerve fiber layer. The swollen end-bulb resembles superficially a cell, hence the term cytoid body. A collection of many cytoid bodies, along with the localized edema, marks the area of the microinfarct or cotton-wool spot.

      3. If the area of coagulative necrosis is more extensive, it appears clinically as a gray retinal area, blotting out the background choroidal pattern.

The clinically seen gray area is due to marked edema of the inner half of the retina. With complete coagulative necrosis of the posterior pole, e.g., after a central retinal artery occlusion, the red choroid shows through the fovea as a *cherry red spot.* The foveal retina has no inner layers and is supplied from the choriocapillaris; therefore, there is no edema or necrosis in the fovea (anatomic foveola).

B. Late (Fig. 11–13)
  1. The outer half of the retina is well preserved.
  2. The inner half of the retina becomes "homogenized" into a diffuse, relatively acellular zone.

Because the glial cells die along with the other retinal elements, gliosis does not occur. Generally, thick-walled retinal blood vessels are present. The boundaries between the different retinal layers in the inner half of the retina become obliterated. In central retinal artery occlusion the inner retinal layers become an indistinguishable homogenized zone. However, in retinal atrophy secondary to glaucoma, to transection of the optic nerve or to descending optic atrophy, the retinal layers, although atrophic, generally are identifiable.

RETINAL HEMORRHAGIC INFARCTION
(Figs. 11–16 and 11–17)

I. Central retinal vein or branch retinal vein or venular occlusion
  A. The many causes include chronic primary open angle glaucoma, atherosclerosis of the central retinal artery, arteriolarsclerosis of the retinal arte-

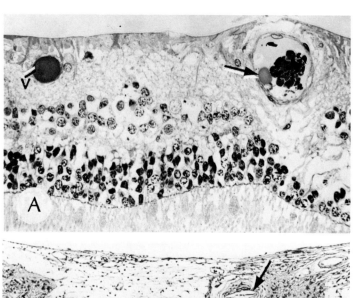

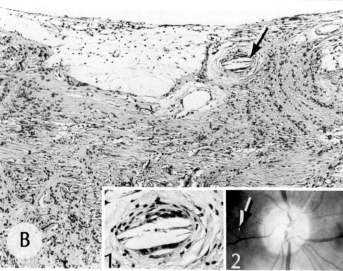

FIG. 11–10. Emboli. **A.** Retinal vessel on left (*v*) is occluded by osmophilic fat globule. Smaller fat globule (*arrow*) is seen in vessel on right. Retinal arteriole fat emboli followed closed-chest cardiac massage. **B.** Cholesterol embolus in retinal artery (*arrow*). **Inset 1** shows higher magnification of embolus. **Inset 2** shows clinical appearance of cholesterol embolus (*arrow*) in same eye prior to enucleation. Multiple cholesterol emboli (Hollenhorst plaques) were present in fundus of 67-year-old man with carotid artery stenosis. **A,** PD ×300; **B,** H&E ×40; **inset 1,** H&E ×101; **inset 2,** clinical.

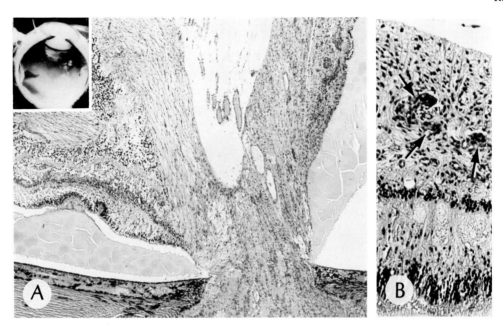

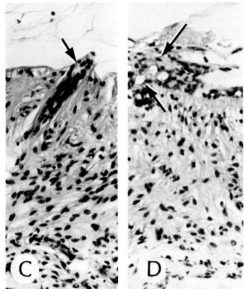

FIG. 11–11. Malignant hypertension in 18-year-old black man with hereditary interstitial nephritis. **A.** Retina detached, disorganized with neovascularization into vitreous. **Inset** shows macroscopic appearance. **B** shows intraretinal neovascularization (*arrows*). **C.** New vessels are leaving retina (*arrow*) to enter subvitreal space. **D.** Neovascularization is budding out of retina (*arrows*) into subvitreal space. **A,** H&E, ×16; **inset,** macroscopic; **B,** H&E, ×69; **C,** H&E, ×101; **D,** H&E, ×101.

rioles, diabetes mellitus, polycythemia vera, mediastinal syndrome with increased venous pressure, dysproteinemias and collagen diseases.

    B. In central retinal vein occlusion 8 to 20 percent occur in patients who already have or will develop chronic primary open angle glaucoma.

  II. Complications

    A. A hemorrhagic infarction of the macular area may result in a permanent loss of vision.

    B. Rubeosis iridis

      1. Rubeosis iridis occurs mainly with central retinal vein occlusion; it occurs much less frequently with a branch vein or venular occlusion.

      2. It follows central retinal vein occlusion in 20 to 30 percent of patients over 40 years of age; generally it does not appear before 6 weeks following occlusion, usually is established before 6 months and causes neovascular glaucoma.

      3. It is rare in people who are under 40 years of age at the time of their central retinal vein occlusion.

    C. Retinal neovascularization and retinitis proliferans also can occur.

  III. Histology of retinal hemorrhagic infarction (Figs. 11–16 and 11–17)

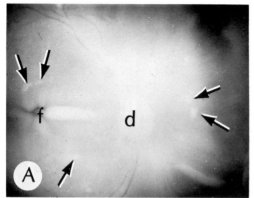

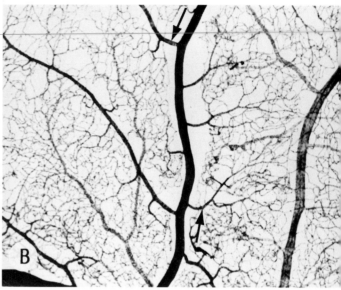

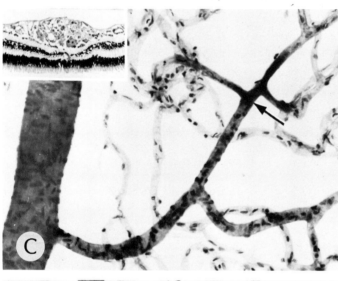

FIG. 11–12. Fatal systemic lupus erythematous in 26-year-old black woman. **A.** Macroscopic appearance of posterior aspect of globe showing cotton-wool spots (*arrows*). *d,* optic disc; *f,* fovea. **B.** Trypsin-digested preparation of retina. Areas at *arrows* shown in higher magnification in C and D. **C.** Area where arteriole becomes capillary (*arrow*) shows fibrinoid necrosis. **Inset** shows cytoid bodies in nerve fiber layer of retina in other eye. **D.** Smallest arteriole (*arrow*) shows fibrinoid necrosis. **Inset** shows cytoid bodies in nerve fiber layer of retina in other eye. **A,** macroscopic. **B,** PAS—H&E, ×16. **C,** PAS—H&E, ×101; inset, H&E, ×28. **D,** PAS—H&E, ×101; inset, PAS, ×28.

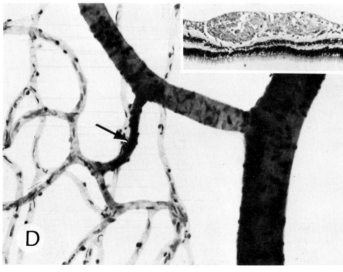

FIG. 11–14. Retinal ischemia, early changes. **A.** Microinfarct of nerve fiber layer (*nfl*) produces aggregates of ruptured and enlarged axons (cytoid bodies). Collection of cytoid bodies is observed clinically as cotton-wool spot lying just deep to internal limiting membrane (*arrow*). **B.** Axon (*Ax*) is enlarged grossly at its ruptured end. Presence of eosinophilic mass within enlarged axon (*arrow*) superficially resembles nucleus within cell, hence term cytoid. **C.** Electron micrograph of cytoid body. Nucleoid consists of dense mass of filamentous material, edge of which can be observed in more detail in enlarged **inset. A,** 1.5 μ section, PD, ×100; **B,** 1.5 μ section, PD, ×675; **C,** ×9,000; **inset,** ×20,000.

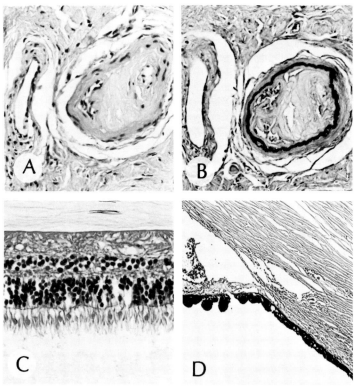

FIG. 11–13. Central retinal artery occlusion.
A. Occluded artery shows recanalization. **B.** Special stain demonstrates internal elastic lamina identifying vessel as artery. **C.** Retina shows homogeneous, diffuse, acellular zone. **D.** Rubeosis iridis developed following occlusion. **A,** H&E, ×101; **B,** elastica, ×101; **C,** H&E, ×136; **D,** H&E, ×40.

int. el. lamina = is artery

Arteriole
① No int. elastic lamina
② loss of continuity of muscle coat

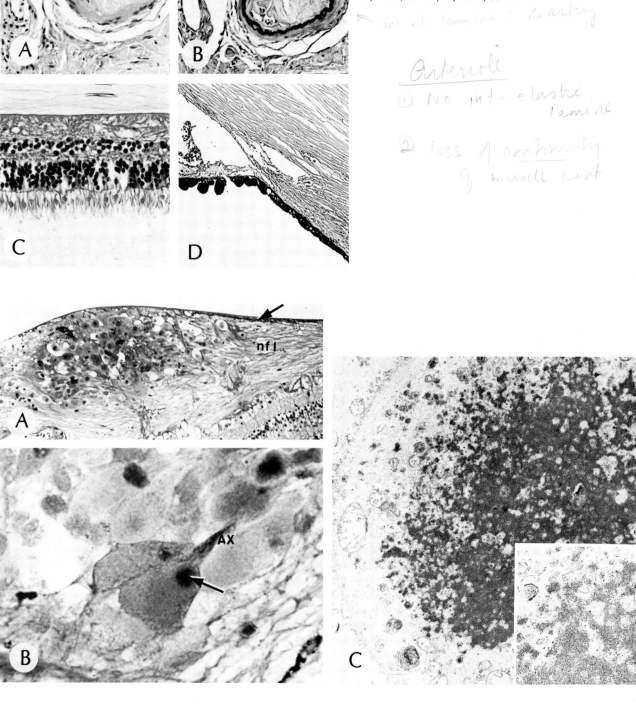

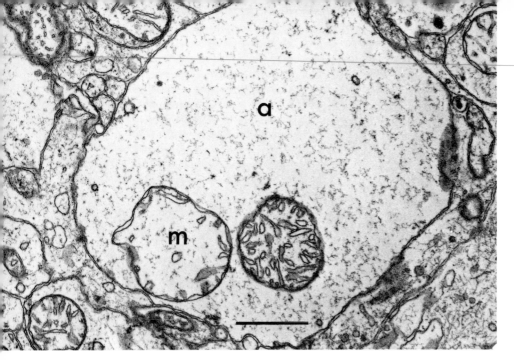

FIG. 11–15. Marked swelling of axon (a) in nerve fiber layer 2 hours after experimental central retinal artery occlusion. *m*, axonal mitochondrion. ×20,000.

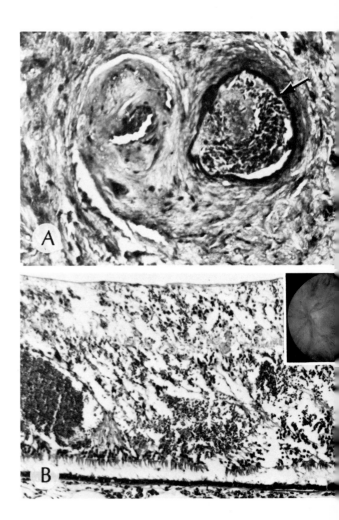

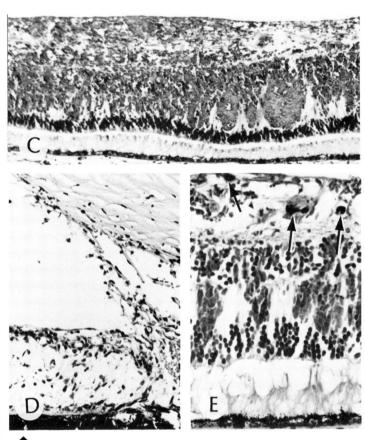

▲
◀ **FIG. 11–16.** Retinal hemorrhagic infarction.
A. Central retinal vein occluded and
recanalized. Artery identified by internal
elastic lamina (*arrow*). **B.** Hemorrhagic
infarction causing disorganization of retina
in individual with polycythemia vera and
central retinal vein occlusion. **Inset** shows
fundus following central retinal vein
occlusion in otherwise healthy 18-year-old
white girl; no cause for occlusion was found.
C. Sheets of blood in inner retinal layers
produce characteristic fundus appearance.
Note preservation of photoreceptors. **D.**
Rubeosis iridis is present in same patient
with polycythemia vera. **E.** Pigment (*arrows*)
is hemosiderin in long-standing occlusion.
A, elastica, ×136; **B,** H&E, ×69; **inset,**
fundus; **C,** H&E, ×69; **D,** H&E, ×101; **E,**
Prussian blue, ×176.

FIG. 11–17. Hemorrhage within nerve fiber
layer (*arrow*) tends to "track" along nerve
fibers producing flame-shaped hemorrhage
observed clinically. Accumulation of blood
in potential space between internal limiting
membrane (*ilm*) and nerve fiber layer
produces submembranous intraretinal
hemorrhage, which is generally restrained
from entering vitreous compartment by
strength of overlying thick basement
membrane (*ilm*). Pockets of blood accumulating within bipolar cell layer or between
Henle fibers (photoreceptor axons) of
extramacular outer plexiform layer produce
dot and blot hemorrhages seen clinically.
H&E, ×115.

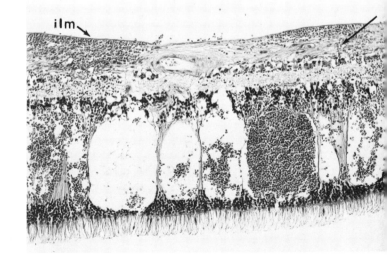

A. Early
1. There is a hemorrhagic necrosis of the retina with massive intraretinal hemorrhage involving all the retinal layers.

The hemorrhage frequently spreads within the nerve fiber layer of the retina appearing clinically in sheets or as "flame shaped." Rarely the hemorrhage will spread into the potential submembranous (between the internal limiting membrane and the nerve fiber layer) space and appear clinically as anteriorly placed retinal pockets of blood ("subhyaloid" hemorrhage).

2. Cytoid bodies are common histologically but may be masked by the hemorrhages clinically.
3. As the hemorrhages resorb, hard waxy exudates may appear (see p. 574 in Chap. 15 and p. 405 in this chapter).
4. Papilledema generally accompanies the hemorrhagic necrosis of the retina in the acute phase.
B. Late (Fig. 11–16)
1. The architectural pattern of the retina is disrupted frequently, especially the inner retinal layers.
2. Gliosis generally is present in the inner retinal layers.
3. Hemosiderosis of the retina (see p. 158 in Chap. 5) is present with the hemosiderin located mainly within macrophages.
4. Thick-walled retinal blood vessels generally are seen.
5. Neovascularization

HYPERTENSIVE AND ARTERIOLARSCLEROTIC RETINOPATHY

I. It is easier to understand the underlying histopathology if the hypertensive and arteriolarsclerotic retinopathy are graded separately.
II. Hypertensive retinopathy (Fig. 11–18)
A. Grade I consists of a generalized narrowing of the arterioles.
B. Grade II consists of a generalized narrowing of the arterioles plus focal arteriolar spasms.
C. Grade III consists of all the changes present in Grade II plus hemorrhages

and exudates (see pp. 574–578 in Chap. 15).
1. "Flame-shaped" or "splinter" hemorrhages (Figs. 11–16, 11–17 and 15–20) are characteristic and are located in the nerve fiber layer.
2. "Dot" and "blot" hemorrhages (Figs. 11–17 and 15–19) may be seen and are located in the inner nuclear layer with spreading to the outer plexiform layer.
3. "Cotton-wool" spots (Figs. 11–12, 11–14 and 11–18) (see p. 397 in this chapter) characteristically are seen and are due to microinfarction of the nerve fiber layer, which produces aggregates of cytoid bodies, i.e., swollen axons of ganglion cells.

Cotton-wool spots may be seen in many conditions such as collagen dis-

FIG. 11–18. Cotton-wool spots are seen in **inset 1** in grade III hypertensive retinopathy. **Inset 2** shows papilledema in grade IV hypertensive retinopathy. Trypsin-digested preparation of retina from hypertensive patient shows narrowing of arteriole. (*A*). Note arteriolar-venular crossing defect (*arrow*). **Main figure,** PAS—H&E, ×28; **inset 1,** fundus; **inset 2,** fundus.

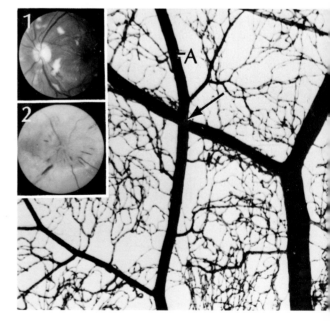

eases, central retinal vein occlusion, blood dyscrasias and multiple myeloma.

4. *"Hard" or "waxy" exudates* may be seen and are lipophilic exudates located in the outer plexiform layer (Figs. 11–19 and 15–15, 15–16 and 15–17).

When the exudates are numerous in the macula and lie within the obliquely oriented and radially arranged fiber layer of Henle, they appear as a *"macular star."*

D. Grade IV consists of all the changes present in Grade III plus papilledema (see pp. 489–490 in Chap. 13).

With malignant hypertension necrosis, thinning, clumping and proliferation of the retinal pigment epithelium may occur as a result of obliterative changes in the choriocapillaris. Four types of fundus lesions associated with choroidal vascular changes have been recognized clinically: 1) pale yellow or reddish patches bordered to a varying extent by pigment deposits; 2) black isolated spot of pigment with a surrounding yellow or red halo (*Elschnig's spot*); 3) chains of pigment flecks arranged linearly along the course of a yellow-white sclerosed choroidal vessel (*Siegrist's spots*); and 4) yellow or red patches of chorioretinal atrophy.

III. Arteriolarsclerotic retinopathy (Figs. 11–20 through 11–22)

A. Grade I consists of an increase in the arteriolar light reflex.

A subintimal hyalin deposition and a thickened arteriolar media and adventitia causes the normally transparent arteriolar wall to become semiopaque with an increased light reflex.

B. Grade II consists of an increased arteriolar light reflex plus arteriolar-venular crossing defects.

The semiopaque wall of the arteriolarsclerotic arteriole, which shares a common adventitia with the venule where they cross, obscures the view of the underlying venule. This results in the clinically seen arteriolar-venular (A-V) crossing defects or "nicking."

C. Grade III consists of all the changes present in Grade II plus *"copper-wire"* arterioles.

The arteriolar wall becomes sufficiently opaque so that the blood column can be seen only by looking perpendicularly through the surface of the wall, i.e., looking through the thinnest area. The arteriole has a burnished or "copper" appearance due to reflection of light from the thickened and partially opacified arteriolar wall.

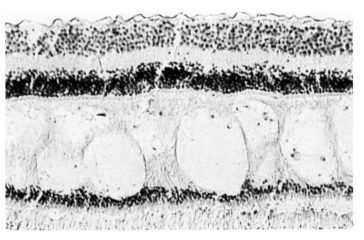

FIG. 11–19. Cystoid spaces in outer plexiform layers are filled with eosinophilic coagulum. Clinically these appear as hard or waxy exudates. Patient had renal-induced hypertension. H&E, ×69.

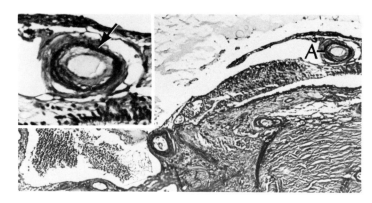

FIG. 11–20. Subintimal hyalin deposition in artery (*A*) is shown at higher magnification in **inset.** Internal elastic lamina of artery (*arrow*) is seen easily. **Main figure,** PAS, ×40; **inset,** PAS, ×101.

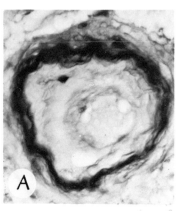

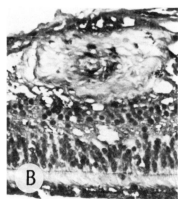

Atherosclerosis   arteriolarsclerosis

FIG. 11–21. Thickened retinal artery in **A** is identified by internal elastic lamina; it shows atherosclerosis. Thickened retinal vessel in **B** has no internal elastic lamina and is arteriole showing arteriolarsclerosis. **A,** PAS, ×252; **B,** PAS, ×101.

FIG. 11–22. Arteriole (*arrow*) is completely obliterated. Cystic space at right is microaneurysm; patient had hypertension and diabetes mellitus. PAS, ×252.

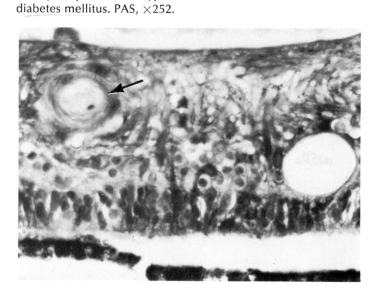

D. Grade IV consists of all the changes present in Grade II plus *"silver-wire"* arterioles.

The wall becomes completely opaque so that the blood column in its lumen cannot be seen. The light then is reflected completely from the surface of the thickened vessel giving a white or "silver" appearance. The lumen of the arteriole then may or may not be patent. The patency can be determined best by fluorescein angiography.

HEMORRHAGIC RETINOPATHY (Fig. 11–23)

I. Retinal hemorrhages may be caused by many diseases such as diabetes mellitus (see Chap. 15), sickle cell disease (see pp. 407–409 in this chapter), retinal venous diseases (see pp. 398–404 in this chapter), hypertension, blood dyscrasias, leukemias, polycythemia vera, subacute bacterial endocarditis, lymphomas, idiopathic thrombocytopenia, trauma, multiple myeloma, pernicious anemia, collagen diseases, carcinomatosis, anemia and many others.

Anemia alone or thrombocytopenia alone rarely causes retinal hemorrhages. The combination of anemia and thrombocytopenia, however, not infrequently results in retinal hemorrhages; and when the two are severe (hemoglobin less than 8 g/100 ml and platelets less than 100,000/mm³), retinal hemorrhages may occur in 70 percent of patients.

II. Histologically the size and morphologic location of the hemorrhage determine its clinical appearance (see p. 404 in this chapter and p. 578 in Chap. 15).

EXUDATIVE RETINOPATHY (Figs. 11–19 and 15–15, 15–16 and 15–17)

I. Retinal exudates may be caused by the same things that cause hemorrhagic retinopathy: the so-called hard, waxy exudates may occur simultaneously with the hemorrhages, alone or as a result of the hemorrhage as the hemorrhage resorbs; the cotton-wool exudate ("cytoid bodies") generally is found in ischemic retinal conditions and represents a microinfarct of the innermost retinal layers.

II. Circinate retinopathy consists of masses of hard, waxy exudate deposited in a circular fashion around a clear area, which often is the foveal area.
   A. It is a degeneration secondary to ischemic vascular disease due to many causes, e.g., diabetes mellitus and hypertension.
   B. Histologically the exudates are identical to isolated, smaller, hard, waxy exudates.
III. Histology
   A. Hard, waxy exudates—see p. 574 in Chapter 15.
   B. Cotton-wool exudates ("cytoid bodies")—see p. 397 in this chapter and p. 574 in Chapter 15.

DIABETES MELLITUS

See Chapter 15.

COATS'S DISEASE AND LEBER'S MILIARY ANEURYSMS

See p. 699 in Chapter 18.

RETINAL ARTERIAL AND ARTERIOLAR MACROANEURYSMS (Fig. 11–24)

I. Macroaneurysms of the retinal arteries and arterioles may occur congenitally or in association with angiomatosis retinae and the diseases of Eales, Leber and Coats; or they may develop in elderly individuals.
II. Histologically, spherical to fusiform aneurysmal dilatations of the arterial or arteriolar walls are seen.

SICKLE CELL DISEASE (Fig. 11–25)

I. The retinopathy is most severe with sickle cell hemoglobin C disease (SC disease) but may also occur in other sickle hemoglobinopathies including sickle thalassemia (Sthal), sickle cell disease (SS) and even in occasional cases of sickle cell trait (SA).
II. Classification of proliferative sickle retinopathy
   A. Stage I: peripheral arteriolar occlusion (generally between the equator and the ora serrata).
   B. Stage II: peripheral arteriolar-venular

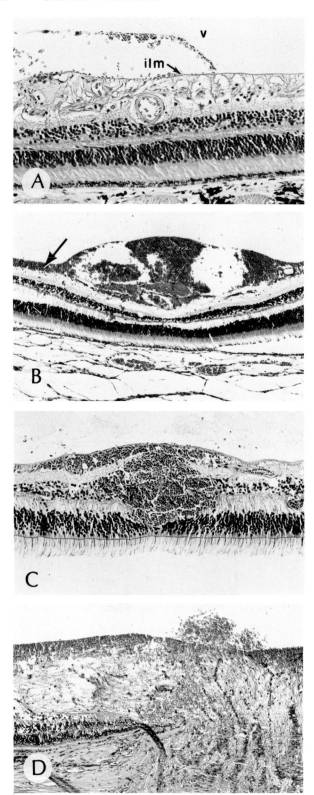

FIG. 11–23. Hemorrhagic retinopathy. **A.** Hemorrhage separating vitreous body (*v*) from internal limiting membrane of retina (*ilm*) is "true" subhyaloid hemorrhage. **B.** Massive accumulation of blood in potential cleft (*arrow*) between internal limiting membrane and nerve fiber layer is submembranous intraretinal hemorrhage. Such hemorrhages may appear with "fluid level" clinically where they are somewhat inaccurately called subhyaloid hemorrhages. **C.** Large submembranous (intraretinal) hemorrhage may extend throughout other layers of retina as here and even rupture through external limiting membrane to gain access to subretinal space. **D.** Hemorrhages may be restrained from entering vitreous compartment by internal limiting membrane of retina (as on left), but this restraint diminishes rapidly whenever thick basement membrane becomes thin (as over optic nerve head on right). **A,** H&E, ×130; **B,** H&E, ×70; **C,** H&E, ×115; **D,** H&E, ×80.

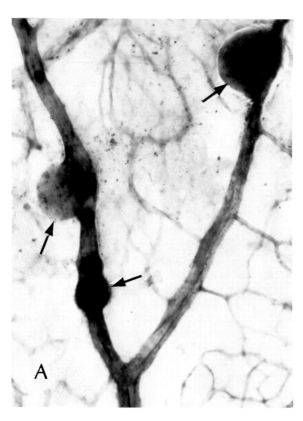

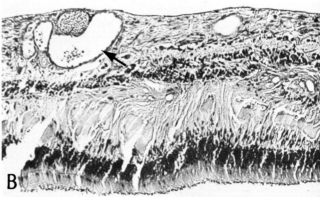

FIG. 11–24. Retinal arteriolar macroanurysms are shown in trypsin-digested preparation in **A** (*arrows*) and in cross-section in **B** (*arrow*). **A,** PAS, ×75; **B,** H&E, ×69.

anastomoses (most commonly in the temporal quadrant).

C. Stage III: neovascular and fibrous proliferations.

In this stage there is fluorescein leakage in many areas of the retina. The new vessels arise from preexisting arteriolar venular anastomoses. When a neovascular patch remains relatively isolated from neighboring patches and coalescence does not occur, the characteristic *sea-fan* anomaly may be observed, most commonly in SC disease. Areas of retinal pigment epithelial hyperplasia ("*sunbursts*") may be seen most commonly in SS disease but also in SC disease.

D. Stage IV: vitreous hemorrhage (generally arising from a neovascular patch).

E. Stage V: retinal detachment (the ultimate and most severe stage).

III. The pathogenesis of sickle cell retinopathy is unknown but probably is related to local hypoxia in a fashion similar to that believed to occur in diabetes mellitus, retrolental fibroplasia, carotid occlusive disease and Takayasu's disease.   → macrophagic arteriolitis.

EALES'S DISEASE (Primary Perivasculitis of the Retina)

I. Eales's disease occurs typically in young men, generally in their third decade.
II. Over 90 percent of the cases are bilateral.
III. The disease tends to progress slowly with rapid progression common as a late event.

Initially there is a slight localized edema of the peripheral retina involving only the small venous branches. Exudates around the involved vessels or sheathing of the vessels can be seen. Next the larger venules become involved; then neovascularization develops within the retina. New vessels enter the subvitreal space where they are vulnerable to hemorrhage. A fibrous component develops, i.e., retinitis proliferans. With shrinkage and traction by fibrovascular membranes a secondary retinal detachment may occur. The total progression is quite similar to that seen in diabetic retinopathy. Rarely there may be a central form with the large central venules affected primarily. Fluorescein has shown that obliteration of the venules of the periphery of the retina seems to be the initiating event.

IV. The cause of the disease is unknown.

SC : sea fans
SS : RPE molif.

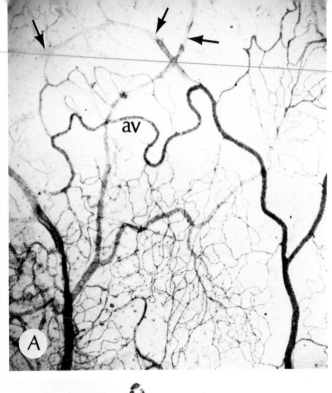

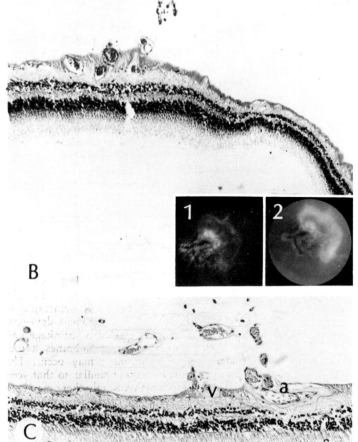

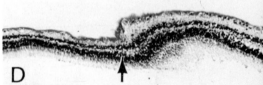

FIG. 11–25. Sickle cell hemoglobin C disease. **A.** Trypsin digestion of retina shows peripheral blood vessels devoid of cells and presumed nonviable (*arrows*), and arteriolar-venular collateral (*av*) in equatorial region. **B.** Neovascular tufts are seen leaving retina and entering vitreous compartment, i.e., sea-fan. Note decrease in thickness and loss of substance in inner retinal layers anterior (to right) of new vessels. **Inset 1** shows photocoagulated sea-fan; **inset 2,** same after fluorescein. **C.** Neovascular tufts of sea-fan can be traced from arteriole (*a*), into vitreous compartment and back into venule (*v*). **D.** Retina anterior (to left) of equator (*arrow*) shows loss of ganglion cells and nerve fiber layer; retina avascular in this area. Note artifactitious fold in retina in region of *arrow*, causing tangential sectioning and apparent thickening of retina. **A,** PAS—H&E, ×25; **B,** H&E, ×75; **inset 1,** fundus; **inset 2,** fundus, fluorescein; **C,** H&E, ×100; **D,** H&E, ×75.

RETROLENTAL FIBROPLASIA

See pp. 698–699 in Chapter 18.

HEMANGIOMA OF THE RETINA

I. Hemangioma of the retina may be associated with similar cavernous hemangiomas of brain as well as with angiomatous hamartomas of skin, or it may occur alone.

II. Histologically a cavernous hemangioma of the retina is seen (see p. 528 in Chap. 14).

HEREDITARY HEMORRHAGIC TELANGIECTASIA
(Rendu-Osler-Weber-Disease)

I. The condition is characterized by multiple dilatations of capillaries and venules in skin, mucous membranes and viscera; the telangiectases tend to bleed wherever they occur. It is inherited as an autosomal dominant.

II. Conjunctival telangiectatic vessels are common.

III. Rarely the retina is involved and the picture can mimic hypertensive or diabetic retinopathy.

INFLAMMATION

NONSPECIFIC RETINAL INFLAMMATIONS

See Chapters 3 and 5.

Secondary retinitis is usually due to a vasculitis (Fig. 11–26).

A. It may be secondary to keratitis, iridocyclitis, choroiditis or scleritis.

B. The condition generally has a perivasculitis around venules with the perivascular infiltrate composed of lymphocytes and plasma cells.

SPECIFIC RETINAL INFLAMMATIONS

See Chapters 2, 3 and 4.

I. A toxic, exudative retinopathy may occur with *carbon monoxide intoxication*.

II. Septic retinitis of Roth (*Roth's spots*) occurs with a bacteremia, especially with subacute bacterial endocarditis.

III. Endogenous mycotic retinitis, e.g., candidiasis and aspergillosis, result from fungus infection (Fig. 11–27).

IV. Viral retinitis, e.g., cytomegalic inclusion disease—see p. 98 in Chapter 4.

V. Acute posterior multifocal placoid pigment epitheliopathy tends to occur in young women and shows multifocal, yellow-white placoid lesions involving predominantly the posterior pole, but occurring anywhere in the fundus.

A. The lesions resolve rapidly but leave permanent pigment epithelial alterations.

B. Presumably the acute process is due to a primary pigment epithelial inflammation, although an acute multifocal choroiditis (choriocapillariitis) cannot be excluded. The histology is unknown.

VI. Acute retinal pigment epitheliitis is characterized by an acute onset with fairly rapid resolution in usually 6 to 12 weeks with involvement mainly of the posterior pole.

A. The acute lesion is a deep, fine, dark gray, sometimes black, spot frequently surrounded by a halo, which may disappear with healing.

B. The cause and histology are unknown.

FIG. 11–26. Retinal vasculitis. Perivascular infiltrate of lymphocytes and plasma cells is secondary to corneal ulcer. H&E, ×101.

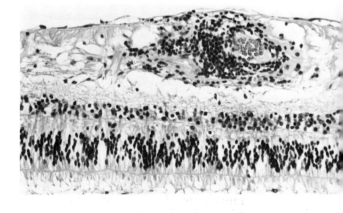

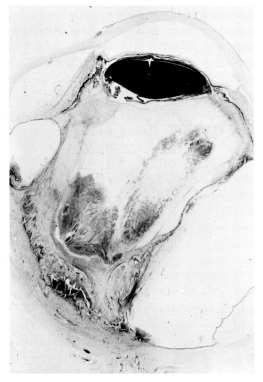

FIG. 11–27. Endogenous intraocular fungus infection. No evidence of infection elsewhere in body could be found. Hyphae considered to be from species of *Aspergillus* were found in microabscesses. Mac Callum gram stain, ×4.

INJURIES

See Chapter 5.

DEGENERATIONS

DEFINITIONS

I. Degenerations are usually unilateral but may be bilateral.
II. They are secondary phenomena, secondary to or a result of previous disease, i.e., ocular "fingerprints" left by prior disease.

MICROCYSTOID DEGENERATION
(Figs. 11–28 through 11–31)

I. Typical microcystoid degeneration (Blessig-Iwanoff cysts; peripheral cystoid degeneration)
  A. Microcystoid degeneration of the retina probably is the most common of all intraocular lesions and appears clinically as a myriad of tiny interconnecting channels in the peripheral retina, especially temporally.
  B. All persons 8 years of age or older

show the lesion, and it may be present at birth with increasing severity of retinal involvement up to the seventh decade of life.
  C. The tendency is toward relatively equal bilateral involvement with the temporal retina involved more than the nasal, the superior sectors affected more than the inferior and relative retinal sparing in the nasal and temporal horizontal meridians (the greatest sparing nasally).
  D. Typical microcystoid degeneration always seems to begin at the ora serrata. From there it extends posteriorly and circumferentially.
  E. Histologically spaces within the neural retina (cysts) are located primarily in the outer plexiform and adjacent nuclear layers.
    1. Early the cysts are limited to the middle layers of the retina. Later they may extend to the external and internal limiting membranes of the retina.
    2. Although they appear empty in H&E-stained sections, generally they contain hyaluronic acid, best seen when stained with special stains. The septa separating the cysts are composed of glial-axonal tissue rich in the cytochrome oxidase enzyme system.
    3. With coalescence of multiple microcysts, an intraretinal macrocyst or *retinoschisis* cavity is formed (see section Degenerative Retinoschisis) when the macrocyst is at least 1.50

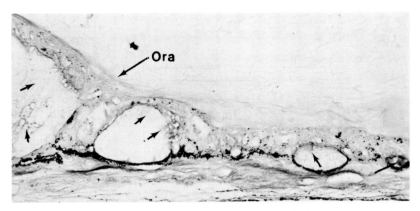

FIG. 11–28. Typical microcystoid degeneration of retina and adjacent cysts of pars plana contain acid mucopolysaccharides (*arrows*) when stained with Hale colloidal iron method. *Ora,* region of ora serrata. AMP, ×50.

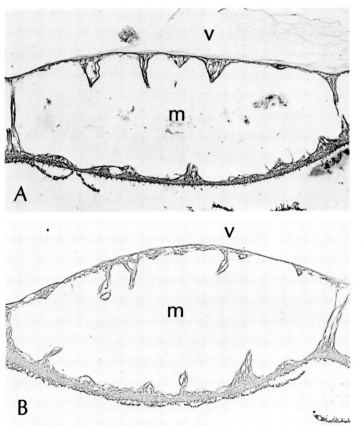

FIG. 11–29. Typical microcystoid degeneration. Both **A** and **B** stained for acid mucopolysaccharides; **B** was digested with hyaluronidase before staining. Note disappearance of positive staining in microcyst (*m*) and in vitreous (*v*). **A,** AMP, ×40; **B,** hyaluronidase—AMP, ×40.

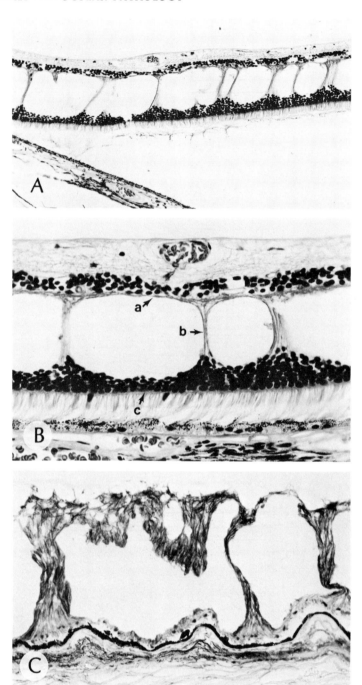

FIG. 11–30. Typical microcystoid degeneration. **A.** Spaces or channels lie initially within outer plexiform layer, i.e., between compressed bundles of photoreceptor axons and remains of Müller glial cells. **B.** Higher magnification shows that middle limiting membrane (a) limits inner boundaries; glial-neuronal columns (b) limit lateral boundaries; and photoreceptor cell bodies (outer nuclear layer) and external limiting membrane (c) limit outer boundaries of microcystoid channels. **C.** Diphosphopyridine nucleotide (DPNH) diaphorase (nitro-blue tetrazolium [BT] method). Glial-neuronal columns show dense precipitate of formazan. **A,** H&E, ×135; **B,** H&E, ×300; **C,** nitro-BT, ×125.

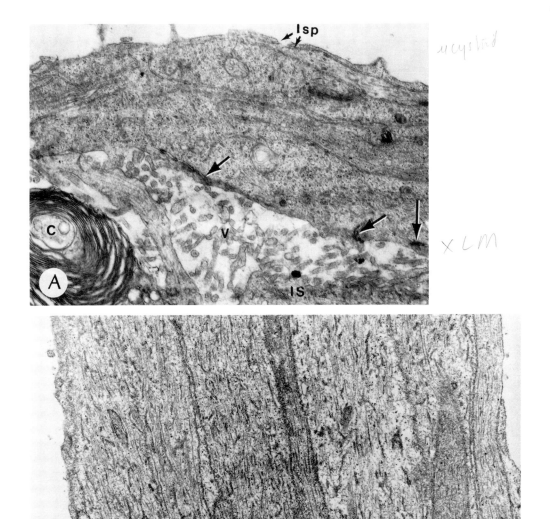

ucystid

↑
int

↓
ext.

× LM

FIG. 11–31. Typical microcystoid degeneration. **A.** Outer attenuated wall of microcystoid degeneration; cystoid space is above. Note continuity of space with adjacent narrow intercellular spaces (*Isp*). Dense attachments forming external limiting membrane are present (*arrows*). Degenerating fragment of cone outer segment (*c*), Müller cell microvilli (*v*) and fragment of photoreceptor inner segment (*IS*) are present external to limiting membrane. **B.** Electron micrograph of column between spaces showing mitochondria in Müller cell cytoplasm. Neuronal processes also present. **A,** ×15,000; **B,** ×10,500.

mm in diameter (one average disc diameter).

Pars plana cysts are intercellular cysts of the nonpigmented layer of ciliary epithelium and may also be filled with hyaluronic acid. They may contain the myeloma protein (IgG type) in *multiple myeloma*. The characteristic milky white appearance of the myeloma cysts on gross examination is an artifact of fixation as they are transparent (clear) clinically.

II. Reticular cystoid degeneration (Fig. 11–32)
   A. Reticular cystoid degeneration appears clinically posterior to microcystoid degeneration. The subsurface retinal vasculature arborizes into fine branches throughout the reticular lesion.
   B. Reticular cystoid degeneration of the retina is seen in about 13 percent of autopsy eyes; it is bilateral about 41 percent of the time.
   C. It can be found in every decade of life and without a clear relationship to aging.
   D. The inferior and superior temporal regions, both involved to about the same extent, are more affected than the inferior and superior nasal regions.

Typical microcystoid degeneration of the retina is always found as an accompanying retinal lesion, most often just anterior to the reticular cystoid degeneration. In some instances the reticular lesion may become partially surrounded by the posterior extension of typical microcystoid degeneration. There are a number of macroscopic features that may distinguish typical microcystoid from reticular cystoid degeneration. The retinal vasculature, when traced from uninvolved retina posteriorly, arborizes into fine branches throughout the reticular lesion; only the larger vessels are apparent in typical microcystoid lesions. In reticular cystoid degeneration the neural retina is less transparent than in typical microcystoid lesions. The lateral and posterior borders of reticular lesions are linear and angular, often coinciding with the course of large retinal arterioles and venules; typical microcystoid lesions usually have a smoothly rounded margin.

E. Histologically the retinal cysts of reticular cystoid degeneration are located primarily in the nerve fiber layer of the retina.
   1. The cysts are located completely within the nerve fiber layer early, but later they may extend from the internal limiting membrane to the inner plexiform layer.
   2. The cysts contain hyaluronic acid.
   3. Similar nerve fiber layer cystic changes can be seen in the retina of *juvenile retinoschisis* in areas adjacent to the retinoschisis cavity.

DEGENERATIVE RETINOSCHISIS

I. Retinoschisis, typical degenerative senile (adult) type* (Fig. 11–33)
   A. Typical degenerative senile retinoschisis is seen in about 4 percent of patients and is bilateral in over 80 percent.
   B. It is rare under the age of 20 years and is much more common beyond the age of 40.
   C. It is found typically in the peripheral inferior temporal quadrant (about 70 percent of cases), with the superior temporal quadrant (about 25 percent) the next most common site; there is little tendency for the retinoschisis to progress posteriorly.

The splitting of retinal tissue in the area of retinoschisis results in an absolute scotoma. Occasionally the retinoschisis involves only the macular area. In most of the macular cases ocular trauma seems to be the initiating factor.

D. The inner layer of schisis has a characteristic beaten metal or pitted appearance and frequently has tiny glistening yellow-white dots.

* Retinoschisis may be defined as an intraretinal tissue loss or splitting at least 1.50 mm in diameter (one average disc diameter). It is differentiated from a retinal cyst by its configuration, i.e., a retinal cyst has about the same diameter in all directions (and usually a narrow neck), whereas the diameter of retinoschisis parallel to the retinal surface is greater than the diameter perpendicular to the surface.

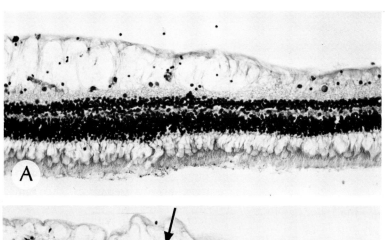

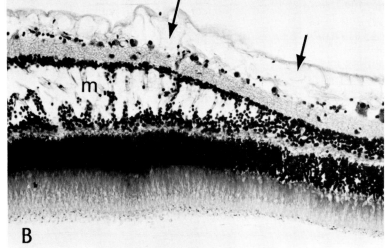

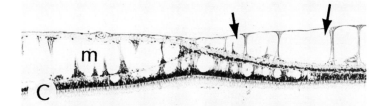

FIG. 11–32. Reticular cystoid degeneration. **A.** Limited to innermost layers of retina. **B** and **C** show reticular cystoid (*arrows*) and typical microcystoid degeneration (*m*) in same regions of retina. **A,** H&E, ×165; **B,** H&E, ×165; **C,** H&E, ×40.

FIG. 11–33. Typical degenerative senile (adult) type of retinoschisis. Rupture of middle limiting membrane and restraining glial-neuronal columns cleaves retina into inner and outer layers, i.e., retinoschisis. H&E, ×80.

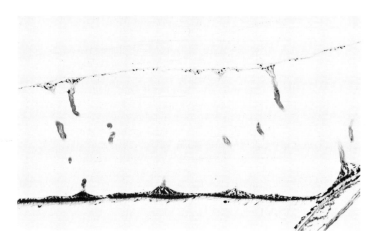

The glistening yellow-white dots have been thought to be reflections from the remnants of ruptured glial septa clinging to the internal limiting membrane of the retina. However, the dots are not found in all cases, and with biomicroscopy they seem to lie internally to the retinal internal limiting membrane. Probably it is the glial remnants that cause an uneven external surface to the inner wall of the schisis cavity that produce the beaten metal appearance.

E. Retinal holes tend to be small and numerous in the inner wall and large and single in the outer wall (just the reverse of juvenile retinoschisis).

F. Histologically there is a splitting in the outer plexiform layers and adjacent nuclear layers, with the cyst filled with a hyaluronidase-sensitive acid mucopolysaccharide, presumably hyaluronic acid.

1. As the area of the retinoschisis extends, much of the involved retina is destroyed (with resultant absolute scotoma).

2. The inner wall in advanced retinoschisis is usually made up of the internal limiting membrane, the inner portions of Müller cells (remnants of ruptured glial septa), remnants of the nerve fiber layer and blood vessels.

3. The outer wall consists mainly of the outer plexiform layer, the outer nuclear layer and the photoreceptors.

4. Bridging the gap between the inner and outer walls are occasional strands or septa composed of compressed and fused remnants of axons, dendrites and Müller cells.

It is tempting to think that the schisis cavity of senile retinoschisis develops from a coalescence of the cysts of microcystoid degeneration. Microcystoid degeneration, however, is present in 100 percent of people over 8 years of age, whereas senile retinoschisis is present in about 4 percent of people. Therefore, if senile retinoschisis does arise from peripheral microcystoid degeneration, it does so only in a small number of cases. The cause of the progression from microcystoid to macrocystoid (i.e., schisis) is unknown but may be genetically determined.

II. Retinoschisis, reticular degenerative (adult) type
   A. Reticular retinoschisis is found in about 2 percent of autopsy cases and is bilateral about 16 percent of the time. A band of typical microcystoid degeneration always separates the schisis from the ora serrata. It may occur concomitant with typical degenerative retinoschisis.
   B. It is rare before the fourth decade and is most common after the fifth decade.
   C. There is a predilection for the inferior temporal quadrant.
   D. Round or ovoid holes may be present in the outer wall but rarely in the inner wall.
   E. Histologically the inner wall of the schisis is composed of the retinal internal limiting membrane and minimal remnants of the nerve fiber layer. The outer wall is made up of receptors and outer nuclear and plexiform layers.

SECONDARY RETINOSCHISIS (Figs. 11–34 and 11–35)

I. Microcystoid degeneration and retinoschisis have been found in a variety of pathologic conditions such as long-standing retinal detachment, choroidal tumors (especially malignant melanomas, hemangiomas and metastatic carcinomas), retrolental fibroplasia, Coats's disease, retinal angiomatosis, diabetic retinopathy, uveitis, parasitic disease and aplastic anemia.

II. Histologically secondary microcystoid degeneration and retinoschisis are quite similar to the primary type, except that the cystoid spaces in the secondary form in most instances do not contain an acid mucopolysaccharide.

Retinoschisis that is secondary to trauma in infants may have a cleavage plane much more internal in the retina than in the typical senile type or the usual secondary type. This internal cleavage plane resembles the area of involvement in reticular retinoschisis and in hereditary juvenile retinoschisis.

FIG. 11–34. Secondary microcystoid degeneration and retinoschisis. **A.** Typical microcystoid degeneration occurring in Henle fiber (outer plexiform) and bipolar cell layers of posterior retina overlying choroidal hemangioma. **B** and **C.** Microcystoid and macrocystoid (retinoschisis) degeneration of macular area of retina secondary to long-standing exudative diabetic retinopathy. Note hole in inner wall of retinoschisis. **A,** H&E, ×50; **B,** H&E, ×40; **C,** H&E, ×40.

OPL

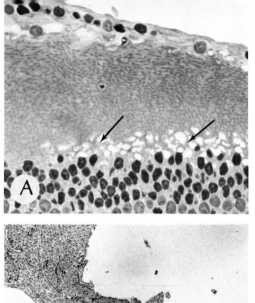

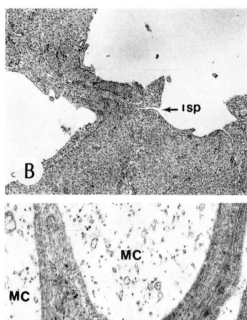

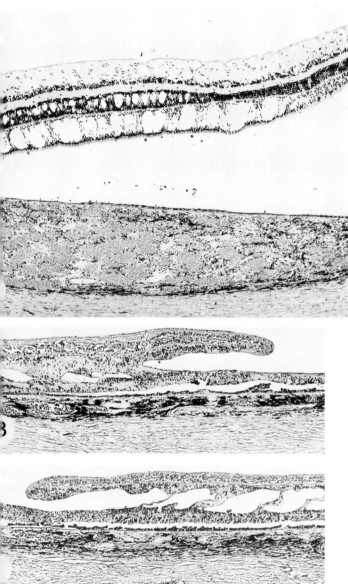

FIG. 11–35. Secondary microcystoid degeneration. **A.** Early macular microcystoid degeneration (*arrows*) produced 1 week following mild argon laser injury to foveal region. Edge of microcystoid changes can be seen tapering off to left. **B.** Separation of neuronal cells by watery spaces produces some of microcystoid spaces seen in **A.** *isp,* intercellular space. **C.** Swelling (edema) of Müller cells (*MC*) accounts for some of lucent spaces in *early* cystoid degeneration in macula. Rhesus monkey. **A,** toluidine blue, ×485; **B,** ×19,200; **C,** ×21,900.

PAVING STONE (COBBLESTONE) DEGENERATION
(Peripheral Chorioretinal Atrophy; Equatorial Choroiditis) (Fig. 11–36)

I. The lesions of paving stone degeneration tend to increase in incidence and in size with age and are present in about 25 percent of autopsy cases, bilateral in about 38 percent.

II. The lesions are located primarily between the ora serrata and equator and separated from the ora serrata by normal retina.

   A. The lesions are nonelevated, sharply demarcated, yellow-white in color, single or multiple and separate or confluent.

   B. Prominent choroidal vessels frequently may be seen at the base of the lesions.

   C. They are most frequent in the inferior temporal quadrant (about 78 percent) with the inferior nasal quadrant the next most frequent site (about 57 percent). The lesions often coalesce and extend in a band with scalloped borders, from temporal to nasal areas in the inferior retina.

III. Histologically the lesions are characterized by

   A. Retinal thinning in an area devoid of pigment epithelium.

   B. An intact Bruch's membrane with the sensory retina closely applied to it.

   With artifactitious detachment of the neural retina (e.g., following fixation) the neural retina in the area of the paving stone degeneration remains attached. Paving stone degeneration, therefore, probably is not a predisposing factor toward retinal detachment and may actually protect against retinal detachment.

   C. An absent choriocapillaris (especially at the center of the lesion) or a partially obliterated choriocapillaris or sometimes only minimal abnormalities such as thickening of the walls of the choriocapillaris; the choroid is otherwise normal.

   D. Hypertrophy and hyperplasia of the pigment epithelium at the margin of the lesion.

DRUSEN

See p. 638 in Chapter 17.

PERIPHERAL RETINAL ALBINOTIC SPOTS

I. Areas of hypopigmentation in the retinal periphery (or in the posterior pole) are due to depigmentation of the retinal pigment epithelium.

II. Although the lesions probably are degenerative, a congenital cause cannot be ruled out.

MYOPIC RETINOPATHY (Fig. 11–37)

I. Myopia of a small or moderate degree generally is not associated with retinal degenerative changes.

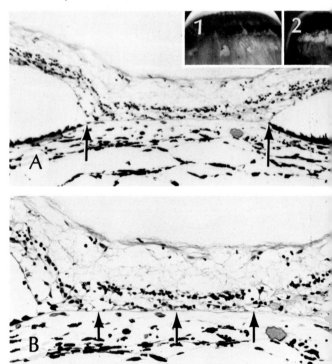

FIG. 11–36. Paving stone degeneration. **A.** RPE ends abruptly in area of degeneration (between *arrows*). **Insets 1** and **2** show typical circumferential lesions of paving stone degeneration. **B.** Higher magnification of **A.** In area of RPE disappearance Bruch's membrane (*arrows*) is intact, but overlying retina (especially outer layers) and underlying choroid show degenerative changes. **A,** H&E, ×69; **inset 1,** macroscopic; **inset 2,** macroscopic; **B,** H&E, ×101.

outer hole in Typ. R.S.
inner " in R. R.S.

II. Progressive or "high" myopia (generally greater than six diopters of myopia) affects the retina most severely in the posterior pole and in the periphery.
   A. The globe is enlarged mainly in its posterior third with thinning of the sclera.
   B. Surrounding the optic disc and extending temporally to involve the posterior pole and sometimes even the equator, the thinned sclera bulges posteriorly forming a *staphyloma*, which is lined by a thin and atrophic choroid.
   C. Bruch's membrane may develop small breaks (*lacquer cracks*) through which connective tissue grows beneath the retina pigment epithelium.

   The breaks in Bruch's membrane in the macular region may lead to a small hemorrhage, which later organizes and becomes pigmented. This may appear clinically as a small, dark, macular lesion, which is sometimes known as *Fuchs's spot* (actually a "mini" disciform degeneration of the macula).

   D. The overlying retina in the posterior pole thins with degeneration affecting mainly the outer layers.
   E. The peripheral retina also becomes thin and atrophic and, therefore, more susceptible to retinal tears.

MACULAR DEGENERATION (See Footnote on p. 391)

I. Senile macular degeneration (Fig. 11–38)
   A. Senile macular degeneration is characterized clinically by a gradual reduction of central vision without apparent cause or inheritance pattern.
   B. Clinically the retinal damage is limited to the foveomacular area where pigment disturbances or retinal cystic degeneration or both are seen.
   C. The changes usually are bilateral and found in people over 50 years of age.
   D. Histologically the following changes may be seen:
      1. Choriocapillaris may be partially or completely obliterated.
      2. Bruch's membrane may be thickened and may show basophilic changes.

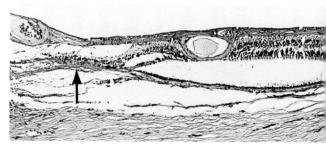

FIG. 11–37. Myopic retinopathy. Retina posteriorly near optic disc is stretched and thin. RPE and outer retinal layers are degenerated (*arrow*). H&E, ×40.

lovely !!!

   3. The pigment epithelium may show atrophy with depigmentation, hypertrophy or even hyperplasia.
   4. The sensory retina may frequently show microcystoid degeneration or even macrocystoid (retinoschisis) degeneration.

   Hole formation may occur in the inner wall of the macrocyst, or rarely total hole formation may occur leaving the macular retinal ends with rounded, smooth edges.

II. Idiopathic central serous choroidopathy (central serous retinopathy; central angiospastic retinopathy) (Figs. 11–39 through 11–41)
   A. Typically, idiopathic central serous choroidopathy occurs in healthy young adults between the ages of 20 and 40 years, most commonly in men.
   B. The symptoms are those of metamorphopsia, positive scotoma and micropsia. They frequently occur following an emotionally stressful event.
   C. The condition recurs in about one-fourth to one-third of patients and occasionally may develop in the other eye.
   D. Types of clinicopathologic entities:
      1. A tiny detachment of the retinal pigment epithelium (RPE) with

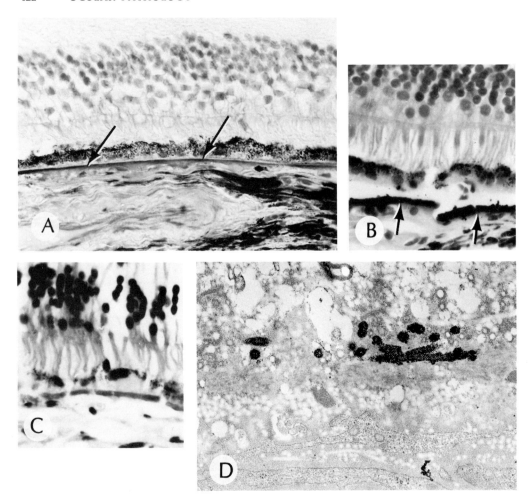

FIG. 11–38. Senile macular degeneration. **A.** Basophilia of region of Bruch's membrane (*arrows*) is common senile change. Note partial obliteration of choriocapillaris. Such aging changes may be precursors to some senile degenerations in macular region. **B** and **C** demonstrate fragility of basophilic Bruch's membrane, which shows numerous cracks. **B** shows positive result (*arrows*) with special stain to demonstrate calcium. **D.** Electron micrograph shows dark areas representing calcification in region of Bruch's membrane. **A,** H&E, ×395; **B,** von Kossa, ×252; **C,** H&E, ×252; **D,** ×20,000.

serous fluid in the sub-RPE space is the simplest form.

    a. The overlying neural retina (NR) is closely applied to the detached RPE.

    b. Fluorescein study shows a tiny bright dot marking the site of the detached RPE.

2. A localized detachment of the NR may be associated with the tiny detachment of the RPE.

    a. Serous fluid is present in the sub-NR space.

    b. If the RPE is intact in the area of the RPE detachment, fluorescein study shows the same as in simple RPE detachment.

    c. If the RPE is not intact, fluorescein study shows fluorescein slowly filling the entire sub-NR space.

3. A large detachment of the RPE is rarer than the above two entities and carries a worse prognosis.

    a. There is an increased chance of hemorrhage with subsequent development of *disciform degeneration of the macula*.

    b. There may or may not be an associated NR detachment, and fluorescein study shows the same results as with a tiny RPE detachment with or without a NR detachment.

E. The basic defect appears to be in Bruch's membrane or the choriocapillaris, or both, but the underlying cause is unknown.

F. Most cases heal spontaneously with restoration of normal vision.

Sometimes the course is prolonged, and irreversible changes in the RPE and NR may result. Such changes may also result from recurrent attacks. If a hemorrhage occurs, however, the condition can be complicated by scarring or disciform degeneration of the macula with a poor visual prognosis. Idiopathic central serous choroidopathy can be simulated by secondary *central serous retinopathy*, secondary to such conditions as a peripheral choroidal malignant melanoma, choroidal hemangioma or pars planitis. Although idiopathic central serous choroidopathy typically involves the posterior pole, it can occur in any part of the posterior half of the eye including regions nasal to the optic disc.

III. Senile disciform macular degeneration (Kuhnt-Junius macular degeneration (Figs. 11–42 through 11–45)

A. Typically, senile disciform macular degeneration occurs in individuals 60 years of age or older. There is no sex predilection, the degeneration is often bilateral, and there is evidence of senile choroidal degeneration in both eyes (drusen, pigment epithelial disturbances and loss of foveal reflex).

B. Evolution of the disciform macular degenerative lesion

1. Early, degenerative changes are seen in the choriocapillaris and in Bruch's membrane in the macular area; collectively these changes are called *senile macular choroidal degeneration.*

2. The hemorrhagic phenomenon may be preceded by any of the above forms of central serous choroidopathy, but most commonly by a large detachment of the RPE with or without an associated NR detachment.

3. The senile macular choroidal degeneration becomes complicated by neovascular invasion from the choroid, through defects in Bruch's membrane, into the sub-RPE space.

4. All of the above factors produce an altered state of the internal choroid and external retina, which predisposes the eye to the development of serous and hemorrhagic phenomena.

5. Ultimately a hemorrhage into the sub-RPE space occurs (*hematoma of the choroid*).

This type of hemorrhage easily may be confused clinically with a malignant melanoma.

6. The hemorrhage may remain localized, but generally breaks into the sub-NR space and rarely into the choroid, the retina or even the vitreous.

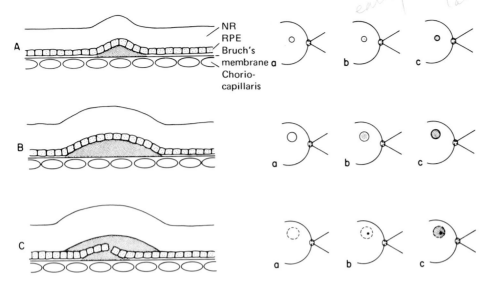

NR
RPE
Bruch's
membrane
Chorio-
capillaris

early   late

FIG. 11–39. Schematic diagram correlates histologic changes on left (**A, B** and **C**) with fundus changes (**a**), very early fluorescein stage (**b**) and late fluorescein stage (**c**). **A.** Simple small detachment of RPE. *NR,* neural retina; *RPE,* retinal pigment epithelium. **B.** Simple large detachment of RPE. **C.** Small detachment of RPE with overlying serous detachment of neural retina, i.e., idiopathic central serous choroidopathy.

FIG. 11–40. Idiopathic central serous choroidopathy. **A.** Patient with diagnosis of possible melanoma superior nasal to disc. **B.** Arteriolar-venular fluorescein phase shows leak (*arrow*) into sub-RPE area. **C.** Late phase shows fluorescein filling subsensory retinal area. Picture is typical of idiopathic central serous choroidopathy even though location is highly unusual. **A,** fundus; **B,** fundus; **C,** fundus, fluorescein.

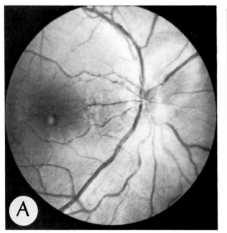

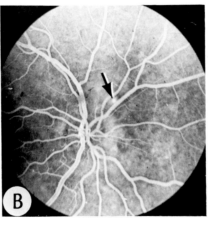

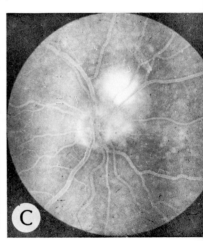

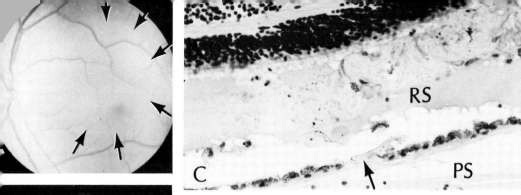

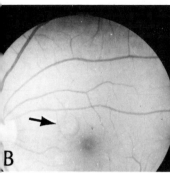

FIG. 11–41. Idiopathic central serous choroidopathy. **A.** Vague outline (*arrows*) delineates subtle central serous choroidopathy. **B.** Sharply outlined RPE detachment (*arrow*) is seen easily. **C.** Eosinophilic fluid is present in sub-RPE space (*PS*) and in subsensory retinal space (*RS*). Fluid presumably goes from sub-RPE space into subsensory retinal space through break in RPE (*arrow*). **A,** fundus; **B,** fundus; **C,** H&E, ×136.

A. Serous detachment stage

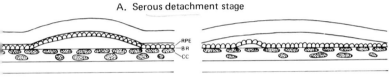

1. Serous detachment of pigment epithelium

2. Extension serous exudate into subretinal space

FIG. 11–42. Schematic drawing of evolutionary stages of senile disciform macular degeneration (disciform detachment of neuroepithelium). *R,* retina; *RPE,* retinal pigment epithelium; *BR,* Bruch's membrane; *CC,* choriocapillaris; *CH,* choroid; *S,* sclera.

B. Hemorrhagic detachment stage

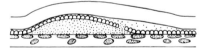

1. Hemorrhagic detachment of pigment epithelium

2. Extension of hemorrhage into subretinal space

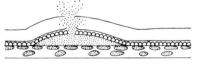

3. Extension of hemorrhage into retina

4. Extension of hemorrhage into vitreous

C. Reparative stage

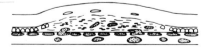

. Degradation and absorption of blood and exudate

2. Organization with secondary degeneration of pigment epithelium and retina

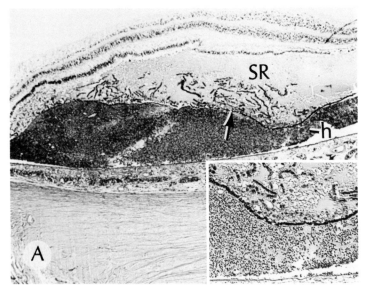

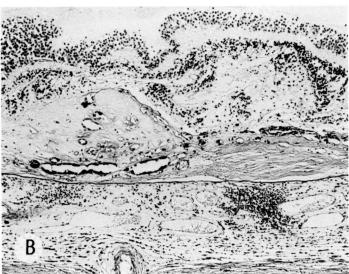

FIG. 11–43. Senile disciform macular degeneration. **A.** Left eye shows hemorrhage (*h*) in sub-RPE space and eosinophilic coagulum in subsensory retinal space (*SR*) in macular area. RPE (*arrow*) has undergone postmortem autolytic changes and is present artifactitiously as short segments in subsensory retinal space (see higher magnification in **inset**). **B.** Other eye from same individual shows RPE proliferation, disciform fibrous scar and chronic nongranulomatous choroiditis in macular area. **A,** H&E, ×16; **inset,** H&E, ×40; **B,** PAS, ×40.

FIG. 11–44. Senile disciform macular degeneration. **A.** Capillary (*arrow*) has grown through Bruch's membrane (*b*) into sub-RPE space. Hemorrhage has occurred and is partially organized. **B.** Another area shows fibrous organization above and below proliferated RPE. Note lymphocytes and plasma cells in choroid and sub-RPE space. **C.** Fibrous nature of disciform plaque better appreciated with special stain that demonstrates collagen. **D.** Another case to illustrate disciform fibrous plaque in macular area. **A,** H&E, ×176; **B,** H&E, ×101; **C,** trichrome, ×40; **D,** H&E, ×16.

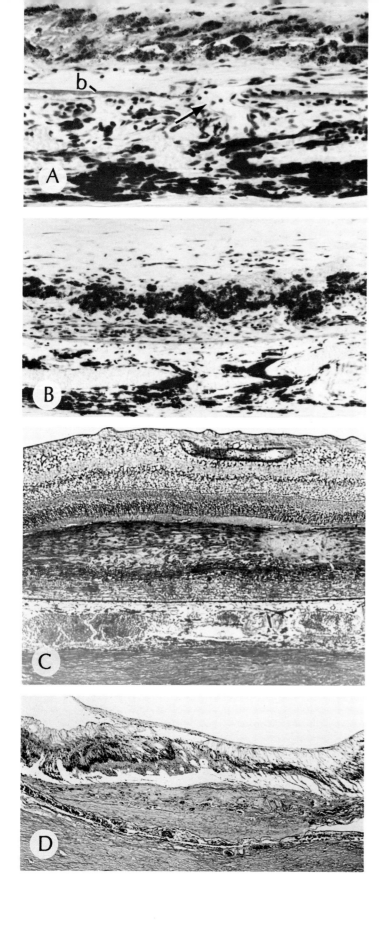

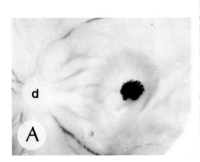

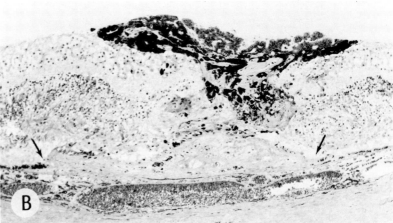

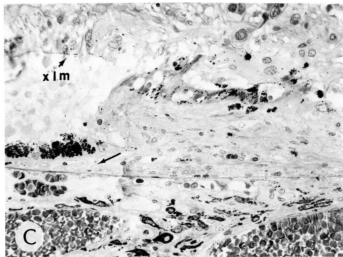

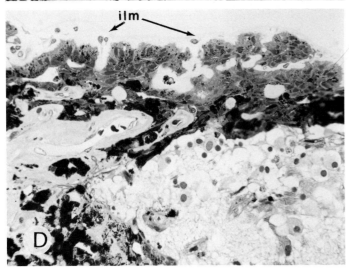

FIG. 11–45. Senile disciform macular degeneration. **A.** Proliferations of RPE may be sufficiently bizarre in region of fovea-macula to pass completely through retina, as here in this postmortem specimen. *d*, optic disc. **B.** Placoid subpigment epithelial macular degeneration with associated adenomatous hyperplasia of RPE. Lateral extent of vascular or connective tissue plaque is indicated by *arrows*. **C.** Edge of subretinal (i.e., subpigment epithelial) plaque. Epithelium is being elevated on left (*arrow*), and abnormal pigment epithelial cells are proliferating on inner surface of plaque. *xlm*, external limiting membrane of retina. **D.** RPE cells proliferating through retinal thickness undergo adenomatous hyperplasia (see Figure 17–78D), proliferating along submembranous cleavage plane of retina. *ilm*, internal limiting membrane. **A,** macroscopic; **B,** 1.5 μ section, PD, $\times$70; **C,** 1.5 μ section, PD, $\times$220; **D,** 1.5 μ section, PD, $\times$220.

7. Organization of the hemorrhage is accompanied by RPE proliferation, RPE fibrous metaplasia and ingrowth of mesenchymal tissue to form granulation tissue.

8. A disciform fibrous scar results in the macular region, causing degeneration of the macular RPE and NR with irreversibly impaired central vision.

IV. Disciform macular degeneration secondary to focal choroiditis (juvenile disciform degeneration of the macula)

A. Most patients with disciform macular degeneration secondary to focal choroiditis are less than 50 years old, represent equally both sexes, have bilateral involvement over 50 percent of the time, show a high incidence of macular hemorrhagic phenomena and usually have irreversible damage to central vision.

B. Probably the vast majority of cases occur secondary to focal inflammatory cell infiltration of the choroid.

C. The group can be subdivided into four divisions:

1. *Disciform macular detachment secondary to multifocal choroiditis (presumed histoplasmic choroiditis)* (Fig. 11–46)—the most common type, occurring in otherwise healthy young adults with the initial onset generally sudden blurring of vision in one eye.

   a. Early a yellowish white or gray, circumscribed, slightly elevated area of choroidal infiltration is present in the macular region soon accompanied by overlying RPE disturbances, resulting in a small dark greenish or blackish macular ring.

   b. Serous and hemorrhagic disciform detachment of the retina ensues.

   c. Multiple, small to tiny, sharply circumscribed, punched-out focal white defects are scattered about the fundus.

   d. An irregular area of peripapillary degeneration of the choroid and RPE frequently is seen.

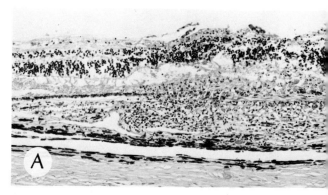

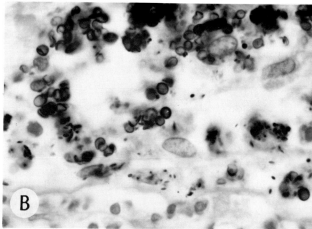

FIG. 11–46. Disciform macular detachment secondary to multifocal choroiditis, presumed histoplasmic choroiditis. **A.** Granulomatous inflammation involving choroid primarily but breaking through Bruch's membrane to involve also retina. **B.** Typical yeast forms of *H. capsulatum* are evident in specially stained preparation. Free-lying RPE melanin granules are also shown. **A,** H&E, ×100; **B,** Grocott's methanamine silver, ×1,000.

Although most patients show a positive skin reaction to intracutaneous injection of 1:1,000 histoplasmin as well as chest x-ray evidence of healed pulmonary histoplasmosis, the fungal organism never has been cultured from a typical retinal lesion or demonstrated satisfactorily in a histologic section. The cause, therefore, is still open to question.

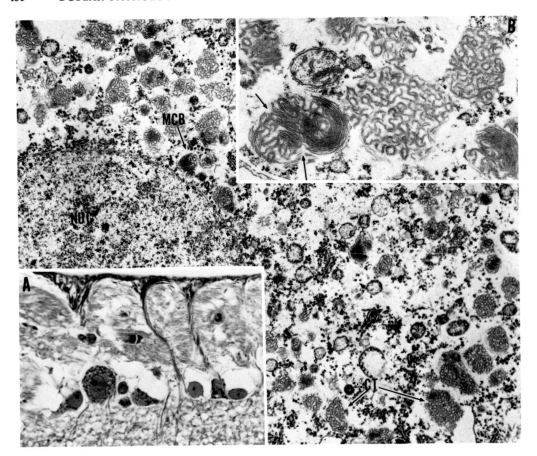

FIG. 11–47. Chloroquine retinal degeneration. Retinal ganglion cell from ganglion
cell layer shown in light micrograph, **inset A.**
Cytoplasm of ganglion cell as seen by
electron microscopy in **main figure** contains
myriad clusters of curvilinear structures (*CT*)
and membranous cytoplasmic bodies (*MCB*).
Bodies are better seen in **inset B;** suggestion
of continuity of curvilinear structure with
membranous body is seen at free *arrows.*
NUC, nucleus of ganglion cell. **Main figure,**
×10,200; **inset A,** 1.5 μ section, toluidine
blue, ×380; **inset B,** ×25,800.

2. *Disciform macular detachment secondary to focal peripapillary choroiditis*—the patients have negative histoplasmin skin tests and no peripheral fundus lesions. Their macular lesions are probably caused by an underlying peripapillary choroiditis.

3. *Disciform macular detachment secondary to focal macular choroiditis*—the patients have negative histoplasmin skin tests, no peripheral fundus lesions and no peripapillary choroiditis. Their macular lesions are probably caused by an underlying, focal, macular choroiditis.

4. *Disciform macular detachment secondary to Toxocara canis*—see pp. 93–94 in Chapter 4 and p. 699 in Chapter 18.

V. Postoperative cystic macular degeneration (Irvine-Gass-Norton Syndrome)—see pp. 136–137 in Chapter 5.

TOXIC RETINAL DEGENERATIONS

I. Chloroquine (Fig. 11–47)
A. The characteristic but nonspecific "bull's eye" macular degeneration appears to be directly related to the total dosage of chloroquine.

The degree of retinopathy and rate of its progression after chloroquine is stopped may reflect individual differences as well as drug dosage. Progression usually continues for varying time periods after the drug is stopped. Occasionally patients show reversible changes after stopping chloroquine.

B. Usually night blindness is the first symptom. Patients may develop extinguished electroretinograms (ERGs) but have normal or only minimally abnormal final dark-adaptation thresholds, thereby differentiating advanced chloroquine retinopathy from retinitis pigmentosa.
C. Histologically there are RPE abnormalities, destruction of rods and cones and of ganglion cells and pigment migration into the neural retina.

Degenerative changes as seen by electron microscopy are widespread occurring in most of the ocular tissues in the human eye. The changes are very prominent in the retinal neurons and appear as curvilinear structures (CT) as well as membranous cytoplasmic bodies (MCB). The MCBs in the acute experimental pig retina are almost restricted to the ganglion cells, whereas in the rat retina they are present in every type of neuron.

II. Many other drugs such as *NP-207, thioridazine, vitamin A, thorazine, indocin, quinine, sparsomycin* and *chloromycetin* may cause a retinopathy, generally of a secondary pigmentary type.

POSTIRRADIATION RETINOPATHY

I. Postirradiation retinopathy may follow months to years after radiation of the eye, usually for cure or control of retinoblastoma, malignant melanoma or orbital neoplasm.

The irradition source may be x rays, ^{60}Co or radon seeds. There is usually a latent period of 12 months or more before a retinopathy develops.

II. The retina can show capillary occlusion and capillary microaneurysms, telangiectatic vessels, neovascularization and signs of arteriolar or venular occlusion, all caused by retinal vascular obliteration secondary to the radiation.

LIGHT ENERGY RETINOPATHY

See pp. 166–170 in Chapter 5.

TRAUMATIC RETINOPATHY

See pp. 151–155 in Chapter 5.

HEREDITARY PRIMARY RETINAL DYSTROPHIES

DEFINITIONS

I. Dystrophies are primary phenomena that are inherited and tend to be bilateral and symmetrical.
II. They may remain stationary or be slowly progressive.

JUVENILE RETINOSCHISIS (Fig. 11–48)
(Vitreous Veils; Congenital Vascular Veils; Cystic Disease of the Retina; Congenital Retinal Detachment)

I. Juvenile retinoschisis generally is a bilateral condition, tends to be slowly progressive, often culminates in extensive chorioretinal atrophy with macular involvement and affects boys.

II. Most often it is inherited as a sex-linked recessive, but occasionally occurs as an autosomal recessive and then usually without macular involvement.

III. Ophthalmoscopically a translucent, veil-like membrane, retinal in origin, bulges into the vitreous, generally in the inferior temporal quadrant.

This membrane, really a retinal schisis cavity, has retinal vessels coursing over its inner wall, which also frequently contains large round or oval holes. The outer wall of the cavity may contain small holes.

IV. Goldmann-Favre vitreotapetoretinal dystrophy consists of
   A. Juvenile retinoschisis.
   B. Vitreous degeneration with liquefaction and the formation of preretinal strands and cords.
   C. Secondary pigmentary and degenerative changes of the retina resembling retinopathia pigmentosa.
   D. Hemeralopia with abolition of the ERG response and a progressive decrease in visual function.
   E. Lens opacities of the cataracta complicata type.
   F. An autosomal recessive heredity.

V. Wagner's vitreoretinal dystrophy consists of
   A. Juvenile retinoschisis plus marked vitreous syneresis.
   B. No posterior pole involvement.
   C. Normal dark adaptation but a subnormal ERG.
   D. Lens opacities of the cataracta complicata type.

The polymorphous ocular signs of this disease also may include myopia, retinal pigmentation, retinal breaks, patchy areas of thinned RPE, chorioretinal atrophy, narrowing and sheathing of retinal vessels, extensive retinal areas of white with pressure, lattice degeneration of the retina, marked retinal meridional folds and optic atrophy.

   E. An autosomal dominant heredity.
VI. Histologically the neural retina shows a cleavage (schisis) at the level of the nerve fiber and ganglion cell layers.

The area of retinal involvement is similar to that found in reticular cystoid degeneration and reticular degenerative retinoschisis, but different from the middle layer retinal involvement of typical microcystoid retinal degeneration and typical degenerative senile retinoschisis. In juvenile retinoschisis the retinal spaces appear empty and do not stain for acid mucopolysaccharides.

CHOROIDAL DYSTROPHIES

See pp. 342–344 in Chapter 9.

STARGARDT'S DISEASE

I. Stargardt's disease is a bilateral, symmetrical, progressive dystrophy initially confined to the posterior pole; it leads eventually to a loss of central vision. It is inherited as an autosomal recessive.

II. Ophthalmoscopically the macula takes on a "beaten bronze atrophy" due to a sharply defined RPE atrophy, and the surrounding area may show white or yellow spots indistinguishable from *fundus flavimaculatus*.

Stargardt's original report described numerous sharkfin-shaped spots around the papillofoveal area characteristic of fundus flavimaculatus. Most likely fundus flavimaculatus and Stargardt's disease represent different ends of a spectrum of the same disease, the former in its pure form consisting of a perifoveal tapetoretinal dystrophy and the latter in its pure form consisting of a central tapetoretinal dystrophy, but generally showing considerable overlap.

III. Dark adaptation and ERG are generally normal or only mildly abnormal in the purely central type but are subnormal in the perifoveal and peripheral retinal type. Fluorescein shows fluorescence of the central retinal focus without leakage, suggesting defects in the RPE with an intact Bruch's membrane.

IV. Histologically there is a complete disappearance of the RPE and of the visual elements in the macular area. The inner layers of the retina may show cystoid degeneration and calcium deposition. Peripheral to the central lesion a layer of vascularized connective tissue may lie between Bruch's membrane and the atrophic outer retinal layers.

FUNDUS FLAVIMACULATUS

I. Fundus flavimaculatus is a bilateral, symmetrical, slowly progressive disease involving the posterior pole, showing ill-defined yellowish spots or dots located at the level of the RPE. The dots often are shaped like crescents, sharkfins, fishtails or fish. It is inherited as an autosomal recessive or occasionally as an autosomal dominant.

About 50 percent of eyes show a Stargardt-type atrophic macular lesion with a decrease in visual acuity. Stargardt's disease and fundus flavimaculatus are probably different forms of the same disease process.

II. Dark adaptation and ERG generally are normal but may be subnormal. Fluorescein does not cause fluorescence of the spots in early lesions, and not all the spots will fluoresce in late lesions. The fluorescein shapes are irregular, soft and fuzzy and show a marked tendency for confluence.

The fluorescein pattern clearly differentiates the spots from drusen.

III. Histologically the RPE is involved solely (and hence the abnormal EOG) and shows
  A. Displacement of the nucleus from near the base of the cell to the center or apical surface.
  B. A peculiar line of condensation of pigment granules in the center or near the apical surface of the cell, frequently at the level of the displaced nucleus.
  C. Accumulations of an acid mucopolysaccharide, largely within the inner half of the cells, in circumscribed areas.
  D. Great variation in cell size from much larger than normal to small, without pigment granules or discernible nuclei.

RETINITIS PUNCTATA ALBESCENS (Albipunctate Dystrophy; Fundus Albipunctatus)

I. Retinitis punctata albescens is a bilateral, symmetrical disease that may extend to the peripheral retina, characterized by white, dotlike lesions with maximum density in the equatorial region. The hereditary pattern is not clear with both dominant and recessive forms suggested.
II. Two types have been described.
  A. *Progressive retinitis punctata albescens* with increasing constriction of visual fields, deterioration of central vision, anomalies of color vision, night blindness, extinguished ERG, mild to moderate optic atrophy and occasionally some retinal pigmentary changes.
  B. *Stationary retinitis punctata albescens* with benign evolution, little or no constriction of visual fields, normal or mildly subnormal ERG, good central vision and the presence of white dots in the fundus without pigmentary changes.   *like drusen*
III. Fluorescein shows multiple areas of fluorescent staining without leakage, corresponding to the dot lesions.
IV. No pathologic specimens have been studied histologically, but the defect is suspected of being at the level of the RPE, perhaps similar to drusen.

DOMINANT DRUSEN OF BRUCH'S MEMBRANE (Doyne's honeycomb dystrophy; malattia leventinese; Hutchinson-Tay choroiditis; guttate choroiditis; Holthouse-Batten superficial choroiditis; family choroiditis; crystalline retinal degeneration; iridescent crystals of the macula; hyaline dystrophies)

I. Dominant drusen of Bruch's membrane is a bilateral, symmetrical, progressive disease with its onset generally between 20 and 30 years of age, involving predominantly the posterior pole and resulting in loss of vision. It is inherited as an autosomal dominant.
II. Dark adaptation and ERG are normal. Fluorescein shows multiple, sharply defined fluorescent spots corresponding to the clinically seen lesions. There is some confluence of fluorescent areas but no leakage of dye.
III. Histologically the lesions are drusen (see p.

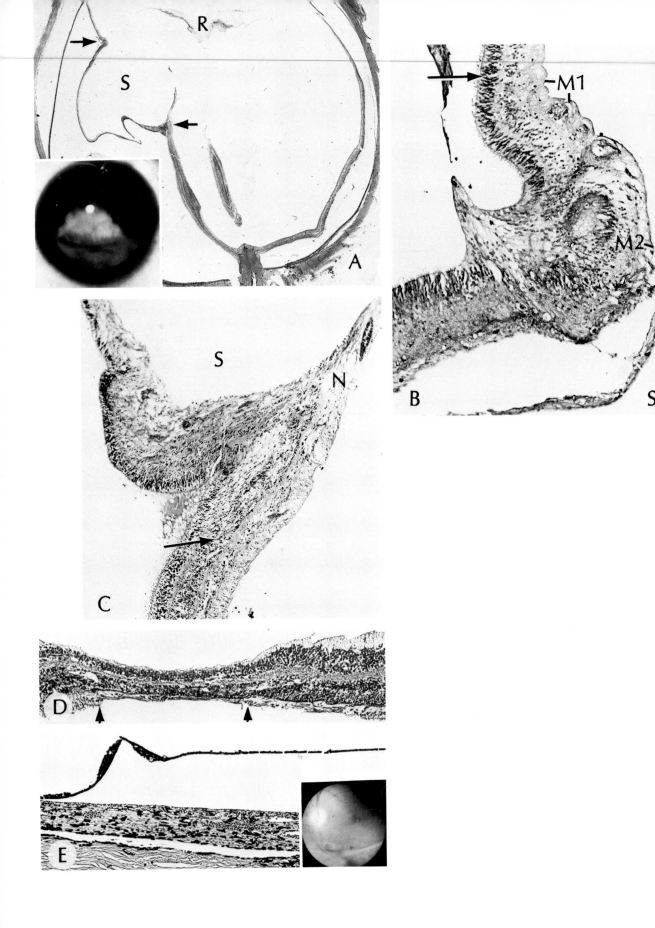

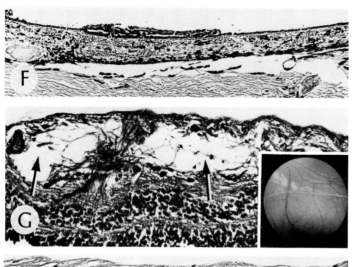

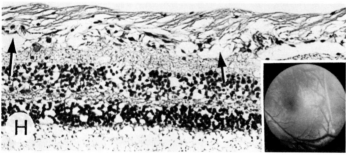

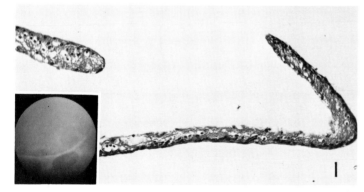

FIG. 11–48. Juvenile retinoschisis. **A. Inset** shows clinical appearance of eye with leukokoria. Temporal peripheral retina has large schisis cavity (*S*). *R,* retrolental mass consisting of organized hematoma. Area of *arrows* shown in higher magnification in **B** and **C. B.** Most peripheral retina (*arrow*) is intact. Internal limiting membrane (*M1* and *M2*) lines inner surface of intact retina and ends in region of M2, but in area of schisis (*S*) there is only a layer of glial tissue. **C,** Central junction of intact retina (*arrow*) with schisis cavity (*S*). Split has taken place within nerve fiber layer (*N*). **D** and **E** show macular area of retina (**D**) and macular area of RPE (**E**). Note loss of photoreceptors (between *arrows*) and RPE proliferation. **Inset** in **E** shows pigmentation in foveomacular region and inferior schisis. **F.** RPE has proliferated in area just nasal to optic disc. **G** and **H.** Areas of retina away from schisis cavity show tendency toward splitting (*arrows*) in ganglion cell and nerve fiber layers. **Inset** in **G** shows normal retinal sheen in intact area, but sheen is lost in schisis area inferiorly. **Inset** in **H** shows normal retinal sheen in intact area, but sheen is lost in schisis area temporal to macula (on right). **I.** Small hole is present in outer wall of schisis cavity. **Inset** shows typical large holes in inner wall. **A,** H&E, ×4; **inset,** clinical; **B,** H&E, ×115; **C,** H&E, ×50; **D,** H&E, ×40; **E,** H&E, ×40; **inset,** fundus; **F,** H&E, ×40; **G,** PAS, ×101; **inset,** fundus; **H,** H&E, ×40; **inset,** fundus; **I,** H&E, ×145; **inset,** fundus.

638 in Chap. 17) between the RPE and Bruch's membrane.

VITELLIFORM FOVEAL DYSTROPHY (Best's disease; vitelliform macular degeneration; vitelliruptive macular degeneration; exudative central detachment of the retina [macular pseudocysts]; cystic macular degeneration; exudative foveal dystrophy)

I. Vitelliform foveal dystrophy is a bilateral, symmetrical, progressive disease involving the macular area with resultant loss of vision. Its onset is generally before 15 years of age. It has an autosomal dominant mode of transmission with diminished penetrance and a highly variable expression.

II. Ophthalmoscopically, early there is an "egg yolk" appearance to the macula, which later becomes "scrambled" and pigmented.

The egg yolk appearance of the macula is not always present and sometimes may never occur. The fundus may show only very slight changes or resemble the terminal stage of extensive central inflammatory chorioretinitis or any stage in between.

III. Dark adaptation and ERG usually are normal. Fluorescein shows marked fluorescence at the time of maximum filling, suggestive of an extensive defect in the RPE and an increased permeability to fluorescein at the site of the abnormality, possibly due to increased permeability of the choroidal vessels.

IV. No pathologic specimens have been examined histologically in the early or intermediate stages. The most plausible site of the lesion is at the level of the RPE, but the nature and exact site of the lesion must await histologic study.

DOMINANT PROGRESSIVE FOVEAL DYSTROPHY

I. The clinical picture of dominant progressive foveal dystrophy is quite similar to Stargardt's disease (which has a recessive inheritance) except that it tends less toward involvement of the peripheral retina, occurs at a later age and generally takes a less progressive course. It is inherited as an autosomal dominant.

II. The one histologic study in a 78-year-old woman showed disappearance of the outer nuclear layer and receptors and pronounced changes in the RPE.

PROGRESSIVE CONE DYSTROPHY

I. Progressive cone dystrophy is characterized by a decrease in previously normal vision with normal or only minimally abnormal fundi. It is inherited as an autosomal dominant.

II. There are no histologic reports, but the pathology most likely involves the cones.

CENTRAL RETINOPATHIA PIGMENTOSA (retinopathia pigmentosa inversa; retinitis pigmentosa inversa)

I. Central retinopathia pigmentosa has the changes of classical retinopathia pigmentosa but is confined to the posterior pole. It is inherited presumably as an autosomal recessive.

II. Dark adaptation and ERG are normal or only minimally subnormal.

III. Histologically the changes are the same as those of classical retinopathia pigmentosa.

FIG. 11–49. Retinopathia pigmentosa, autosomal dominant type, in 46-year-old black man who died from multiple sclerosis. **A.** Foveomacular area (*arrow*) almost devoid of photoreceptors. **B.** Higher magnification of area of *arrow* in **A** shows almost complete degeneration of photoreceptors. **C** and **D** show migration of melanin in macrophages and RPE into retina, mainly around blood vessels (*arrows*). **Inset** in **D** shows characteristic moth-eaten appearance of involved retina and pigment around blood vessels. Choriocapillaris from macular (**E**), just temporal to macular (**F**), temporal equatorial (**G**), nasal equatorial (**H**), just posterior to nasal equatorial (**I**) and nasal posterior (**J**) areas. Note widespread atrophy and obliteration of choriocapillaris. Whether choriocapillaris degeneration is primary or secondary has not been determined. **A**, H&E, ×16; **B**, H&E, ×252; **C**, H&E, ×54; **D**, H&E, ×40; **inset**, fundus; **E**, H&E, ×101; **F**, H&E, ×252; **G**, PAS, ×252; **H**, PAS, ×252; **I**, H&E, ×252; **J**, PAS, ×252.

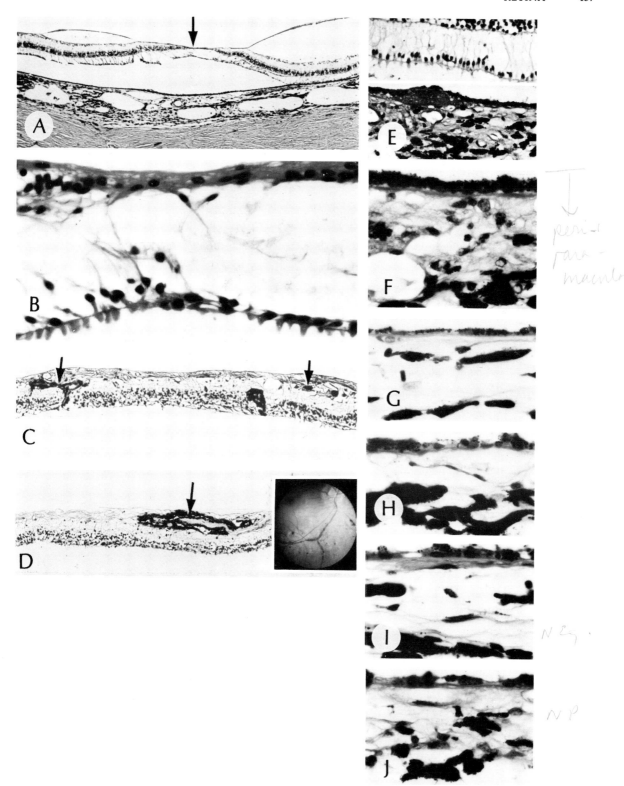

perir-
para-
macula

N 2g.

N P

RETINOPATHIA PIGMENTOSA (retinitis pigmentosa; pigmentary degeneration of the retina) (Fig. 11–49)

I. Retinopathia pigmentosa is a bilateral, symmetrical, progressive disease, with onset in early adult life, which starts in the equatorial area of the retina and spreads centrally and peripherally, but more rapidly in the latter direction. It may be inherited as an autosomal dominant or recessive or as a sex-linked recessive.

II. Clinically night blindness is an early symptom, marked visual impairment a late symptom. The tetrad of bone-corpuscular retinal pigmentation, pale waxy optic disc, attenuation of retinal blood vessels and posterior subcapsular cataract is characteristic.

Hamartomas at the disc or peripapillary retina may be an associated clinical finding.

III. Dark adaptation is markedly abnormal, as is the ERG, which usually is extinguished. Fluorescein study shows a blotchy or mottled hyperfluorescence involving the posterior and preequatorial eyegrounds, even when minimal ophthalmoscopic changes are present.

In most of the cases of secondary retinopathia pigmentosa, fluorescein study shows a blotchy or mottled hyperfluorescence only in areas of abnormal pigmentation, thereby differing from primary retinopathia pigmentosa.

IV. Histologically the earliest changes most likely are in the RPE and receptors, especially the rods. With progression the rods disappear, and the RPE undergoes both degeneration and proliferation. Intrasensory retinal migration of pigment-filled macrophages and of RPE occurs. The pigment tends to collect and remain around blood vessels accounting for the clinical bone-corpuscular appearance. Bruch's membrane remains intact, even in the latest stages of the disease.

Traumatic chorioretinopathy (Fig. 11–50), which can resemble primary retinopathia pigmentosa to a marked degree both clinically and histologically, generally is accompanied by interruptions of Bruch's membrane and true chorioretinal scars. If no chorioretinal scars are present histologically, the diagnosis of primary retinopathia pigmentosa may be made. If, however, chorioretinal scars are present histologically, the diagnosis remains uncertain because eyes blind from primary retinopathia pigmentosa frequently also are traumatized, and, therefore, develop secondary chorioretinal scars.

V. Secondary retinopathia pigmentosa has many causes such as *trauma; viral retinitis,* e.g., congenital rubella; *bacterial or protozoal retinitis,* e.g., congenital or acquired syphilis or toxoplasmosis; *drug-induced retinopathy,* e.g., vitamin A, chloroquine or chlorpromazine intoxication; *organization of retinal hemorrhages; Laurence-Moon syndrome* (mental retardation, hypogenitalism and spastic paraplegia; autosomal recessive); *Bardet-Biedl syndrome* (mental retardation, obesity, hypogenitalism and polydactyly; autosomal recessive); *Bassen-Kornzweig syndrome* (acanthocytosis, heredodegenerative neuromuscular disease and abetalipoproteinemia; autosomal recessive); *Alstrom's syndrome* (obesity, diabetes mellitus and nystagmus; possible autosomal recessive); *Refsum's syndrome* (chronic polyneuritis and cardiac abnormalities with storage in tissue of phytanic acid; autosomal recessive); *Friedreich's ataxia* (posterior column disease, nystagmus and ataxia; autosomal recessive); *Hallervorden-Spatz disease* (extrapyramidal signs related to degenerative changes in the basal ganglia, which are rust brown at autopsy; autosomal recessive); *late infantile and juvenile forms of amaurotic idiocy* (Batten-Spielmeyer-Vogt; autosomal recessive); *Cockayne's syndrome* (progressive infantile deafness, dwarfism, progeria, oligophrenia and changes in Bowman's membrane; autosomal recessive); *Flynn-Aird syndrome* (cataracts, ataxia, dementia, epilepsy and cutaneous changes; autosomal dominant); *Hallgren's syndrome* (congenital deafness, vestibulocerebellar ataxia, mental deficiency, psychoses, nystagmus and cataract; autosomal recessive); *Kartagener's syndrome* (dextrocardia, bronchiectasis and sinusitis; autosomal recessive); *Pelizaeus-Merzbacher syndrome* (diffuse cerebral sclerosis leading to extrapyramidal signs and mental deterioration; sex-linked recessive); *myotonic dystrophy* (Steinert's disease); *Lignac-Fanconi syndrome* (renal dwarfism, osteoporosis and chronic nephritis); *Turner's syndrome* (infertility, short stature, shield chest and low hairline; 45, XO); *hereditary olivopontocerebellar degeneration* (ataxia of all extremities; slurred speech and writhing athetosis; autosomal dominant); *Leber's congenital amaurosis of retinal origin* (usually autosomal recessive but rarely autosomal dominant); *imidazole aminoaciduria* (seizures, mental deterioration, excess carnosine and anserine excretion; autosomal recessive); *Usher's syndrome* (familial congenital deafness; autosomal recessive); and *mucopolysaccharidoses* (see pp. 302–306 in Chap. 8).

RETICULAR DYSTROPHY OF THE RETINAL PIGMENT EPITHELIUM (Sjögren dystrophia reticularis laminae pigmentosae retinae)

I. Reticular dystrophy of the RPE is a bilateral, symmetrical disease, characterized by foveal involvement with a good visual

prognosis. It is inherited as an autosomal recessive.

II. Ophthalmoscopically the fovea shows accumulation of dark pigment, surrounded by a finely meshed network of polygonally arranged pigment granules with densification at the sites of the knots of the network.

III. Dark adaptation and ERG are normal. Fluorescein study dramatically "lights up" the finely meshed polygonal network suggesting pigment lack in the involved RPE cells. There is no fluorescein leakage.

IV. No histologic studies have been performed, but the pathology is presumed to be in the RPE.

BUTTERFLY-SHAPED PIGMENT DYSTROPHY OF THE FOVEA

I. Butterfly-shaped pigment dystrophy of the fovea is a bilateral, symmetrical disease characterized by pigmentation localized in the deeper layers of the central retina taking the shape of a butterfly.

II. Dark adaptation and ERG are normal. Fluorescein study shows the butterfly

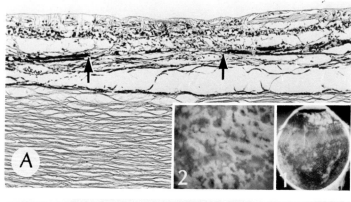

FIG. 11–50. Traumatic retinopathy. **A.** RPE is interrupted (between *arrows*) at site of chorioretinal scar. **Inset 1** shows macroscopic appearance of eye; pigment retinopathy shown at higher magnification in **inset 2. B.** Pigment has migrated into retina around blood vessel (*arrow*). Note almost complete atrophy of retina and RPE proliferation. **A,** H&E, ×40; **insets 1** and **2,** macroscopic of same eye; **B,** H&E, ×101.

abnormality to better advantage. There is no leakage of fluorescein.

III. No histologic studies have been performed, but the pathology is presumed to be in the RPE.

PSEUDOINFLAMMATORY DYSTROPHY (Sorsby's familial pseudoinflammatory macular dystrophy)

I. Pseudoinflammatory dystrophy is a bilateral, symmetrical disease with a late onset, generally in the fifth decade. It is inherited as an autosomal dominant.

II. Clinically there is an acute onset of loss of central vision with an inflammatorylike macular lesion showing edema, hemorrhages and exudates. Healing takes place slowly, and over the next few decades a slow extension of the process toward the periphery takes place, leaving a spreading area of choroidal atrophy and some pigment deposition.

III. Dark adaptation is normal as is the ERG early, but later the ERG becomes subnormal. Fluorescein study shows extensive defects in the RPE.

IV. The histology is uncertain because the two patients studied histologically did not have a history of dominant transmission.

HEREDITARY SECONDARY RETINAL DYSTROPHIES

ANGIOID STREAKS (Fig. 11–51)

I. Angioid streaks may be found in *pseudoxanthoma elasticum* (Grönblad-Stranberg syndrome), *fibrodysplasia hyperelastica* (Ehlers-Danlos syndrome), *osteitis deformans* (Paget's disease), *choriocapillaris atrophy involving the posterior eyegrounds* and *sickle cell anemia;* the mode of hereditary transmission depends on the primary affection.

II. Hemorrhages in and around the macula frequently complicate the condition and may lead to disciform degeneration of the macula.

III. Histologically Bruch's membrane shows basophilia and is broken and interrupted at the sites of the "streaks." Fibrovascular tissue usually fills the break and the contiguous RPE may be abnormal.

SJOGREN-LARSSON SYNDROME

I. The Sjögren-Larsson syndrome consists of congenital low-grade stationary mental deficiency, congenital ichthyosis and symmetrical spastic paresis of the extremities, which tends to involve the legs more than the arms. It is inherited as an autosomal recessive.

II. About 20 to 30 percent of patients have fundus abnormalities consisting predominantly of depigmented, pale areas in the macular region.

III. No histology is available, but the pathology is presumed to be at the level of the RPE.

MUCOPOLYSACCHARIDOSES

See pp. 302–306 in Chapter 8.

Retinopathia pigmentosalike fundus changes may be found in about 20 percent of the patients, types IV (Morquio) and VI (Maroteaux-Lamy) usually excepted.

MUCOLIPIDOSES

I. The mucolipidoses are a group of storage diseases ("*Hurler variants*"), which exhibit signs and symptoms of both the mucopolysaccharidoses and sphingolipidoses (Table 11–1).

II. With the exception of Austin type of sulfatidosis, the urinary excretion of uronic acid containing mucopolysaccharides is normal.

SPHINGOLIPIDOSES (Figs. 11–52 through 11–54)

I. The sphingolipidoses are a group of storage diseases, which share in common a portion of the molecular structure of a complex lipid (distinct for each separate disease) called *ceramide* (the long-chain amino alcohol called sphingosine to which a long-chain fatty acid is joined by an amide bond to the nitrogen atom on carbon 2 of sphingosine; Table 11–2).

II. Assay procedures currently are available for the detection of patients and carriers for all the sphingolipidoses.

OTHER LIPIDOSES

I. *Schilder's disease* and the *Pelizaeus-Merzbacher syndrome*. These primarily affect the white matter (optic nerve) with secondary degeneration of the retina (see Chap. 13).

II. *Goldberg's disease*. Macular cherry red spot, corneal clouding and β-galactosidase deficiency characterize the disease, which is a syndrome that combines clinical features of several storage diseases (mucopolysaccharidoses, sphingolipidoses and mucolipidoses) and is inherited as an autosomal recessive.

III. *Wolman's disease*. Although clinically similar, Wolman's disease differs from Niemann-Pick disease in having a tissue deposition in "foam cells" of cholesterol and triglycerides rather than phospholipids. Wolman's disease is characterized by hepatosplenomegaly, malabsorption, adrenal calcification and death in early infancy and is due to a deficiency of a lysosomal acid esterase. It is inherited as an autosomal recessive. There are no described ocular findings.

DISORDERS OF CARBOHYDRATE METABOLISM

I. Diabetes mellitus—see Chapter 15.

II. Lafora's disease (Fig. 11–55)

A. Lafora's disease is due to a deficiency of an unknown enzyme, which results in tissue storage of polyglucosans in different stages of aggregation. It is inherited as an autosomal recessive.

B. The disease is characterized by *Unverricht's syndrome*, which consists of myoclonic seizures, grand mal attacks, progressive ataxia, dysarthria, dyskinesia, amaurosis and dementia. It starts in the pre- or early adolescence and is relentlessly progressive with death 4 to 10 years after onset.

C. Histologically basophilic, spherical, laminated deposits (*Lafora bodies*) are found in the ganglion cells and inner nuclear layer of the retina and in the brain. An amorphous, basophilic de-

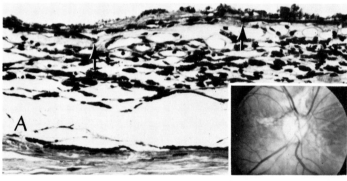

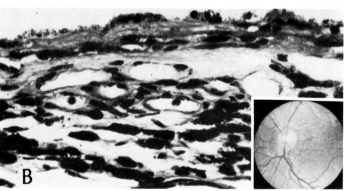

FIG. 11–51. Angioid streaks. Break in Bruch's membrane present between *arrows* in **A** (and at higher magnification in **B**). Patient had Paget's disease of bone and angioid streaks. **Inset** in **A** shows angioid streaks around optic disc. **Inset** in **B** shows massive involvement of posterior eye with angioid streaks. **A,** PAS, ×136; **inset,** fundus. **B,** PAS, ×252; **inset,** fundus.

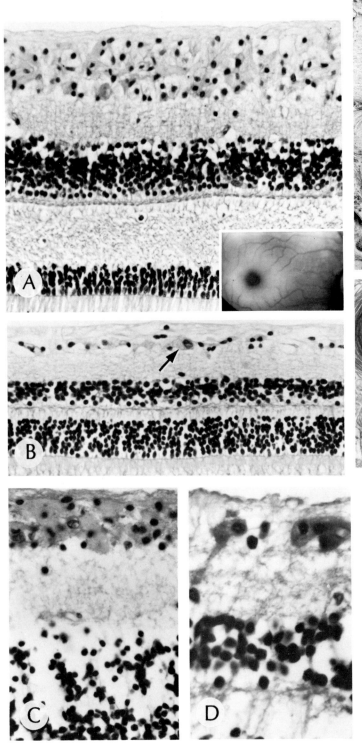

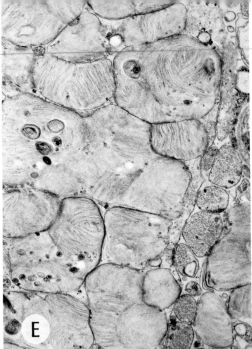

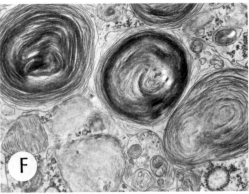

FIG. 11–52. Tay-Sachs disease. **A.** Macular area shows swollen cytoplasm of ganglion cells. **Inset** shows typical cherry red spot fundus appearance. **B.** Peripheral retina of same case shows less involvement, with cytoplasm of one ganglion cell (*arrow*) especially swollen. **C.** Macular area of another case shows marked involvement of ganglion cells, which contain PAS-positive material. **D.** Peripheral retinal ganglion cells also involved. **E.** By electron microscopy of case shown in **C** and **D,** ganglion cells contain whorled, laminated bodies that accumulate to fill cells. Accumulated ganglioside produces opacification of retina wherever there are ganglion cells (most prominent in foveomacular area). **F.** Another area of ganglion cells to show more dense lamination that may be seen in accumulating substance. **A,** PAS, ×176; **inset,** fundus; **B,** PAS, ×176; **C,** H&E, ×252; **D,** PAS, ×441; **E,** ×22,000; **F,** ×20,000.

posit is found in the heart muscle, liver cells and striated muscle cells.

III. Glycogen-storage disease (GSD)

A. *Type I GSD (Von Gierke's disease)* is due to a deficiency of the enzyme glucose-6-phosphatase, which results in tissue storage of glycogen. It is inherited as an autosomal recessive.

 1. Bilateral, symmetrical, yellowish, nonelevated, discrete paramacular retinal lesions resembling drusen are found.

 2. No histopathology is available, but the lesions are presumed to be at the level of the RPE.

B. *Type II GSD (Pompe)* is due to a deficiency of the enzyme α-1,4-glucosidase (acid maltase), which results in tissue storage of glycogen. It is inherited as an autosomal recessive.

 1. No clinical ocular signs are present.

 2. Histologically glycogen is found in retinal ganglion cells, retinal pericytes and ocular smooth and striated muscles.

Type III GSP (Forbes) due to amylo-1,6-glucosidase (debrancher) deficiency; *type IV GSP* (Anderson) due to amylo-1,4-1,6-transglucosidase (brancher) deficiency; *type V GSP* (McArdle Schmidt-Pearson) due to muscle phosphorylase deficiency; *type VI GSP* (Hers) due to hepatic phosphorylase deficiency; *type VII GSP* due to phosphoglucomutase deficiency; *type VIII GSP* due to hepatic phosphorylase deficiency (normal after glucagon or epinephrine); and *type IX GSP* is due to hepatic deficiency (no change after glucagon or epinephrine) have no known ocular findings.

OSTEOPETROSIS

I. Osteopetrosis is due to an inborn error of metabolism (enzyme deficiency unknown) in which the basic metabolic defect is unknown.

II. Clinically optic atrophy, exophthalmos, ptosis, squint, nystagmus and papilledema have been described.

III. The hereditary pattern consists of a lethal autosomal recessive congenital or infantile

type and a milder autosomal dominant type with a later onset.

IV. Histologically degeneration of rods and cones and of the outer nuclear layer and atrophy and gliosis of the ganglion cell, nerve fiber layers and the optic nerve may be found.

Retinal degeneration may occur in the absence of any bone pressure on the optic nerves. The retinal degeneration, therefore, probably is a primary dystrophy and an integral part of the disease.

HOMOCYSTINURIA

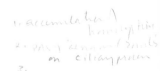

See p. 380 in Chapter 10.

I. Homocystinuria is due to a deficiency in the enzyme cystathionine synthetase resulting in an increased concentration of homocysteine, homocystine or a derivative of homocysteine. It is inherited as an autosomal recessive.

II. A peripheral retinal pigmentary dystrophy may be seen ophthalmoscopically in the far periphery near the equator.

III. Histologically the peripheral retina may show atrophy of its outer layers with inward migration of pigment-filled macrophages (Fig. 10–37).

SYSTEMIC DISEASES INVOLVING THE RETINA

HEREDITARY SECONDARY RETINAL DYSTROPHIES

See pp. 440–443 in this chapter.

DIABETES MELLITUS

See pp. 574–582 in Chapter 15.

HYPERTENSION AND ARTERIOLARSCLEROSIS

See pp. 404–407 in this chapter.

COLLAGEN DISEASES

See pp. 195–199 in Chapter 6.

Rheumatoid arthritis, scleroderma, periarteritis nodosa, systemic lupus erythe-

TABLE 11-1.
Mucolipidoses

Disease	Eponym	Enzyme defect	Tissue storage	Ocular signs	Inheritance
Gm_1-gangliosidosis, type I	Generalized gangliosidosis; Norman-Landing's disease	β-Galactosidase A, B and C	Keratan sulfate (cornea); Gm_1-ganglioside in retinal ganglion cells and elsewhere	Corneal clouding; macular cherry red spot	Autosomal recessive
Gm_1-gangliosidosis, type II	Late onset Gm_1 gangliosidosis	β-Galactosidase B and C	Keratan sulfate (viscera); Gm_1-ganglioside (brain only)	Not important	Autosomal recessive
Fucosidosis	—	α-Fucosidase	Fucose-containing glycolipids	None	Not known
Mannosidosis	—	α-Mannosidase	Mannose-containing glycolipids	None	Not known
Juvenile sulfatidosis, Austin type	—	Arylsulfatases A, B and C	Sulfated mucopolysaccharides (Alder-Reilly granules in leukocytes and Buhot cells in bone marrow)	Pale optic disc; retinal hypopigmentation	Autosomal recessive
Mucolipidosis I	Lipomucopolysaccharidosis	Not known	Acid mucopolysaccharides and glycolipids	Corneal opacities; macular cherry red spot	Autosomal recessive
Mucolipidosis II	I-cell disease	β-galactosidase	Acid mucopolysaccharides and glycolipids (derived from lysosomes?); peculiar fibroblast inclusions	Corneal opacities; macular cherry red spots	Autosomal recessive
Mucolipidosis III	Pseudo-Hurler polydystrophy	Not known	Acid mucopolysaccharides and glycolipids	Corneal clouding	Autosomal recessive
Lipogranulomatosis	Farber's disease	Ceramidase	Ceramide and hematoside	Macular cherry red spot	Autosomal recessive
Sea blue histiocyte syndrome	Chronic Niemann-Pick disease (Silverstein's syndrome)	Not known	Di- and trihexosylceramide, sphingomyelin and psychosine	Macular cherry red spot	Autosomal recessive

TABLE 11–2.
Sphingolipidoses

Disease	Eponym	Enzyme defect	Tissue storage	Ocular signs	Inheritance
Gm_2-gangliosidosis, type I	Tay-Sachs disease	Hexosaminidase A	Gm_2-ganglioside and ceramide trihexoside	Macular cherry red spot	Autosomal recessive
Gm_2-gangliosidosis, type II	Sandhoff's disease	Hexosaminidase A and B	Gm_2-ganglioside	Not important	Autosomal recessive
Gm_2-gangliosidosis, type III	Late onset Gm_2 gangliosidosis; late infantile or juvenile amaurotic idiocy	Partial deficiency hexosaminidase A	Gm_2-ganglioside	Not important	Autosomal recessive
Neuronal ceroidlipofuscinosis	Late infantile or juvenile Batten-Spielmeyer-Vogt syndrome (Sjögren, Mayou, Jansky-Bielschowsky, Kufs)	Peroxidase deficiency	Lipofuscin	Macular abnormalities (*not* cherry red spot), optic atrophy, secondary retinopathia pigmentosa	Autosomal recessive
Essential lipid histiocytosis	Infantile Niemann-Pick disease	Sphingomyelinase	Sphingomyelin and cholesterol	Macular cherry red spot	Autosomal recessive
Primary splenomegaly	Gaucher's disease	β-Glucosidase	Ceramide glucoside (glucocerebroside)	None	Autosomal recessive*
Angiokeratoma corporis diffusum universale	Fabry's disease	α-Galactosidase	Ceramide trihexoside	Corneal lesions; tortuous retinal blood vessels containing lipid deposits	Sex-linked recessive
Globoid leukodystrophy	Krabbe's disease; infantile diffuse cerebral sclerosis	Galactocerebroside β-galactosidase	Ceramide galactoside (galactocerebroside)	Optic atrophy; nystagmus	Autosomal recessive
Infantile metachromatic leukodystrophy	Sulfatide lipidosis	Lysosomal sulfate enzyme(s) (sulfatidase)	Sulfated glycolipids; metachromatic granules in retinal ganglion cells (mainly the large ones)	Grayness of macula; macular cherry red spot	Autosomal recessive
Ceramide lactoside lipidosis	—	β-Galactosidase	Ceramide lactoside	None	Autosomal recessive

* An adult type may also have an autosomal dominant type of inheritance.

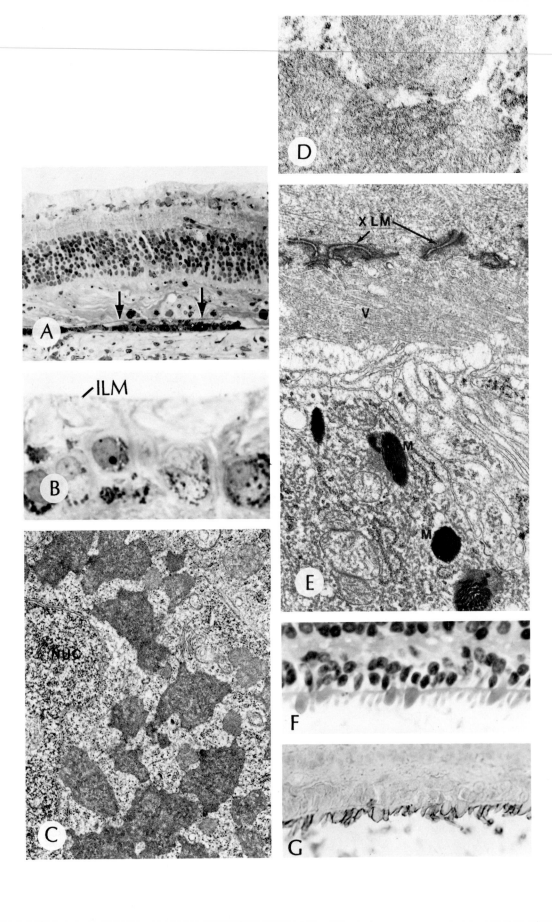

◀ **FIG. 11–53.** Batten-Spielmeyer-Vogt syndrome. **A.** Retina from region of macula. Small number of ganglion cells are present. Photoreceptor cells are entirely absent, but most of pigment epithelium has remained. External limiting membrane (*arrows*) is present near pigment epithelium. Pigment-filled macrophages have migrated into outer retinal layers. Choriocapillaris is present. **B.** Ganglion cell cytoplasm is filled with numerous granules. *ILM,* internal limiting membrane of retina. **C.** Cytoplasmic granules as seen by electron microscopy are irregular in shape, membrane bound and have membranous appearance to their content. *NUC,* nucleus of ganglion cell. **D.** Cytoplasmic inclusions possess irregular membrane content (i.e., multilaminar cytosome). **E.** Loss of photoreceptor cells results in nonspecific reformation of terminal bars or external limiting membrane (*XLM*) of retina by Müller glial cells where apical villi (*V*) now occupy much of subretinal space. Villi frequently interdigitate with apical villi of pigment epithelial cells. *M,* melanin granules of pigment epithelium. **F.** Nasal equatorial retina. Photoreceptor inner segments persist while outer segments have degenerated. **G.** Residual photoreceptor inner segments are coated with acid mucopolysaccharides (dark outlines limited to outer segments). **A,** 1.5 μ section, toluidine blue, ×165; **B,** 1.5 μ section, toluidine blue, ×750; **C,** ×19,200; **D,** ×60,000; **E,** ×21,000; **F,** ×700; **G,** PAS-AMP, ×530.

Multiple sclerosis, neuromyelitis optica and diffuse cerebral sclerosis (Schilder, Krabbe, Pelizaeus-Merzbacher, metachromatic leukodystrophy) generally cause primary white matter (optic nerve) disease with secondary retinal atrophy.

Many other systemic diseases may have retinal manifestations.

TUMORS

GLIA

I. Ordinary retinal gliosis
  A. Ordinary retinal gliosis may be intra-retinal (Fig. 11–56), preretinal (Figs. 11–57 and 11–58) or postretinal (subneural retina) (Fig. 11–59).
  B. It is found in such diverse conditions as chronic retinal detachment, most types of chronic secondary glaucoma, chronic retinitis or chorioretinitis, central retinal vein occlusion and diabetic retinopathy.
  C. Histologically there is an increased number of glial cells with or without preservation of the normal retinal architecture.

  If the retina becomes atrophic and the normal retinal architecture becomes replaced totally by glial cells (e.g., in toxoplasmosis where there may be complete segmental replacement of the retina by glial tissue), the retina becomes thinned. Conversely, with massive gliosis the retina becomes thickened.

II. Massive gliosis (Fig. 11–60)
  A. Criteria for massive gliosis are
    1. Segmental or total replacement of the retina by glial tissue.
    2. Abnormal blood vessels within the glial mass.
    3. A resultant thickening of the retina in the involved area.
  B. Massive gliosis is a benign, nonneoplastic proliferation of retinal glia in response to diverse pathologic states initiated by a variety of causative factors, e.g., congenital malformations, trauma, chronic inflammatory processes resulting in atrophia bulbi and retinal vascular disorders.

matosus, dermatomyositis and temporal arteritis can all cause retinal vasculitis with secondary retinal hemorrhages and exudates.

BLOOD DYSCRASIAS

Leukemia, lymphoma, aplastic anemia, sickle cell anemia and macroglobulinemia can all cause retinal vascular problems or infiltrates (leukemia and lymphoma).

DEMYELINATING DISEASES

See p. 441 in this chapter and p. 491 in Chapter 13.

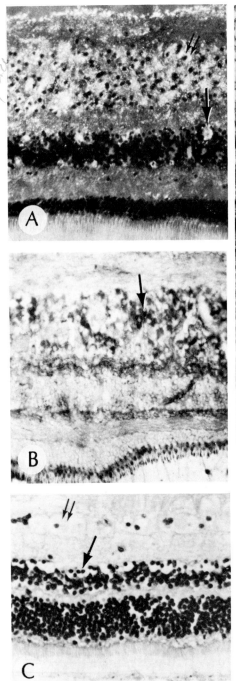

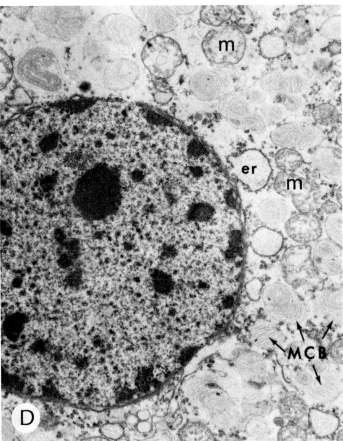

FIG. 11–54. Niemann-Pick disease (type A).
A. Frozen section of retina adjacent to fovea
shows birefringent material in ganglion cells
(*double arrow*) and in several amacrine cells
(*arrow*). Lesser amounts of birefringent
material are in nerve fiber, inner plexiform
and photoreceptor layers. **B.** Fat-stained,
frozen sections of perifoveal retina show
lipid in ganglion cells (*arrow*) and to lesser
extent in inner plexiform layer, synaptic
portion of outer plexiform layer and inner
segments of rods and cones. **C.** Routinely
stained paraffin-embedded sections to show
distended ganglion cells (*double arrow*) and
amacrine cells (*arrow*). **D.** Electron micrograph shows ganglion cell containing
numerous membranous cytoplasmic bodies
(*MCB*). Mitochondria (*m*) and dilated
endoplasmic reticulum (*er*) also are evident.
A, H&E, polarized, ×100; **B,** Sudan black B,
×100; **C,** H&E, ×160; **D,** ×15,000.

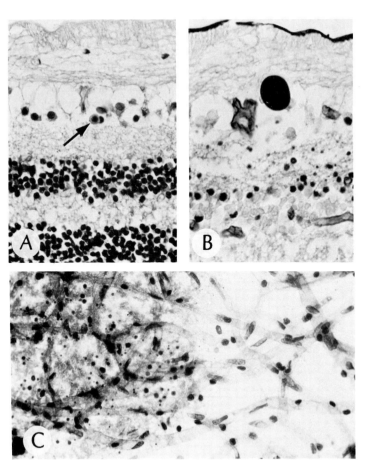

FIG. 11–55. Lafora's disease. **A.** Laminated Lafora body is seen within ganglion cell (*arrow*). **B.** Retinal Lafora bodies (black deposits) are seen in ganglion cells and in neurons of inner nuclear layer. **C.** Lafora bodies are seen as small black bodies in areas of incomplete digestion on left half of retinal trypsin digest preparation. **A,** H&E, ×300; **B,** PAS, ×440; **C,** H&E—PAS, ×305.

FIG. 11–56. Intraretinal gliosis. Small, spindle-shaped glial nuclei, mainly in nerve fiber layer, can be distinguished easily from larger ganglion cells (*arrows*). H&E, ×176.

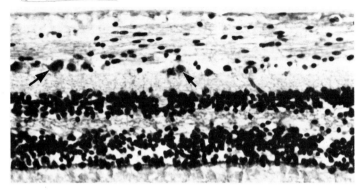

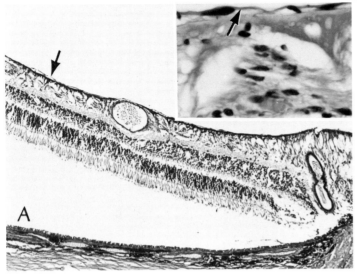

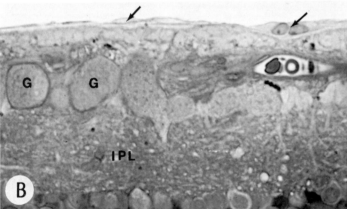

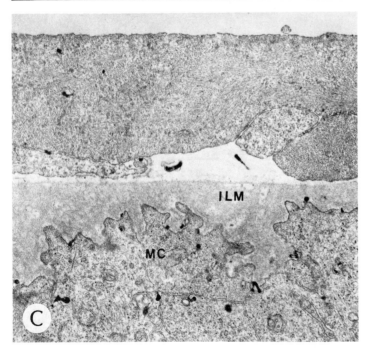

FIG. 11–57. Preretinal gliosis. **A.** Fine glial membrane (*arrow*) lines surface of retina internal to internal limiting membrane. Shrinkage of such membranes can produce multiple tiny folds of internal retina appearing clinically as cellophane retina. **Inset** shows glial membrane (*arrow*) at higher magnification. **B.** Light micrograph of preretinal glial membrane (*arrows*) growing over internal limiting membrane of retina just temporal to macula. Thickness of internal limiting membrane can be discerned by space between glial sheet and retina. Note that there is almost no space between glial cells in one area overlying large retinal vessel. *G*, ganglion cells; *IPL*, inner plexiform layer. **C,** Layer of fibrous astrocytes (packed with filaments) has grown along flat inner surface of internal limiting membrane (*ILM*). *MC*, Müller glial cells containing less prominent intracytoplasmic filaments. **D.** Preretinal membrane consists of both filament-containing (*Fil*) and nonfilament-containing cells indicating that astrocytes here are of both fibrous and protoplasmic varieties, respectively. Dense, maculalike attachments (*arrows*) are present between villous ends of cells as may be seen between astroglia normally in such tissues as optic nerve head. *ILM*, internal limiting membrane; *MC*, basal footplates of Müller cells. **E.** Glial cell (*GC*) beginning its migration out of retina directly through internal limiting membrane (*ILM*). *Arrows* indicate sites where glial cell is squeezing past Müller cell footplates. *NF*, nerve fibers in nerve fiber layer (axons of ganglion cells). **A,** H&E, ×40; **inset,** H&E, ×252; **B,** 1.5 μ section, PD, ×615; **C,** ×21,000; **D,** ×21,000; **E,** ×21,000.

FIG. 11–58. Preretinal RPE membrane formation in midperiphery of experimentally detached retina. *ilm,* internal limiting membrane; *r,* retina; *v,* vitreous. Presumably RPE cells become loose from RPE layer and float in subretinal fluid through retinal hole into vitreous compartment where they settle or become implanted on surfaces such as retinal and vitreal. Monolayer of RPE cells such as this takes at least 4 weeks to develop after experimental production of retinal detachment. ×5,850.

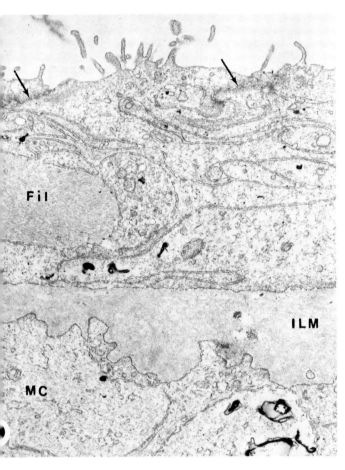

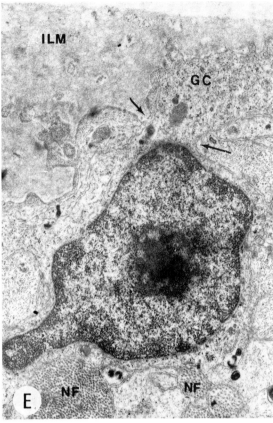

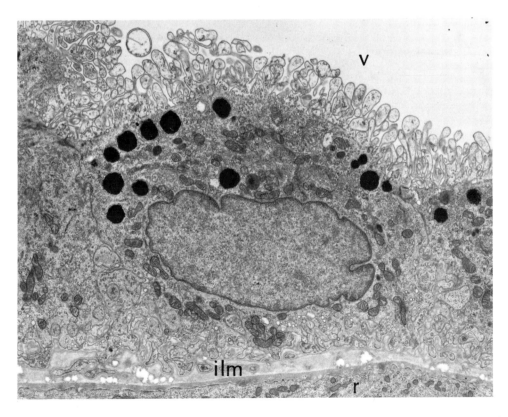

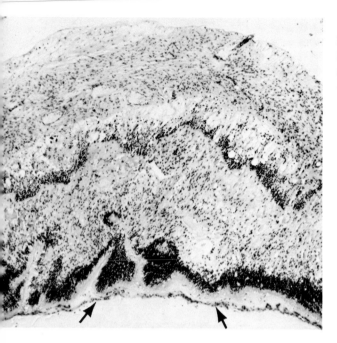

FIG. 11–59. Postretinal (subretinal) membrane. Membranes on outer surface of neural retina (*arrows*) may be glial or RPE in origin. H&E, ×28.

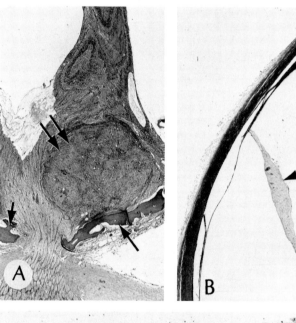

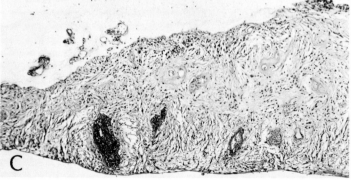

FIG. 11–60. Massive gliosis. **A.** Segmental replacement and thickening of posterior retina (*double arrow*) by glial tissue. Note intraocular ossification (*arrows*). **B** (and higher magnification in **C**) shows segmental replacement and thickening of anterior retina (*arrow* in **B**) by glial tissue. **D.** Retina is totally replaced by glial tissue (*G*), which fills vitreous compartment. Note marked intraocular ossification (*arrows*). **E.** Abnormal vessels are found throughout areas of massive gliosis. Vessels show dilatation, engorgement, varicosities, hyalinization and mineralization. **F.** Laminated calcific concretions may be present. **G.** Glial cells are elongated, contain pale eosinophilic fibrillated cytoplasm with indistinct borders, show rather uniform nuclei and course in all directions. **H.** Fatty marrow, or active hematopoietic marrow as shown here, is observed in areas of osseous metaplasia. **A,** H&E, ×14; **B,** H&E, ×7; **C,** H&E, ×60; **D,** H&E, ×5; **E,** H&E, ×50; **F,** H&E, ×305; **G,** H&E, ×305; **H,** H&E, ×100.

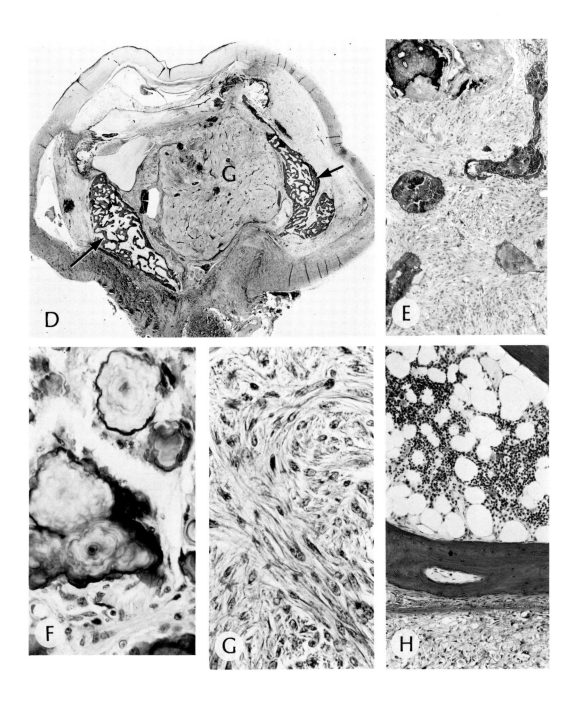

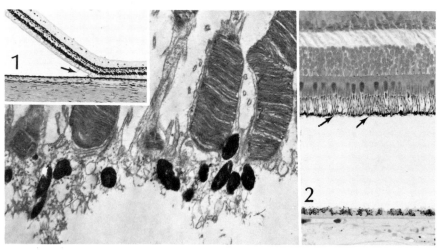

FIG. 11–61. Artifactitious retinal separation (detachment) (*arrow* in **inset 1**) separates neural (sensory) retina from its pigment epithelium. Higher magnification (**inset 2**) of thinner section shows pigment granules (*arrows*) remaining attached to tips of photoceptors. Note loss of apical villi of pigment epithelial cells. Electron micrograph shows adherence of apical villi and cytoplasmic portions of pigment epithelial cells with mostly ovoid melanin granules. Zonular (terminal bar) attachments of pigment epithelial cells remain with cell bodies. Antemortem disturbances, conversely, generally cause "clean" separation of photoreceptors from entire pigment epithelial cell. **Main figure,** ×7,500; **inset 1,** H&E, ×55; **inset 2,** 1.5 μ section, PD, ×180.

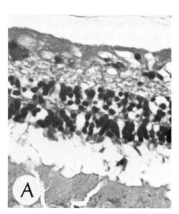
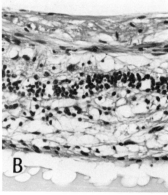

FIG. 11–62. True retinal detachment. **A.** Recent retinal detachment shows degeneration of photoreceptors and fluid in subretinal space. **B.** Chronic retinal detachment shows marked degeneration of outer retinal layers and fluid in subretinal space. **A,** H&E, ×176; **B,** H&E, ×101.

C. Histologically the tumors are composed of 1) interweaving groups of large, pale, spindle cells containing rather uniform nuclei and abundant, faintly eosinophilic, fibrillated cytoplasm and having indistinct cell borders; 2) dilated, large abnormal blood vessels with thin walls and an anastomosing pattern; and 3) frequently calcium deposits in walls of blood vessels, in the tumor and in contiguous drusen.

III. True glioma
True gliomas of the retina are exceedingly rare and behave much like juvenile pilocytic astrocytomas of the optic nerve (see pp. 502–505 in Chap. 13).

PHAKOMATOSIS

See Chapter 2.

RETINAL PIGMENT EPITHELIUM

See Chapter 17.

RETINOBLASTOMA AND PSEUDOGLIOMAS

See Chapter 18.

RETINAL DETACHMENT

DEFINITIONS

I. A retinal "detachment" is a retinal separation, i.e., a separation between the neural (sensory) retina and the retinal pigment epithelium rather than a true retinal detachment.

II. An artifactitious retinal detachment (Fig. 11–61), a frequent finding following formaldehyde fixation, can be differentiated histologically from a true retinal detachment (Fig. 11–62) by
A. An "empty" subretinal space.
B. Good preservation of rods and cones.
C. Pigment granules (derived from apexes of RPE cells) adherent to the external ends of the rods and cones.

The use of glutaraldehyde, or a formaldehyde-glutaraldehyde mixture, as the initial ocular fixative helps to prevent the formation of an artifactitious retinal detachment.

MAJOR CAUSES

I. Accumulation of fluid beneath an intact sensory retina, e.g., in Harada's disease, Coats's disease, malignant hypertension, eclampsia, choroidal malignant melanomas or subretinal hemorrhages.

II. Traction bands in the vitreous due to many causes, e.g., posttraumatic vitreous condensation and fibrosis, complications following cataract extraction (especially with vitreous loss) with an inferior detachment or vitreous bands in diabetes mellitus.

III. Accumulation of fluid beneath a broken sensory retina associated with vitreous traction, e.g., a rhegmatogenous retinal detachment.

CLASSIFICATION OF RETINAL DETACHMENT

I. Rhegmatogenous—due to a retinal hole usually associated with vitreous traction.
A. Equatorial type (mainly in age group over 40 years)—pathologic cause occurs at the equatorial area.
   1. Myopia—about one-third of all nontraumatic retinal detachments occur in myopic patients, and about 1 to 3 percent of all patients with high myopia develop a retinal detachment.
   2. Secondary to lattice degeneration.
   3. Secondary to other perivascular degenerations.
   4. Secondary to retinal horseshoe tears (Fig. 11–63) or round holes.
B. Oral type (mainly in age group over 40 years but somewhat younger than equatorial type)—pathologic cause occurs at the ora serrata area.
   1. Aphakic—about 20 percent of all retinal detachments occur in aphakes, and about 2 to 5 percent of all aphakes develop a retinal detachment.
   2. Dialysis in young—congenital and usually located inferotemporally.
   3. Traumatic dialysis (Fig. 11–64)—usually superonasally.
   4. Giant retinal break (a retinal break greater than 90 degrees).
C. Macular type (Figs. 11–65 and 11–66) (most rare)—pathologic cause occurs at the macular area.
   1. High myopia.

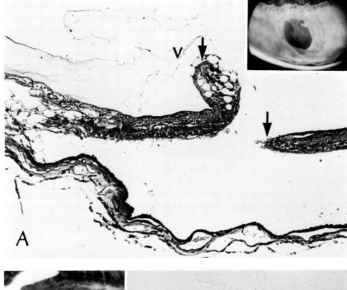

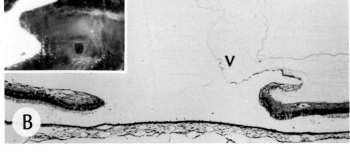

FIG. 11–63. Horseshoe tear of retina. **A.** Rounded edges (*arrows*) show tear is true retinal tear (artifact shows sharp edges). Note vitreous (*v*) adherent to anterior lip of tear causing traction. **Inset** shows macroscopic appearance. **B.** Another case similar to **A.** Again vitreous (*v*) adherent to anterior lip of tear causing traction. **Inset** shows macroscopic appearance. **A,** PAS, ×40; **inset,** macroscopic. **B,** H&E, ×16; **inset,** macroscopic.

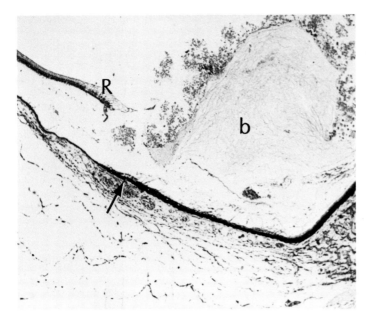

FIG. 11–64. Traumatic retinal dialysis shows peripheral retina (*R*) torn from nonpigmented ciliary epithelium at ora serrata (*arrow*). *b,* blood in vitreous. H&E, ×16.

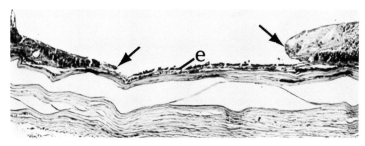

FIG. 11–65. Macular hole between rounded edges (*arrows*) of torn retina. Base of hole lined by RPE (*e*). Patient had ocular injury 20 years and 1 year previously. Compare to hole in inner wall of macular cyst shown in Figure 11–34. H&E, ×40.

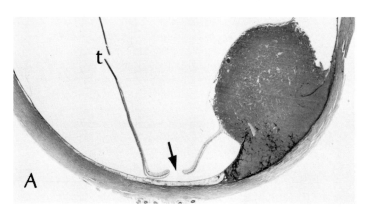

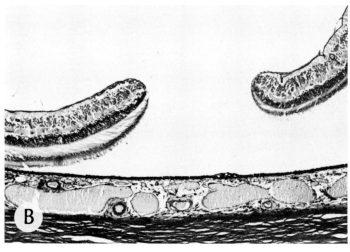

FIG. 11–66. A. Macular hole (*arrow*) in eye with melanoma (hole shown at higher magnification in **B**). Origin of hole not clear but thought to be secondary to intraretinal edema caused by melanoma. Compare with Figures 11–34 and 11–65. Note sharp edges of artifactitious retinal tear (*t*). **A,** PAS, ×8; **B,** PAS, ×28.

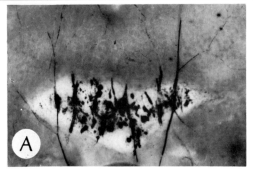

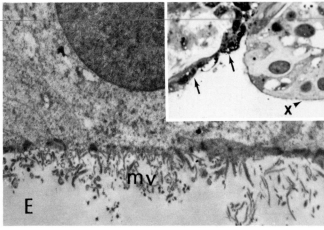

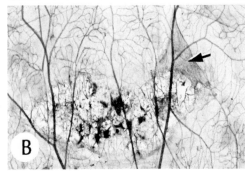

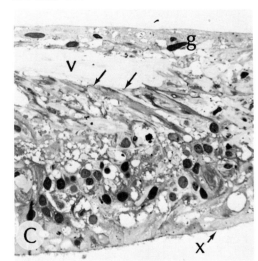

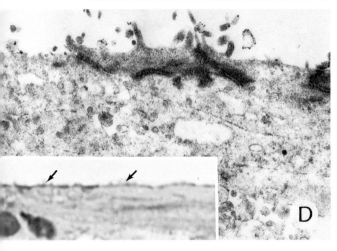

FIG. 11–67. Lattice degeneration of retina.
A. Heavily pigmented ovoid lesion in retinal periphery parallels ora serrata. **B.** Retinal digest of lesion in **A.** Note increased density of vitreous attachments particularly anteriorly (*arrow*). **C.** Section of anterior part of lesion. Vitreous base (*v*) is contracted anteriorly. Glial cells (*g*) proliferating within inner retinal layers have grown along retracted vitreal surface. *Arrows* indicate side of delicate original internal limiting membrane of peripheral retina (poorly visualized by light microscopy). Note loss of photoreceptors along external limiting membrane (*x*). **D. Inset** is light micrograph of glia proliferating along "opened" inner surface of lesion. Note formation of surface "membrane" beyond which project delicate villi (*arrows*). Electron micrograph shows glial cells, their characteristic dense attachments (see Figure 11–57) and their villous projections. **E. Inset** is light micrograph of outer retinal surface approximately midlesion. There is loss of photoreceptors, and external limiting membrane (*x*) of retina is interrupted by ingrowing proliferating pigment epithelial cells (*arrows*). Electron micrograph illustrates terminal barlike arrangement of external glial (i.e., Müller) cells. Glial microvilli (*mv*) project into subretinal space. **A,** macroscopic; **B,** trypsin digest; **C,** 1.5 μ section, toluidine blue, $\times 300$; **D,** $\times 12,378$; **inset,** 1.5 μ section, toluidine blue, $\times 1,260$; **E,** $\times 5,232$; **inset,** 1.5 μ section, toluidine blue, $\times 525$.

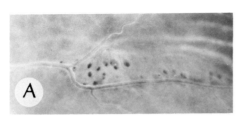

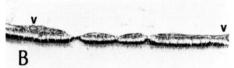

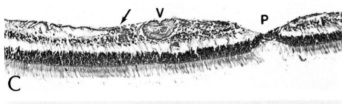

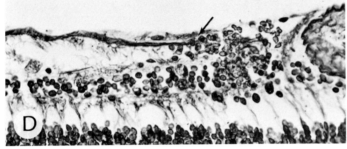

FIG. 11–68. Retinal pits. **A.** Macroscopic appearance of retinal pits arranged along thickened and sheathed vessel. Optic disc is to left. **B.** Several retinal pits in vicinity of sclerotic blood vessels (*v*). **C.** Internal limiting membrane ends abruptly (*arrow*) as it approaches sclerotic vessel (*v*) and associated retinal defect or pit (*P*). **D.** Higher magnification of **C** to show termination of internal limiting membrane (*arrow*) and proliferation of glial membrane onto its inner surface (preretinal glial membrane). **A,** macroscopic; **B,** H&E, ×36; **C,** Wilder's reticulum stain, ×90; **D,** Wilder's reticulum stain, ×325.

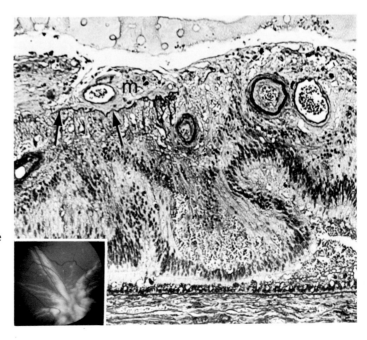

FIG. 11–69. Fixed folds, noted by folding of internal limiting membrane (*arrows*), are due to shrinkage of membrane (*m*) on internal surface of retina. **Inset** shows massive vitreous retraction and total retinal detachment due to shrinkage of internal surface membranes. **Main figure,** PAS, ×69. **inset,** fundus.

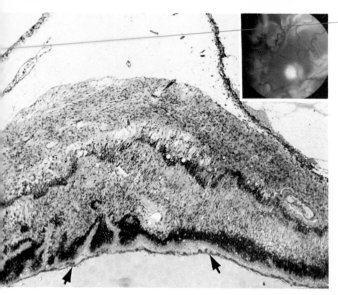

Fig. 11–70. Fixed folds of outer retina, noted by external nuclear layer's being thrown into folds, are due to shrinkage of membrane (*arrows*) on outer retinal surface. **Inset** shows massive membrane formation on inner surface of detached retina. **Main figure,** H&E, ×16; **inset,** fundus.

FIG. 11–71. Proliferation of RPE (*double arrow*) at ora serrata (*R*) at site of detached retina's "tugging" on RPE is called ringschwiele. Note break of RPE (*arrows*) due to traction. Material (*m*) in space shows that break probably is not artifact. Note also blood vessel extending from choroid, through RPE, just posterior (below) to ora serrata, into upper aspect of ringschwiele. PAS, ×40.

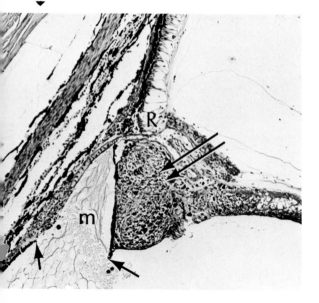

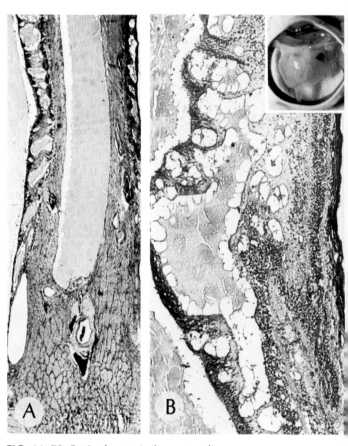

FIG. 11–72. Retinal cysts in long-standing retinal detachment (**A** and **B**). **Inset** in **B** shows that neck or connection of cyst with retina is of smaller diameter than largest diameter of cyst. Neck of cyst is difficult to see in microscopic sections unless serial sections are compared. Note in **B** that cysts contain PAS-positive material. **A,** H&E, ×16; **B,** PAS, ×40; **inset,** macroscopic.

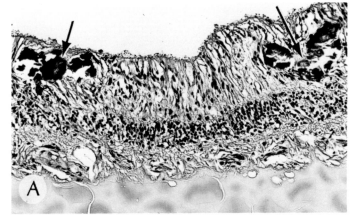

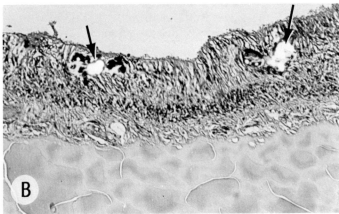

FIG. 11–73. Calcium oxalate crystals (*arrows* in **A**) are present in inner layers of retina, which has been detached for some time. Note total degeneration of photoreceptors and outer nuclear layer and fluid in subretinal space. **B.** Crystals (*arrows*) are birefringent to polarized light. **A,** H&E, ×100; **B,** H&E, polarized, ×80.

2. Posttraumatic.

II. Nonrhegmatogenous—may be transudative, exudative (Figs. 11–11, 11–41 and 11–43) or hemorrhagic.

 A. Uveitis, e.g., pars planitis, sympathetic uveitis, Harada's disease, uveal effusion, posttraumatic or eclampsia.

 B. Scleritis.

 C. Choroidal tumor; about 75 percent of uveal malignant melanomas have an associated retinal detachment, most of which (about 84 percent) are segmental.

 D. Traction of vitreous bands, e.g., with retrolental fibroplasia, diabetic retinopathy, sickle cell retinopathy or posttraumatic.

*75% o̅ m.m.
have R.D.*

PREDISPOSING FACTORS TO RETINAL DETACHMENT

I. Juvenile and senile retinoschisis (see section Degenerative Retinoschisis above).

P. 417, 418.

II. Lattice (palisade) degeneration (Fig. 11–67).

 A. Lattice degeneration can occur in any decade of life with the average age between 40 and 50 years, affects the sexes equally, generally is bilateral and involves the retina circumferentially between the equator and the ora serrata.

 B. It consists of criss-crossing white lines (latticework), which represent the branching pattern of thickened, hyalinized blood vessels. Pigmentation and depigmentation are common in the involved area, and the overlying vitreous is liquefied.

 C. Condensations of vitreous are adherent to the edges or margins of the area of lattice; subsequent shrinkage or vitreous detachment may cause retinal tears.

D. Lattice degeneration causes retinal detachments in 20 to 30 percent of the retinal detachment patients. However, less than 1 percent of patients with lattice degeneration develop a retinal detachment.

E. Histologically the retina is thinned and gliosed (especially the inner layers), and thick, hyalinized blood vessels are present. There is no perceptible basement membrane (internal limiting membrane of the retina) over the area of lattice. Vitreoretinal adhesions are seen mainly on the anterior side of the area of lattice degeneration.

III. Retinal pits (Fig. 11–68)

A. Retinal pits are small defects in the inner retinal layers most often found in the peripheral retina.

B. They probably are caused by minute vitreoretinal adhesions adjacent to sclerotic blood vessels. The adhesions may tear off a partial thickness piece of retina at the time of a vitreous detachment. An alternate theory is that the pit is formed initially by focal atrophy of the Müller cells in the paravascular regions.

C. Histologically a small, funnel-shaped defect occupies most of the thickness of the inner retina, often leaving only the receptors and the external part of the outer nuclear layer behind.

IV. Vitreoretinal adhesions—see p. 470 in Chapter 12.

V. Trauma and cataract surgery—see pp. 129, 155 in Chapter 5.

VI. Myopia—see pp. 420–421 in this chapter and pp. 488–489 in Chapter 13.

VII. Paving Stone Degeneration (probably not a predisposing factor to retinal detachment)—see p. 420 in this chapter.

PATHOLOGIC CHANGES FOLLOWING RETINAL DETACHMENT

I. *Retinal atrophy* (Fig. 11–62). The outer retinal layers mainly are affected because they are removed from their source of nourishment, i.e., the choriocapillaris, whereas the inner retinal layers retain their blood supply from the central retinal artery.

II. The subretinal space is filled with material (Fig. 11–62) (serous fluid, blood, inflammatory cells or neoplasm).

The material may be quite watery so that it runs out of the tissue during processing. The subretinal space then appears empty histologically.

III. *Glial* or RPE membranes can occur on the internal or external surface of the neural retina as well as within the retina. Shrinkage of these membranes causes *fixed retinal folds* (Figs. 11–57 through 11–59, 11–69 and 11–70).

IV. RPE may proliferate at the anterior (usually ora serrata) or posterior (advancing edge) site where the detached retina remains attached. The proliferated RPE may lay down considerable amounts of basement membrane* and is seen clinically and pathologically as a *demarcation line*. A similar proliferation of the RPE just posterior to the ora serrata is known as a *ringschwiele* (Fig. 11–71).

V. Large intraretinal cysts may form. They contain a PAS-positive but acid mucopolysaccharide-negative fluid.

A *retinal cyst* (Fig. 11–72) is defined as an intraretinal space with a "neck" of smaller diameter than the largest diameter of the cyst. If there is no neck, then the space is called microcystic if small (under 1.50 mm) and retinoschisis if large (1.50 mm or greater). With reattachment of the retina the cysts may resorb rapidly.

VI. Calcium oxalate crystals may form in the retina (Fig. 11–73).

PATHOLOGIC COMPLICATIONS FOLLOWING RETINAL DETACHMENT SURGERY

See section Complications of Retinal Detachment Surgery in Chapter 5.

* The basement membrane material clinically should be clear or white. The proliferated RPE cells may accentuate the demarcation line by giving it a brown color.

BIBLIOGRAPHY

CONGENITAL ANOMALIES

Blume RS, Wolff SM: The Chediak-Higashi syndrome: studies in four patients and a review of the literature. Medicine (Baltimore) 51:247, 1972

Deutman AF: The Hereditary Dystrophies of the Posterior Pole of the Eye. Assen, The Netherlands, Van Gorcum, 1971, pp. 26–28

Forgacs J, Bozin I: Manifestations familiale de pigmentations groupées de la région maculaire. Ophthalmologica 152:364, 1966

Johnson DL, Jacobson LW, Toyama R, Monahan RH: Histopathology of eyes in Chediak-Higashi syndrome. Arch Ophthalmol 75:84, 1966

Kalina RE: A histopathologic postmortem and clinical study of peripheral retinal folds in infant eyes. Am J Ophthalmol 71:446, 1971

Lahav M, Albert DM, Wyand S: Clinical and histopathologic classification of retinal dysplasia. Am J Ophthalmol 75:648, 1973

Maumenee AE, Emery JM: An anatomic classification of diseases of the macula. Trans Am Acad Ophthalmol Otolaryngol 74:594, 1972

Scheie HG, Yanoff M: Peters' anomaly and total posterior coloboma of retinal pigment epithelium and choroid. Arch Ophthalmol 87:525, 1972

Shields JA, Tso MOM: Histopathology of congenital grouped pigmentation of retina. In preparation

Spencer WH, Hogan MJ: Ocular manifestations of Chediak-Higashi syndrome: report of a case with histopathologic examination of ocular tissue. Am J Ophthalmol 50:1197, 1960

Winn S, Tasman W, Spaeth G, McDonald PR, Justice J Jr: Oguchi's disease in Negroes. Arch Ophthalmol 81:501, 1969

Zimmerman LE, Fine BS: Myelin artifacts in the optic disc and retina. Arch Ophthalmol 74:394, 1965

VASCULAR DISEASE

Archer DB, Ernest JT, Newell FW: Classification of branch retinal vein obstruction. Trans Am Acad Ophthalmol Otolaryngol 78:148, 1974

Ashton N: The eye in malignant hypertension. Trans Am Acad Ophthalmol Otolaryngol 76:17, 1972

Ball CJ: Atheromatous embolism to the brain, retina, and choroid. Arch Ophthalmol 76:690, 1966

Bilchik RC, Muller-Bergh HA, Freshman ME: Ischemic retinopathy due to carbon monoxide poisoning. Arch Ophthalmol 86:142, 1971

Brownstein S, Font RL, Alper MG: Atheromatous plaques of the retinal blood vessels. Arch Ophthalmol 90:49, 1973

Cohen DN: Temporal arteritis: an improvement in visual prognosis and management with repeat biopsies. Trans Am Acad Ophthalmol Otolaryngol 77:74, 1973

Cohen DN, Smith TR: Skip areas in temporal arteritis: myth versus fact. Trans Am Acad Ophthalmol Otolaryngol 78:772, 1974

Dahrling BE: The histopathology of early central retinal artery occlusion. Arch Ophthalmol 73:506, 1965

David NJ, Gilbert DS, Gass JDM: Fluorescein angiography in retinal arterial branch obstructions. Am J Ophthalmol 69:43, 1970

Davis DG, Smith JL: Retinal involvement in hereditary hemorrhagic telangiectasia. Arch Ophthalmol 85:618, 1971

Dryden RM: Central retinal vein occlusion and chronic simple glaucoma. Arch Ophthalmol 73:659, 1965

Eagle RC, Yanoff M, Fine BS: Hemoglobin SC retinopathy and fat emboli to the eye. A light and electron microscopical study. Arch Ophthalmol 92:28, 1974

Ferry AP, Leopold IH: Marginal (ring) corneal ulcer as presenting manifestations of Wegener's granuloma: a clinicopathologic study. Trans Am Acad Ophthalmol Otolaryngol 74:1276, 1970

Font RL, Naumann G: Ocular histopathology in pulseless disease. Arch Ophthalmol 82:784, 1969

Friedman E, Smith TR, Kuwabara T, Beyer CK: Choroidal vascular patterns in hypertension. Arch Ophthalmol 71:842, 1964

Gass JDM: A fluorescein angiographic study of macular dysfunction secondary to retinal vascular disease. I. Embolic retinal artery obstruction. Arch Ophthalmol 80:535, 1968

Gass JDM: A fluorescein angiographic study of macular dysfunction secondary to retinal vascular disease. II. Retinal vein occlusion. Arch Ophthalmol 80:550, 1968

Gass JDM: A fluorescein angiographic study of macular dysfunction secondary to retinal vascular disease. III. Hypertensive retinopathy. Arch Ophthalmol 80:569, 1968

Gass JDM: A fluorescein angiographic study of macular dysfunction secondary to retinal vascular disease. IV. Diabetic retinal angiopathy. Arch Ophthalmol 80:583, 1968

Gass JDM: A fluorescein angiographic study of macular dysfunction secondary to retinal vascular disease. V. Retinal telangiectasis. Arch Ophthalmol 80:592, 1968

Gass JDM: A fluorescein angiographic study of macular dysfunction secondary to retinal vascular disease. VI. X-ray irradiation, carotid artery occlusion, collagen vascular disease, and vitritis. Arch Ophthalmol 80:606, 1968

Gass JDM: Cavernous hemangioma of the retina: A neuro-oculocutaneous syndrome. Am J Ophthalmol 71:799, 1971

Gold DH, Morris DA, Henkind P: Ocular findings in systemic lupus erythematosus. Br J Ophthalmol 56:800, 1972

Goldberg MF: Classification and pathogenesis of proliferative sickle retinopathy. Am J Ophthalmol 71:649, 1971

Goldberg MF, Charache S, Acacio I: Ophthalmologic manifestations of sickle cell thalassemia. Arch Intern Med 128:33, 1971

Gutman FA, Zegarra H: The natural course of temporal retinal branch occlusion. Trans Am Acad Ophthalmol Otolaryngol 78:178, 1974

Hayreh SS: Pathogenesis of occlusion of the central retinal vessels. Am J Ophthalmol 72:998, 1971

Hayreh SS: Occlusion of the posterior ciliary arteries. Trans Am Acad Ophthalmol Otolaryngol 77:300, 1973

Henkind P: Radial peripapillary capillaries: Past—Present–Future, in Fluorescein Angiography. Edited by K Shimizu. Tokyo, Igaku Shoin Ltd, 1974, pp 91–95

Jampol LM, Wong AS, Albert DM: Atrial myxoma and central retinal artery occlusion. Am J Ophthalmol 75:242, 1973

Karjalainen K: Occlusion of the central retinal artery and retinal branch arterioles. Acta Ophthalmol [Suppl] (Kbh) 109:9, 1971

Kimura T: Arteriolar sclerosis of the human retina. Eye Ear Nose Throat Mon 53:52, 647, 1974

Klien BA: Sidelights on retinal venous occlusion. Am J Ophthalmol 61:25, 1966

Konner EM, Dollery CT, Shakib M, Henkind P, Patterson JW, de Oliveira LNF, Bulpitt CJ: Experimental retinal branch vein occlusion. Am J Ophthalmol 69:778, 1970

Kroll AJ: Experimental central retinal artery occlusion. Arch Ophthalmol 79:453, 1968

Maumenee AE, Emery JM: An anatomic classification of diseases of the macula. Trans Am Acad Ophthalmol Otolaryngol 74:594, 1972

Michels RG, Gass JDM: The natural history of retinal branch vein obstruction. Trans Am Acad Ophthalmol Otolaryngol 78:166, 1974

Michelson PE, Knox DL, Green WR: Ischemic ocular inflammation: a clinicopathologic case report. Arch Ophthalmol 86:274, 1971

Morse PH: Elschnig's spots and hypertensive choroidopathy. Am J Ophthalmol 66:844, 1968

Penner R, Font RL: Retinal embolism from calcified vegetations of aortic valve. Spontaneous complications of rheumatic heart disease. Arch Ophthalmol 81:565, 1969

Robertson DM: Macroaneurysms of the retinal arteries. Trans Am Acad Ophthalmol Otolaryngol 77:55, 1973

Romayananda N, Goldberg MF, Green WR: Histopathology of sickle cell retinopathy. Trans Am Acad Ophthalmol Otolaryngol 77:652, 1973

Ross R, Glomset JA: Atherosclerosis and the arterial smooth muscle cell. Science 180:1332, 1973

Rothstein T: Bilateral central retinal vein closure as the initial manifestation of polycythemia. Am J Ophthalmol 74:256, 1972

Rubenstein RA, Yanoff M, Albert DM: Thrombocytopenia, anemia, and retinal hemorrhage. Am J Ophthalmol 65:435, 1968

Sandok BA: Temporal arteritis. J Am Med Assoc 222:1405, 1972

Schneider HA, Weber AA, Ballen PH: The visual prognosis in temporal arteritis. Ann Ophthalmol 3:1215, 1971

Serjeant GR, Serjeant BE, Condon PI: The conjunctival sign in sickle cell anemia. J Am Med Assoc 219:1428, 1972

Shults WT, Swan KC: Pulsatile aneurysms of the retinal arterial tree. Am J Ophthalmol 77:304, 1974

Stein MR, Gay AJ: Acute chorioretinal infarction in sickle cell trait. Report of a case. Arch Ophthalmol 84:485, 1970

Theodossiadis G: Fluorescein angiography in Eales' disease. Am J Ophthalmol 69:271, 1970

Ts'o MOM, Bettman JW: Occlusion of choriocapillaris in primary nonfamilial amyloidosis. Arch Ophthalmol 86:281, 1971

Williams DF, Drance SM, Harris GS, Fairclough M: Diabetic cotton-wool spots: evaluation using perimetric and angiographic techniques. Can J Ophthalmol 5:68, 1970

Wilson RS, Ruiz RS: Bilateral central retinal artery occlusion in homocystinuria. A case report. Arch Ophthalmol 82:267, 1969

Wolter JR: Double embolism of the central retinal artery and one long posterior ciliary artery followed by secondary hemorrhagic glaucoma. Am J Ophthalmol 73:651, 1972

Yanoff M: Ocular pathology of diabetes. Am J Ophthalmol 67:21, 1969

INFLAMMATION

Deutman AF, Oosterhuis JA, Boen-Tan TN, Aan De Kerk AL: Acute posterior multifocal placoid pigment epitheliopathy. Pigment epitheliopathy or choriocapillaritis. Br J Ophthalmol 56:863, 1972

Dobbie JG: Toxoplasma retinochoroiditis. Successful isolation of Toxoplasma gondii from subretinal fluid of the living human eye. Ann Ophthalmol 2:509, 1970

Fine BS: Intraocular mycotic infections. Lab Invest 11:1161, 1962

Fitzpatrick PJ, Robertson DM: Acute posterior multifocal placoid pigment epitheliopathy. Arch Ophthalmol 89:373, 1973

Gass JDM: Acute multifocal placoid pigment epitheliopathy. Arch Ophthalmol 80:177, 1968

Gills JP Jr, Buckley CE III: Cyclophosphamide therapy of Behçet's disease. Ann Ophthalmol 2:399, 1970

Krill AE, Deutman AF: Acute retinal pigment epitheliitis. Am J Ophthalmol 74:193, 1972

Maumenee AE, Emery JM: An anatomic classification of diseases of the macula. Trans Am Acad Ophthalmol Otolaryngol 74:594, 1972

Nelson DA, Weiner A, Yanoff M, DePeralta J: Retinal lesions in subacute sclerosing panencephalitis. Arch Ophthalmol 84:613, 1970

Ryan SJ, Maumenee AE: Acute posterior multifocal placoid pigment epitheliopathy. Am J Ophthalmol 74:1066, 1972

Yanoff M: The Retina in rubella, in Retinal Diseases in Children. Edited by W Tasman. New York, Harper & Row, 1971, pp 223–232

DEGENERATIONS

Beyer NE: Clinical study of senile retinoschisis. Arch Ophthalmol 79:36, 1968

Carr RE, Siegel IM: Retinal function in patients treated with indomethacin. Am J Ophthalmol 75:302, 1973

Curtin BJ, Karlin DB: Axial length measurements and fundus changes of the myopic eye. Am J Ophthalmol 71:42, 1971

Fine BS: Retinal structure: light- and electron-microscopic observations, in New and Controversial Aspects of Retinal Detachment. Edited by A McPherson. New York, Harper & Row, 1968, pp 16–52

Foos RY, Feman SS: Reticular cystoid degeneration of the peripheral retina. Am J Ophthalmol 69:392, 1970

Frayer WC: Elevated lesions of the macular area. A histopathologic study emphasizing lesions similar to disciform degeneration of the macula. Arch Ophthalmol 53:82, 1955

Ganley JP, Smith RE, Knox DL, Cornstock GW: Presumed ocular histoplasmosis. III. Epidemiologic characteristics of people with peripheral atrophic scars. Arch Ophthalmol 83:116, 1970

Gass JDM: Pathogenesis of disciform detachment of the neuroepithelium. I. General concepts and classification. Am J Ophthalmol 63:573, 1967

Gass JDM: Pathogenesis of disciform detachment of the neuroepithelium. II. Idiopathic central serous choroidopathy. Am J Ophthalmol 63:587, 1967

Gass JDM: Pathogenesis of disciform detachment of the neuroepithelium. III. Senile disciform macular degeneration. Am J Ophthalmol 63:617, 1967

Gass JDM: Pathogenesis of disciform detachment of the neuroepithelium. V. Disciform macular degeneration secondary to focal choroiditis. Am J Ophthalmol 63:661, 1967

Gass JDM: Pathogenesis of disciform detachment of the neuroepithelium. VI. Disciform detachment secondary to heredodegenerative, neoplastic and traumatic lesions of the choroid. Am J Ophthalmol 63:689, 1967

Gass JDM: Drusen and disciform macular detachment and degeneration. Arch Ophthalmol 90:206, 1973

Green WR, Gass JDM: Senile disciform degeneration of the macula. Retinal arterialization of the fibrous plaque demonstrated clinically and histopathologically. Arch Ophthalmol 86:487, 1971

Hayreh SS: Postradiation retinopathy: fluorescence fundus angiographic study. Br J Ophthalmol 54:705, 1970

Henkes HE, vanLith GHM, Canta LR: Indomethacin retinopathy. Am J Ophthalmol 73:846, 1972

Hodgkinson BJ, Kobb H: A preliminary study of the effect of chloroquine on the rat retina. Arch Ophthalmol 84:509, 1970

Inomata H: Electron microscopic observations on cystoid degeneration in the peripheral retina. Jap J Ophthalmol 10:26, 1966

Johnson BL, Storey JD: Proteinaceous cysts of the ciliary epithelium. I. Their clear nature and immuno-electrophoretic analysis in a case of multiple myeloma. Arch Ophthalmol 84:166, 1970

Klintworth GK, Hollingsworth AS, Lusman PA, Bradford WD: Granulomatous choroiditis in a case of disseminated histoplasmosis. Arch Ophthalmol 90:45, 1973

Krill AE, Deutman AE: Dominant macular degeneration. Am J Ophthalmol 73:352, 1972

Krill AE, Potts AM, Johnson BS: Cloroquine retinopathy. Investigation of discrepancy between dark adaptation and electro-retinographic findings in advanced stages. Am J Ophthalmol 71:530, 1971

Maumenee AE, Emery JM: An anatomic classification of diseases of the macula. Trans Am Acad Ophthalmol Otolaryngol 74:594, 1972

Mazow ML, Ruiz RS: Eccentric disciform degeneration. Trans Am Acad Ophthalmol Otolaryngol 77:68, 1973

McFarlane JR, Yanoff M, Scheie HG: Toxic retinopathy following sparsomycin therapy. Arch Ophthalmol 76:532, 1966

O'Malley PF, Allen RA: Peripheral cystoid degeneration of the retina: incidence and distribution in 1,000 autopsy eyes. Arch Ophthalmol 77:769, 1967

O'Malley PF, Allen RA, Straatsma BR, O'Malley CC: Paving stone degeneration of the retina. Arch Ophthalmol 73:169, 1965

Ramsey MS, Fine BS: Chloroquine toxicity in the human eye. Histopathologic observations by electron microscopy. Am J Ophthalmol 73:229, 1972

Sarks SH: New vessel formation beneath the retinal pigment epithelium in senile eyes. Br J Ophthalmol 57:951, 1973

Schlernitzauer DA, Green WR: Peripheral retinal albinotic spots. Am J Ophthalmol 72:729, 1971

Straatsma BR, Foos RY: Typical and reticular degenerative retinoschisis. Am J Ophthalmol 75:551, 1973

Teeters VW, Bird AC: The development of neovascularization of senile disciform macular degeneration. Am J Ophthalmol 76:1, 1973

Yanoff M, Rahn EK, Zimmerman LE: Histopathology of juvenile retinoschisis. Arch Ophthalmol 79:49, 1968

Yanoff M, Tsou K-C: Tetrazolium studies of the whole eye: effect of chloroquine in the incubation medium. Am J Ophthalmol 59:808, 1965

Zimmerman LE, Naumann G: The Pathology of retinoschisis, in New and Controversial Aspects of Retinal Detachment. Edited by A McPherson. St. Louis, Mosby, 1968, pp 400–423

Zimmerman LE, Spencer WH: The pathologic anatomy of retinoschisis, with a report of two cases diagnosed clinically as malignant melanomas. Arch Ophthalmol 63:10, 1960

HEREDITARY PRIMARY RETINAL DYSTROPHIES

Albert DM, Beltzer AI: Retinitis punctata albescens in a Negro child studied with fluorescein angiography. Arch Ophthalmol 81:170, 1969

Babel J, Stangos N: Progressive degeneration of the photopic system. Am J Ophthalmol 75:511, 1973

Betten MG, Bilchik RC, Smith ME: Pigmentary retinopathy of myotonic dystrophy. Am J Ophthalmol 72:720, 1971

Brodrick JD, Dark AJ: Corneal dystrophy in Cockayne's syndrome. Br J Ophthalmol 57:391, 1973

Burns RP, Lovrien EW, Cibis AB: Juvenile sex-linked retinoschisis: clinical and genetic studies. Trans Am Acad Ophthalmol Otolaryngol 75:1011, 1971

Cherry PM: Usher's syndrome. Ann Ophthalmol 5:743, 1973

Cross HE: Systemic disorders associated with retinitis pigmentosa-like fundus abnormalities. Personal communication.

Deutman AF: The Hereditary Dystrophies of the Posterior Pole of the Eye. Springfield, Thomas, 1971

Edwards WC, Price WD, Macdonald R: Congenital amaurosis of retinal origin (Leber). Am J Ophthalmol 72:724, 1971

François J: The diagnostic importance of functional electrooculography in some hereditary dystrophies of the eye fundus. Ann Ophthalmol 3:929, 1971

Fraser HB, Wallace DC: Sorsby's familial pseudo-inflammatory macular dystrophy. Am J Ophthalmol 71:1216, 1971

Gelber PF, Shah A: Fluorescein study of albipunctate dystrophy. Arch Ophthalmol 81:164, 1969

Gouras P, Carr RE, Gunkel RD: Retinitis pigmentosa in abetalipoproteinemia: effects of vitamin A. Invest Ophthalmol 10:784, 1971

Hirose T, Lee KY, Schepens CL: Wagner's hereditary vitreoretinal degeneration and retinal detachment. Arch Ophthalmol 89:176, 1973

Holland MG, Cambie E, Kloepfer W: An evaluation of genetic carriers of Usher's syndrome. Am J Ophthalmol 74:940, 1972

Kandori F, Tamai A, Kurimoto S, Fukunaga K: Fleck retina. Arch Ophthalmol 73:673, 1972

Kolb H, Gouras P: Electron microscopic observations of human retinitis pigmentosa, dominantly inherited. Invest Ophthalmol 13:487, 1974

Krill AE, Archer D: Classification of the choroid atrophies. Am J Ophthalmol 72:562, 1971

Krill AE, Archer D, Newell FW: Fluorescein angiography in retinitis pigmentosa. Arch Ophthalmol 69:826, 1970

Krill AE, Deutman AF: Dominant macular degenerations. The cone dystrophies. Am J Ophthalmol 73:352, 1972

MacVicar JE, Wilbrandt HR: Hereditary retinoschisis and early hemeralopia. Arch Ophthalmol 83:629, 1970

Manschot WA: Pathology of hereditary juvenile retinoschisis. Arch Ophthalmol 88:131, 1972

Maumenee AE, Emery JM: An anatomic classification of diseases of the macula. Trans Am Acad Ophthalmol Otolaryngol 74:594, 1972

Mausolf FA, Burns CA, Burian HM: Morphologic and functional retinal changes in myotonic dystrophy unrelated to quinine therapy. Am J Ophthalmol 74:1141, 1972

McLeod AC, McConnell FE, Sweeny A, Cooper M, Nance WE: Clinical variation in Usher's syndrome. Arch Otolaryngol 94:321, 1971

Newell FW, Krill AE, Farkas TG: Drusen and fundus flavimaculatus: clinical, functional and histologic charac-

teristics. Trans Am Acad Ophthalmol Otolaryngol 76:88, 1972

Nishida S, Misuno K: Electron microscopy of pigmentary degeneration of the human retina (in Japanese). Acta Soc Ophthalmol Jap 75:1779, 1971

Reinstein NM, Chalfin AI: Inverse retinitis pigmentosa, deafness and hypogenitalism. Am J Ophthalmol 72:332, 1971

Robertson DM: Hamartomas of the optic disc with retinitis pigmentosa. Am J Ophthalmol 74:526, 1972

Roth AM, Hepler RS, Mukoyama M, Cancilla PA, Foos RY: Pigmentary retinal dystrophy in Hallervorden-Spatz disease: clinicopathological report of a case. Survey Ophthalmol 16:24, 1971

Ryan SJ, Smith RE: Retinopathy associated with hereditary olivopontocerebellar degeneration. Am J Ophthalmol 71:838, 1971

Sperling MA, Hiles DA, Kennerdell JS: Electroretinographic responses following vitamin A therapy in A-beta-lipoproteinemia. Am J Ophthalmol 73:342, 1972

Toussaint D, Danis P: An ocular pathologic study of Refsum's syndrome. Am J Ophthalmol 72:342, 1971

Yanoff M, Rahn EK, Zimmerman LE: Histopathology of juvenile retinoschisis. Arch Ophthalmol 79:49, 1968

HEREDITARY SECONDARY RETINAL DYSTROPHIES

Armstrong D, Dimitt S, Van Wormer DE: Studies in Batten disease. I. Peroxidase deficiency in granulocytes. Arch Neurol 30:144, 1974

Brady RO, Johnson WG, Uhlendorf BW: Identification of heterozygous carriers of lipid storage diseases. Current status and clinical applications (editorial). Am J Med 51:423, 1971

Cogan DG: Retinal architecture and pathophysiology: the Sanford R. Gifford lecture. Am J Ophthalmol 54:347, 1962

Cogan DG, Kuwabara T: The sphingolipidoses and the eye. Arch Ophthalmol 79:437, 1968

Cogan DG, Kuwabara T, Moser H: Metachromatic leukodystrophy. Ophthalmologica 160:2, 1970

Cotlier E: Tay-Sachs' retina: deficiency of acetyl hexosaminidase A. Arch Ophthalmol 86:352, 1971

Cotlier E: Biochemical detection of inborn errors of metabolism affecting the eye. Trans Am Acad Ophthalmol Otolaryngol 76:1165, 1972

Emery JM, Green WR, Huff DS: Krabbe's disease. Histopathology and ultrastructure of the eye. Am J Ophthalmol 74:400, 1972

Emery JM, Green WR, Huff DS, Sloan HR: Niemann-Pick disease (type C). Histopathology and ultrastructure. Am J Ophthalmol 74:1144, 1972

Fine RN, Wilson WA, Donnell GN: Retinal changes in glycogen storage disease type I. Am J Dis Child 115:328, 1968

Font RL: Fine BS: Ocular pathology in Fabry's disease. Histochemical and electron microscopic observations. Am J Ophthalmol 73:419, 1972

Gambetti P, DiMauro S, Hirt L, Blume RP: Myoclonic epilepsy with Lafora bodies: some ultrastructural, histochemical and biochemical aspects. Arch Neurol 25:483, 1971

Garner A: Ocular pathology of GM$_2$ gangliosidosis type 2 (Sandhoff's disease). Br J Ophthalmol 57:514, 1973

Gass JDM, Clarkson JG: Angioid streaks and disciform macular detachment in Paget's disease (osteitis deformans). Am J Ophthalmol 75:576, 1973

Gilbert WR, Smith JL, Nylan WL: The Sjögren-Larsson syndrome. Arch Ophthalmol 80:308, 1968

Goebel HH, Fix JD, Zeman W: Retinal pathology in GM$_1$ gangliosidosis, type II. Am J Ophthalmol 75:434, 1973

Goebel HH, Fix JD, Zeman W: The fine structure of the retina in neuronal ceroid-lipofuscinosis. Am J Ophthalmol 77:25, 1974

Goldberg MF, Cotlier E, Fichenscher LG, Kenyon K, Enat R, Borowsky SA: Macular cherry-red spot, corneal clouding, and β-galactosidase deficiency. Arch Intern Med 128:387, 1971

Harcourt B, Ashton N: Ultrastructure of the optic nerve in Krabbe's leucodystrophy. Br J Ophthalmol 57:885, 1973

Hug G, Garancis JC, Schubert WK, Kaplan M: Glycogen storage disease, Types II, III, VII, and IX. Am J Dis Child 111:457, 1966

Ishii T, Gonatas NK: The multilamellar cytosome in late infantile amaurotic idiocy. Acta Neuropathol (Berl) 19:265, 1971

Keith CG: Retinal atrophy in osteopetrosis. Arch Ophthalmol 79:234, 1968

Kenyon KR, Sensenbrenner JA: Mucolipidosis II (I-cell disease): ultrastructural observations of conjunctiva and skin. Invest Ophthalmol 10:568, 1971

Maumenee AE, Emery JM: An anatomic classification of diseases of the macula. Trans Am Acad Ophthalmol Otolaryngol 74:594, 1972

Miller WL, Reimann BEF: Childhood variant of Niemann-Pick disease: report of a case with biochemical, histochemical and electron microscopic observations. Am J Clin Pathol 58:450, 1972

O'Brien JS: Five gangliosidoses (letter to the editor). Lancet 2:805, 1969

Quigley HA, Goldberg MF: Conjunctival ultrastructure in mucolipidosis III (pseudo-Hurler polydystrophy). Invest Ophthalmol 10:568, 1971

Raafat F, Hashemian MP, Abrishami MA: Wolman's disease: report of two cases, with a review of the literature. Am J Clin Pathol 59:490, 1973

Rahman AN: The ocular manifestations of hereditary dystopic lipoidosis (angiokeratoma corporis diffusum universale). Arch Ophthalmol 69:708, 1963

Rahn EK, Yanoff M, Tucker S: Neuro-ocular considerations in the Pelizaeus-Merzbacher syndrome: a clinicopathologic study. Am J Ophthalmol 66:1143, 1968

Ramsey MB, Yanoff M, Fine BS: Ocular histopathology in homocystinuria. Am J Ophthalmol 74:377, 1972

Robb RM, Kuwabara T: The ocular pathology of type A Niemann-Pick disease. A light and electron microscopic study. Invest Ophthalmol 12:366, 1973

Rywlin AM, Lopez-Gomez A, Tachmes P, Pardo V: Ceroid histiocytosis of the spleen in hyperlipemia: relationship to the syndrome of sea-blue histiocyte. Am J Clin Pathol 56:572, 1971

Schwarz GA, Yanoff M: Lafora bodies, corpora amylacea and Lewey bodies—a morphologic and histochemical study. Arch Neurobiol (Madr) 28:801, 1965

Seringe P, Dhermy P, Aaron J-J: Les manifestations oculaires de la gengliosidose généralisée à G$_{M1}$ (maladie de Norman-Landing). Arch Ophthalmol (Paris) 30:113, 1970

Smith RS, Reinecke RD: Electron microscopy of ocular muscle in type II glycogenosis (Pompe's disease). Am J Ophthalmol 73:965, 1972

Spaeth GL: Ocular manifestations of the lipidoses, in Retinal Diseases in Children. Edited by W Tasman. New York, Harper & Row, 1971, pp. 127–206

Spranger JW, Wiedemann H-R: The genetic mucolipidoses: diagnoses and differential diagnosis. Humangenetik 9:113, 1970

Sugita M, Dulaney JT, Moser HW: Ceramidase deficiency in Farber's disease (lipogranulomatosis). Science 178:1100, 1972

Toussaint D, Denis P: Ocular histopathology in generalized glycogenosis (Pompe's disease). Arch Ophthalmol 73:342, 1965

Towfighi J, Baird HW, Gambatti P, Gonatas NK: The significance of cytoplasmic inclusions in late infantile and juvenile amaurotic idiocy. Acta Neuropathol (Berl) 23:32, 1973

Tremblay M, Szots F: GM$_2$ type 2-gangliosidosis (Sandhoff's disease): ocular and pathological manifestations. Am J Ophthalmol 9:338, 1974

Weiss MJ, Krill AE, Dawson G, Hindman J, Cotlier E: GM$_1$ gangliosidosis type I. Am J Ophthalmol 76:999, 1973

Weiter J, Farkas TG: Retinal abnormalities in lactosyl ceramidosis. Am J Ophthalmol 76:804, 1973

Witzleben CL, Smith K, Nelson JS, Monteleone PL, Livingston D: Ultrastructural studies in late-onset amaurotic idiocy: lymphocyte inclusions as a diagnostic marker. J Pediatr 79:285, 1971

Yanoff M, Schwarz GA: The retinal pathology of Lafora's disease: a form of glycoprotein-acid mucopolysaccharide dystrophy. Trans Am Acad Ophthalmol Otolaryngol 69:701, 1965

Zeman W: Neuronal ceroid-lipofuscinosis (Batten's disease); relationship to amaurotic family idiocy? Pediatrics 44:570, 1969

SYSTEMIC DISEASES INVOLVING THE RETINA

See bibliography above under Vascular Disease, Hereditary Primary Retinal Dystrophies and Hereditary Secondary Retinal Dystrophies.

TUMORS

Ganley JP, Streeten BW: Glial nodules of the inner retina. Am J Ophthalmol 71:1099, 1971

Yanoff M, Zimmerman LE, Davis R: Massive gliosis of the retina. A continuous spectrum of glial proliferation. Int Ophthalmol Clin 11:211, 1971

RETINAL DETACHMENT

Apple DJ, Goldberg MF, Wyhinny G: Histopathology and ultrastructure of the argon laser lesion in human retinal and choroidal vasculature. Am J Ophthalmol 75:595, 1973

Boniuk M, Butler FC: An autopsy study of lattice degeneration, retinal breaks, and retinal pits, in New and Controversial Aspects of Retinal Detachments. Edited by A McPherson. New York, Harper & Row, 1968, pp 59–75

Byer NE: Changes in and prognosis of lattice degeneration of the retina. Trans Am Acad Ophthalmol Otolaryngol 78:114, 1974

Davis MD: The natural history of retinal breaks without detachment. Trans Am Ophthalmol Soc 71:343, 1973

Meyer E, Kurz GH: Retinal pits: a study of pathologic findings in two cases. Arch Ophthalmol 70:102, 1963

Powell JO, Bresnick GH, Yanoff M, Frisch GD, Chester JE: Ocular effects of argon laser radiation. II. Histopathology of chorioretinal lesions. Am J Ophthalmol 71:1267, 1971

Roth AM, Foos RY: Surface wrinkling retinopathy in eyes enucleated at autopsy. Trans Am Acad Ophthalmol Otolaryngol 75:1047, 1971

Schepens CL, Elzeneiny II, Moura P, Morse P, Kraushar MF: Aphakic and phakic retinal detachment. Arch Ophthalmol 89:476, 1973

Spencer LM, Foos RY, Straatsma BR: Meridional folds, meridional complexes, and associated abnormalities of the peripheral retina. Am J Ophthalmol 70:697, 1970

Straatsma BR, Zeegen PD, Foos RY, Feman SS, Shabo AL: Lattice degeneration of the retina. Trans Am Acad Ophthalmol Otolaryngol 78:87, 1974

Streeten BW, Bert M: The retinal surface in lattice degeneration of the retina. Am J Ophthalmol 74:1201, 1972

Yanoff M: Formaldehyde-glutaraldehyde fixation. Am J Ophthalmol 76:303, 1973

chapter 12

Vitreous

CONGENITAL ANOMALIES

PERSISTENT PRIMARY VITREOUS

Remnants of the primitive hyaloid vascular system can persist into adulthood as anterior or posterior remnants, or the entire hyaloid vessel from the optic disc to its lenticular attachment can remain (it may or may not contain blood).

I. Anterior remnants (Figs. 9–1 and 12–1)
   A. The lenticular portion of the hyaloid artery may hang free in the vitreous from its lens attachment site.
   B. Mittendorf dot is an opacity just below and nasal to the posterior pole of the lens marking the lenticular attachment site of the hyaloid artery.
II. Posterior remnants (Figs. 12–1 and 12–2)
   A. Vascular loops from the optic disc may remain within Cloquet's canal.
   B. Bergmeister's papilla is the glial remnant of the hyaloid system in the region of the optic disc.

   The papilla may appear as solid masses of whitish tissue, as delicate ragged strands or as a well-defined membrane stretching over the disc (*prepapillary membrane*).

   C. Congenital cysts are the cystic remains of the hyaloid system, which are usually pearly gray, wrinkled and translucent.

   They generally are free floating but may be attached to the optic disc or suspended by a pedicle.

PERSISTENT HYPERPLASTIC PRIMARY VITREOUS (PHPV)

See p. 698 in Chapter 18.

INFLAMMATION

ACUTE

See Chapter 3.

CHRONIC

See Chapters 3 and 4.

VITREOUS ADHESIONS

POSTTRAUMATIC AND POSTSURGICAL

See Chapter 5.

I. Vitreocorneal adhesions may cause corneal "touch" syndrome.
II. Iridovitreal adhesions may lead to total posterior synechias (*seclusion of pupil*) with resultant iris bombé, or they may form a membrane across the pupil (*occlusion of pupil*), or both.
III. Cyclovitreal adhesions may lead to a cyclitic membrane and subsequent retinal detachment.
IV. Vitreoretinal adhesions may lead to the macular vitreous traction syndrome (*Irvine-Gass-Norton syndrome*) or to wrinkling of the internal limiting membrane, i.e., "cellophane" retina.

   Vitreal traction of the attached vitreous on normal paravascular vitreoretinal attachment sites in an eye with a posterior vitreous detachment can cause retinal tears (Figs. 12–3 and 12–4). Retinal tears tend to occur in clusters between the equator and the posterior border of the vitreous base.

POSTINFLAMMATION

See Chapters 3 and 4.

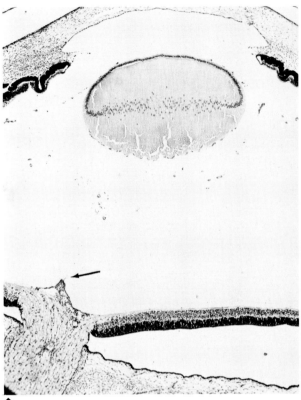

FIG. 12–1. Twelve-week-old fetus. Vessels of primary (or vascularized) vitreous are visible clearly in zone around posterior lens surface. Portion of hyaloid vessel (*arrow*) projects from glial tissue (papilla of Bergmeister) on optic nerve head. H&E, ×35.

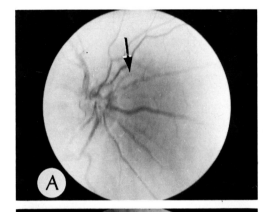

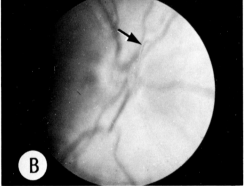

FIG. 12–2. Posterior remnants. **A.** Fundus photograph with focus just anterior to optic disc to show persistent hyaloid vessel (*arrow*) in 22-year-old man. **B.** Focus in posterior part of vitreous to show hyaloid vessel (*arrow*) running anteriorly where it inserts on posterior aspect of lens. **C.** Bergmeister's papilla, glial remnant of hyaloid system, persists (*arrow*) in eye from adult. **A,** fundus; **B,** fundus; **C,** H&E, ×16.

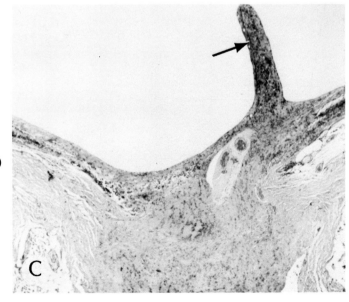

IDIOPATHIC

Idiopathic vitreous adhesions may follow partial vitreoretinal separation (posterior vitreous detachment).

VITREOUS OPACITIES

HYALOID VESSEL REMNANTS

Muscae volitantes are minute remnants of the hyaloid vascular system or detachments of small folds of poorly differentiated retinal tissue, usually present in the anterior vitreous.

Muscae volitantes also is an historical, obsolete term for acquired vitreous floaters.

ACQUIRED VITREOUS STRANDS AND FLOATERS

I. Collapse and condensation of vitreous sheets with aging, especially in myopes, frequently cause the formation of strands and floaters.
II. Separation of the vitreous attachment to the optic disc following posterior vitreoretinal separation may cause a complete or incomplete ringlike floater (partial or complete vitreous "peephole").

INFLAMMATORY CELLS

I. "Snowball" opacities (microabscesses) may occur with mycotic infections (especially with the mold fungi).

II. Diffuse whitish masses ("white balls") inferiorly may be seen with vitritis, e.g., with sarcoidosis.

RED BLOOD CELLS

Red blood cells in the vitreous compartment most often are due to retinal tears but may have many other causes.

Red blood cells may be subvitreal, i.e., between vitreous body and internal limiting membrane of the retina, or intravitreal, i.e., within the vitreous body. The relative hypoxia of the vitreous body may be illustrated dramatically when blood enters it in a patient with sickle cell trait or disease (Fig. 12–5). Sickling and hemolysis of the erythrocytes occur with increased incidence toward the most hypoxic, i.e., central, vitreous. Occasionally the diagnosis of sickle cell trait or disease is made by such histologic evidence in a person not known previously to be so affected.

IRIDESCENT PARTICLES

I. Asteroid hyalosis (Benson's disease) (Figs. 12–6 and 12–7). Asteroid hyalosis consists of crystals embedded in an amorphous matrix containing calcium, sulfur and phosphorus and attached to the vitreous framework. The condition is of unknown cause with the following clinical properties.
 A. Gold colored balls with edge illumi-

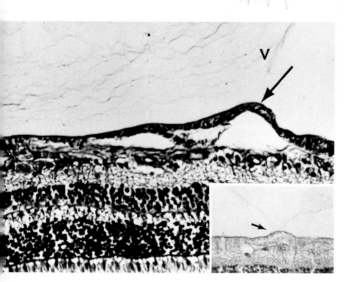

FIG. 12–3. Partially detached vitreous (*v*) causes traction and tenting up of retina (*arrow*) at point of attachment. **Inset** shows traction on retina (*arrow*) at site of vitreous attachment. **Main figure**, trichrome, ×101; **inset**, H&E, ×50.

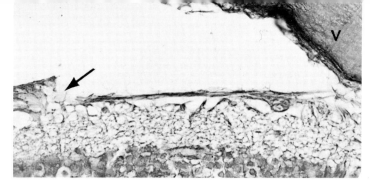

FIG. 12–4. Vitreous (*v*) detachment (retraction) has torn inner layers of retina (*arrow*). Although possibly an artifactitious tear, it demonstrates what vitreous adherence followed by retraction can do. AMP, ×305.

FIG. 12–5. Hemorrhage into eye. **A.** Erythrocytes beneath retina (*r*) appear normal, while those in vitreous (*arrows*) are grossly sickled. Deepest part of vitreous is occupied by red blood cell ghosts (*g*) due to intense hemolysis in this relatively hypoxic region (see **B**). **B. Inset** shows grossly sickled red blood cells (*arrows*) in vitreous. Deeper region contains hemolyzed red blood cells (ghosts, *g*). Electron micrograph shows almost complete hemolysis of red blood cells (ghosts), free clumps of hemoglobin outside cells (*arrows*) and tip of sickled, nonhemolyzed cell (*rbc*) nearby. **A,** H&E, ×85; **B,** ×15,000; **inset,** H&E, ×530.

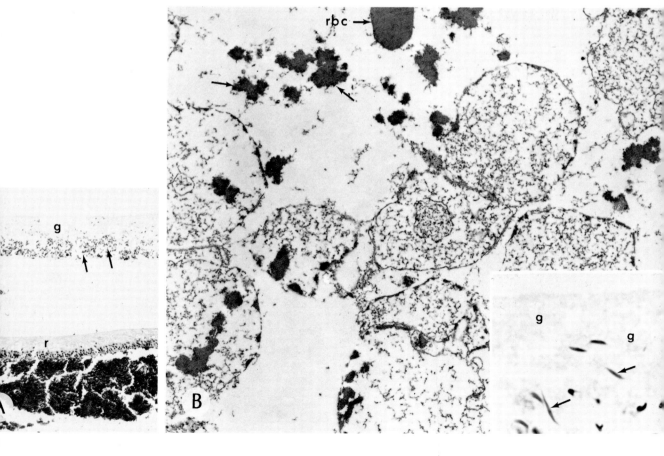

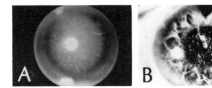

FIG. 12–6. Asteroid hyalosis. **A.** Fundus reflex view of white balls in vitreous. **B.** White balls in vitreous in anterior chamber in aphakic eye. **A,** fundus reflex; **B,** clinical.

FIG. 12–7. Asteroid hyalosis. **A.** Myriad tiny white spherules are suspended throughout vitreous framework. **B.** Bodies appear composed of outer dense ring and central homogeneous zone. **C.** Central zone contains birefringent material as seen in polarized light. **D.** Asteroid body is composed of round particles of equal size in symmetrical arrangement, growing more dense towards center. Particles appear embedded in matrix which merges with surrounding vitreous and seems to be of same substance. **A,** macroscopic; **B,** H&E, ×130; **C,** H&E, polarized, ×130; **D,** ×50,000.

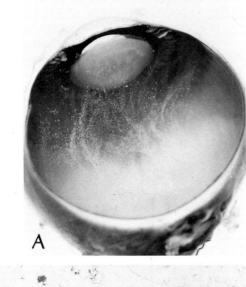

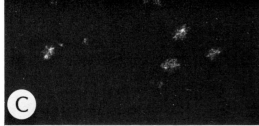

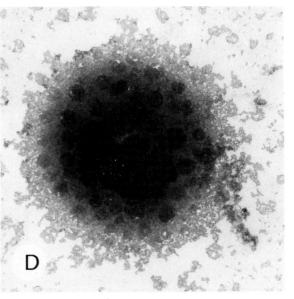

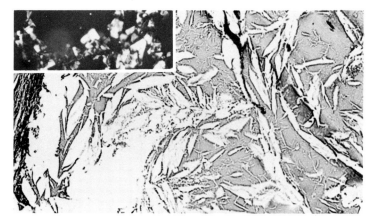

FIG. 12–8. Clefts in vitreous represent areas where cholesterol crystals had resided before processing of tissue dissolved them out. **Inset** shows birefringent cholesterol crystals obtained from anterior chamber fluid in eye with cholesterolosis bulbi. **Main figure,** H&E, ×40; **inset,** unstained, polarized, ×101.

(synchisis)

nation and white colored with direct view.

B. Remains attached to collagenous framework and only moves with oscillation of the collagenous framework.

C. Most are unilateral and commonest in seventh and eighth decades of life.

D. Infrequently associated with retinal detachment.

E. Histologically, asteroid bodies consist of an amorphous matrix which is PAS- and acid-mucopolysaccharide-positive and contains birefringent, small crystals when viewed with polarized light. Electronmicroscopically, the bodies are composed of electron-opaque particles arranged symmetrically.

II. Synchisis scintillans (Fig. 12–8). This disorder consists of degenerative material not attached to the vitreous framework with the following clinical properties:

A. Vitreous usually fluid.

B. Material appears as flat, angular crystalline particles.

When vitreous gains access into the anterior chamber, e.g., as in aphakia or with a dislocated lens, a synchisis scintillans of the anterior chamber results.

C. Golden in color both to retroillumination and to direct view.

D. Material settles inferiorly when the eye is immobile.

E. Usually bilateral and commonest in people under 35 years of age.

F. Frequently follows an intravitreal (within vitreous body) hemorrhage.

G. Histologically clefts are present within the vitreous, representing the sites of dissolved out cholesterol crystals.

TUMOR CELLS

I. Retinoblastomas frequently shed their cells into the vitreous body.

II. Malignant melanomas, metastatic carcinomas, and medulloepitheliomas (embryonal type) rarely shed their cells into the vitreous body.

PIGMENT DUST

I. Pigment dust follows intraocular trauma (nonsurgical or surgical); most frequently it is seen after cataract extraction and probably is derived from the posterior surface of the iris.

II. It also follows intraocular inflammation.

CYSTS

I. Congenital (see p. 470 above).

II. Cysticercus—see p. 93 in Chapter 4.

III. Echinococcus—see p. 97 in Chapter 4.

IV. Embryonal medulloepithelioma (diktyoma), on occasion, may shed cells into the vitreous body. The cells then may grow in a cystic fashion.

V. Retinoblastoma not infrequently may seed into the vitreous body. The tumor cells then tend to grow into cysts.

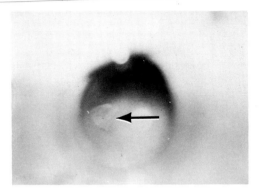

FIG. 12–9. Posterior vitreous detachment often recognized clinically in fundus reflex as ring opacity (*arrow*) in central part of vitreous compartment.

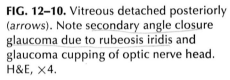

FIG. 12–11. Vitreous detached posteriorly (*arrows*) everywhere except over optic nerve (*o*). Retina (*r*) also is detached. H&E, ×5.

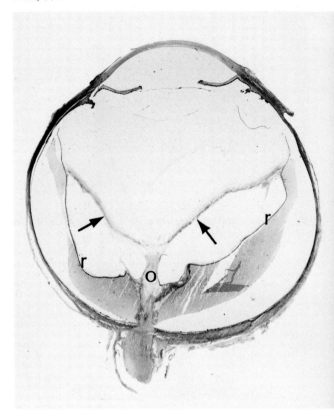

FIG. 12–10. Vitreous detached posteriorly (*arrows*). Note secondary angle closure glaucoma due to rubeosis iridis and glaucoma cupping of optic nerve head. H&E, ×4.

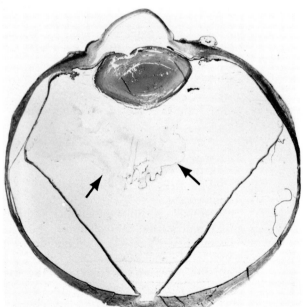

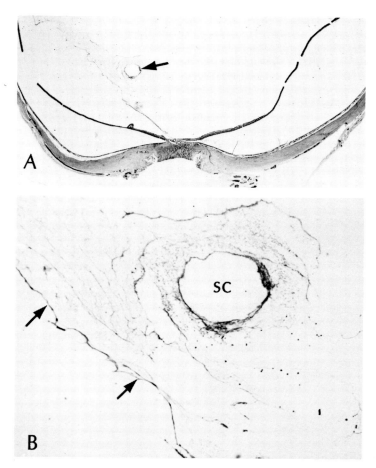

FIG. 12–12. Syneresis. **A.** Large area of cortical liquefaction and degeneration appears as hole (*arrow*) in cortical vitreous. **B.** Higher magnification to show edge of posteriorly detached vitreous (*arrows*) and syneresis cavity (*sc*). **A,** PAS, ×8; **B,** PAS, ×16.

RETINAL FRAGMENTS

A free-floating operculum is the nonattached or separated retinal tissue overlying and derived from a retinal hole.

TRAUMATIC AVULSION OF VITREOUS BASE

Traumatic avulsion of the vitreous base is rare and usually due to trauma or shrinkage of vitreal fibrous membranes.

ANTERIOR VITREOUS DETACHMENT

Anterior vitreous detachment (hyaloideocapsular separation) occurs in about 0.1 percent of the population. It has a greater incidence in phakic eyes with retinal detachment.

POSTERIOR VITREOUS DETACHMENT
(Figs. 12–9 through 12–11)

I. Posterior vitreous detachment is present in about 65 percent of people over 65 years of age and more than 50 percent of people over 50 years of age.
II. Partial posterior vitreous detachment is less common than the complete form.
III. The most common cause of posterior vitreous detachment is senescence; other causes include diabetes mellitus, ocular inflammation and aphakia.

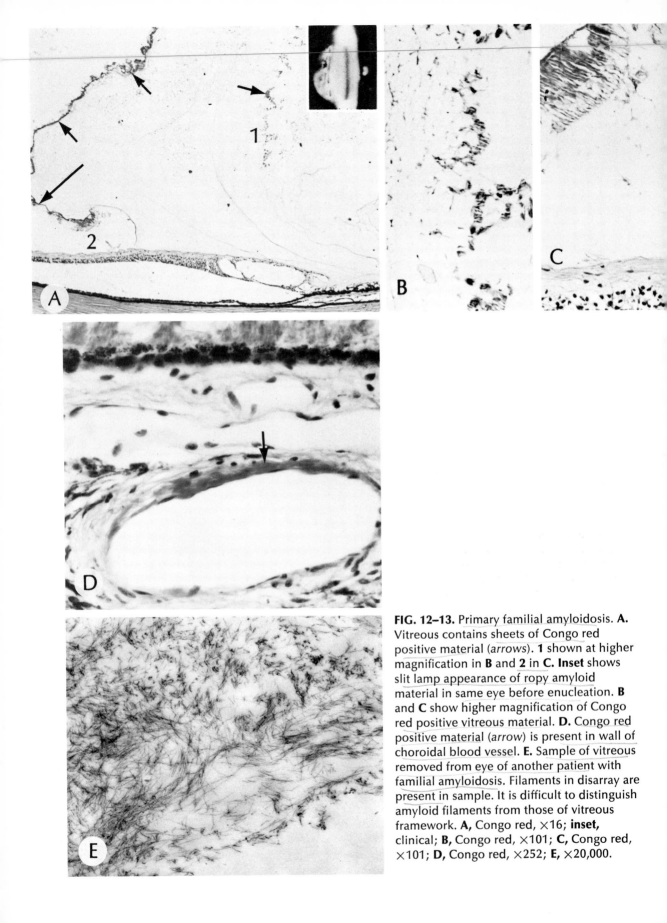

FIG. 12–13. Primary familial amyloidosis. **A.** Vitreous contains sheets of Congo red positive material (*arrows*). **1** shown at higher magnification in **B** and **2** in **C. Inset** shows slit lamp appearance of ropy amyloid material in same eye before enucleation. **B** and **C** show higher magnification of Congo red positive vitreous material. **D.** Congo red positive material (*arrow*) is present in wall of choroidal blood vessel. **E.** Sample of vitreous removed from eye of another patient with familial amyloidosis. Filaments in disarray are present in sample. It is difficult to distinguish amyloid filaments from those of vitreous framework. **A,** Congo red, ×16; **inset,** clinical; **B,** Congo red, ×101; **C,** Congo red, ×101; **D,** Congo red, ×252; **E,** ×20,000.

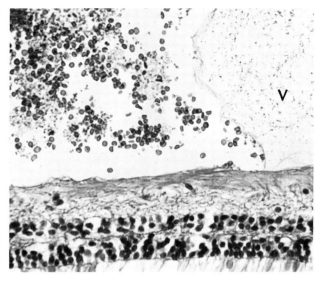

FIG. 12–14. Subvitreal hemorrhage is present between internal surface of retina and detached vitreous (*v*). Vitreous also contains blood products. H&E, ×265.

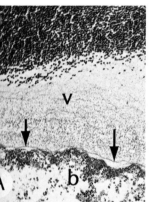 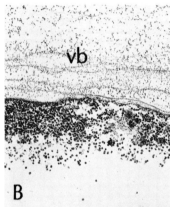

FIG. 12–15. Intravitreal and subvitreal hemorrhage. **A.** Blood is present within vitreous (*v*), i.e., intravitreal hemorrhage, as well as between vitreous and retina (*b*), i.e., subvitreal hemorrhage. *Arrows* show posterior surface of vitreous. **B.** Red blood cell fragments in vitreous (*vb*) as well as intact erythrocytes between vitreous and retina. **A,** H&E, ×100; **B,** H&E, ×100.

FIG. 12–16. Intraretinal submembranous hemorrhage shows blood between retinal internal limiting membrane and nerve fiber layer. **Arrow** shows surface of posteriorly detached vitreous (posterior hyaloid). H&E, ×70.

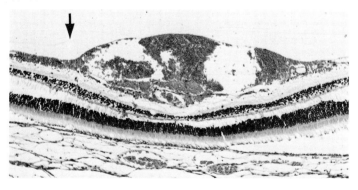

IV. The most important complication of vitreous detachment, aside from the creation of floaters, is retinal tear(s).

V. Syneresis. Syneresis, i.e., one or more areas of central degeneration and liquefaction of the vitreous body (Fig. 12–12), may occur with or without posterior vitreous detachment.

VI. Histologically the vitreous filaments are collapsed anteriorly so as to form a condensed posterior vitreous layer ("membrane"). The new subvitreal space posteriorly contains a watery fluid but lacks collagenous filaments.

PROTEINACEOUS DEPOSITS ← II° to inflammation

I. Proteinaceous deposits may form diffuse dustlike or cloudlike opacities.

II. They are analogous to plasmoid aqueous and occur chiefly with cyclitis, chorioretinitis or trauma.

AMYLOID

See p. 248 in Chapter 7.

I. Primary familial amyloidosis (Fig. 12–13)
   A. Vitreous opacities, frequently in the form of bilateral, sheetlike, vitreous veils, are seen along with a retinal perivasculitis.
   B. Amyloid may gain access to vitreous via direct extension from affected retinal blood vessels.
   C. Ecchymosis of lids, proptosis, ocular palsies, internal ophthalmoplegia and neuroparalytic keratitis result from amyloid deposition in the lid and orbital connective tissues, muscles, nerves and ganglia.
   D. Glaucoma may be caused by amyloid deposition in the aqueous outflow areas.
   E. Widespread systemic amyloid deposition is present.
   F. Histologically there is a pale, eosinophilic material in the vitreous that binds iodine and Congo red, demonstrates metachromasia with metachromatic dyes such as toluidine blue and crystal violet, shows fluorescence after exposure to Thioflavin-T and has a filamentous ultrastructure; it is dif-

ficult to identify filaments of amyloid separately from normal vitreous filaments. The walls of retinal and choroidal blood vessels may be thickened by the amyloid material.

FAMILIAL EXUDATIVE VITREORETINOPATHY (FEV)

I. FEV is characterized by organized membranes in all quadrants (peripheral and central) of the vitreous.
   A. Vitreoretinal traction results from the pull of the membranes.
   B. Snowflakelike opacities are present in the vitreous body.
   C. Vitreous usually is detached posteriorly.

II. Peripheral retinal exudates, localized retinal detachment often forming a broad fold temporally from the disc and peripheral retinal neovascularization with recurrent vitreous hemorrhages are frequently encountered.

III. Slowly progressive ocular changes may ultimately lead to a condition that mimics certain aspects of retrolental fibroplasia, Coats's disease and peripheral uveitis.

IV. FEV has an irregular mode of inheritance via an autosomal dominant gene.

VITREOUS HEMORRHAGE

DEFINITIONS

I. Subvitreal hemorrhage (Figs. 12–14 and 12–15). Blood is present between the internal limiting membrane of the retina and the posterior "face" of the vitreous and takes weeks to months to clear.

II. Intravitreal hemorrhage (Figs. 12–14 and 12–15). Blood is present within the vitreous body and takes many months to years to clear.

III. Subhyaloid hemorrhage. This is identical to subvitreal hemorrhage, but clinical use of the term may be confusing.

Sometimes the term subhyaloid hemorrhage is used clinically to describe an *intraretinal submembranous hemorrhage*, i.e., a hemorrhage located mainly between the nerve fiber layer and the internal limiting membrane of the retina (Fig. 12–16). *Gunn's dots*, i.e., basement membrane facets of internal limiting

smaller than normal and the optic nerve tissue is "heaped up" on the surface of the optic disc.

CONGENITAL CRESCENT OR CONUS

I. A white, semilunar area lies at the margin of the optic disc.
   A. Usually the inferior or inferotemporal margin of the disc is involved.
   B. The conus often is associated with an oval disc with its long axis parallel to the crescent.

II. The vision generally is defective.

III. There usually is an associated hypermetropia, and there may be an associated *pit of the optic disc.*

IV. A congenital crescent is not to be confused with a *myopic crescent,* which unlike the former is not present at birth, is progressive, has a temporal or annular location about the optic disc, is associated with other retinal degenerative changes and of course is associated with myopia.

V. Histologically there is a lack of retinal pigment epithelium and choroid in the area of the conus.

A lack of embryonic development of retinal pigment epithelium may be the primary defect.

OPTIC PIT (Fig. 13–2)

I. An optic pit is a small, circular or triangular pit about one-eighth to one-half the diameter of the optic disc, generally located in the inferiortemporal quadrant of the disc.
   A. It usually is unilateral, and there may be more than one optic pit present.
   B. The optic disc may be of greater size than in the uninvolved fellow eye.

   Less frequently a *centrally placed pit* of the optic disc may occur. With such a defect the presenting symptom may be decreased vision or a defect in the visual field, which generally remains unchanged. Central serous retinopathy has not been described with a central pit of the disc.

II. In about one-third of cases the optic pit

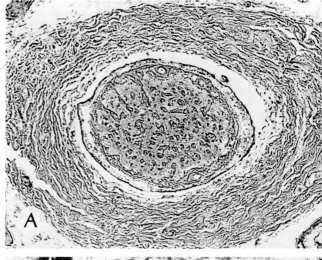

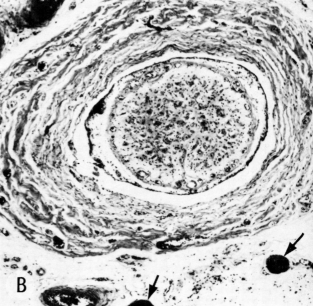

FIG. 13–1. Hypoplasia of optic nerve in case of tetraploid–diploid mosaicism. **A.** Marked atrophy of optic nerve is present. **B.** Special stain shows almost complete loss of myelin from optic nerve. Note normal amount of myelin in ciliary nerves (*arrows*). **A,** H&E, ×40; **B,** luxol fast blue, ×40.

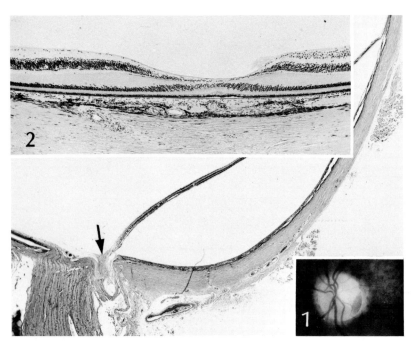

FIG. 13–2. Optic pit. **Inset 1** is clinical picture of congenital pit of optic nerve head. Note typical lower temporal location. **Inset 2** shows macula of similar case. Ganglion cells are decreased noticeably between fovea and optic disc toward left, whereas ganglion cells are normal in number temporal (to right) of fovea. Coloboma of optic disc (*arrow*) shows atrophic retinal tissue lining space adjacent to optic nerve. Note detachment of temporal retina from pit almost to equator. **Main figure,** H&E, ×8; **inset 1,** fundus; **inset 2,** H&E, ×48.

may be associated with macular changes such as central serous retinopathy, hemorrhages, pigmentary changes, cysts and holes.

A. Serous detachment of the macula (central serous retinopathy) probably is the basic lesion that causes the other macular changes.

1. The serous detachment of the macula usually occurs between 20 and 40 years of age and carries a poor visual prognosis.

2. There is no angiographic evidence of leakage of fluorescein dye into the area of the detached retina.

3. Subretinal fluid may consist of

vitreous fluid leaked into the area through the pit or cerebrospinal fluid leaked around the pit into the subretinal space.

III. The optic pit probably is caused by an anomalous development of the primordial optic nerve papilla and failure of complete resolution of peripapillary neuroectodermal folds, which are part of the normal development of the optic nerve head.

IV. Histologically the pit is an outpouching of neuroectodermal tissue surrounded by a connective tissue capsule. The pit passes posteriorly through a defect in the lamina cribrosa and protrudes into the subarachnoid space.

CONGENITAL OPTIC ATROPHY

See p. 502 in Chapter 13.

COLOBOMA (Fig. 13–3)

I. Coloboma may involve the optic disc alone or may be part of a complete coloboma involving the entire embryonic fissure.

A. It may have a clinical appearance that varies from a deep physiologic cup to

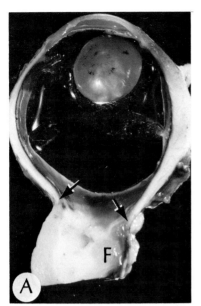

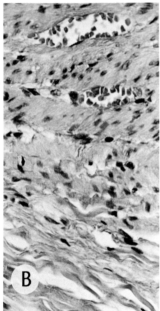

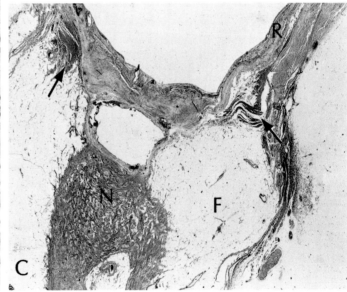

FIG. 13–3. Coloboma of optic nerve. **A.** There is large depression and defective area of sclera at optic nerve entrance (between *arrows*). Small dysplastic optic nerve is situated centrally within mantle of fatty tissue (*F*). **B.** Fusiform smooth muscle cells with centrally placed spindle-shaped nuclei may be found in surrounding atrophic optic nerve in region of defective sclera. Scleral fibers are present in lower part of picture. **C.** Gliosed optic nerve (*N*) shows tenuous connection anteriorly with gliosed retina (*R*). Thick cuff of fat (*F*) surrounds abnormal nerve and is itself invested partially by dura. Small, darkly stained area of smooth muscle (*arrows*) is evident anteriorly at margins of scleral defect and projects into adjacent choroid. **A,** macroscopic; **B,** H&E, ×350; **C,** H&E, ×10.

a large hole associated with a retro-bulbar cyst.

  B. The surrounding retina may or may not be involved.

  II. It usually is unilateral and due to either a failure in fusion of the proximal end of the embryonic fissure or aplasia of the primitive papilla of Bergmeister.

  III. Coloboma of the optic disc may be associated with other ocular anomalies such as congenital nonattachment of the retina, coloboma of the retina and choroid and persistent hyaloid artery.

  IV. The vision may be normal but usually is defective.

  V. Histologically the coloboma appears as a large defect at the side of the nerve usually involving the retina, choroid and sclera.

    A. The defect is lined by fibrous tissue. Frequently it contains retina that may be well formed, hypoplastic or gliotic. The gliosis may be massive so as to simulate a neoplasm.

    B. Its wall may contain adipose tissue and even smooth muscle fibers.

The smooth muscle fibers may give rise to a *contractile peripapillary staphyloma*.

    C. The coloboma may protrude into the surrounding retrobulbar tissue giving rise to a *coloboma with cyst* (see pp. 516–517 in Chap. 14).

MYOPIA (Fig. 13–4)

  I. In myopia the optic disc is oblique with exaggeration of the normally raised nasal and flattened temporal edges. A surrounding white scleral crescent is present temporally.

  II. The optic nerve head is ovoid with its long axis vertical.

  III. Histologically the optic nerve passes obliquely through the scleral canal.

    A. Temporal side of optic disc

      1. The retinal pigment epithelium and Bruch's membrane do not extend to the temporal margin of the optic disc.

      2. The choroid extends farther toward the temporal margin of the disc than does the retinal pigment epithelium and Bruch's membrane, but

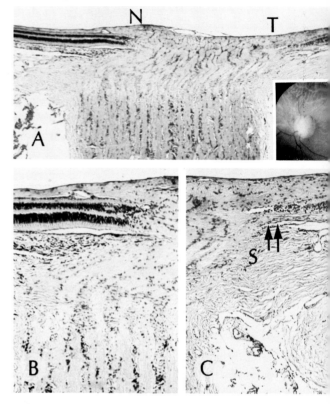

FIG. 13–4. Myopia. **A.** Optic disc is oblique with exaggeration of normally raised nasal (*N*) and flattened temporal (*T*) edges. **Inset** shows typical myopic disc with temporal crescent. **B.** Higher magnification of nasal side of disc shows overlapping tissue, i.e., sensory retina, RPE, Bruch's membrane and choroid, extending over nasal aspect of scleral opening of optic nerve. **C.** Higher magnification of temporal side of disc shows RPE and Bruch's membrane (*single arrow*) stopping short of disc. Choroid (*double arrow*) also stops short of disc, allowing sclera (*S*) to be seen through transparent sensory retina as white scleral crescent. **A,** H&E, ×16; **inset,** fundus; **B,** H&E, ×40; **C,** H&E, ×40.

it also does not reach the temporal edge of the disc.

The sclera exposed just temporal to the margin of the optic disc is seen through the transparent sensory retina as a white scleral crescent.

B. Nasal side of disc
Overlapping tissue, i.e., sensory retina, retinal pigment epithelium, Bruch's membrane and choroid, may extend as far as halfway over the nasal half of the scleral opening.

PAPILLEDEMA

Generally visual acuity is affected not at all or minimally.

CAUSES

I. Relative or absolute increase in venous pressure at or posterior to the lamina cribrosa (Figs. 13–5 and 13–6), e.g., acute glaucoma, optic nerve tumors, orbital tumors, brain tumors, subarachnoid hemorrhage, meningitis, encephalitis, malignant hypertension and drugs such as tetracycline and possibly oral contraceptives.
II. Relative increase in venous pressure at or anterior to the lamina cribrosa (hypotony) (Fig. 13–7), e.g., accidental penetrating wounds, intraocular surgery, uveitis, central retinal vein thrombosis and ocular hypotony due to any cause (acute or chronic).
III. Local phenomena, e.g., the Irvine-Gass-Norton syndrome, iron deficiency anemia, gastrointestinal hemorrhage, papillitis, juxtapapillary choroiditis and perhaps birth control pills.

PSEUDOPAPILLEDEMA

Papilledema may be simulated by hypermetropic optic disc; drusen of optic nerve head, congenital developmental abnormalities; optic neuritis and perineuritis; and myelinated (medullated) nerve fibers.

HISTOLOGY OF PAPILLEDEMA
(Figs. 13–5 through 13–8)

I. Acute
A. Edema and vascular congestion of the nerve head result in an increased volume of tissue. Hemorrhages may be seen in the optic nerve or in the retinal nerve fiber layer. The increased mass of tissue causes a narrowing of the physiologic cup.
B. The above changes result in a displacement of the sensory retina away from the edge of the optic disc.
1. The outer layers of the retina may be buckled (retinal and choroidal folds are seen clinically).
2. The rods and cones are displaced away from the end of Bruch's membrane.

The lateral displacement of the rods and cones results in enlargement of the blind spot on visual field testing. A peripapillary retinal detachment can add to the density of the scotoma. The pigment epithelial cells sometimes also are pushed laterally so that the peripapillary RPE is flattened and the cells farther away are "squeezed" together.

3. There may be a peripapillary retinal detachment.
II. Chronic
A. Degeneration of nerve fibers may occur, especially with chronic papilledema.
B. Gliosis and optic atrophy are most likely to occur with long-standing or chronic papilledema rather than with short-term or acute papilledema, which is reversed in a short period of time.

With papilledema secondary to increased intraocular pressure, e.g., acute narrow angle glaucoma, necrosis of optic nerve fibers may occur resulting ultimately in optic atrophy and even cavernous optic atrophy. The fibers in the optic nerve are more susceptible to injury by high intraocular pressure than are the retinal ganglion cells.

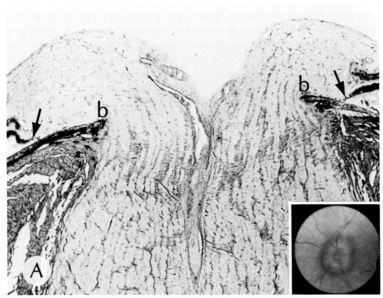

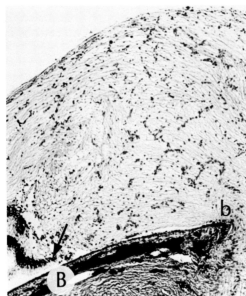

FIG. 13–5. Papilledema. **A.** Papilledema secondary to increased cerebrospinal fluid pressure. There is increased mass, tissue edema (shown better at higher magnification in **B**), vascular congestion and lateral displacement of photoreceptors (*arrows* in **A** and **B** show photoreceptors displaced laterally from ends of Bruch's membrane, *b*). **Inset** shows papilledema in patient with pseudotumor cerebri. **A,** H&E, ×16; **inset,** fundus; **B,** H&E, ×40.

FIG. 13–6. Papilledema secondary to acute glaucoma in patient with phacolytic glaucoma. Note hemorrhage (*h*) in nerve fiber layer. H&E, ×40.

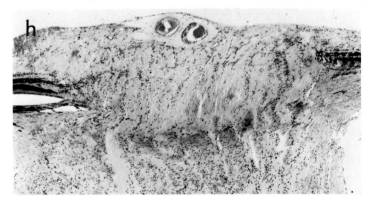

OPTIC NEURITIS

Generally visual acuity is affected severely.

CAUSES

I. Secondary to ocular disease, e.g., keratitis, especially acute corneal ulcer; anterior or posterior uveitis; endophthalmitis or panophthalmitis; and chorioretinitis or retinochoroiditis.

II. Secondary to orbital disease (Figs. 13–9 and 13–10), e.g., cellulitis (may be primary, but more commonly secondary to sinusitis); thrombophlebitis; arteritis; Wegener's granulomatosis; and midline lethal granuloma.

III. Secondary to intracranial disease, e.g., meningitis; encephalitis; and meningoencephalitis.

IV. Secondary to spread of distant infection, e.g., syphilis; tuberculosis; coccidioidomycosis; and bacterial endocarditis.

V. Secondary to vascular disease (Fig. 13–11), e.g., cranial arteritis; periarteritis nodosa; pulseless (Takayasu's) disease; and arteriosclerosis.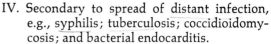

VI. Secondary to demyelinating disease
    A. Multiple sclerosis (Figs. 13–12 through 13–14)
        1. Retrobulbar neuritis
            a. Retrobulbar neuritis has an acute onset in one eye with a sudden loss of vision, generally preceded by orbital pain (especially with ocular movement). There is a tendency to recover vision in a few weeks to months.

With loss of vision a central

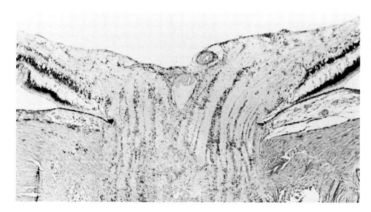

FIG. 13–7. Papilledema secondary to hypotony in eye with perforating corneal injury. H&E, ×21.

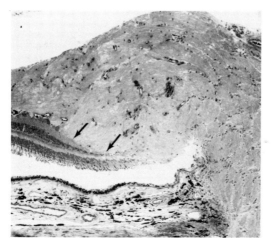

FIG. 13–8. Papilledema. Markedly swollen nerve fibers of optic nerve are displacing retinal layers outward and peripherally (*arrows*). 1.5 μ section, toluidine blue, ×50.

scotoma can be demonstrated on central visual field examination. Frequently the second eye is involved after the first eye has recovered.

b. The ophthalmoscopic appearance may be normal with a papillitis or may simulate papilledema. An associated sheathing of the temporal veins may be seen.

2. Ocular muscle palsies may occur (conjugate movements may be involved) along with nystagmus, frequently of the cerebellar type. Internuclear ophthalmoplegia also may occur.

Pupillary changes that are variable and not characteristic may be noted. In one study 13 to 15 percent of patients with multiple sclerosis presented with optic neuritis, and 27 to 37 percent of multiple sclerosis patients showed evidence of optic neuritis during the course of the disease. Approximately 17 percent of patients with optic neuritis ultimately developed multiple sclerosis; younger patients would have a much higher incidence.

B. Neuromyelitis optica (Encephalomyelitis optica; Devic's disease) (Figs. 13–15 and 13–16)
1. Bilateral optic atrophy
a. The loss of vision is acute in onset and rapid in progression, even to complete blindness.

Unlike multiple sclerosis pain precedes loss of vision in very few cases. The loss of vision precedes onset of paraplegia in about 80 percent of cases.

b. The ophthalmoscopic appearance may be normal or if a papillitis is present may simulate papilledema.
c. Bilaterality of optic atrophy along with paraplegia are characteristic.

2. Extraocular muscle palsies may be present, but nystagmus is found in-

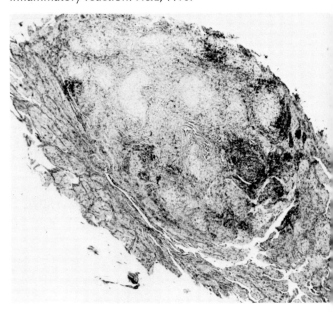

FIG. 13–9. Granulomatous optic neuritis caused by sarcoidosis. Optic nerve is replaced to large extent by granulomatous inflammatory reaction. H&E, ×16.

frequently. Pupillary changes are variable and not characteristic.
3. Paraplegia generally follows loss of visual acuity in days to weeks, but may follow in months or, rarely, in years.

C. Diffuse cerebral sclerosis involves primarily white matter of the central nervous system and includes Schilder's disease (Fig. 13–17), Krabbe's disease, Pelizaeus-Merzbacher syndrome (Fig. 13–18) and metachromatic leukodystrophy.

VII. Secondary to nutritional and/or toxic and/or metabolic disease, e.g., starvation (nutritional); tobacco–alcohol toxicity; methyl alcohol; diabetes mellitus; hyperthyroidism; disulfiram (Antabuse); iodochlorhydroxyquinoline (Enterovioform); ethambutol; and chloramphenicol.

VIII. Secondary to hereditary conditions—see p. 502 in this chapter.

IX. Secondary to idiopathic or unknown causes.

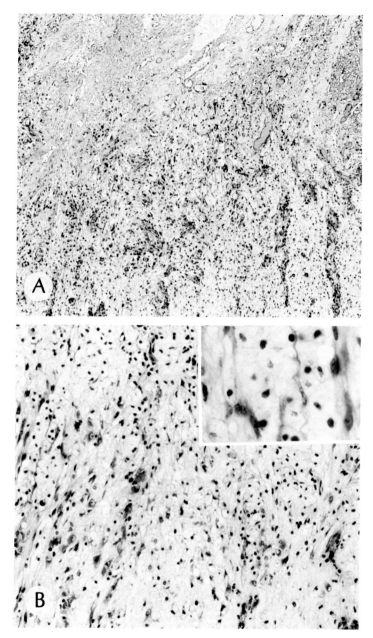

FIG. 13–10. Optic neuritis secondary to orbital aspergillosis. **A.** Optic nerve is undergoing necrosis. **B.** Macrophages are phagocytosing disintegrating myelin. Fat-laden macrophages (gitter cells) are shown at higher magnification in **inset**. Hyphae compatible with aspergillus fungi were found in optic nerve (see Figure 4–20). **A,** giemsa, ×40; **B,** giemsa, ×101; **inset,** giemsa, ×252.

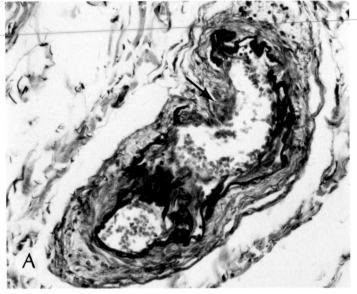

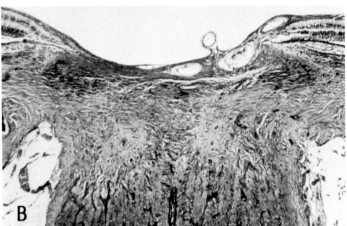

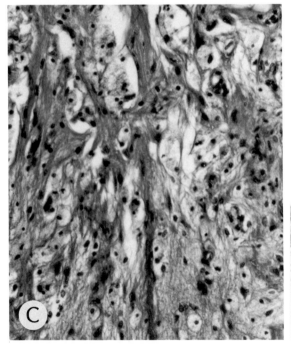

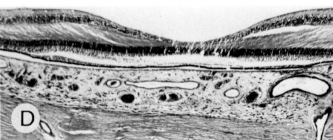

FIG. 13–11. Fatal temporal arteritis with unilateral ischemic optic neuropathy in 67-year-old woman. **A.** Ciliary artery behind involved eye shows fragmented internal elastic lamina (*arrow*) and some round inflammatory cells in adventitia and periadventitia. **B.** Optic nerve shows atrophy of retinal layer and atrophy and gliosis of choroidal and scleral layers. **C.** Fat-laden (foamy) histiocytes (gitter cells) are present in scleral layer of optic nerve. **D.** Macular area shows marked atrophy of ganglion and nerve fiber layers. **A.** Verhoeff elastic, ×320; **B,** Verhoeff elastic, ×50; **C,** H&E, ×320; **D,** Verhoeff elastic, ×50.

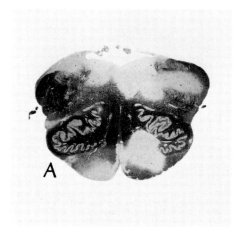

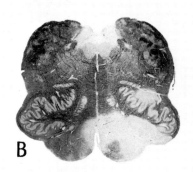

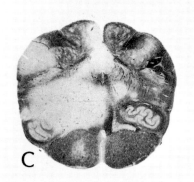

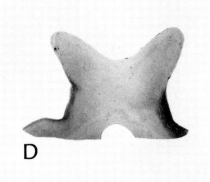

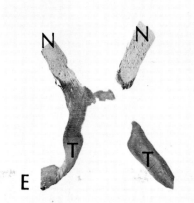

FIG. 13–12. Multiple sclerosis. **A, B** and **C** show large astrocytic plaques in different areas of brain stem. Note irregular distribution of plaques at different levels. **D** shows almost total demyelination of chiasm. **E** is from another case to show demyelination of optic nerves (N) but preservation of myelin in optic tracts (T). **A,** Klüver-Barerra, ×3; **B,** Klüver-Barerra, ×3; **C,** Klüver-Barerra, ×3; **D,** Klüver-Barerra, ×3; **E,** Klüver-Barerra, ×3.

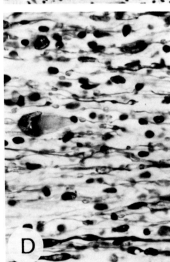

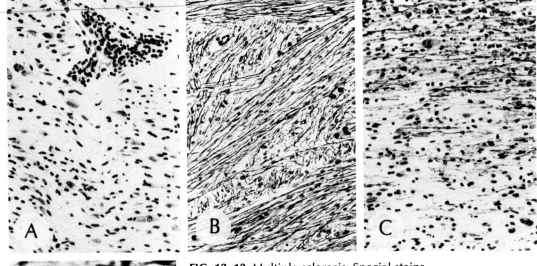

FIG. 13–13. Multiple sclerosis. Special stains of chiasm shown in Figure 13–12D demonstrate almost complete loss of myelin (**A**) but preservation of axons (**B**). **C.** Lower half of picture shows complete loss of myelin, whereas in upper half some myelin preservation is present. Astrocytic response in **C** demonstrated at higher magnification in **D.** **A,** Klüver-Barerra, ×101; **B,** Bodian, ×101; **C,** Klüver-Barerra, ×101; **D,** Klüver-Barerra, ×252.

FIG. 13–14. Multiple sclerosis. **A.** Late stage shows marked optic atrophy. **B.** Special stain for myelin shows complete loss of myelin. **C.** Special stain for nerve fibers shows preservation of some axonal processes. **A,** PAS, ×16; **B,** Klüver-Barerra, ×40; **C,** Bodian, ×850.

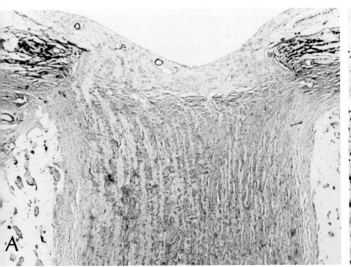

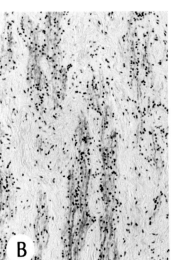

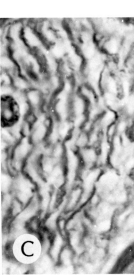

HISTOLOGY OF OPTIC NEURITIS

I. General information
   A. The terms optic neuritis, retrobulbar neuritis, papillitis and neuroretinitis are clinical terms and do not connote specific causes. Actually there are many causes, e.g., inflammatory, vascular and degenerative.

   "Itis," therefore, as generally used here is not necessarily synonymous with inflammation.

   B. Topographic histologic classification of optic neuritis
      1. Perineuritis—leptomeninges involved, e.g., extension of intracranial meningitis or direct extension from orbital inflammation or from intraocular inflammations.
      2. Periaxial neuritis—leptomeningeal involvement spreads to the optic nerve parenchyma, usually in its peripheral portions.
      3. Axial neuritis—inner or central portions of the optic nerve involved, e.g., multiple sclerosis, toxic factors, malnutrition and vascular factors.
      4. Transverse neuritis—total cross-sectional destruction of a variable length of optic nerve, e.g., Devic's disease and purulent infection.

II. Specific types of tissue reaction
   A. Inflammatory disease
   The types of inflammatory disease of the optic nerve depends on the etiologic agent (see section Inflammation in Chapters 1, 3 and 4).
   B. Vascular disease
   The clinicpathologic picture depends on the type of vascular disease involving the optic nerve.
      1. Temporal (cranial) arteritis—a granulomatous arteritis (may have giant cells) with necrosis of the arterial wall and a splitting and destruction of the inner elastic lamina (Figs. 11–9 and 13–11).
      2. Periarteritis nodosa—a fibrinoid necrosis of muscular arteries and arterioles with acute and chronic nongranulomatous intraarterial wall inflammatory reaction (Fig. 6–28).
      3. Pulseless disease and arteriosclerosis—coagulative or ischemic type of necrosis (Fig. 11–8).
   C. Demyelinating diseases
      1. Demyelinating stage (Figs. 13–10 and 13–16).
         a. Early there is a breakdown of myelin sheaths.
         b. Macrophages phagocytose the disintegrated myelin. The "fat-laden" phagocytes then move to perivascular locations.
         c. A perivascular "cuffing" or exudation of fluid, lymphocytes and plasma cells around blood vessels in areas remote from the acute reaction is seen frequently.
      2. Healing stage (Figs. 13–13 and 13–14)
         a. Astrocytic response in areas of demyelination occurs.
         b. Ultimately the area of involvement shows gliosis.
   D. Nutritional and/or toxic and/or metabolic diseases
      1. Very little is known of the acute reaction.
      2. Ultimately these conditions may cause considerable destruction of optic nerve parenchyma with resultant secondary optic atrophy.

OPTIC ATROPHY*

CAUSES

I. Ascending optic atrophy
   A. The primary lesion is in the retina or optic disc, e.g., glaucoma* (Fig. 16–28); retinochoroiditis†; retinopathia pigmentosa†; traumatic or secondary retinopathia pigmentosa†; central retinal artery occlusion* (Fig. 11–13); chronic papilledema†; and toxic or nutritional causes, e.g., chloroquine*.
   B. The secondary effects are on the optic nerve and white tracts in the brain.

* Generally very little if any gliotic reaction on surface of optic disc, hence "white" or primary optic atrophy.
† Generally gliotic reaction on surface of optic disc, hence "dirty" or secondary optic atrophy.

TABLE 13–1.
Familial Optic Atrophies*

	Congenital		Juvenile		Leber's	Behr's
	Dominant	Recessive	Dominant	Recessive		
Inheritance	Dominant	Recessive	Dominant	Recessive	? x-linked, ? dominant, ? cytoplasmic, ? slow virus	Recessive
Systemic signs and symptoms	—	—	—	Diabetes, decreased hearing	Headache, vertigo, nervousness, palpitations	Increased tendon reflexes, + Babinski, ataxia, + Romberg, muscular rigidity, mental debility
Onset	Congenital or neonatal	Congenital or neonatal	Insidious onset 6- to 12-years-old	Insidious onset 6- to 12-years-old	Acute onset 16- to 30-years-old	1- to 9-years-old
Nystagmus	Yes	Yes	No	No	No	Possibly
Vision	20/100 to hand movements	Marked loss	20/20 to 3/400	May be hand movements or light perception	Usually 10/200	Usually 10/200
Fields	Constricted peripheral; no characteristic scotoma	—	Central scotoma; possibly bitemporal defect; blue inside red	—	Central scotoma; peripheral fields normal	Central scotoma; peripheral fields normal
Fundi	Marked atrophy of entire disc; narrow arteries	Total atrophy	Temporal atrophy	Total atrophy	Hyperemia or papilledema at onset; white disc develops after neuritis; arteries are narrow	Temporal atrophy
Color testing	May be reduced	—	Possible blue-green defect	—	Red-green defect	—
ERG	—	—	Normal	Normal	Normal	Normal
(VECP) Visually evoked cortical potential	—	—	Possibly diminished	—	—	—
Dark adaptation	—	—	Possibly diminished	Normal	Diminished	Normal
Clinical course	May progress slowly; usually in school for blind	—	Atrophy is stationary or may progress	—	Acute course may progress, or regress to essentially normal vision	Evolution of neurological symptoms for years, then stabilization
Pathology	—	—	Optochiasmatic arachnoiditis seen at surgery	—	Atrophy of retinal ganglion cells, especially about fovea, demyelination in optic nerve and temporal lobe	Degeneration of second retinal neuron

* From Caldwell et al., 1971.

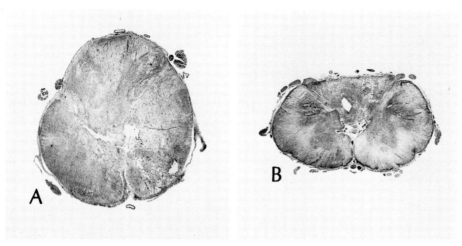

FIG. 13–15. Neuromyelitis optica. Caudal medulla (**A**) and upper cervical cord (**B**) of 26-year-old man show peripheral demyelination (especially in cervical cord) and extensive necrosis. **A,** Klüver-Barerra, ×3; **B,** Klüver-Barrera, ×3.

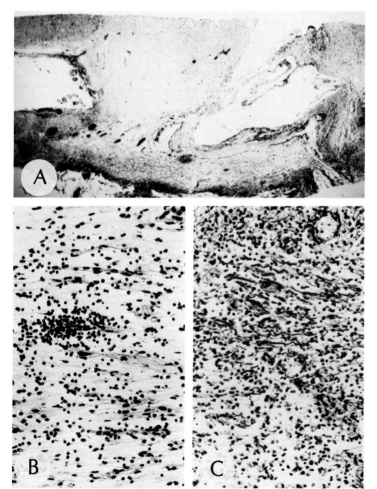

FIG. 13–16. Neuromyelitis optica (same case as Figure 13–15). **A.** Chiasm shows inflammation and extensive loss of myelin (**B**) with relative preservation of axons (**C**). **A,** Klüver-Barerra, ×4; **B,** Klüver-Barerra, ×101; **C,** Bodian, ×101.

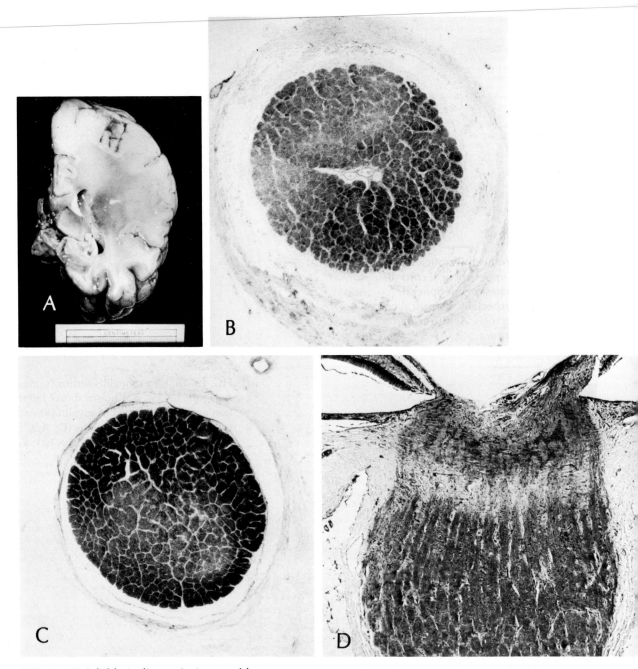

FIG. 13–17. Schilder's disease in 8-year-old white boy. **A.** Macroscopic coronal section of occipital lobe shows giant plaque. **B.** Distal left optic nerve (near globe) shows descending optic atrophy involving mainly upper left periphery of nerve. **C.** Proximal left optic nerve (near chiasm) shows descending optic atrophy involving mainly central portion of nerve. **D.** Scleral portion of optic nerve shows mild atrophy. **A,** macroscopic; **B,** Klüver-Barerra, ×9; **C,** Klüver-Barerra, ×9; **D,** Weil, ×21.

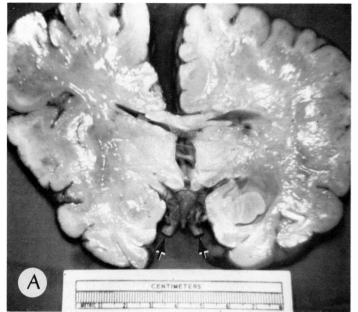

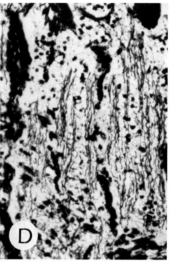

FIG. 13–18. Pelizaeus-Merzbacher syndrome in 7½-year-old white boy. **A.** Coronal section of brain showing large, brownish discolored optic nerves (*arrows*). **B.** There is severe demyelination of optic chiasm and optic tracts (*T*) and moderate demyelination of optic nerves (*N1, N2*). **C.** Cross-section of optic nerve at anterior portion of *N2* in **B** shows demyelination most evident in central portion of optic nerve. **D.** There is extensive loss and fragmentation of axonal processes in optic nerve. **E.** Macular area of retina shows descending atrophy manifested by atrophy of ganglion cell and nerve fiber layers. **A,** macroscopic; **B,** Klüver-Barerra, ×15; **C,** Klüver-Barerra, ×15; **D,** Bodian, ×160; **E,** H&E, ×218.

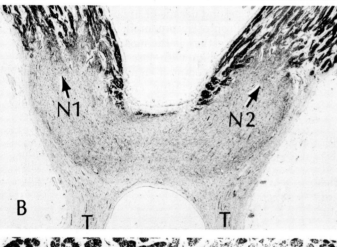

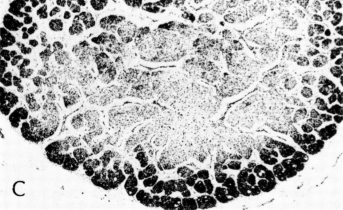

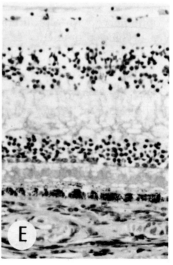

II. Descending optic atrophy (Figs. 13–14, 13–17 and 13–18)
   A. The primary lesion is in the brain or optic nerve, e.g., tabes dorsalis*; hydrocephalus*; meningioma*; optic nerve glioma*; traumatic transection of the optic nerve*; and toxic or nutritional causes, e.g., methyl alcohol.*
   B. The secondary effects are on the optic disc and retina.
III. Inherited optic atrophy
   A. Familial optic atrophies (congenital, juvenile, Leber's and Behr's optic atrophies—see Table 13–1).
   B. G-6-PD Worcester
      1. G-6-PD Worcester is a variant of *glucose-6-phosphate dehydrogenase deficiency* with congenital, nonspherocytic hemolytic anemia, absent erythrocyte G-6-PD activity and optic atrophy.
      2. It is inherited as a sex-linked recessive.
   C. Friedreich's ataxia

HISTOLOGY OF OPTIC ATROPHY (Fig. 13–19)

I. There is a shrinkage or loss of parenchyma, with a loss of both myelin and axis cylinders. With shrinkage a widening of the subarachnoid space results and the dura becomes redundant. There is loss of the normal spongy texture of the optic nerve.
II. Widening of pial septa occurs in order to occupy the space made by the loss of parenchyma.
III. Gliosis of optic nerve with a proliferation of astrocytes becomes prominent.
IV. A widening or deepening of the physiologic cup with a baring of the lamina cribrosa occurs.
V. Secondary changes
   A. Glial proliferation on the surface of the disc results in a "secondary" type of optic atrophy.
   B. Accumulation of hyaluronic acid in the anterior portion of the optic nerve, i.e., *cavernous (Schnabel's) optic atrophy* (Fig. 13–20), occurs following long-standing glaucoma (see p. 613 in Chap. 16).

* Generally very little if any gliotic reaction on surface of optic disc, hence "white" or primary optic atrophy.

INJURIES

See Chapter 5.

TUMORS

PRIMARY

I. Juvenile pilocytic astrocytoma ("glioma") of optic nerve (Fig. 13–21)
   A. There is a slight preponderance of optic nerve juvenile pilocytic astrocytomas in girls. The median age at onset is about 5.2 years with over 80 percent of patients under 15 years of age; 71 percent occur during the first decade of life. It is quite rare after the second decade of life.
   B. Proptosis, predominantly temporal in direction, is the most common presenting sign with loss of vision the next most common sign. Nystagmus, headache, vomiting and convulsions may be the presenting sign with intracranial involvement.

      A central retinal vein occlusion occasionally may be the presenting sign clinically. More commonly, it occurs as a late phenomenon.

   C. Neurofibromatosis is present in at least 10 percent of patients.
   D. Papilledema early and optic atrophy late are frequent clinical findings.
   E. The astrocytoma most often is located in the orbital portion of the optic nerve alone, with combined involvement of both orbital and intracranial portions next most common (Table 13–2).

TABLE 13–2.
Juvenile Pilocytic Astrocytoma of the Optic Nerve: Location of Astrocytoma

Location	Number	Percent
Orbital	27	47
Intracranial and orbital	15	26
Intracranial	6	10
Intracranial and chiasm	7	12
Chiasm	3	5
Total	58	100

F. The optic foramen may be enlarged if the astrocytoma is limited to the orbital portion of the optic nerve or limited to the intracranial portion. Also the optic foramen may be normal with an astrocytoma limited to the intracranial optic nerve.

Secondary meningeal hyperplasia probably travels proximally (or distally) and is responsible for the enlargement of the optic foramen. An enlarged optic foramen, therefore, is not necessarily proof of intracranial extension of an orbital astrocytoma. Conversely, the optic foramen may be normal in the face of intracranial or chiasmal juvenile pilocytic astrocytoma.

G. There is a significant mortality rate in some series.
   1. If the astrocytoma is limited to the orbital portion of the optic nerve, the prognosis is excellent.
   2. With involvement of the intracranial optic nerve, the prognosis is guarded.
   3. If only the orbital portion of the optic nerve is involved, surgical removal, even when incomplete, generally cures.
H. Histology
   1. Three main patterns may all be present in different parts of the same tumor:
      a. Transitional area—the tumor merges into the normal optic nerve. It is difficult to differentiate this area from reactive gliosis.
         1) Glial nuclei are more numerous and less orderly than in the normal nerve.
         2) Nerve bundles are enlarged by the increased number and size of glial cells.
         3) The area has a finely reticulated appearance.
      b. Coarsely reticulated and myxomatous area—microcystoid spaces within the tumor probably are secondary to necrosis of the tumor. The spaces contain acid mucopolysaccharides that are partially sensitive to hyaluronidase.

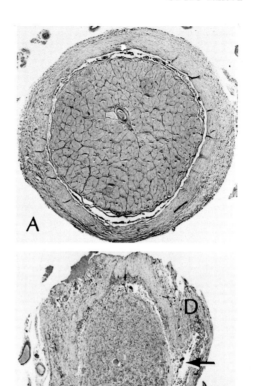

FIG. 13–19. Optic atrophy. **A.** Normal optic nerve in cross section. **B.** Atrophic optic nerve at same magnification to show shrinkage of parenchyma, widening of pial septa, gliosis, widening of subarachnoid space (*arrow*) and redundant dura. (*D*). **Inset** shows optic atrophy in child. **A,** H&E, ×8; **B,** H&E, ×8; **inset,** fundus.

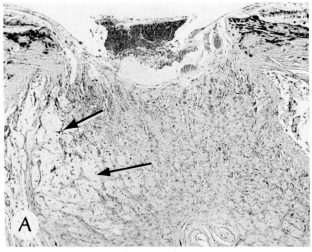

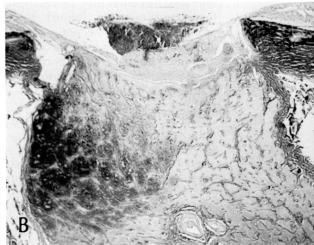

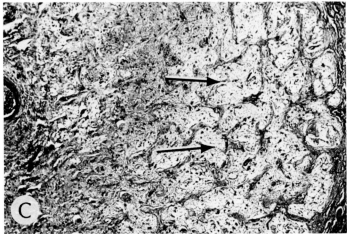

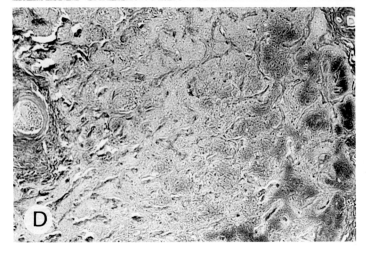

FIG. 13–20. Cavernous (Schnabel's) optic atrophy. Clear cystic spaces (*arrows*), in longitudinal section (**A**) and cross-section (**C**) of optic nerve, contain hyaluronidase-sensitive acid mucopolysaccharides (**B, D**) seen when stained with special stains. **A,** H&E, ×16; **B,** AMP, ×16; **C,** elastica, ×40; **D,** AMP, ×40.

(c̄ chronic glaucoma)

c. *"Fibrous"* or *astrocytic* *areas*—the areas resemble juvenile astrocytomas of the cerebellum and probably are the same type of tumor. The cellular areas show spindle cell formation. Intracytoplasmic, eosinophilic structures within astrocytes called *Rosenthal fibers* may be prominent.

Although Rosenthal fibers are found characteristically in optic nerve juvenile pilocytic astrocytomas, they are not pathognomonic. The fibers may be found within astrocytes in a number of inflammatory and neoplastic processes involving the central nervous system.

2. Secondary effects
   a. Infiltration of the juvenile pilocytic astrocytoma through the pia with resultant arachnoid hyperplasia is seen frequently.

   Secondary or reactive arachnoid (meningothelial) hyperplasia may become quite extensive and extend well beyond the limits of the astrocytoma. The hyperplasia may mimic a meningioma of the optic nerve sheath.

   b. The tumor itself may enlarge the optic foramen (as may proliferating meninges).
   c. The optic nerve astrocytoma may cause papilledema or optic atrophy.
   d. There may be infiltration of the optic nerve head by the astrocytoma.
   e. The tumor may cause compression or occlusion of the central retinal vein.

II. Other astrocytic neoplasms
   A. Malignant astrocytic neoplasms on rare occasions may involve primarily the optic nerve, most commonly in adults.
   B. Histologically the neoplasms are marked by areas of anaplasia.

III. Meningioma (Fig. 13–22)
   A. Primary meningioma of the intra-orbital meninges of the optic nerve is more common in women (5:1).
   B. The average age at onset is 32 years (range 3.5 to 73 years) with the median 38 years.

   About 40 percent of the tumors occur in patients under 20 years of age and 25 percent in patients under 10 years.

   C. The main clinical presentations are loss of vision and progressive exophthalmos.
   D. There may be associated neurofibromatosis in approximately 16 percent of patients.
   E. The prognosis for life depends somewhat on age at onset.

   With an onset in childhood the meningiomas tend to be much more aggressive and to have a much worse prognosis than with an onset at an older age. In one series, out of eight patients under 20 years of age, two patients were alive without recurrence (follow-up under 2 years), four had recurrent tumor (one with intracranial extension and three without) and one died during the attempt to excise the recurrent tumor. In the same series, out of 13 patients over 20 years of age, ten were alive and well without recurrent tumor (follow-up 3 to 21 years), and three patients had died (one an operative death).

   F. Histologically the tumors have either a meningotheliomatous or a mixed type of pattern.
      1. Fibroblastic and angioblastic types of meningiomas rarely, if ever, occur primarily in the orbit.
      2. Frequently meningiomas extend extradurally to invade the orbital tissue.
      3. Uncommonly they invade the optic nerve and sclera and may even invade into the choroid and retina.

IV. Melanocytoma—see pp. 679–681 in Chapter 17.
V. Hemangioma is usually associated with the phakomatoses (see pp. 30, 37 in Chap. 2).

   Hemangiomas, usually cavernous, extremely rarely may occur as a primary optic nerve tumor unassociated with the phakomatoses.

transitional

cystic

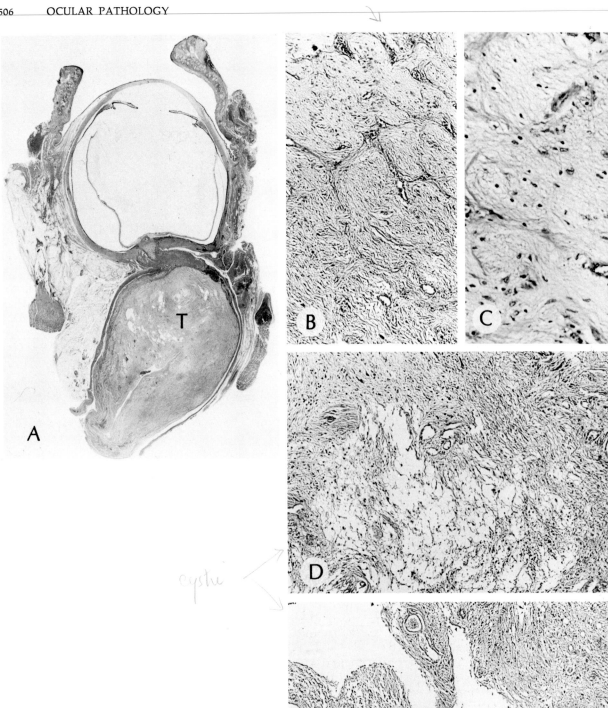

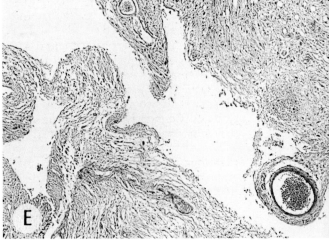

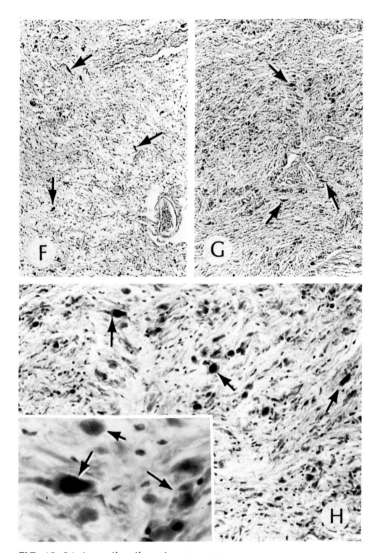

[handwritten margin note: astrocytic: spindle cells c̄ Rosenthal fibrils]

FIG. 13–21. Juvenile pilocytic astrocytoma (glioma) of optic nerve. **A.** Large tumor (*T*) involves optic nerve. **B** and **C.** Transitional area between tumor and nerve shows numerous large glial cells that are less ordered than normal, enlarged nerve bundles and finely reticulated appearance. Myxomatous microcystoid spaces (**D**) and macrocystoid spaces (**E**) contain hyaluronidase-sensitive (partially) acid mucopolysaccharides and are probably due to secondary necrosis of tumor. **F, G** and **H** show fibrous or astrocytic areas that contain intracytoplasmic astrocytic eosinophilic structures (*arrows*), shown at highest magnification in **inset** in **H,** called Rosenthal fibers. **A.** H&E, ×3; **B,** H&E, ×40; **C,** H&E, ×136; **D,** H&E, ×40; **E,** H&E, ×40; **F,** H&E, ×40; **G,** H&E, ×40; **H,** H&E, ×101; **inset,** H&E, ×252.

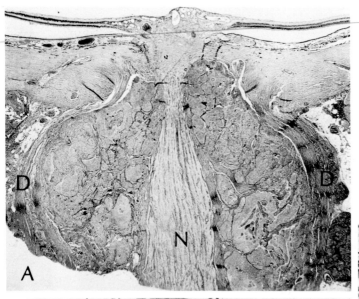

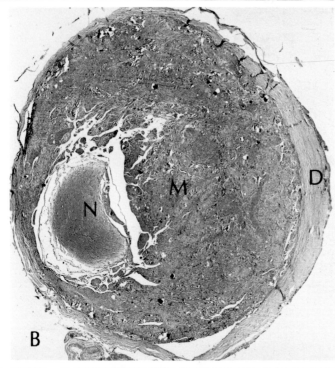

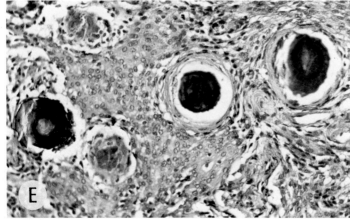

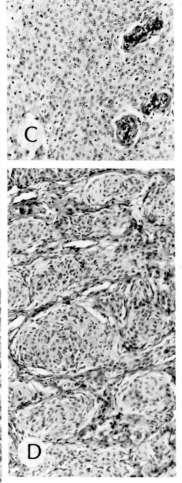

FIG. 13–22. Meningioma of optic nerve. **A.** Primary intradural meningioma surrounds optic nerve (*N*). *D*, dura. **B.** Cross-section to show compression of optic nerve (*N*) by primary intradural meningioma (*M*). *D*, dura. **C.** Meningotheliomatous (syncytial) meningioma. **D.** Mixed (transitional) meningioma. **E.** Psammoma bodies in mixed (transitional) meningioma. **A,** H&E, ×15; **B,** H&E, ×14; **C,** H&E, ×100; **D,** H&E, ×115; **E,** H&E, ×165.

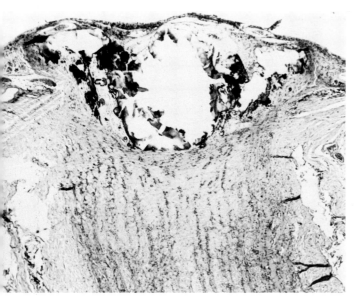

FIG. 13–23. Giant drusen occupy retinal layer of optic nerve in case of tuberous sclerosis. H&E, ×21.

astrocytic hamartoma

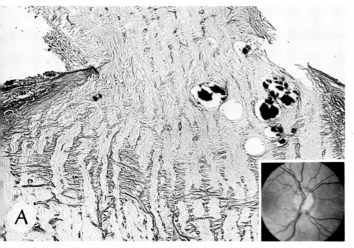

FIG. 13–24. Ordinary drusen of optic nerve. Dark bodies in retinal layer of optic nerve stain positive for acid mucopolysaccharides (**A**) and are PAS-positive (**B**). **Inset** in **A** shows drusen most marked at nasal edge of optic disc. **C.** Massive drusen occupy most of retinal layer of optic nerve in individual who did not have tuberous sclerosis. **Inset** shows massive drusen of optic disc in another individual without tuberous sclerosis. **A,** AMP, ×40; **inset,** fundus; **B,** PAS, ×54; **C,** H&E, ×40; **inset,** fundus.

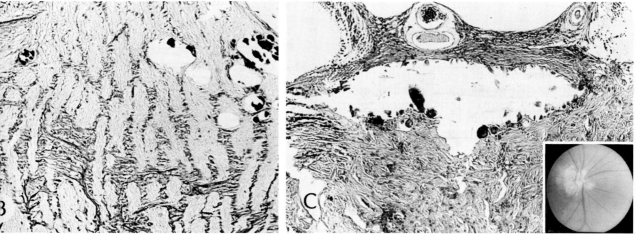

VI. Medulloepithelioma may arise rarely from the distal end of the optic nerve (see p. 642 in Chap. 17 and p. 702 in Chap. 18).

VII. Giant drusen of the optic nerve (anterior portion) are astrocytic hamartomas usually associated with tuberous sclerosis (Fig. 13–23) (see pp. 35–36 in Chap. 2).

VIII. Ordinary drusen of the optic nerve (anterior portion) (Fig. 13–24).

    A. Ordinary drusen of the optic nerve can present clinically as a pseudopapilledema.

    B. Although field defects are common (87 percent in one series), very rarely does a patient lose central vision.

    C. Hemorrhage of the optic disc is a rare complication. The hemorrhage may extend into the vitreous or under the surrounding retina.

    D. Histologically basophilic, calcareous, laminated acellular bodies of different sizes and shapes are located within the substance of the optic disc anterior to the scleral lamina cribrosa.

IX. Drusen of the adjacent retinal pigment epithelium (Fig. 13–25) may protrude into the lateral aspect of the retinal layer of the optic nerve head.

Although drusen of the RPE and of the optic nerve have the same name, they are quite different as to cause and to structure. RPE drusen are homogeneous secretions of the RPE, whereas optic nerve drusen are structurally as described above and may be secretory products of optic nerve glial cells, presumably astrocytes anterior to the scleral lamina cribrosa.

X. Corpora amylacea (Fig. 13–26) ("brain dust"). These are intracellular and extracellular, basophilic, PAS-positive structures observed with great regularity in the white matter of the brain, including optic nerve and retina (mainly nerve fiber layer). The structures appear to be composed of a glycoprotein–acid mucopolysaccharide complex produced within glial cells (astrocytes). They have no clinical significance and can be considered as an aging phenomena.

XI. Corpora arenacea (Fig. 13–27) (psammoma bodies). These are laminated, basophilic bodies produced by the meningothelial

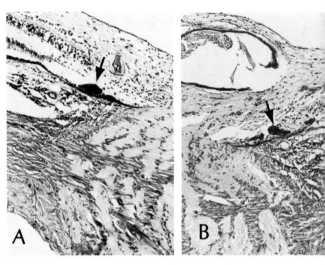

FIG. 13–25. Drusen (*arrows*) of juxtapapillary RPE are seen on both sides of optic nerve (**A** and **B**). **A,** PAS, ×40; **B,** PAS, ×40.

FIG. 13–26. Corpora amylacea (*arrows* in **A**) are PAS-positive (**B**) and lie in tissue of retinal layer of optic nerve head. **A,** PAS, ×100; **B,** PAS, ×530.

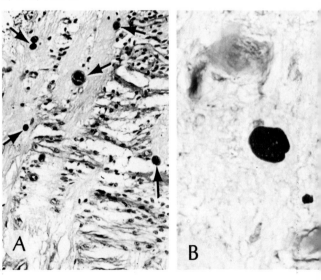

cells of the arachnoid matter. They are of no clinical significance and can be considered as an aging phenomena.

Morphologically identical structures called psammoma bodies may be found in meningiomas and in a variety of papillary carcinomas.

XII. Buscaiano bodies resemble corpora amylacea and are fixation artifacts.

SECONDARY

I. Retinoblastoma.
II. Malignant melanoma of choroid.
III. Pseudotumor of retinal pigment epithelium.
IV. Intracranial meningioma.
V. Metastatic carcinoma.
   A. Metastatic to parenchyma.
   B. Metastatic to meninges.
VI. Glioblastoma multiforme of brain.
VII. Artifacts may simulate macroscopically secondary (or primary) optic nerve tumors, e.g., myelin (Fig. 13–28).

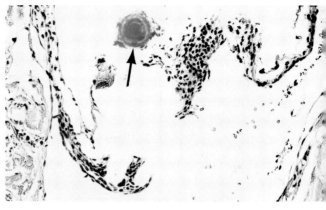

FIG. 13–27. Corpus arenaceus (psammoma body) is seen as laminated, basophilic body (*arrow*) produced by meningothelial cells of arachnoid. H&E, ×200.

FIG. 13–28. Myelin artifact. **A.** Major retinal vessel filled with myelin debris. **Inset** shows macroscopic appearance of white mass (i.e., myelin) protruding from vicinity of optic nerve head and several retinal vessels that are similarly white. **B.** Electron micrograph shows content of vessel to be debris of whole optic nerve fibers that have been squeezed into vessels due to severe compression of optic nerve during enucleation. Note laminations (*arrow*) of relatively intact myelin sheath. **C.** Macroscopic view of myelin extruding artifactitiously from optic nerve head. This might be misinterpreted in laboratory as tumor. **A,** 1.5 μ section, PD, ×220; **B,** ×53,200; **C,** macroscopic.

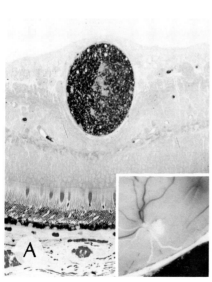

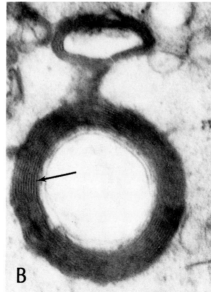

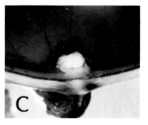

BIBLIOGRAPHY

CONGENITAL DEFECTS AND ANATOMIC VARIATIONS

Curtin BJ, Karlin DB: Axial length measurements and fundus changes of the myopic eye. Am J Ophthalmol 71:42, 1971

Edwards WC, Layden WE: Optic nerve hypoplasia. Am J Ophthalmol 70:950, 1970

Ferry AP: Macular detachment associated with congenital pit of the optic nerve head—pathology findings in two cases simulating malignant melanoma of the choroid. Arch Ophthalmol 70:346, 1963

Font RL, Zimmerman LE: Intrascleral smooth muscle in coloboma of the optic disc. Electron microscopic verification. Am J Ophthalmol 72:452, 1971

Gass JDM: Serous detachment of the macula secondary to congenital pit of the optic nerve head. Am J Ophthalmol 67:821, 1969

Grear JN: Pits, or crater-like holes, in the optic disc. Arch Ophthalmol 28:467, 1942

Hamada S, Ellsworth RE: Congenital retinal detachment and the optic disc anomaly. Am J Ophthalmol 71:460, 1971

Hogan MJ, Zimmerman LE (eds): Ophthalmic Pathology: An Atlas and Textbook (2nd ed). Philadelphia, Saunders, 1962, p 586

Jack MK: Central serous retinopathy with optic pit treated with photocoagulation. Am J Ophthalmol 67:519, 1969

Pfaffenbach DD, Walsh FB: Central pit of the optic disc. Am J Ophthalmol 73:102, 1972

Savir H, Rosen ES: Congenital pit of the optic disc with acquired retinal cyst. Ann Ophthalmol 4:756, 1972

Scheie HG, Adler FH: Aplasia of the optic nerve. Arch Ophthalmol 26:61, 1941

Willis R, Zimmerman LE, O'Grady R, Smith RS, Crawford B: Heterotopic adipose tissue and smooth muscle in the optic disc. Arch Ophthalmol 88:139, 1972

Yanoff M, Rorke LB: Ocular and central nervous system findings in tetrapolid-diploid mosaicism. Am J Ophthalmol 75:1036, 1973

PAPILLEDEMA

Bird AC, Sanders MD: Choroidal folds in association with papilloedema. Br J Ophthalmol 57:89, 1973

Drill VA: Oral contraceptives and thromboembolic disease. I. Prospective and retrospective studies. J Am Med Assoc 219:583, 1972

Drill VA, Calhoun DW: Oral contraceptives and thromboembolic disease. II. Estrogen content of oral contraceptives. J Am Med Assoc 219:593, 1972

Lazaro EJ, Cinotti AA, Eichler PN, Khawaja AA: Amaurosis due to massive gastrointestinal hemorrhage. Am J Gastroenterol 55:50, 1971

Trujillo MH, Desenne JJ, Pinto HB: Reversible papilledema in iron deficiency anemia. Two cases with normal spinal fluid pressure. Ann Ophthalmol 4:378, 1972

OPTIC NEURITIS

Appen RE, Allen JC: Optic neuritis under 60 years of age. Ann Ophthalmol 6:143, 1974

Blackwood W, McMenemey WH, Meyer A, Norman RM, Russell DS: Greenfield's Neuropathology. London, Arnold, 1963, pp 475–519

Brownstein S, Jannotta FS: Sarcoid granulomas of the retina and optic nerve. Canad J Ophthalmol 9:372, 1974

Cogan DG, Truman JT, Smith TR: Optic neuropathy, chloramphenicol, and infantile genetic agranulocytosis. Invest Ophthalmol 12:534, 1973

Hayreh SS: Optic disc vasculitis. Br J Ophthalmol 56:652, 1972

Henkind P, Charles NC, Pearson J: Histopathology of ischemic optic neuropathy. Am J Ophthalmol 69:78, 1970

Kean BH: Subacute myelo-optic neuropathy. A probable case in the United States. J Am Med Assoc 220:243, 1972

Knox DL, Duke JR: Slowly progressive ischemic optic neuropathy. A clinicopathologic case report. Trans Am Acad Ophthalmol Otolaryngol 75:1065, 1971

Miller BW, Frankel M: Report of a case of tuberculous retrobulbar neuritis and osteomyelitis. Am J Ophthalmol 71:751, 1971

Norton AL, Walsh FB: Disulfiram-induced optic neuritis. Trans Am Acad Ophthalmol Otolaryngol 76:1263, 1972

Percy AK, Nobregan FT, Kurland LT: Optic neuritis and multiple sclerosis. An epidemiologic study. Arch Ophthalmol 87:135, 1972

Phillips CI, Wang MK, VanPeborgh PF: Some observations on mechanism of tobacco amblyopia and its treatment with sodium thiosulfate. Trans Ophthalmol Soc UK 90:809, 1971

Saraux H, Biais B: Optic neuritis caused by Disulfiram (in French). Ann Ocul (Paris) 203:769, 1970

OPTIC ATROPHY

Anderson DR: Ascending and descending optic atrophy produced experimentally in squirrel monkeys. Am J Ophthalmol 76:693, 1973

Caldwell JBH, Howard RO, Riggs LA: Dominant juvenile optic atrophy. Arch Ophthalmol 85:133, 1971

Emery JM, Green WR, Huff DS: Krabbe's disease. Histopathology and ultrastructure of the eye. Am J Ophthalmol 74:400, 1972

Harcourt B, Ashton N: Ultrastructure of the optic nerve in Krabbe's leucodystrophy. Br J Ophthalmol 57:885, 1973

Knox DL, Duke JR: Slowly progressive ischemic optic neuropathy. A clinicopathologic case report. Trans Am Acad Ophthalmol Otolaryngol 75:1065, 1971

Krill AE, Smith VC, Pokorny J: Further studies supporting the identity of congenital tritanopia and hereditary dominant optic atrophy. Invest Ophthalmol 10:457, 1971

Rahn EK, Yanoff M, Tucker S: Neuro-ocular considerations in the Pelizaeus-Merzbacher syndrome: a clinicopathologic study. Am J Ophthalmol 66:1143, 1968

Seedorff T: Leber's disease. Acta Ophthalmol (Kbh) 48:186, 1970

Smith JL, Hoyt WF, Susac JO: Ocular fundus in acute Leber optic neuropathy. Arch Ophthalmol 90:349, 1973

Snyder LM, Necheles TF, Reddy WJ, Calcagni K, Reed F: G-6-PD Worcester: a new variant, associated with X-linked optic atrophy. Am J Med 49:125, 1970

Wallace DC: Leber's optic atrophy: a possible example of vertical transmission of a slow virus in a man. Aust Ann Med 3:259, 1970

TUMORS

Brandt DE, Beisner DH: Meningioma of the optic nerve. Arch Ophthalmol 84:477, 1970

Cogan DG, Kuwabara T: Myelin artifacts. Am J Ophthalmol 64:622, 1967

Ellis W, Little HL: Leukemic infiltration of the optic nerve head. Am J Ophthalmol 75:867, 1973

Fine BS, Yanoff M: Ocular Histology: A Text and Atlas. New York, Harper & Row, 1972, p 87

Gibberd FB, Miller TN, Morgan AD: Glioblastoma of the optic chiasm. Br J Ophthalmol 57:788, 1973

Gudas PP Jr: Optic nerve myeloma. Am J Ophthalmol 71:1085, 1971

Hamilton AM, Garner A, Tripathi RC, Sanders MD: Malignant optic nerve glioma. Report of a case with electron microscopic study. Br J Ophthalmol 57:253, 1973

Kamin DF, Hepler RS, Foos RY: Optic nerve drusen. Arch Ophthalmol 89:359, 1973

Karp LA, Zimmerman LE, Borit A, Spencer W: Primary intraorbital meningiomas. Arch Ophthalmol 91:24, 1974

Lloyd LA: Gliomas of the optic nerve and chiasm in childhood. Trans Am Ophthalmol Soc 71:488, 1973

Schwarz GA, Yanoff M: Lafora bodies, corpora amylacea, and Lewy bodies. A morphologic and histochemical study. Arch Neurobiol (Madr) 28:803, 1965

Shuangshoti S: Meningioma of the optic nerve. Br J Ophthalmol 57:265, 1973

Susac JO, Smith JL, Powell JO: Carcinomatous optic neuropathy. Am J Ophthalmol 76:672, 1973

Wise GN, Henkind P, Alterman M: Optic disc drusen and subretinal hemorrhage. Trans Am Acad Ophthalmol Otolaryngol 78:212, 1974

Yanoff M, Davis R, Zimmerman LE: Juvenile pilocytic astrocytoma ("glioma") of optic nerve: clinicopathologic study of 63 cases. In preparation

Zimmerman LE, Fine BS: Myelin artifacts in the optic disc and retina. Arch Ophthalmol 74:394, 1965

chapter 14

Orbit

EXOPHTHALMOS

The main clinical manifestation of orbital disease is exophthalmos (proptosis).*

The extent and direction of the exophthalmos depends on four main factors:
 I. The size of the lesion.
 II. The character of the lesion.
   A. Expansile versus infiltrative growth.
   B. Rapid versus slow growth.
 III. The location of the lesion within the orbit.
   A. A small lesion within the muscle cone causes more exophthalmos than a lesion of the same size outside of the muscle cone.
   B. Lesions anterior to the septum orbitale do not produce exophthalmos unless they also grow posteriorly.
 IV. The effect of the lesion on the extraocular muscles.
      Complete paralysis of all muscles by itself can cause 2 mm of exophthalmos.

Exophthalmos may be simulated by
 I. Lid retraction due to any cause, most commonly lid retraction of *Graves's disease.*
 II. Unilateral enlargement of the globe.
   A. *High myopia.*
   B. *Buphthalmos.*
 III. A sagging lower lid.
 IV. Relaxation of the rectus muscle(s).
 V. Enophthalmos or microphthalmos of the opposite eye.
 VI. Asymmetry of the bony orbits.
 VII. Shallow orbits.

The most common causes of exophthalmos are
 I. Thyroid disease. This is the most common cause of unilateral *and* bilateral exophthalmos.
 II. Hemangioma.

---

* Exophthalmos refers specifically to protrusion of the eyes, whereas proptosis refers to protrusion of any part of the body, including the eyes.

 III. Combined group of inflammatory pseudotumors and benign and malignant lymphoid tumors.
 IV. Dermoid.

Although dermoids are one of the most common orbital tumors, if not the most common, they rarely cause exophthalmos because of their position, which generally is anterior to the septum orbitale.

DEVELOPMENTAL ABNORMALITIES

DEVELOPMENTAL ABNORMALITIES OF BONY ORBIT

Developmental abnormalities of the bony orbit usually are associated with abnormalities of the cranial and facial bones such as tower skull or hypertelorism.

Although most of the developmental anomalies of the skull affecting the eyes have no known cause, they may have a chromosomal abnormality such as a trisomy 21 mosaic.

MICROPHTHALMOS WITH CYST (Figs. 2–21 and 14–1)

 I. Microphthalmos with cyst is usually a unilateral condition but may be bilateral.
 II. The cyst may be so large as to obscure the microphthalmic eye.
 III. Proliferated neuroectodermal tissue, i.e., pseudogliomatous hyperplasia, may simulate an orbital neoplasm.
 IV. The condition is due to an incomplete closure of the fetal cleft.

Although microphthalmos with cyst usually has no known cause, it may be associated with the *18 chromosomal deletion defect (partial 18 monosomy).*

V. Histologically the eye may range from relative normality to complete disorder containing such structures as smooth muscle and cartilage. The cyst may be lined by gliotic retina or it may be filled with proliferated glial tissue that can reach massive amounts (massive gliosis) and simulate a glial neoplasm.

CEPHALOCELES (Fig. 14–2)

I. Cephaloceles are due to a developmental malformation in which brain tissue and/or meninges are present in the orbit:
   A. Meningocele—only meninges are present.
   B. Encephalocele—only brain tissue is present.
   C. Meningoencephalocele—meninges and brain tissue are present.
   D. Hydroencephalocele — considerable fluid is present in the cyst. *Brain tissue*
   E. All of the above may communicate with the brain.
      1. It may have communicated initially, but the continuity became closed later.
      2. It may remain in communication, but this is a rare occurrence.
II. Most cephaloceles are developmental displacements of brain tissue and are now generally referred to as *ectopic brain tissue*.
III. Histologically most cases show a structure similar to that of the optic nerve with white matter separated by pial septa.

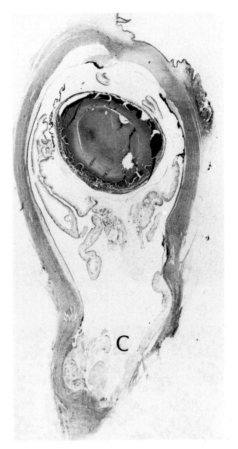

FIG. 14–1. Microphthalmos with cyst. Multiple anomalies, including hypoplasia of iris and ciliary body, cataract and non-attachment and dysplasia of retina, are present. Note cystic structure (C) lined by glia and poorly formed retinal tissue at site of scleral coloboma. H&E, ×4.

ORBITAL INFLAMMATION

ACUTE INFLAMMATION

I. Nonsuppurative (see section Nonsuppurative, Chronic, Nongranulomatous Uveitis and Endophthalmitis in Chap. 3).
   Orbital cellulitis most commonly is caused by extension of an inflammation from the paranasal sinuses (Fig. 14–3).
II. Suppurative (see section Suppurative Endophthalmitis and Panophthalmitis in Chap. 3).
   A. Purulent infection (e.g., with *Staphylococcus aureus*) occurs commonly secondary to trauma.

encephalocele

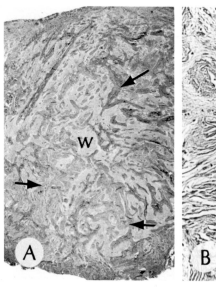
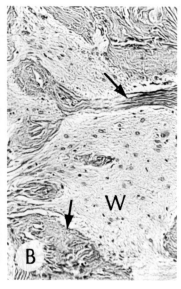

FIG. 14–2. Ectopic brain tissue from 4-year-old boy with mass below right eye since birth. **A** and **B** show low and high magnification of white matter (*W*) divided by septa (*arrows*). **A**, H&E, ×6; **B**, H&E, ×69.

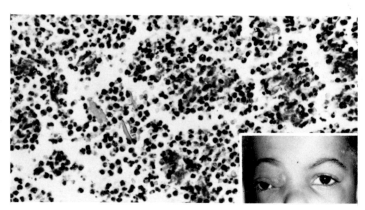

FIG. 14–3. Orbital cellulitis secondary to acute ethmoiditis. Acute purulent inflammatory infiltrate is present in orbital and ethmoidal tissue removed from 48-year-old man. **Inset** shows similar reaction on right side in child. **Main figure,** H&E, ×176; **inset,** clinical.

B. Phycomycosis (mucormycosis) is an increasing cause of suppurative orbital inflammation in recent years (Fig. 14–4).
   1. It usually is associated with other disease, especially when acidosis is present, e.g., diabetes mellitus, renal disease and malignancies.
   2. Thrombotic complications may dominate the clinical picture.

CHRONIC INFLAMMATION

I. Nongranulomatous (Fig. 14–5)
   A. Chronic nongranulomatous inflammation is the most common inflammatory lesion of the orbit and is of unknown cause (see pp. 552–556 in this chapter).
   B. A rare cause of nongranulomatous orbital inflammation is the *benign lymphoepithelial lesion* (so-called *Mikulicz's disease**) (Fig. 14–6).

* Mikulicz's disease is the old term used for *benign lymphoepithelial lesion.* Mikulicz's syndrome is a confusing term that has been used to describe secondary diseases of the lacrimal or salivary glands as may occur in tuberculosis, sarcoidosis, metastatic cancer, malignant lymphomas and leukemia. Because it is uncertain what Mikulicz originally described, it now is advisable to avoid completely the terms Mikulicz's disease and Mikulicz's syndrome. The avoidance will eliminate much future confusion, which now exists in the literature and in clinical terminology.

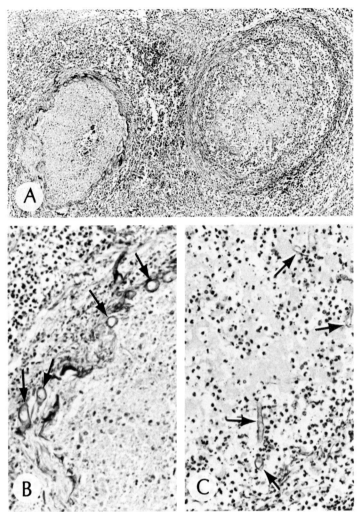

FIG. 14–4. Orbital phycomycosis. **A.** Two large orbital vessels are thrombosed and surrounded by acute suppurative inflammation. **B** and **C** show higher magnification of left and right vessels in **A,** respectively. *Arrows* show hematoxylinophilic, large, nonseptate fungal hyphae. **A,** H&E, ×40; **B,** H&E, ×202; **C,** H&E, ×202.

FIG. 14–5. Chronic nongranulomatous orbital myositis. Muscle fibers (*arrows*) are separated by lymphocytes and plasma cells. H&E, ×101.

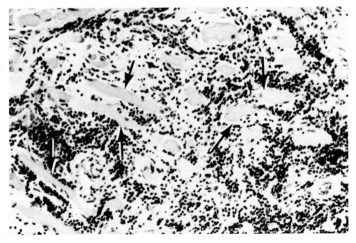

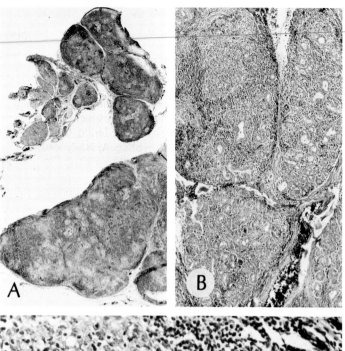

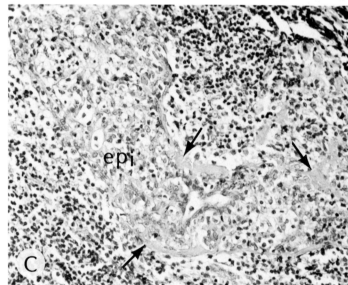

FIG. 14–6. Benign lymphoepithelial lesion is characterized by replacement of glandular parenchyma by benign lymphoid infiltrate (**A, B** and **C**), general preservation of glandular lobular architecture (**A** and **B**) and epimyoepithelial islands of proliferation within glandular ducts (*epi* in **C**). *Arrows* in **C** show thickened ductal basement membrane. **A,** H&E, ×4; **B,** H&E, ×50; **C,** H&E, ×145.

FIG. 14–7. Endogenous sporotrichosis of orbital margin in 58-year-old woman on long-term antiinflammatory therapy is characterized by granulomatous inflammatory infiltrate with multinucleated giant cells. **Inset** shows cigar-shaped and round forms of sporotrichia in specially stained section. **Main figure,** H&E, ×101; **inset,** Gomori's methenamine silver, ×250.

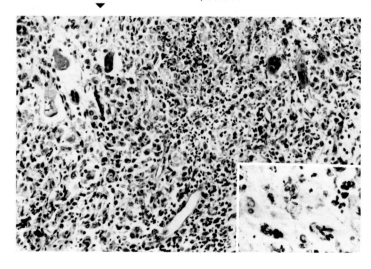

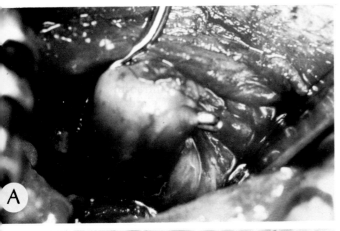

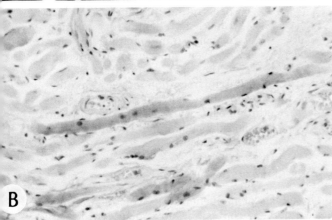

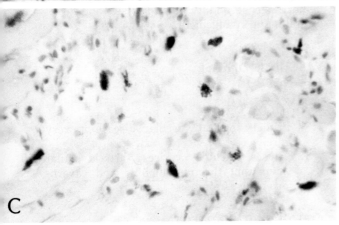

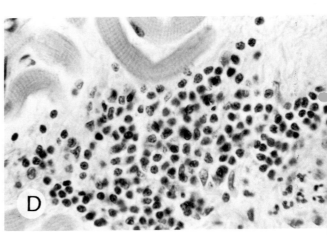

Fɪɢ. 14–8. Graves's disease. **A.** View at time of Krönlein orbital decompression shows muscle hook under lateral rectus muscle, which is thickened and rubbery and measures 13 mm at its narrowest available width (normal muscle measures about 5 mm). **B.** Muscle fibers are separated by interstitial edema. **C.** Special stain demonstrates increased numbers of mast cells (very dark-staining cells). **D.** Many lymphocytes and some plasma cells and polymorphonuclear leukocytes are present between striated muscle fibers. **A,** clinical; **B,** H&E, ×200; **C,** toluidine blue, ×500; **D,** H&E, ×500.

1. It is characterized by painless unilateral or bilateral enlargement of the salivary or, rarely, the lacrimal glands.
2. The condition may be part of *Sjögren's syndrome.*
3. Rarely it may become malignant.
4. Histologically benign lymphoepithelial lesion is characterized by
   a. Replacement of the glandular parenchyma by a benign lymphoid infiltrate.
   b. General preservation of the lobular architecture of the lacrimal gland.
   c. *Epimyoepithelial islands* of proliferation within the glandular ducts.
C. Inflammatory pseudotumor (see pp. 552–556 in this chapter).

II. Granulomatous
   A. Granulomatous inflammations rarely involve the orbit.
   B. Causes include tuberculosis, sarcoidosis, syphilis, fungi (Fig. 14–7), parasites (trichinosis, schistosomiasis, etc.), Wegener's granulomatosis and midline lethal granuloma.
   C. Inflammatory pseudotumor (see pp. 552–556 in this chapter).

INJURIES

PENETRATING WOUNDS

I. Direct effect on whatever tissue may be wounded by the injury.
II. Complications
   A. Infection
      1. Organisms may be introduced at the time of injury.
         a. Bacteria cause an acute purulent inflammation.
         b. Fungi cause a delayed, chronic, granulomatous inflammation.
   B. Inflammation
      1. The inflammation may be secondary to toxic products of tissue destruction.
      2. Thrombophlebitis of orbital veins

may be a complication of the inflammation.
3. A retained intraorbital foreign body may induce inflammation.
   a. Frequently cilia, pieces of skin, wood, bone, etc. may be introduced into orbit at the time of injury and cause a secondary foreign body granulomatous inflammatory reaction.
   b. Fungi may enter as a coincidental saprophyte along with the penetrating foreign body, which causes an inflammatory reaction, usually granulomatous in type, or even superimposed infection if the organism proliferates.
C. Orbital inflammation may lead to other complications such as cavernous sinus thrombosis, central retinal vein thrombosis, glaucoma and proptosis with corneal exposure.

NONPENETRATING WOUNDS

The effects of nonpenetrating wounds are those secondary to contusion and concussion, mainly hemorrhage, secondary muscle palsies and infraorbital nerve involvement.

VASCULAR DISEASE

PRIMARY

I. Primary orbital vascular disease is very rare.
II. Causes include varices, arteriovenular aneurysm, thrombophlebitis and cavernous sinus thrombosis.

PART OF SYSTEMIC DISEASE

I. Collagen diseases—see pp. 195–199 in Chapter 6, p. 525 in this chapter and p. 397 in Chapter 11.
II. Wegener's granulomatosis—see p. 196 in Chapter 6.
III. Allergic vasculitis—see p. 196 in Chapter 6.
IV. Temporal (cranial) arteritis—see p. 395 in Chapter 11.

OCULAR MUSCLE INVOLVEMENT IN SYSTEMIC DISEASE

GRAVES'S DISEASE

I. Classification of eye changes of Graves's disease (see Table 14–1).

II. Mild form ("thyrotoxic" exophthalmos).
 A. The mild form of Graves's disease has its onset in early adult life with women predominating (approximately 9:1).
 B. It may present initially with unilateral involvement but generally becomes bilateral.
 C. Clinically and chemically the individual is hyperthyroid.
 D. Proptosis may be apparent due to lid retraction or may be real (mild to moderate).
 E. Prognosis for vision is good.

III. Severe form ("thyrotropic" or "malignant" exophthalmos) (Fig. 14–8)
 A. The severe form of Graves's disease affects individuals in middle age (average 50 years).
 B. There is an equal sex incidence except for postoperative cases where men predominate (approximately 4:1).
 C. The disease usually is bilateral and asymmetrical.
 D. Clinically and chemically the individual may be hyperthyroid, hypothyroid or euthyroid.
  1. Ophthalmic Graves's disease
   a. The term ophthalmic Graves's disease describes ocular manifestations of Graves's disease in individuals who are euthyroid and have no past history suggesting hyperthyroidism, i.e., malignant exophthalmos in a euthyroid individual.
   b. The eye signs frequently are asymmetrical.
   c. The individuals may have a family history of thyroid disease or pernicious anemia.
   d. The 6-hour radioiodine uptake is not suppressed by triiodothyronine about half of the time.
   e. About half of the individuals show a rise in radioiodine uptake after administration of thyroid-stimulating hormone.
   f. *Long-acting thyroid stimulator (LATS)* may be present in the serum, but it is unlikely that it is a major factor in the pathogenesis of the ocular manifestations.
 E. The proptosis is severe and associated frequently with *pretibial myxedema* (Fig. 14–9). Along with the proptosis often there is chemosis, dilated vessels (especially over the rectus muscles) and limitation of ocular motility.
 F. The prognosis for vision is poor.
 G. Histologically the orbital tissue is characterized by edema, lymphocytic infiltration (with some plasma cells and mast cells) and increased mucin content.

 With time, the extraocular muscles may degenerate and become fibrotic.

The inferior rectus muscle especially is prone to becoming fibrotic. If the patient is asked to look up while sitting during Schiøtz tonometry, abnormally high readings may be obtained. It is important, therefore, to have the patient lying down and looking straight ahead when doing indentation tonometry, or to do applanation tonometry.

MYASTHENIA GRAVIS

I. Myasthenia gravis involves the extraocular

TABLE 14–1.
Eye Changes in Graves's Disease*

Class	Ocular symptoms and signs
0	No signs or symptoms
1	Only signs, no symptoms
2	Soft tissue involvement with symptoms and signs
3	Proptosis
4	Extraocular muscle involvement
5	Corneal involvement
6	Optic nerve involvement with some loss of vision

* Modified from Table 2 in Werner, 1969.

muscles, especially the levator palpebrae superioris.

II. Ptosis of the eyelid is the most common clinical manifestation.

As a rough test, the ptosis often can be aggravated by having the individual elevate and depress his eyes 10 to 30 times in rapid succession. The normal patient can do this easily with no ptosis or accentuation of a ptosis afterward.

III. Histologically the ocular muscles are edematous and infiltrated by lymphocytes.

MYOTONIA DYSTROPHICA (Steinert's disease)

I. Myotonia dystrophica is characterized by myotonia, i.e., failure to voluntarily relax a contracted muscle. It has an autosomal dominant inheritance pattern.

II. Its onset is between 20 and 30 years of

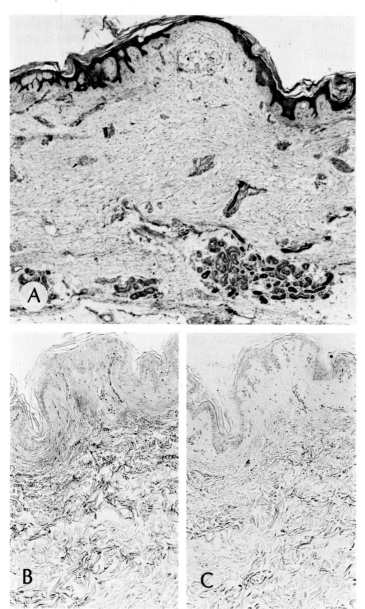

FIG. 14–9. Pretibial myxedema in 45-year-old woman with "thyrotoxic goiter" and exophthalmos. **A.** Pretibial skin shows basophilic deposit in thickened dermis, especially in upper third. **B.** Abdominal skin shows similar but less marked changes. **C.** Adjacent section to that shown in **B.** Acid mucopolysaccharide material present to greatest degree in upper third (see **B**) disappears if section is pretreated with hyaluronidase. **A,** H&E, ×35; **B,** AMP, ×80; **C,** hyaluronidase-AMP, ×80.

age, and the patients rarely live beyond 40 or 50.

III. Frontal baldness and endocrinopathy, especially testicular atrophy, are common.

IV. Ocular findings include cataracts consisting of iridescent dots in the anterior and posterior cortex, a foveal dystrophy that hardly affects vision, a pigmentary retinopathy and ocular hypotension.

V. Histologically selective atrophy of muscle fibers is seen.

MYOTONIA CONGENITA (Thomsen's disease)

I. Myotonia congenita is characterized by myotonia. It has an autosomal dominant or recessive inheritance pattern.

II. Its onset is early in life and may involve muscles of the face and eyelids.

III. It does not cause death and rarely causes severe disability.

IV. Histologically the muscles are not atrophic and the individual muscle fibers may be larger than normal with an increase in sarcolemmal nuclei.

OCULAR MYOPATHY
(Progressive External Ophthalmoplegia)

I. Ocular myopathy is a slowly progressive, bilaterally symmetrical, ocular muscle dystrophy that starts in childhood and has an autosomal dominant inheritance pattern.

II. A pigmentary retinopathy may be present.

III. Histologically there is atrophy of muscle fibers, absence of glycogen from the muscle, loss of cross-striations and the myofibrillar structure, large variation in muscle diameter, granular and vacuolar degeneration of muscle fibers, fibrous and fatty replacement of tissue, loss of succinic dehydrogenase and preservation of myelinated nerve fibers and myoneural junctions.

DERMATOMYOSITIS (Fig. 14–10)

I. Dermatomyositis is one of the collagen diseases of unknown cause with a poor prognosis and death a frequent outcome.

II. Men predominate and may acquire the disease in childhood.

III. Conjunctivitis, iritis, ptosis, paralysis of external ocular muscles, horizontal nystagmus and exophthalmos may be present.

Erythematous, edematous patches of skin frequently are seen. There is a predilection for the face and periorbital region.

IV. A retinitis with superficial whitish exudates in the macula and round and flame-shaped hemorrhages may be seen.

V. Histologically lymphocytes are present in the muscles (myositis) and in the walls of blood vessels (vasculitis), in general giving a picture of a nonspecific chronic nongranulomatous inflammation.

FIG. 14–10. Dermatomyositis. **A.** Atrophy and fibrosis of muscle fibers is associated with lymphocytic infiltrate. **B.** Higher magnification to show lymphocytes and plasma cells in clusters (*arrow*) and individually scattered about. **A,** H&E, ×69; **B,** H&E, ×101.

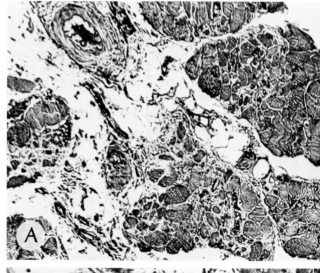

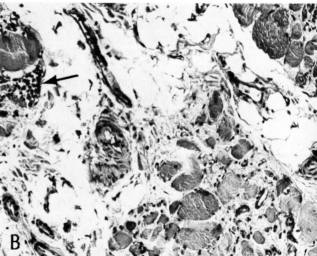

NEOPLASMS AND OTHER TUMORS*

PRIMARY ORBITAL TUMORS

I. Choristomas. These are congenital tumors composed of elements normally not present in the location under consideration.
- A. Dermoid cyst† (Figs. 14–11 and 14–12)
    1. A dermoid cyst most often is found in the upper outer part of the orbit.
    2. It usually has a pedicle attached to the periorbita and may produce bony changes detectable upon x ray.
    3. Histologically a dermoid cyst is composed of ectoderm, i.e., stratified squamous epithelium with *epidermal appendages* (hair follicles, sebaceous glands, sweat glands, etc.), in the wall lining a cavity containing keratin, hair shafts and debris.
- B. Epidermoid cyst† (Fig. 14–13B)
    1. An epidermoid cyst is composed of epidermis, i.e., stratified squamous epithelium with no epidermal appendages in the wall of the cyst.
    2. The cyst cavity contains keratin debris.
- C. Teratoma‡ (Fig. 14–13)
    1. A teratoma is composed of ectoderm, endoderm and mesoderm.
    2. It may contain stratified squamous epithelium, colonic mucosa, central nervous system tissue, etc.
    3. It has malignant potential.
- D. Ectopic lacrimal gland‡ (Fig. 14–14)
    1. Ectopic lacrimal gland consists of lacrimal gland tissue anywhere outside of the lacrimal fossa.
    2. It may be associated with other choristomatous tissues such as muscle, nerve, cartilage or various dermal appendages, or it may occur alone.
    3. It generally causes symptoms only when inflamed; the origin of the inflammation is unknown.
    4. Histologically it is composed of relatively normal-looking lacrimal gland tissue with a mild inflamma-

---

*A † following the name of the tumor denotes that the tumor is common, important or both. A ‡ denotes that the tumor is uncommon, unimportant or both.

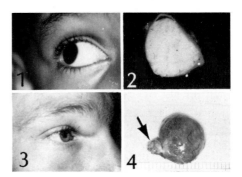

FIG. 14–11. Dermoid cyst. Typical location at upper outer rim of orbit is shown in **1.** In **2** note characteristic "cheesy" center of specimen from **1.** Atypical location nasally is shown in **3;** dermoid, as seen in **4,** was clear cyst with dermal structures present in pedicle (*arrow*). **1,** clinical; **2,** macroscopic; **3,** clinical; **4,** macroscopic.

FIG. 14–12. Dermoid cyst shows epidermis lining lumen (*L*). Glandular structures are present in wall of cyst. H&E, ×40.

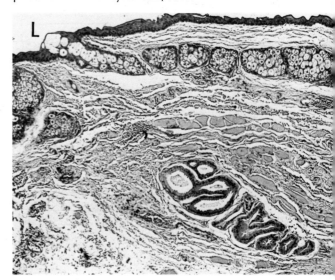

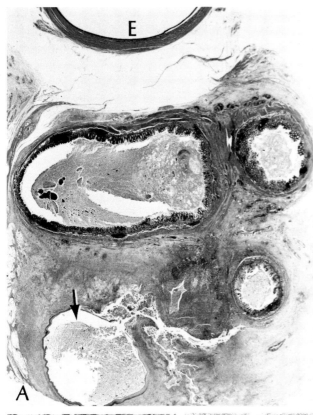

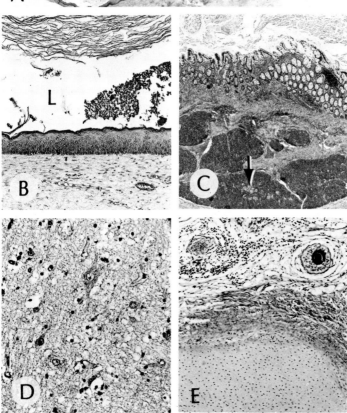

FIG. 14–13. Teratoma. **A.** Large teratoma present behind eyeball (*E*) contains glandular tissue and ruptured epidermoid cyst (*arrow*). **B.** Higher magnification shows epidermoid cyst lined by epidermis with keratin debris in lumen (*L*). **C.** Pancreatic tissue with islets of Langerhans (*arrow*) is present in wall of intestinal tissue. **D.** Brain tissue containing neurons is seen. **E.** In this area hair follicles and cartilage are present. **A,** H&E, ×4; **B,** H&E, ×55; **C,** H&E, ×26; **D,** H&E, ×165; **E,** H&E, ×35.

tory infiltrate of lymphocytes and plasma cells.

II. Hamartomas. These are congenital tumors composed of elements normally found at the involved site.

A. Phakomatoses—see Chapter 2.

B. Hemangioma

1. Hemangioblastoma‡ (Figs. 2–1 and 14–15)

   a. Hemangioblastoma is found in *angiomatosis retinae* (see p. 30 in Chap. 2).

   b. Histologically it is composed of a fine mesh of blood spaces and channels of capillary structures intimately associated with pale, foamy, polygonal, *stromal* cells.

2. Hemangioendothelioma ("strawberry" hemangioma)† (Fig. 14–16)

   a. A hemangioendothelioma is a benign, diffuse hemangioma, which clinically may have a "strawberry" appearance.

   b. About 20 percent are noted at birth with most of the remainder noted within the first month of life. They generally remain stationary or progress during the first year of life, but then almost always regress spontaneously.

   c. No treatment is needed in the vast majority of cases, if not in all.

   d. Histologically it is composed of endothelial cells with very few capillary lumens.

   The nature of the lesion is such that it may arise simultaneously in a number of areas, thereby simulating invasion and malignancy. The lesion is benign but does have a tendency toward multifocal origin.

3. Capillary hemangioma ("cherry" hemangioma)† (Fig. 14–17)

   a. A capillary hemangioma is generally a solitary, bright red, smooth hemangioma.

   b. Usually it begins within the first 5 years of life and tends to spontaneously regress.

Another form of capillary hemangioma occurs in middle-aged or older individuals, often in persons with cardiovascular problems.

   c. Histologically it is composed primarily of capillaries.

4. Cavernous hemangioma† (Figs. 14–18 and 14–19)

   a. Cavernous hemangioma is the *most common primary orbital tumor producing exophthalmos.*

   b. In addition to frequently producing exophthalmos, it may give rise, through pressure on the coats of the eye, to chorioretinal striae.

   c. It is a well-encapsulated tumor, generally within the muscle cone, and usually can be shelled out easily with little or no bleeding.

   d. Generally no feeder vessels can be demonstrated by dye study techniques.

   e. Histologically it is composed of large blood-filled spaces, lined by endothelium and separated by fibrous septal walls ranging from quite thin to fairly thick.

5. Arteriovenous communication‡

   a. Arteriovenous communication (arteriovenous aneurysm; cirsoid, serpentine, plexiform, racemose and cavernous angioma) is rare.

   b. It is found in *arteriovenous communication of retina and brain* (see pp. 37–38 in Chap. 2) or as an incidental finding.

   c. Histologically the tumor is composed of mature blood vessels, which may be hypertrophied. The malformation, rather than hemangioma or angioma, seems to be a mature artery (albeit hypertrophied) becoming a mature vein (again frequently hypertrophied) without passing through a vascular (i.e., capillary) bed.

6. Telangiectasia‡

   a. Telangiectasia of the orbit is rare.

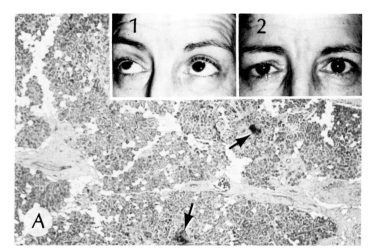

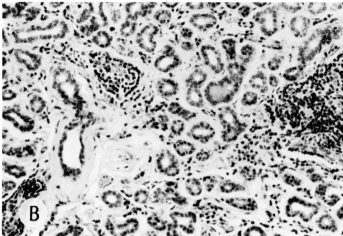

FIG. 14–14. Ectopic lacrimal gland. **A.** Proptosis of left eye is present (**insets 1** and **2**). Biopsy of mass behind the eye, in no way connected to lacrimal gland, shows glandular tissue, resembling lacrimal gland, with foci of chronic nongranulomatous inflammation (*arrows*). **B.** Higher magnification to show lymphocytic (predominantly) and plasma cell infiltrates. **A,** H&E, ×16; **inset 1,** clinical; **inset 2,** clinical; **B,** H&E, ×101.

FIG. 14–15. Hemangioblastoma is characterized by fine mesh of blood spaces and channels of capillary structures intimately associated with pale, foamy, polygonal, stromal cells. **Inset** shows higher magnification of capillaries (*arrows*) and stromal cells. **Main figure,** H&E, ×101; **inset,** H&E, ×200.

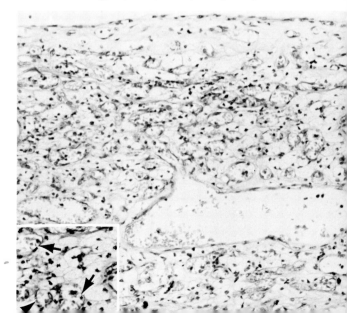

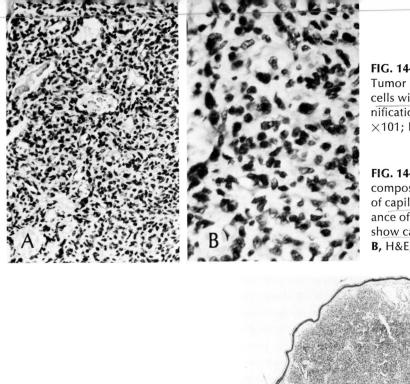

strawberry

FIG. 14–16. Hemangioendothelioma. **A.** Tumor is composed primarily of endothelial cells with few capillaries. **B.** Higher magnification to show endothelial cells. **A,** H&E, ×101; **B,** H&E, 252.

FIG. 14–17. Capillary hemangioma. **A.** Tumor composed of blood vessels predominantly of capillary size. **Inset** shows clinical appearance of tumor. **B.** Higher magnification to show capillaries. **A,** H&E, ×4; **inset,** clinical; **B,** H&E, ×101.

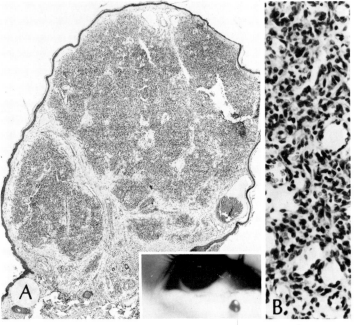

cherry-red

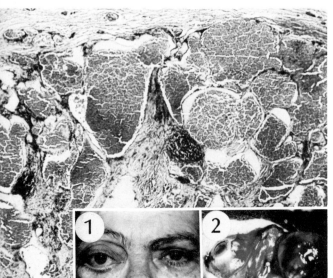

FIG. 14–18. Cavernous hemangioma is characterized by large blood-filled spaces, lined by endothelium and separated by fibrous septal walls of different thickness. **Insets** show clinical appearance of lesion before (**1**) and during (**2**) surgery. **Main figure,** H&E, ×16; **inset 1,** clinical; **inset 2,** clinical at surgery.

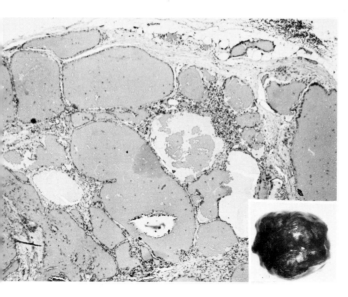

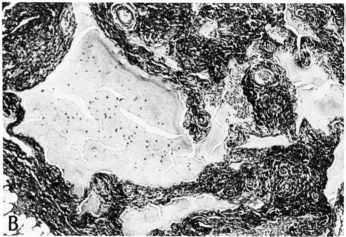

FIG. 14–19. Cavernous hemangioma. Mild nongranulomatous inflammatory reaction present between large blood-filled spaces. **Inset** shows macroscopic appearance of tumor. **Main figure,** H&E, ×21; **inset,** macroscopic.

FIG. 14–20. Lymphangioma. **A.** Tumor is composed of lymph-filled spaces of different sizes. Note lymphoid collections (*arrows*) in walls of tumor. **B.** Special stain shows collagenous nature of septa. **A,** H&E, ×16; **B,** trichrome, ×40.

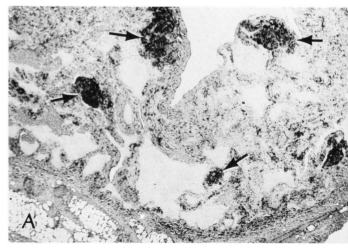

b. Telangiectasia is found in *meningocutaneous angiomatosis* (see pp. 30–32 in Chap. 2), *ataxia-telangiectasia* (see p. 37 in Chap. 2) and *hereditary and familial telangiectasia* (*Osler-Rendu-Weber disease*—see p. 411 in Chap. 11).

c. Histologically it is composed of dilated and tortuous capillaries.

C. Lymphangioma† (Fig. 14–20)
1. Frequently the clinical onset of lymphangioma is in children under 10 years of age.
2. It may diffusely involve the orbit, conjunctiva and lids.
3. The tumor probably regresses in time but easily becomes infected.
4. Histologically it is composed of lymph-filled spaces of different sizes, lined by endothelium and separated by thin, delicate walls.

III. Mesenchymal tumors
A. Vascular
1. Hemangiopericytoma‡ (Fig. 14–21)
a. This rare orbital tumor is most common in the fourth decade.
b. It may be malignant in 12 to 57 percent of cases (varies according to author's series).

It seems that the longer the follow-up, the greater the mortality from the tumor.

c. The clinical course cannot necessarily be predicted from its histologic appearance, especially when its cytology "appears" benign.
d. Hemangiopericytoma probably arises from pericytes, although some authors believe that it arises from endothelial cells.
e. Histologically an increased number of thin-walled vascular channels separated by tumor cells (pericytes) in a network of extracellular material is seen.
1) There is perivascular massing of pericytes.
2) Silver-stained material reveals characteristic appearance of reticulin segregating cells into groups.

3) There is a rather uniform cell morphology.

2. Hemangiosarcoma‡
a. A hemangiosarcoma is an extremely rare orbital tumor.
b. Histologically it is composed of intercommunicating channels or irregular vascular spaces lined by atypical endothelial cells confined within a thin reticulin network.
1) The lining endothelial cells may form a single layer, proliferate in focal areas or produce papillary projections.
2) There is a marked histologic variation within the same tumor and from tumor to tumor.

3. Kaposi's sarcoma‡ (Fig. 14–22)
a. Kaposi's sarcoma is an extremely rare orbital tumor. It occurs in individuals over 40 years of age in 90 percent of cases. There is an overwhelming preponderance in men (approximately 4:1).
b. An association between Kaposi's sarcoma and other cancers exists.

The second primary neoplasm frequently has a higher mortality rate than the disease itself.

c. Classically it originates as a bluish red skin macule that multiplies, coalesces and spreads eventually to internal viscera.
d. Histologically it is composed of many foci of capillary clusters in a stroma of malignant spindle-shaped cells.

Commonly the tumor is admixed with lymphocytes, hence the term *malignant granulation tissue*.

B. Fatty
1. Lipoma† (Fig. 14–23)
a. It is easier to determine clinically than histologically whether a tumor is a primary orbital lipoma or a herniation of orbital fat.
b. Histologically a lipoma is composed of groups of mature fat

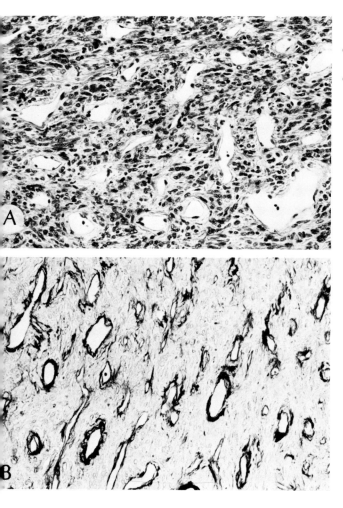

FIG. 14–21. Hemangiopericytoma. **A.** Tumor (nonorbital) shows thin-walled vascular channels separated by masses of pericytes. **B.** Silver stain shows reticulin segregating cells into groups. **A,** H&E, ×101; **B,** reticulum, ×101.

FIG. 14–22. Kaposi's sarcoma. **A.** Conjunctival tumor is composed of many loci of capillary clusters in stroma of malignant-appearing spindle cells. **B.** Higher magnification to show slitlike capillary spaces, malignant-appearing spindle cells and lymphocytes (malignant granulation tissue). **A,** H&E, ×40; **B,** H&E, ×252.

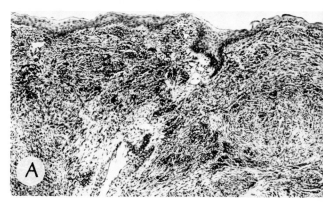

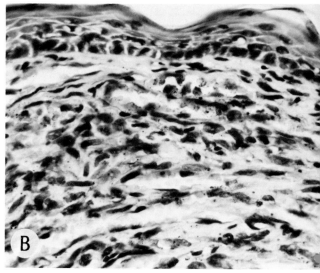

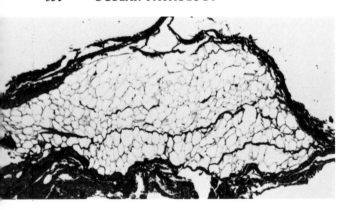

FIG. 14–23. Lipoma is composed of lobules of mature fat separated from each other by delicate fibrovascular septa. H&E, ×28.

cells separated from other groups by delicate fibrovascular septae.

1) Coarser septa divide the tumor into lobules.
2) A true lipoma generally has a thin fibrous capsule.

2. Liposarcoma‡ (Fig. 14–24)
   a. Liposarcoma is an extremely rare orbital tumor.
   b. It may be primary or secondary to radiation therapy (e.g., as for retinoblastomas).
   c. Histologically it is composed of malignant lipoblast cells.

C. Fibrous
   1. Reactive fibrous proliferations
      a. Nodular fasciitis† (Fig. 14–25)
         1) Nodular fasciitis is a benign proliferation of connective tissue.

         The tumor also is called subcutaneous pseudosarcomatous fibromatosis, pseudosarcomatous fasciitis and nodular fibrositis.

         2) Clinically it presents as a rapidly growing mass.
         3) Histologically it is composed of nodular proliferations of plump, stellate or spindle-shaped fibroblasts arranged either in parallel bundles or haphazardly, resembling tissue culture fibroblasts.
            a) A variable amount of intercellular myxoid ground substance is present.
            b) Abundant reticulin fibers and moderate numbers of collagen fibers can be demonstrated.
            c) Proliferation of slitlike vascular spaces or well-formed capillaries is characteristic.
      b. Juvenile fibromatosis‡ (Fig. 14–26)
         1) Juvenile fibromatosis is usually seen in children.

         This group of tumors includes keloids, desmoids, fibromatoses of palmar and plantar fascias and of sternomastoid muscle, radiation fibromatosis and congenital progressive polyfibromatosis.

         2) It may recur after excision and frequently is mistaken for fibrosarcoma.
         3) Histologically it is composed of interlacing fibrous tissue with numerous mature capillaries.
      c. Fibrous histiocytoma† (xanthoma) (Fig. 14–27)

         premalignant

         1) In the past fibrous histiocytoma has been misdiagnosed as sclerosing hemangioma, dermatofibrosarcoma protuberans and even neurofibroma, and when associated with multinucleated giant cells and lipid-filled histiocytes, as synovial giant-cell tumor and villonodular synovitis.

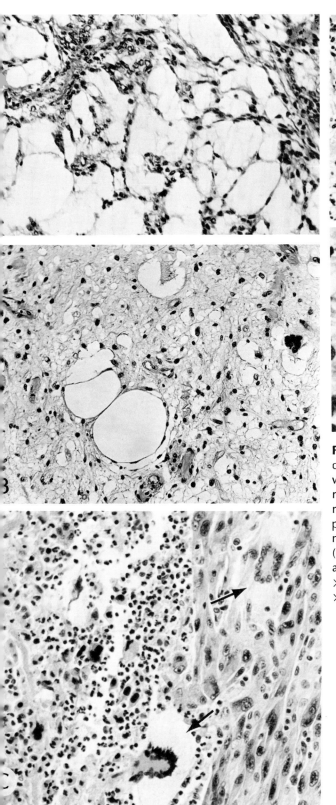

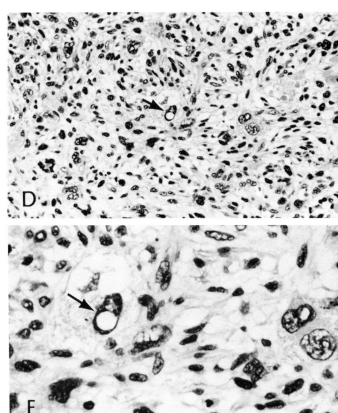

FIG. 14–24. Liposarcoma. Examples (non-orbital) of well-differentiated myxoid tumors with predominance of myxoid cells and mature lipocytes (**A**), poorly differentiated myxoid tumors with bizarre nuclei and paucity of mature lipocytes (**B**), and non-myxoid tumors with Touton giant cells (*arrows* in **C**) and signet cells (*arrows* in **D** and **E**) are shown. **A,** H&E, ×200; **B,** H&E, ×150; **C,** H&E, ×250; **D,** H&E, ×101; **E,** H&E, ×252.

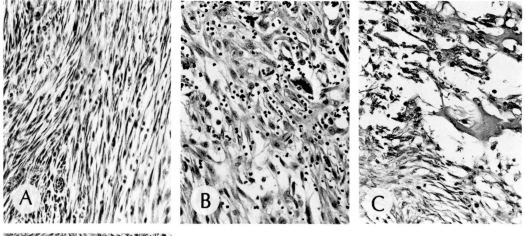

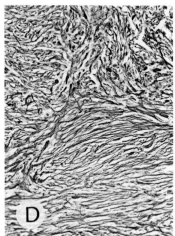

FIG. 14–25. Nodular fasciitis. **A.** Proliferations of plump or spindle-shaped fibroblasts are arranged in parallel bundles and fascicles. **B.** Plump fibroblasts arranged in loose stroma resemble tissue culture growth. **C.** Serous exudate contained in multiple cystlike spaces is surrounded by spindle-shaped fibroblasts. **D.** Special stain shows abundance of reticulin fibers arranged in interlacing fascicles around small slitlike vascular spaces. **A,** H&E, ×180; **B,** H&E, ×180; **C,** H&E, ×145; **D,** Wilder's reticulum, ×90.

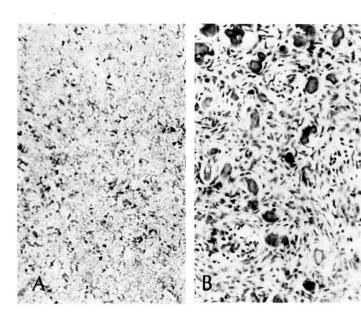

FIG. 14–26. Juvenile ossifying fibroma in 2½-year-old child with proptosis. **A.** Tumor is composed of fibroblasts and calcific concretions, better seen at higher magnification in **B. A,** H&E, ×16; **B,** H&E, ×101.

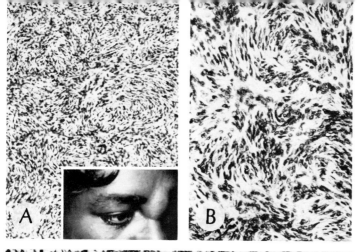

FIG. 14–27. Fibrous histiocytoma in 50-year-old woman. Tumor first excised from nasal orbit in 1965. Recurrences excised in 1970, 1971 and 1973 (**inset** in **A** shows 1973 recurrence). Histologically primary tumor and three recurrences appear identical. **A.** Note matted, "storiform" pattern, shown at higher magnification in **B. C.** Tumor is composed of foamy histiocytes (left side) and fibrous spindle cells. Foamy histiocytes stained positively for fat. **A,** H&E, ×40; **inset,** clinical; **B,** H&E, ×101; **C,** H&E, ×101.

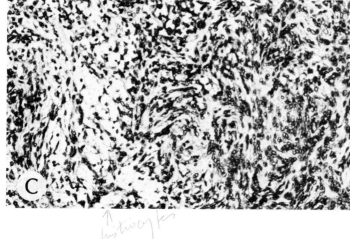

FIG. 14–28. Fibrosarcoma. **A. Insets 1** and **2** show clinical (proptosis of left eye) and macroscopic appearance of orbital tumor in 66-year-old woman. Note characteristic interlacing bundles of spindle-shaped cells forming "herringbone" pattern. **B.** Well-differentiated fibrosarcoma in 60-year-old man in 1961. Tumor recurred in 1964 and was excised. Recurrence (**C** and **D**) is much more cellular and less well-differentiated than primary (**B**). Patient alive with no evidence of tumor in 1973. **A,** H&E, ×130; **inset 1,** clinical; **inset 2,** macroscopic; **B,** H&E, ×260; **C,** H&E, ×60; **D,** H&E, ×260.

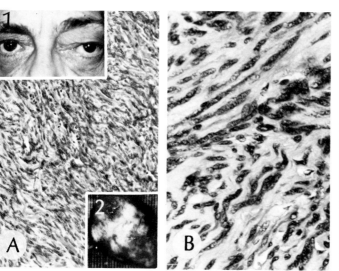
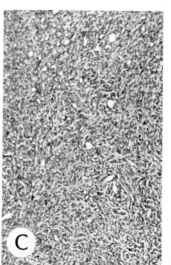
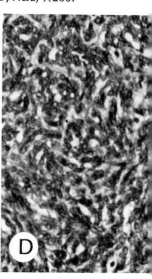

2) It presumably arises from histiocytes.
   a) A pure *histiocytoma* forms no fibers.
   b) Fibrous histiocytoma has a fibrous component; the latter may predominate.
3) It may be reactive but probably is a true neoplasm.
   a) The tumor has a malignant potential.
   b) It should be distinguished from xanthomas and xanthelasmas, which are probably not neoplastic and have no malignant potential.
4) Histologically it has a characteristic "storiform" (matted) pattern composed of fibrous spindle cells with single, or clumps of, foamy histiocytes.
d. Fibroma and fibrosarcoma‡ (Figs. 14–28 and 14–29)
   1) True orbital fibroma is extremely rare, if it exists at all.
   2) Fibrosarcoma is a very rare orbital tumor, which grows slowly.
   3) Histologically it is composed of interlacing bundles of spindle-shaped cells forming a "herring-bone" pattern.

D. Muscle
   1. Leiomyoma‡ is a very rare orbital tumor, and leiomyosarcoma‡ probably does not occur in the orbit.
      Histologically leiomyoma consists of interlacing fascicles of smooth muscle cells (Fig. 9–22).
   2. Rhabdomyoma‡ probably does not occur in the orbit.
   3. Rhabdomyosarcoma†
      a. Rhabdomyosarcoma is the most common malignant mesenchymal orbital neoplasm and is the most common primary malignant orbital tumor in children.
      b. Although found in many parts of the body, rhabdomyosarcoma has a predilection for the orbit.
      c. The average age of onset is about 6 years with the majority

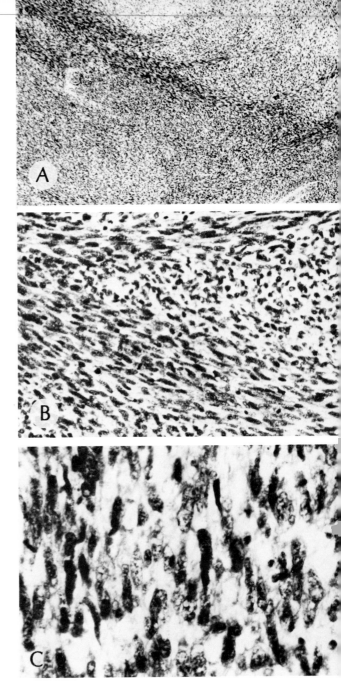

FIG. 14–29. Fibrosarcoma. Orbital tumor developed in 9-year-old child. **A.** Interlacing bundles of spindle-shaped cells form herring-bone pattern, shown at higher magnification in **B. C.** Special stain shows collagen fibers between spindle-shaped nuclei. **A,** H&E, ×28; **B,** H&E, ×101; **C,** trichrome, ×340.

younger than 10 years; it is extremely rare after 25 years of age.

d. The tumor is characterized clinically by a very rapid onset, often simulating an orbital cellulitis.

e. Three types exist:

1) Embryonal (Figs. 14–30 and 14–31)

a) The embryonal form of rhabdomyosarcoma is the most common type.

b) When it arises subconjunctivally, it is identical to the vaginal submucosal tumor of infancy called *sarcoma botryoides.*

c) Histologically it is composed of malignant embryonal cells, *rhabdomyoblasts,* in a loose syncytial arrangement generally with frequent mitotic figures.

(1) The cells are round, oval, elongate or stellate with nuclei rich in chromatin and cytoplasm rich in glycogen.

(2) A ribbon of eosinophilic cytoplasm may be seen around the nucleus.

Generally most of the microscopic fields consist of rather undifferentiated embryonal cells with large hyperchromic nuclei and a scant amount of cytoplasm.

In some areas, however, cells with a ribbon of pink cytoplasm can be seen. It is in these areas where cross-striations are most likely to be found.

(3) Striations sometimes cannot be found in the primary tumor but are found easily in the metastases.

2) Differentiated (adult pleomorphic) (Figs. 14–32 and 14–33)

a) The differentiated form of rhabdomyosarcoma is the least common type but seems to have the best prognosis.

b) Unlike the embryonal and alveolar types where cross-striations are hard to find, cross-striations are found easily in the differentiated type.

3) Alveolar (Fig. 14–34)

a) The alveolar form of rhabdomyosarcoma seems to have the worst prognosis.

b) The individual cell type is similar to the cells found in the embryonal type, but the tumor has a distinct alveolar pattern rather than the undifferentiated or embryonal pattern seen in the embryonal type of rhabdomyosarcoma.

Rhabdomyoblastic cell processes fuse to make the

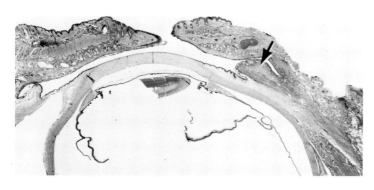

FIG. 14–30. Rhabdomyosarcoma. Subconjunctival embryonal rhabdomyosarcoma (*arrow*) is identical to vaginal submucosal sarcoma botryoides of infants. H&E, ×8.

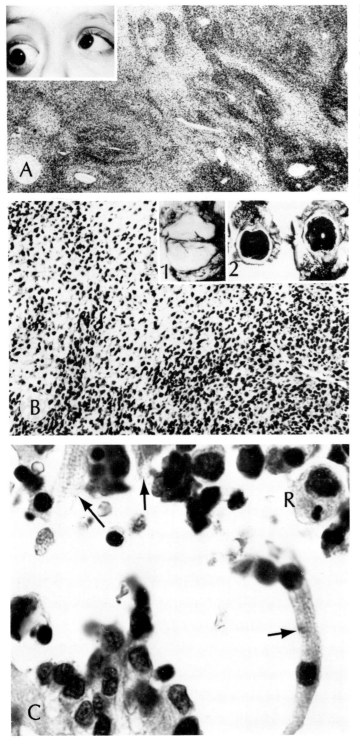

FIG. 14–31. Embryonal rhabdomyosarcoma in 3-year-old girl. **A. Inset** shows clinical appearance of proptosis of right eye. Very cellular tumor shows light or "loose" (less cellular) areas and dark (more cellular) areas. **B.** Higher magnification shows embryonic cellular pattern with more cellular areas darker than less cellular areas. **Insets** show exenteration specimen whole (**1**) and sectioned (**2**). **C.** Note rhabdomyoblast (*R*) and three strap cells (*arrows*) with characteristic cross-striations. **A,** H&E, ×16; **inset,** clinical; **B,** H&E, ×101; **inset 1,** whole macroscopic; **inset 2,** sectioned macroscopic; **C,** H&E, ×630.

walls of the alveolae, whereas other cells lie free in the lumen of the alveolae.

   c) It is the most difficult tumor in which to find cross-striations.

f. Prognosis

   1) The mortality is between 40 and 60 percent with the alveolar type having the worst prognosis and the differentiated the best.

   2) Most deaths occur within the first 3 years so that a 5-year cure probably is a valid one.

E. Cartilage

  1. Chondroma‡ and chondrosarcoma‡

   a. Chondromas and chondrosarcomas are extremely rare orbital tumors.

   b. Chondrosarcoma may arise primarily without antecedent cause, but more frequently it follows radiation for retinoblastoma.

F. Bone

  1. Nonneoplastic and neoplastic diseases of bone generally cause exophthalmos by decreasing orbital volume.

   a. Fibrous dysplasia† (Fig. 14–35).

   b. Juvenile fibromatosis‡ (Fig. 14–26).

   c. Leontiasis ossea‡.

   d. Osteopetrosis‡.

   e. Osteitis fibrosa cystica†.

   f. Paget's disease†.

   g. Osteoma‡ and osteosarcoma‡

    1) Both are extremely rare orbital tumors.

    2) Osteosarcoma may follow radiation for retinoblastomas.

IV. Neural tumors

A. Amputation neuroma‡ (Fig. 14–36)

  1. An amputation neuroma is quite rare in the orbit.

  2. It is not a neoplasm but rather a benign proliferation of Schwann cells.

  3. Histologically it is composed of a haphazard entanglement of regenerated nerve fibers from the cut end of the peripheral ciliary nerve(s).

B. Neurofibromas† (Figs. 2–3 through 2–6 and 14–37)—see section Neurofibromatosis in Chapter 2.

C. Neurilemmoma (Schwannoma)† (Fig. 14–38)

  1. A neurilemmoma is a rare orbital tumor.

  2. The tumor is composed of a neoplastic proliferation of Schwann cells.

  3. Histologically it consists of spindle-shaped Schwann nuclei with a tendency toward palisading.

   a. When the texture is compact and composed of interwoven bundles of long bipolar spindle cells, frequently with ribbons of palisading cells alternating with relatively acellular areas, the *Antoni type A* pattern is present.

    1) Areas of the tumor may mimic tactile corpuscles and are called *Verocay bodies*.

    2) The tumor may have a more haphazard arrangement with a loose texture and microcystoid areas of necrosis; this type of degenerative pattern is called the *Antoni type B* pattern.

   b. The tumor generally is encapsulated.

  4. Malignant Schwannoma (malignant neurilemmoma, neurogenic sarcoma)‡ is extremely rare and when present is associated with neurofibromatosis in 50 percent of cases.

V. Miscellaneous tumors (probably) of neurogenic origin

A. Juvenile pilocytic astrocytoma (glioma) of optic nerve†—see pp. 502–505 in Chapter 13.

B. Meningioma†—see p. 505 in Chapter 13.

C. Nonchromaffin paraganglioma (carotid body tumor)‡

  1. A nonchromaffin paraganglioma is a rare, benign orbital tumor probably of neurogenic origin.

The tumor chiefly occurs outside of the orbit at the bifurcation of the common carotid artery.

best Px , least common

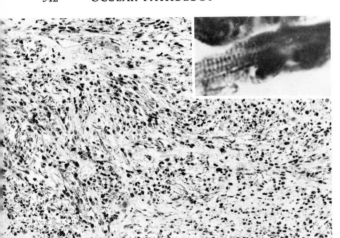

FIG. 14–32. Differentiated rhabdomyo-sarcoma. Most cells have ribbon of eosino-philic cytoplasm. **Inset** shows cross-striation, which is easy to find in this type of tumor. **Main figure,** H&E, ×115; **inset,** phospho-tungstic acid hematoxylin (PTAH), ×850.

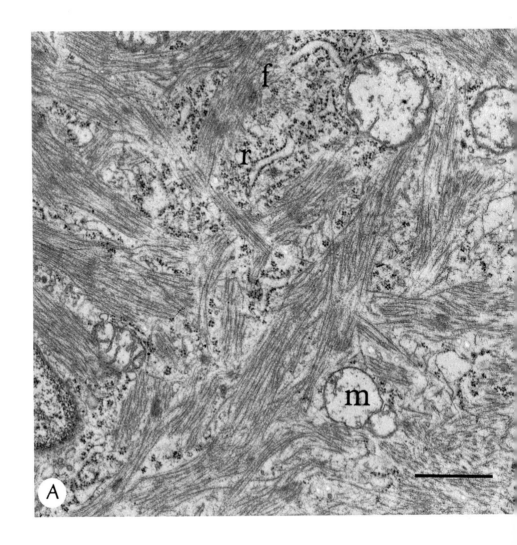

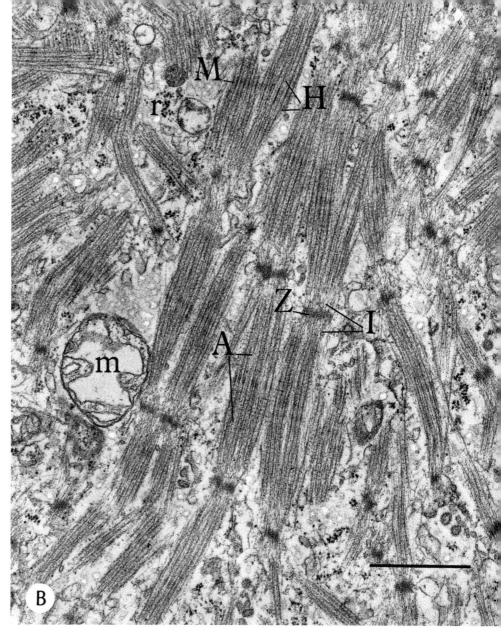

◄ FIG. 14–33. Differentiated rhabdomyosarcoma. **A.** Cytoplasm of poorly differentiated muscle cell ("myofilamentous"). Filaments (*f*) are of thick (~ 150 A diameter) and thin (~ 60 A diameter) varieties. *r*, ribosomes and segment of granular endoplasmic reticulum; *m*, mitochondrion. **B.** Well-differentiated tumor cell ("myofibrillar"). Thick and thin filaments are organized into parallel groupings crossed by dense Z bands (cross-striations) as well as by recognizable A band, I band, H band and M bands. *r*, cluster of ribonucleoprotein particles; *m*, mitochondrion. **A,** ×21,000; **B,** ×27,900.

→ want Px

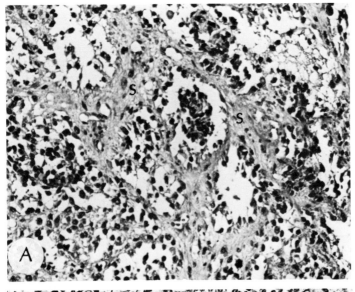

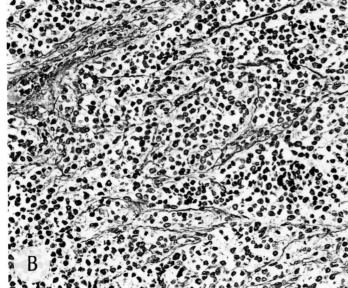

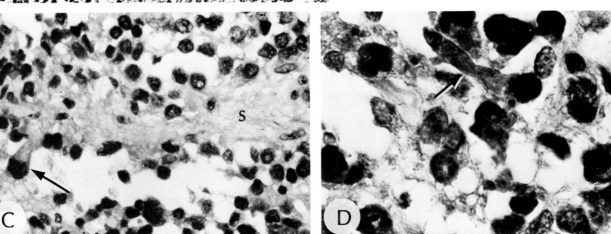

FIG. 14–34. Alveolar rhabdomyosarcoma in 21-year-old man with proptosis of left eye. **A.** Septa (s) separate tumor into compartments resulting in alveolated appearance. **B.** Septa appear delicate with special stain for reticulin. **C.** Cytoplasm of rhabdomyoblasts make up in part septa (s). Note rhabdomyoblast in shape of tadpole cell (arrow). **D.** Typical cross-striations (arrow) present. **A,** trichrome, ×101; **B,** reticulum, ×101; **C,** H&E, ×252; **D,** trichrome, ×630.

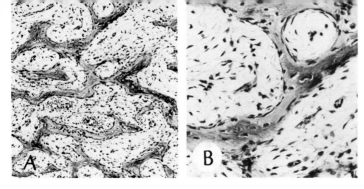

FIG. 14–35. Fibrous dysplasia. **A.** Highly characteristic bone structure composed of moderately cellular and loosely textured fibrous connective tissue that encloses poorly formed spicules of bone, which show both formative and resorptive changes (higher magnification shown in **B**). **A,** H&E, ×40; **B,** H&E, ×101.

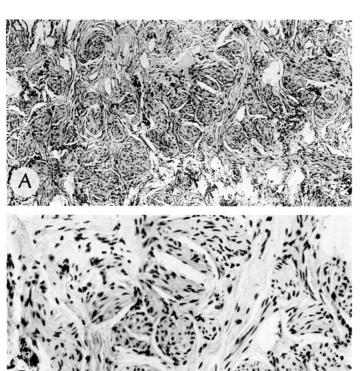

FIG. 14–36. Amputation neuroma. **A.** Haphazard entanglement of regenerated ciliary nerve fibers is seen in orbital tissue. **B.** Higher magnification shows nonordered regenerated nerves. **A,** H&E, ×40; **B,** H&E, ×101.

FIG. 14–37. Plexiform neurofibroma consists of diffuse proliferation of Schwann cells within nerve sheath, producing thickened, tortuous nerves. H&E, ×40.

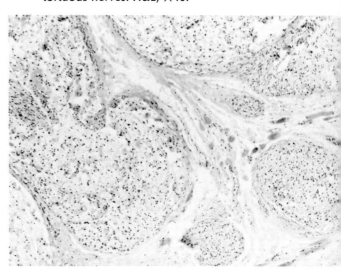

schwannoma

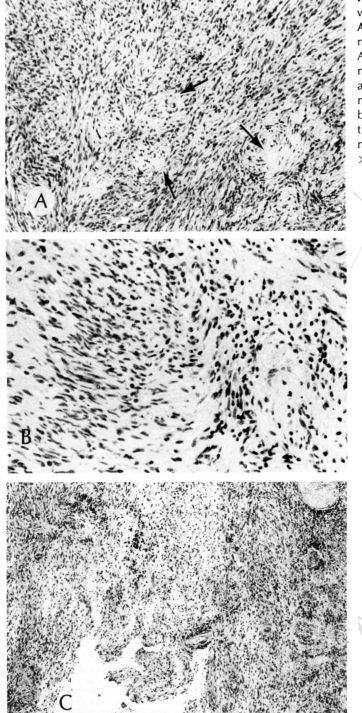

A

B

C

Antoni A

Antoni B

FIG. 14–38. Neurilemmoma in 67-year-old white woman with unilateral exophthalmos. **A.** Ribbons of spindle-shaped Schwann nuclei show tendency toward palisading in Antoni type A pattern. Areas of tumor mimicking tactile corpuscles (*arrows* and areas of relative acellularity seen at higher magnification in **B**) are called Verocay bodies. **C.** Tumor shows marked degeneration with microcystoid changes due to necrosis in Antoni Type B pattern. **A,** H&E, ×69; **B,** H&E, ×136; **C,** H&E, ×40.

2. Histologically it is composed of nests, or aggregates, of clusters of relatively clear (epithelioid) or dark (chief) cells surrounded by a connective tissue stroma containing many capillaries.
   a. Typically silver stains show that reticulin separates or surrounds tumor cell clusters but does not surround individual cells.
   b. By electron microscopy two cellular elements are present:
      1) Central chief cells containing membrane-bound *neurosecretory granules* in great abundance.
      2) Fibroblastlike sustentacular cells at the periphery of cell clusters.
D. Granular cell myoblastoma‡ (Fig. 14–39)
   1. Granular cell myoblastoma is a rare, benign, orbital tumor probably of neurogenic (Schwannian) origin.

   Myofilaments have been found in tumor cells in a granular cell myoblastoma of the urinary bladder, documenting the myogenous derivation of that tumor. The pattern of the common variety of granular cell tumors as seen by transmission electron microscopy (TEM), however, indicates a Schwannian histogenesis. The *granules* of these tumors are similar in appearance by TEM regardless of the location of the neoplasm and are reminiscent of lysosomes and cytosegresomes. Granular cell myoblastoma, therefore, may derive from different cell types, i.e., Schwannian and myogenous.

   2. Histologically it is composed of relatively solid groups and cords, occasionally alveolated collections, of round to polygonal cells frequently contiguous with adjacent skeletal muscle.
      a. The nuclei are round and relatively small in relation to the voluminous, finely granular, eosinophilic cytoplasm, which is diastase-resistant, PAS-positive.
      b. Silver stains frequently show

reticulin surrounding individual cells.
   c. By TEM oval and round membrane-bound *cytoplasmic bodies* are found.
E. Alveolar soft part sarcoma‡ (Fig. 14–40)
   1. An alveolar soft part sarcoma is a rare malignant orbital tumor.
   2. Histologically it is composed of alveolated groups of round and polygonal cells circumscribed by bands of connective tissue some of which contain delicate vascular channels.
      a. Cytoplasm of tumor cells contains scattered eosinophilic and PAS-positive granules as well as larger refractile bodies.
      b. By electron microscopy *intracytoplasmic crystalline inclusions* exhibiting a variety of geometric configurations are found.

   The cytoplasmic crystalloids are similar to the rods observed in benign rhabdomyoma cells. The tumor, therefore, has been thought by some to be a unique type of rhabdomyosarcoma rather than being of neural derivation.

VI. Epithelial tumors of lacrimal gland
   A. General information
      1. Characteristically lacrimal gland tumors cause a "down and in" type of proptosis.
      2. The lacrimal gland is the only epithelial structure in the orbit.
      3. Approximately 50 percent of lacrimal gland tumors are epithelial, and approximately 50 percent are lymphoid tumors and inflammatory pseudotumors. The lymphoid tumors and pseudotumors are identical to those occurring elsewhere in orbit (see pp. 552–556 in this chapter).
      4. *Benign mixed tumor* is the most common benign neoplasm of the salivary glands and of the lacrimal gland.
      5. *Mucoepidermoid carcinoma,* the

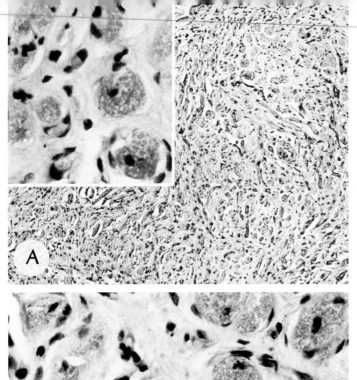

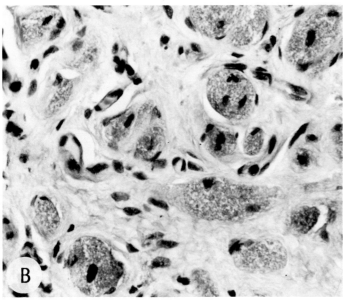

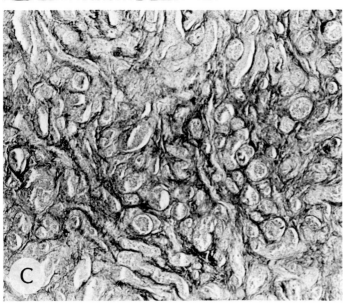

FIG. 14–39. Granular cell myoblastoma in 48-year-old woman with hard tumor of right eyebrow. **A.** Solid groups and cords of cells are seen. **Inset** is higher magnification to show small nuclei and granular eosinophilic cytoplasm of round and polygonal cells. **B.** Granular cytoplasm is diastase-resistant, PAS-positive. **C.** Section stained with colloidal iron (to show acid mucopolysaccharides) demonstrates "neural" appearance. **A,** H&E, ×54; **inset,** H&E, ×252; **B,** PAS, ×252; **C,** AMP, ×101.

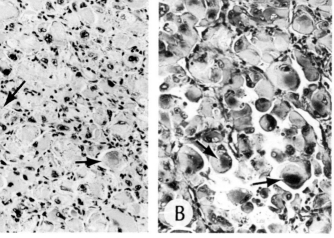

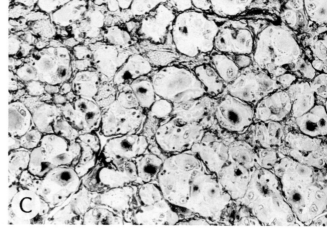

most common carcinoma of the salivary gland, almost never occurs in the lacrimal gland.

6. Simplified classification of tumors of the lacrimal gland.

   a. Lymphoid tumors and inflammatory pseudotumors—approximately 50 percent.

   b. Benign epithelial tumors—approximately 25 percent (all are benign mixed tumors).

   c. Malignant epithelial tumors (carcinomas)—approximately 25 percent.

     1) Malignant mixed tumor—about 20 percent. *1/5*

     2) Adenoid cystic carcinomas—about 60 percent. *3/5*

     3) Other types of carcinoma—about 20 percent. *1/5*

       a) Adenocarcinoma.

       b) Mucinous carcinoma.

       c) Undifferentiated carcinoma.

       d) Mucoepidermoid carcinoma (possibly).

B. Benign mixed tumor† (Fig. 14–41) *25% / all*

   1. Benign mixed tumor occurs in young adults with a median age of 35 years.

   2. Males predominate 2:1.

   3. It is a locally invasive tumor and may infiltrate its own pseudocapsule to involve adjacent periosteum.

     a. With incomplete removal it may recur in the soft tissues or in the bony wall.

     b. If removed surgically in piecemeal fashion, multiple recurrences may occur.

FIG. 14–40. Alveolar soft part sarcoma (nonorbital). **A.** Abundant eosinophilic cytoplasm frequently contains inclusions (*arrows*), which are PAS-positive (*arrows* in **B**). **C.** Special stain shows that alveolated groups of round and polygonal cells are separated by delicate connective tissue fibers or septa (seen as black lines), some of which contain vascular channels. **A**, H&E, ×101; **B**, PAS, ×101; **C**, reticulum, ×101.

   4. Histologically the tumor shows marked structural variation from case to case and from part to part in the same tumor.

     a. Almost all, at least in some areas, have tubular structures arranged in an irregularly anastomosing pattern, lying in a myxoid stroma.

     b. The tubes or ducts are lined by a double layer of epithelium.

       1) The inner layer of epithelium may secrete mucus or undergo squamous metaplasia.

       2) The outer layer of epithelium may undergo metaplasia to form a myxoid, fibrous or cartilaginous stroma.

       The stroma is rich in a hyaluronidase-resistant type of acid mucopolysaccharide.

     c. The pseudocapsule of the tumor is formed by the tumor's pressure on surrounding tissue; the tumor almost always infiltrates its pseudocapsule in some area.

C. Malignant mixed tumor† (Fig. 14–42)

   1. Malignant mixed tumor occurs in an

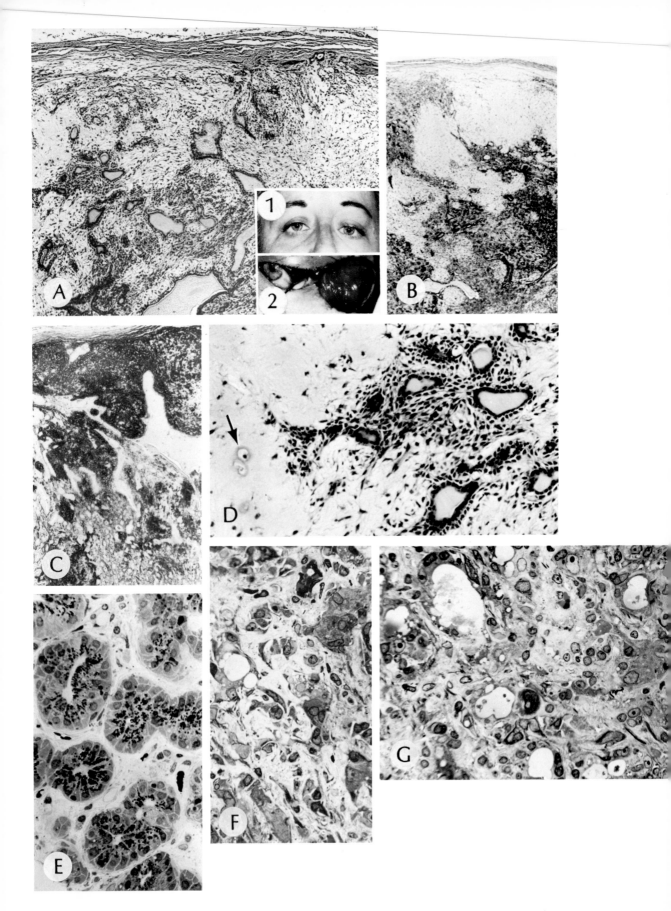

◀ **FIG. 14–41.** Benign mixed tumor. **A.** Marked structural variations are present within tumor. **Insets** show preoperative proptosis of left eye (**1**) and operative (**2**) appearance. Background myxomatous stroma has pale amorphous appearance in H&E-stained sections (**B**) but stains positively for hyaluronidase-resistant acid mucopolysaccharides with colloidal iron stain (**C**). **D.** Ductal structures lined by two layers of epithelium are characteristic. Outer layer may undergo myxoid and cartillagenous (*arrow*) metaplasia; inner layer may secrete mucous as noted here or may undergo squamous metaplasia. **E.** 1.5 μ section of normal lacrimal gland to compare to 1.5 μ sections of benign tumor (**F** and **G**) from same tumor as shown in **A–D**. **A,** H&E, ×40; **inset 1,** clinical preoperative; **inset 2,** clinical operative; **B,** H&E, ×16; **C,** AMP, ×16; **D,** H&E, ×101; **E,** 1.5 μ section, toluidine blue, ×300; **F,** 1.5 μ section, toluidine blue, ×30; **G,** 1.5 μ section, toluidine blue, ×300.

---

older age group than does the benign mixed tumor, with a median age of 51 years.
2. There is no sex predilection.
3. It probably arises from a benign mixed tumor.
4. Histologically areas resembling a benign mixed tumor are seen along with adenocarcinomatous areas.
D. Adenoid cystic carcinoma† (malignant cylindroma) (Fig. 14–43)
1. Adenoid cystic carcinoma occurs in young adults with a median age of about 38 years.
2. There is no sex predilection.
3. Very early the tumor invades perineural lymphatics and has an extremely poor prognosis.
4. Histologically under lower power it has a characteristic "*swiss cheese*" pattern.
   a. Aggregates or islands of poorly differentiated, small, tightly packed, epithelial cells are outlined sharply from the surrounding characteristic, hyalinelike stroma.
   1) Aggregates may be very

small, moderate or quite large, but they always are sharply outlined.
   2) Aggregates contain mucin-filled, cystic spaces of different sizes, hence the "swiss cheese" type of pattern.

The hyaline stroma surrounding the nests of neoplastic cells is an important finding in differentiating adenoid cystic carcinoma from the similarly appearing basal cell or adnexal cell carcinomas. Rather than having a hyaline, relatively acellular stroma, the basal cell and adnexal cell carcinomas have a highly cellular, sarcomatouslike, "desmoplastic" stroma surrounding the nests of neoplastic cells.

E. Other types of carcinoma‡
1. Adenocarcinomas, mucinous carcinomas, undifferentiated carcinomas and possibly mucoepidermoid carcinomas occur.
2. Median age group is about 53 years with a 3:1 predominance in men.
3. All have a very poor prognosis.
F. Prognosis
1. Benign mixed tumors—the mortality is well under 10 percent with the deaths due mainly to multiple recurrences and intracranial extension.
2. All malignant tumors—the mortality is around 50 percent or more.
VII. Reticuloendothelial system, lymphatic system and myeloid system
A. This group is considered together because of overlap in some of the tumors.
B. Classification
1. Reticuloendotheliosis (xanthogranulomatous lesions; histiocytosis X)
   a. Eosinophilic granuloma.
   b. Hand-Schüller-Christian disease.
   c. Letterer-Siwe disease.
   d. Juvenile xanthogranuloma (nevoxanthoendothelioma).
2. Inflammatory pseudotumor
   a. Chronic granulomatous.

b. Chronic nongranulomatous.
  1) Obviously inflammatory.
  2) Reactive lymphoid or plasma cell hyperplasia.
3. Malignant lymphoma
4. Leukemia ("chloroma")

C. Reticuloendotheliosis *(Histiocytosis X)*
1. Eosinophilic granuloma† (Fig. 14–44)
  a. An eosinophilic granuloma is a relatively benign tumor that usually involves a single bone in a destructive process. It is found frequently in the outer part of the upper orbital rim.
  b. Histologically the tumor is composed of histiocytes admixed with eosinophils; histiocytes are essential for the diagnosis.
2. Hand-Schüller-Christian disease†
  a. Characteristic triad
    1) Bony lesions in the skull seen on x ray.
    2) Exophthalmos.
    3) Diabetes insipidus.
  b. The disease may be lethal.
  c. Histologically the orbit is infiltrated by atypical histiocytes.
3. Letterer-Siwe disease‡ (Figs. 14–45 and 14–46)
  a. Letterer-Siwe disease affects infants and very young children.
  b. It is a rapidly progressive disease that is almost always fatal.
  c. The disease rarely involves the orbit.
  d. Histologically nonlipoidal, atypical histiocytes infiltrate the involved tissues.

    Rarely the uveal tract may be involved in Letterer-Siwe disease. When it is involved, the process generally is restricted to the posterior uveal tract.

4. Juvenile xanthogranuloma (nevoxanthoendothelioma)†—see pp. 338–339 in Chapter 9.
    Some authors believe this is not one of the histiocytoses X.

D. Inflammatory pseudotumor†—any nonneoplastic space occupying orbital lesion, which presents clinically like a neoplasm.

1. Chronic granulomatous
  a. Foreign body.
  b. Ruptured dermoid.
  c. Fat necrosis or lipogranuloma.
  d. Sarcoidosis.
  e. Tuberculosis.
  f. Many others (see Chap. 4).
2. Chronic nongranulomatous
  a. Obviously inflammatory (Figs. 14–47 and 14–48)
    1) Histologic triad:
      a) Cellular polymorphism, i.e., different types of inflammatory cells, e.g., lymphocytes, plasma cells and eosinophils.
      b) Lymphoid follicles with germinal centers.

        Mitotic figures are normally found within the germinal centers of lymphoid follicles. *(not outside)*

      c) Ancillary evidence of inflammation, e.g., plasmacytoid cells, Russell bodies and proliferation of capillaries with swollen, enlarged endothelial cells.
    2) Histology may be quite varied:
      a) Very cellular.
      b) Predominantly collagen and relatively acellular.
      c) Myositis if the ocular muscles are involved.
      d) Dacryoadenitis if the lacrimal gland is involved.
      e) Vasculitis if vessels are involved.
      f) Hemangioma with hemorrhage, organization and inflammation.
    3) May be part of systemic disease:
      a) Endocrine exophthalmos.
      b) Sjögren's syndrome.
      c) Abnormalities of IgA, IgG or IgM immunoglobulin fractions of serum may be associated with inflammation and intranuclear, PAS-positive inclusions (Fig. 14–49)

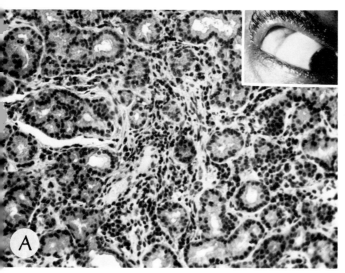

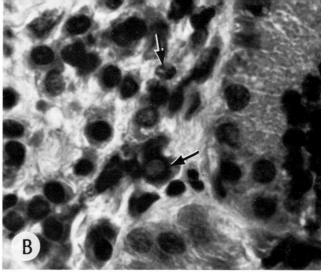

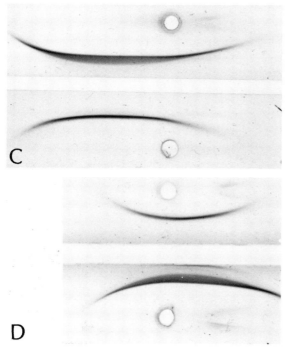

FIG. 14–49. Chronic nongranulomatous inflammation of both lacrimal glands associated with diffuse γ-globulin elevation. **A.** Lacrimal gland is infiltrated by lymphocytes and plasma cells. **Inset** shows clinical appearance of enlarged lacrimal gland. **B.** Higher magnification demonstrates PAS-positive intranuclear inclusion bodies (*arrows*). **C.** Immunoelectrophoresis of patient's serum (**upper**) as compared with normal control (**lower**). Rabbit antiserum specific against γ-chain of human IgG is in trough. Anode is to right. **D.** Patient's serum (**lower**) as compared with normal control (**upper**). Rabbit antiserum specific against α-chain of human IgA is in trough. Note that both IgG and IgA bands are diffusely thickened, but there is no distortion to indicate paraprotein. **A,** H&E, ×340; inset, clinical; **B,** H&E, ×1,050; **C** and **D,** immunoelectrophoresis.

E. Malignant lymphoma†
   1. Nodular (giant follicular) or diffuse (lymphosarcoma) lymphocytic (well or poorly differentiated), histiocytic (reticulum cell sarcoma), mixed cellularity and undifferentiated malignant lymphomas rarely present initially with orbital involvement but may have orbital involvement late in the course of the diseases (Figs. 14–51 and and 14–52).
   2. *Hodgkin's disease* almost never presents initially with orbital in-volvement, and orbital involvement is rare in any stage of the disease (Fig. 14–53).
   3. Burkitt's lymphoma (Fig. 14–54)
      a. Burkitt's lymphoma, a type of undifferentiated malignant lymphoma, is the most common malignant tumor among children in tropical Africa. By far it is the most common orbital tumor regardless of age in Uganda. It does, however, have a worldwide distribution.

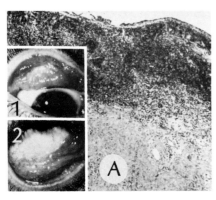

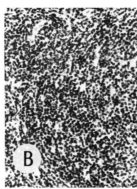

FIG. 14–50. Reactive lymphoid hyperplasia. **A.** Pure lymphocytic infiltrate is present in subconjunctival tissue. **Insets 1** and **2** show clinical appearance. **B.** Higher magnification demonstrates monotonous infiltrate of mature lymphocytes. Occasional mitotic figures are seen. **A,** H&E, ×16; **inset 1,** clinical; **inset 2,** clinical; **B,** H&E, ×101.

FIG. 14–51. Nodular malignant lymphoma. **A.** Extensive nodular lymphoid infiltrate of orbital tissue is present. **Inset** shows clinical appearance with proptosis of left eye. **B.** Higher magnification shows monotonous uniform lymphocytic infiltrate with mitotic figures. **C.** Lymphomatous cells infiltrate orbital fat. **D.** Same nodular lymphomatous infiltrate replaces kidney parenchyma; glomerulus present on left. **A,** H&E, ×25; **inset,** clinical; **B,** H&E, ×400; **C,** H&E, ×220; **D,** H&E, ×160.

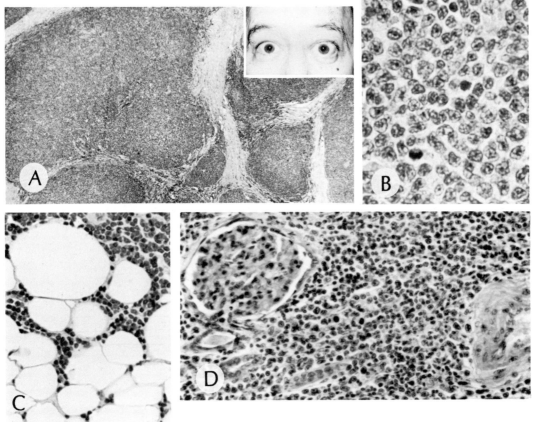

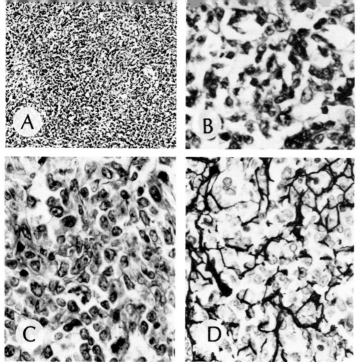

FIG. 14–52. Histiocytic malignant lymphoma (reticulum cell sarcoma) with primary orbital presentation and no systemic involvement in 75-year-old woman with proptosis of left eye. **A.** Diffuse pattern is present. **B.** Cells vary but predominant cells have large vesicular nuclei, prominent nucleoli and well-defined nuclear membranes. **C.** Mitotic figures are present. **D.** Special stain shows increased reticulin formation within cellular areas and in compressed intervening stroma. **A,** H&E, ×40; **B,** H&E, ×252; **C,** PAS, ×252; **D,** reticulum, ×252.

FIG. 14–53. Hodgkin's disease presenting initially as left exophthalmos in 59-year-old man. Autopsy one year later revealed Hodgkin's disease, mixed cellularity (granulomatous) type. **A.** Orbital tissue showing marked cellular infiltrate. **B** and **C.** Higher magnification shows fibroblasts, monocytes, lymphocytes, histiocytes and eosinophils. Sternberg-Reed cells (*arrows*) and mitotic figures are present. **D.** Liver shows identical cellular infiltrate. **A,** H&E, ×136; **B,** H&E, ×340; **C,** H&E, ×340; **D,** H&E, ×176.

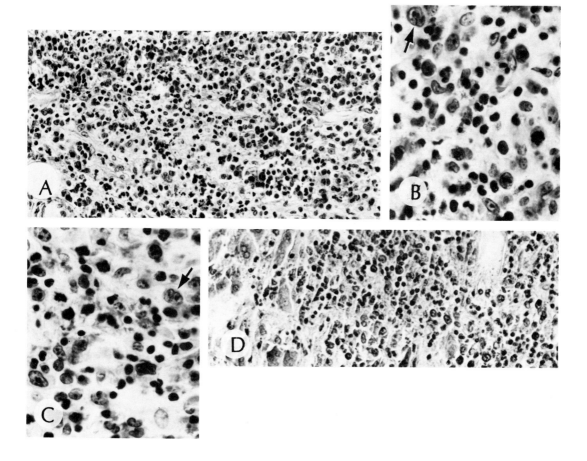

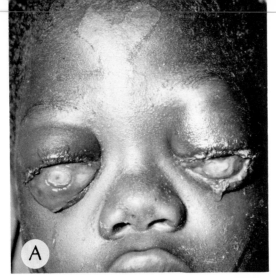

FIG. 14–54. Burkitt's (undifferentiated) lymphoma. **A.** Massive bilateral infiltration of orbits by malignant lymphoma is shown. **B.** Histiocytes, which often display phagocytosis, are scattered among tumor cells, giving characteristic "starry-sky" appearance. **C.** Undifferentiated anaplastic lymphoid cells containing ovoid vesicular or basophilic nuclei with prominent nucleoli compose tumor. **A,** clinical; **B,** H&E, ×60; **C,** H&E, ×525.

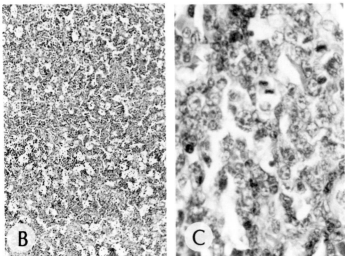

FIG. 14–55. Acute granulocytic leukemia presenting with exophthalmos of left eye in 9-year-old boy who died about 2 years after disease was diagnosed. **A.** Diffuse cellular infiltrate in orbital tissue. **Inset 1** shows clinical appearance. **Inset 2** shows bone marrow smear with blast cells. **B** and **C.** Primitive granulocytic leukemic cells present in orbital tissue. **A,** H&E, ×40; **inset 1,** clinical; **inset 2,** bone marrow, ×850; **B,** H&E, ×252; **C,** H&E, ×630.

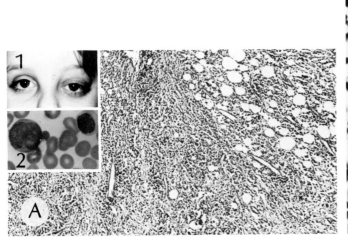

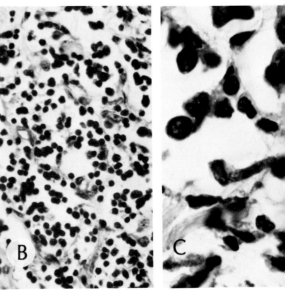

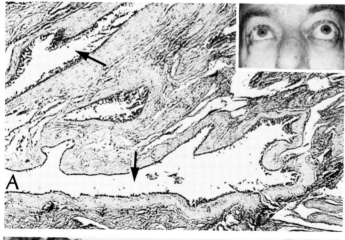

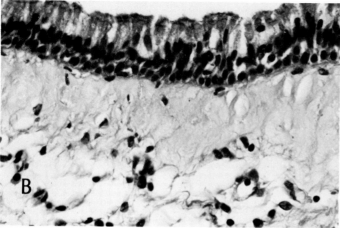

FIG. 14–56. Orbital mucocele. **A.** Mucocele (*arrows*) surrounded by mild inflammatory reaction. **Inset** shows clinical appearance with proptosis of left eye. **B.** Higher magnification shows cyst lined by respiratory-type pseudostratified, ciliated, columnar epithelium and containing scattered round inflammatory cells in its wall. **A,** H&E, ×40; **inset,** clinical; **B,** H&E, ×252.

b. The tumor, which has a predilection for the face and jaws, may be induced by an insect-vectored agent.

c. The prognosis for life is extremely grave.

d. Histologically it is composed of tightly packed undifferentiated lymphoid cells with scattered large histiocytes containing abundant almost clear cytoplasm with phagocytosed cellular debris. The histiocytes give a characteristic "*starry sky*" appearance to the tumor.

F. Leukemia† (Fig. 14–55)

1. Acute leukemia, usually granulocytic (myeloid or myelogenous) or stem cell, occasionally may present initially with exophthalmos.

a. The blood count initially may be normal or low with no circulating leukemic cells.

b. The bone marrow initially may be normal or hypocellular.

c. Exophthalmos is due to the orbital infiltrate of leukemic cells (*chloroma*).

d. About two-thirds of patients with myeloid leukemia present with some blurring of vision and accompanying fundus changes.

2. Orbital leukemic infiltrates most commonly occur late in the disease.

3. Histologically there is an orbital infiltrate of leukemic cells.

SECONDARY ORBITAL TUMORS

I. Direct Extension†:

A. Intraocular neoplasms, especially

malignant melanoma and retinoblastoma.

B. Eyelid neoplasms, especially basal cell carcinoma, squamous cell carcinoma, malignant melanoma and sebaceous gland carcinoma.

C. Conjunctival neoplasms, especially squamous cell carcinoma and malignant melanoma.

D. Paranasal sinus cysts (mucoceles) (Fig. 14–56) and neoplasms, especially squamous cell carcinoma, adenoid cystic carcinoma (malignant cylindroma) and mucoepidermoid carcinoma.

E. Intracranial, especially meningioma

II. Metastatic†

A. Neuroblastoma in children.

Metastatic neuroblastoma in children generally occurs as a late manifestation of the disease. Frequently the orbital metastases are heralded by the onset of lower lid ecchymosis (unilateral or bilateral).

B. Lung carcinoma in adult men.

C. Breast carcinoma in adult women.

D. All other sites of primary neoplasms are rare.

BIBLIOGRAPHY

EXOPHTHALMOS

Abboud IA, Hanna LJ: Intermittent exophthalmos. Br J Ophthalmol 55:628, 1971

Reese AB: Tumors of the Eye, 2nd ed. New York, Hoeber, 1963, pp. 529–537

Wright JE: Proptosis. Ophthalmol Surg 2:62, 1971

DEVELOPMENTAL ABNORMALITIES

Blodi FL: Developmental anomalies of the skull affecting the eye. Arch Ophthalmol 57:593, 1957

Chohan BS, Parmar IPS, Bhatia JN: Anterior orbital meningoencephalocele. Am J Ophthalmol 68:144, 1969

Hoepner J, Yanoff M: Craniosynostosis and syndactylism (Apert's syndrome) associated with a trisomy 21 mosaic. J Pediatr Ophthalmol 8:107, 1971

Krueger JL, Ide CH: Acrocephalosyndactyly (Apert's syndrome). Ann Ophthalmol 6: 787, 1974

Roy FH, Summitt RL, Hiatt RL, Hughes JG: Ocular manifestations of Rubinstein-Taybi syndrome. Case report and review of the literature. Arch Ophthalmol 79:272, 1968

Yanoff M, Rorke LB, Niederer BS: Ocular and cerebral abnormalities in 18 chromosome deletion defect. Am J Ophthalmol 70:391, 1970

ORBITAL INFLAMMATION

Chandler JR, Langenbrunner DJ, Stevens ER: The pathogenesis of orbital complications in acute sinusitis. Laryngoscope 70:1414, 1970

Font RL, Yanoff M, Zimmerman LE: Benign lymphoepithelial lesion of the lacrimal gland and its relationship to Sjögren's syndrome. Am J Clin Pathol 48:365, 1967

Gravanis MB, Giansanti DMD: Malignant histopathologic counterpart of the benign lymphoepithelial lesion. Cancer 26:1332, 1970

Hale LM: Orbital-cerebral phycomycosis. Report of a case and a review of the disease in infants. Arch Ophthalmol 86:39, 1971

Hughes GRV, Whaley K: Sjögren's syndrome. Br Med J 4:533, 1972

Jarrett WH, Gutman FA: Ocular complications of infection in the paranasal sinuses. Arch Ophthalmol 81:683, 1969

Meyer D, Yanoff M, Hanno H: Differential diagnosis in Mikulicz's syndrome, Mikulicz's disease and similar disease entities. Am J Ophthalmol 71:516, 1971

Streeten BW, Rabuzzi DD, Jones DB: Sporotrichosis of the orbital margin. Am J Ophthalmol 77:750, 1974

INJURIES

See Chapter 5 for Bibliography.

VASCULAR DISEASE

Crummy CS, Perlin E, Ross MB: Microangiopathic hemolytic anemia in Wegener's granulomatosis. Am J Med 51:544, 1971

McCord CD, Spitalny LA: Localized orbital varices. Arch Ophthalmol 80:455, 1968

Rubinstein MK, Wilson G, Levin DC: Intraorbital aneurysms of the ophthalmic artery. Report of a unique case and review of the literature. Arch Ophthalmol 80:42, 1968

Zimmerman LE, Rodgers JB: Idiopathic thrombophlebitis of orbital veins simulating primary tumor of orbit. Trans Am Acad Ophthalmol Otolaryngol 61:609, 1957

OCULAR MUSCLE INVOLVEMENT IN SYSTEMIC DISEASE

Allen JH, Barer CG: Cataract of dystrophia myotonica. Arch Ophthalmol 24:867, 1940

Caughey JE: Relationship of dystrophia myotonica (myotonic dystrophy) and myotonia congenita (Thomsen's disease). Neurology (Minneap) 8:469, 1958

Chopra IJ, Solomon DH: Graves' disease with delayed hyperthyroidism. Onset after several years of euthyroid ophthalmopathy, dermopathy and high serum LATS. Ann Intern Med 73:985, 1970

deVries S: Retinopathy in dermatomyositis. Arch Ophthalmol 46:432, 1951

Drachman DB: Ophthalmoplegia plus: the neurodegenerative disorders associated with progressive external ophthalmoplegia. Arch Neurol 18:654, 1968

Eustace P: Corneal lesions in myotonic dystrophy. Br J Ophthalmol 53:633, 1969

Foxx SA: Surgery for progressive familial myopathic ptosis. Ann Ophthalmol 3:1033, 1971

Frenkel M: Myasthenia gravis: current trends. Am J Ophthalmol 61:522, 1966

Hall R, Doniach D, Kirkham K, Kabir DE: Ophthalmic Graves' disease. Diagnosis and pathogenesis. Lancet 1:375, 1970

Johnson CC, Kuwabara T: Oculopharyngeal muscular dystrophy. Am J Ophthalmol 77:872, 1974

Koerner F, Schlote W: Chronic progressive external ophthalmoplegia. Arch Ophthalmol 88:155, 1972

Kroll AJ, Kuwabara T: Dysthyroid myopathy. Anatomy, histology and electron microscopy. Arch Ophthalmol 76:244, 1966

Lessell S, Coppeto J, Samet S: Ophthalmoplegia in myotonic dystrophy. Am J Ophthalmol 71:1231, 1971

Lyons DE: Postural changes in IOP in dysthyroid exophthalmos. Trans Ophthalmol Soc UK 91:799, 1971

Metz HS, Cohen M: Progressive external ophthalmoplegia. Ann Ophthalmol 5:775, 1973

Moses L, Heller GL: Ocular myopathy. Am J Ophthalmol 59:1051, 1965

Werner SC: Classification of the eye changes of Graves' disease. Am J Ophthalmol 68:646, 1969

Yanoff M: Pretibial myxedema, a case report. Med Ann DC 34:319, 1965

ORBITAL TUMORS

Albert DM, Rubenstein RA, Scheie HG: Tumor metastasis to the eye. I. Incidence in 213 adult patients with generalized malignancy. Am J Ophthalmol 63:723, 1967

Albert DM, Rubenstein RA, Scheie HG: Tumor metastasis to the eye. II. Clinical study in infants and children. Am J Ophthalmol 63:727, 1967

Archer DB, Deutman A, Ernest JT, Krill AE: Arteriovenous communications of the retina. Am J Ophthalmol 75:224, 1973

Backwinkel KD, Diddams JA: Hemangiopericytoma. Report of case and comprehensive review of literature. Cancer 25:896, 1970

Barber JC, Barber LF, Guerry D III, Geeraets WJ: Congenital orbital teratomas. Arch Ophthalmol 91:45, 1974

Blodi FC, Gass JDM: Inflammatory pseudotumor of the orbit. Trans Am Acad Ophthalmol Otolaryngol 71:303, 1967

Brooks HW, Evans AE, Glass RM, Pang EM: Chloromas of head and neck in childhood, initial manifestation of myeloid leukemia in 3 patients. Arch Otolaryngol 100:304, 1974

Cárdenas-Ramírez L, Albores-Saavedra J, deBuen S: Mesenchymal chondrosarcoma of the orbit: report of the first case in orbital location. Arch Ophthalmol 86:410, 1971

Cassan SM, Divertie MG, Hollenhorst RW, Harrison EG: Pseudotumor of the orbit and limited Wegener's granulomatosis. Ann Intern Med 72:687, 1970

Christ ML, Ozzello L: Myogenous origin of a granular cell tumor of the urinary bladder. Am J Clin Pathol 56:736, 1971

Dorfman RF: Relationship of histology to site in Hodgkin's disease. Cancer Res 31:1786, 1971

Dorfman RF: Histopathologic classification of malignant lymphomas other than Hodgkins' disease, in Proceedings of the 7th National Cancer Conference, September 1972. Philadelphia, Lippincott, 1973, p 261

Enterline HT, Culberson JD, Rochlin DB, Brady LW: Liposarcoma: a clinical and pathological study of 53 cases. Cancer 13:932, 1960

Enzinger FM, Shiraki M: Alveolar rhabdomyosarcoma. Cancer 24:18, 1969

Ferry AP: Teratoma of the orbit: a report of two cases. Survey Ophthalmol 10:434, 1965

Ferry AP: Metastatic carcinoma of the eye and ocular adnexa. Int Ophthalmol Clin 7:615, 1967

Ferry AP: The biological behavior and pathological features of carcinoma metastatic to the eye and orbit. Trans Am Ophthalmol Soc 71:373, 1973

Ferry AP, Sherman SE: Nodular fasciitis of the conjunctiva apparently originating in the fascia bubli (Tenon's capsule). Am J Ophthalmol 78:514, 1974

Fisher ER, Reidbord H: Electron microscopic evidence suggesting the myogenous derivation of the so-called alveolar soft part sarcoma. Cancer 27:150, 1971

Fisher ER, Zawadzki AZ: Ultrastructural features of plasma cells in patients with paraproteins. Am J Clin Pathol 54:779, 1970

Font RL, Zimmerman LE: Nodular fasciitis of the eye and adnexa. Arch Ophthalmol 75:475, 1966

Foos R: Fibrosarcoma of the orbit. Am J Ophthalmol 67:244, 1969

Forrest AW: Tumors following radiation about the eye. Int Ophthalmol Clin 2:543, 1962

Forrest AW: Pathologic criteria for effective management of epithelial lacrimal gland tumors. Am J Ophthalmol 71:178, 1971

Frayer WC, Enterline HT: Embryonal rhabdomyosarcoma of the orbit in children and young adults. Arch Ophthalmol 62:203, 1959

Friedman Z, Eden E, Neumann E: Granular cell myoblastoma of the eyelid margin. Br J Ophthalmol 57:757, 1973

Gass JDM: Orbital and ocular involvement in fibrous dysplasia. South Med J 58:324, 1965

Gaynes PM, Cohen GS: Juvenile xanthogranuloma of the orbit. Am J Ophthalmol 63:755, 1967

Gibson MJ, Middlemiss JH: Fibrous dysplasia of bone. Br J Radiol 44:1, 1971

Green WR, Zimmerman LE: Ectopic lacrimal gland tissue. Arch Ophthalmol 78:318, 1967

Grinberg MA, Levy NS: Malignant neurilemoma of the supraorbital nerve. Am J Ophthalmol 78:489, 1974

Haegert DG, Wang NS, Farrer PA, Seemayer TA, Thelmo W: Non-chromaffin parangliomatosis manifesting as a cold thyroid nodule. Am J Clin Pathol 61:561, 1974

Hogan MJ, Zimmerman LE (eds): Ophthalmic Pathology: An Atlas and Textbook. Philadelphia, Saunders, 1962, p 778

Honrubia FM, Davis WH, Moore MK, Elliott JH: Carcinoid syndrome with bilateral orbital metastasis. Am J Ophthalmol 72:1118, 1972

Jakobiec FA, Ellsworth R, Tannenbaum M: Primary orbital melanoma. Am J Ophthalmol 78:24, 1974

Jakobiec FA, Howard GM, Jones IS, Tannenbaum M: Fibrous histiocytomas of the orbit. Am J Ophthalmol 77:333, 1974

Jakobiec FA, Howard GM, Jones IS, Wolff M: Hemangiopericytoma of the orbit. Am J Ophthalmol 78:816, 1974

Jakobiec FA, Jones IS, Tannenbaum M: Leiomyoma. An unusual tumor of the orbit. Br J Ophthalmol 57:825, 1973

Jha BK, Lamba PA: Proptosis as a manifestation of acute myeloid leukemia. Br J Ophthalmol 55:844, 1971

Jones IS, Reese AB, Krout J: Orbital rhabdomyosarcoma. Am J Ophthalmol 61:721, 1966

Kapelow SM, Foos RY, Straatsma BR, Hepler RS, Pearlman JT: Cavernous hemangioma of the orbit. Int Ophthalmol Clin 11:113, 1971

Karp LA, Zimmerman LE, Payne T: Intraocular involvement in Burkitt's lymphoma. Arch Ophthalmol 85:295, 1971

Kim H, Heller P, Rappaport H: Monoclonal gammopathies associated with lymphoproliferative disorders: a morphologic study. Am J Clin Pathol 59:282, 1973

Kirk RC, Zimmerman LE: Rhabdomyosarcoma of the orbit. Arch Ophthalmol 81:559, 1969

Kroll AJ, Kuwabara T, Howard GM: Electron microscopy of rhabdomyosarcoma of the orbit. A study of two cases. Invest Ophthalmol 2:523, 1963

Lagios MD, Friedlander LM, Wallerstein RO, Bohannon RA: Atypical azurophilic crystals in chromic lymphocytic leukemia. Am J Clin Pathol 62:342, 1974

Levitt JM, de Veer JA, Oguzhan MC: Orbital nodular fasciitis. Arch Ophthalmol 81:235, 1969

Lieberman PH, Llovera IN: Kaposi's sarcoma of the bulbar conjunctiva. Arch Ophthalmol 88:44, 1972

Macoul KL: Hemangiopericytoma of the lid and orbit. Am J Ophthalmol 66:731, 1968

Meacham CT: Pseudosarcomatous fasciitis. Am J Ophthalmol 77:747, 1974

Meyer D, Yanoff M, Hanno H: Differential diagnosis in Mikulicz's syndrome, Mikulicz's disease and similar disease entities. Am J Ophthalmol 71:516, 1971

Mittleman D, Apple DJ, Goldberg MF: Ocular involvement in Letterer-Siwe disease. Am J Ophthalmol 75:261, 1973

O'Brien JE, Stout AP: Malignant fibrous xanthomas. Cancer 17:1445, 1964

O'Brien PH, Brasfield RD: Kaposi's sarcoma. Cancer 19:1497, 1966

Olson JR, Abell MR: Nonfunctional, nonchromaffin paragangliomas of the retroperitoneum. Cancer 23:1358, 1969

Palutke M, McDonald JM: Monoclonal gammopathies associated with malignant lymphomas. Am J Clin Pathol 60:157, 1973

Pearlstein AD, Flom L: Letterer-Siwe's disease. J Pediatr Ophthalmol 7:103, 1970

Pfaffenbach DD, Green WR: Ectopic lacrimal gland. Int Ophthalmol Clin 11:149, 1971

Polack FM, Kanai A, Hood CI: Light and electron microscopic studies of orbital rhabdomyosarcoma. Am J Ophthalmol 71:75, 1971

Porterfield JF, Zimmerman LE: Orbital rhabdomyosarcoma: a clinicopathologic study of 55 cases. Virchows Arch [Pathol Anat] 335:329, 1962

Ramchander P, Satyendran OM: Neurilemmoma of the orbit—a case report. J All India Ophthalmol Soc 10:45, 1962

Ramsey HJ: Fine structure of hemangiopericytoma and hemangioendothelioma. Cancer 19:2005, 1966

Rappaport H, Bernard C, Butler JJ, Dorfman RF, Lukes RJ, Thomas LB: Report of the committee on histopathological criteria contributing to staging of Hodgkin's disease. Cancer Res 31:1864, 1971

Reese AB: Tumors of the Eye, 2nd ed. New York, Hoeber, 1963, pp 529–580

Rodman HI, Font RL: Orbital involvement in multiple myeloma. Review of the literature and report of three cases. Arch Ophthalmol 87:30, 1972

Schatz H: Benign orbital neurilemmoma. Sarcomatous transformation in von Recklinghausen's disease. Arch Ophthalmol 86:268, 1971

Sen DK, Mohan H: Fibroxanthoma of the orbit. Orient Arch Ophthalmol 8:150, 1970

Sen DK, Mohan H, Chatterjee PK: Hodgkin's disease in the orbit. Int Surg 55:183, 1971

Slem G, Ilcayto R: Hemangioma of lacrimal gland in an adult. Ann Ophthalmol 4:77, 1972

Stout AP: Hemangio-endothelioma: a tumor of blood vessels featuring vascular endothelial cells. Ann Surg 118:445, 1954

Strong EW, McDivitt RW, Brasfield RD: Granular cell myoblastoma. Cancer 25:415, 1970

Yanoff M, Nix R, Arvan D: Bilateral lacrimal gland enlargement associated with a diffuse gamma globulin elevation: a case report. Ophthalmol Res 1:245, 1970

Yanoff M, Scheie HG: Fibrosarcoma of the orbit: report of two cases. Cancer 19:1711, 1966

Yanoff M, Scheie HG: Malignant lymphoma of the orbit. Difficulties in diagnosis. Survey Ophthalmol 12:133, 1967

Ziegler JL, Wright DH, Kyalwazi SK: Differential diagnosis of Burkitt's lymphoma of the face and jaws. Cancer 27:503, 1971

Zimmerman LE: Ocular lesions of juvenile xanthogranuloma. Trans Am Acad Ophthalmol Otolaryngol 69:412, 1965

Zimmerman LE, Sanders TE, Ackerman LV: Epithelial tumors of the lacrimal gland: prognostic and therapeutic significance of histologic types. Int Ophthalmol Clin 2:337, 1962

chapter 15

Diabetes Mellitus

NATURAL HISTORY

Diabetes mellitus is the second leading cause of blindness in the United States with over three-quarters of the blind being women. The duration of the disease is the most important factor influencing the occurrence of clinical retinopathy.

Although 60 percent or more of patients develop retinopathy after 15 years of diabetes, the risk of actual legal blindness in a given diabetic is only about 7 to 9 percent even after 20 to 30 years of diabetes. There is a good positive correlation between the presence of diabetic retinopathy and of the nephropathy (*Kimmelsteil-Wilson* disease). Once blindness develops, the average life expectancy is less than 6 years. Ocular symptoms occur in about 20 to 40 percent of diabetics at the clinical onset of the disease, but these symptoms are mainly due to refractive changes rather than to retinopathy. The low frequency of the retinopathy in secondary diabetes, e.g., chronic pancreatitis, pancreatectomy, hemochromatosis, Cushing's syndrome and acromegaly, may be due to the comparative rarity of long survival among these secondary diabetics.

CONJUNCTIVA AND CORNEA

CONJUNCTIVAL MICROANEURYSMS

   I. Conjunctival microaneurysms may be found, but they are of questionable diagnostic significance because they also occur in nondiabetics.

      Irregular deposition of pigment on the posterior cornea and folds in Descemet's membrane may be found, but they are nonspecific findings.

  II. Transmural lipid imbibition may occur in conjunctival capillaries in diabetic lipemia retinalis.

      Histologically lipid-laden cells, either endothelial cells or subintimal macrophages, are present projecting into and encroaching upon conjunctival capillary lumens.

LENS

"SNOWFLAKE" CATARACT OF JUVENILE DIABETIC

   I. The cataract consists of subcapsular opacities with vacuoles and chalky white flake deposits.

  II. The whole lens may become a milky white cataract (at times the process is reversible completely).

 III. The histopathology has not been defined.

ADULT ONSET DIABETIC CATARACT (see Fig. 15–28)

   I. The cataract (cortical and nuclear) is indistinguishable clinically and histopathologically from the senile cataracts seen in the general population.

  II. Diabetics may have transient lens opacities with induced myopia during hyperglycemia.

IRIS

VACUOLATION OF IRIS PIGMENT EPITHELIUM
(Figs. 15–1 and 15–2)

   I. Vacuolation of the iris pigment epithelium is present in 40 percent of diabetic enucleated eyes. The vacuoles contain glycogen.

      Rupture of the vacuoles when the intraocular pressure is suddenly reduced, e.g., entering the anterior chamber during cataract surgery, results in release of pigment into the posterior chamber. This pigment is visible clinically as a pigment stream flowing through the pupil into the anterior chamber. Many diabetics show poor or delayed dilatation of the iris

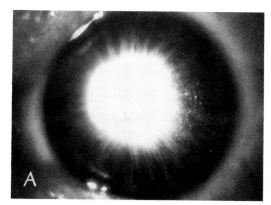

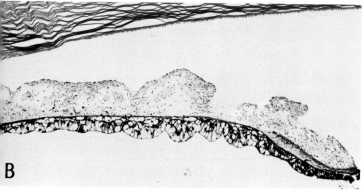

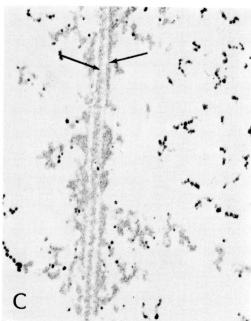

FIG. 15–1. Lacy vacuolation of iris pigment epithelium. **A.** Myriad pinholes of transillumination of iris may be seen clinically on transpupillary retroillumination. Fine points of light generally tend to follow circumferential ridges and furrows of posterior pigment epithelial layer. Transmission is due to swelling of epithelial cells with displacement of pigment rather than to loss of pigment from cells. **B.** Note abrupt cessation of vacuolation at iris root and also that there is great accentuation of circumferential ridges (cut here meridionally). Although pupillary portion is not here involved, it may become so and has been noted clinically in region of pupil. **C.** Glycogen particles (very dark dots) are present throughout vacuoles of pigment epithelium. Plasma membranes and intercellular space between adjacent cells are present at *arrows.* Irregular clumps are cytoplasmic debris. Remainder of space presumably occupied mostly by water. **A.** clinical; **B,** H&E, ×38; **C,** thiosemicarbazide (TSC) only without counterstain, ×33,000.

after attempted dilatation with mydriatics. The cause of the sluggish dilatation may be related to the lacy vacuolation with "damage" to the overlying dilator muscle.

II. Pinpoint "holes" may be seen clinically with the slit lamp, using transpupillary retroillumination in light-colored irises (as high as 25 percent in known diabetics with blue irises).

RUBEOSIS IRIDIS (Figs. 15–3 and 15–4)

I. Rubeosis iridis is present in less than 5 percent of diabetic patients without proliferative retinopathy but approaches 43 to 65 percent of patients with proliferative retinopathy.

II. Neovascularization of the anterior surface of the iris may start in the anterior chamber angle, the pupillary border, midway between or all three.

Infrequently the anterior iris stroma, between the pupil and the colarette, may show a very

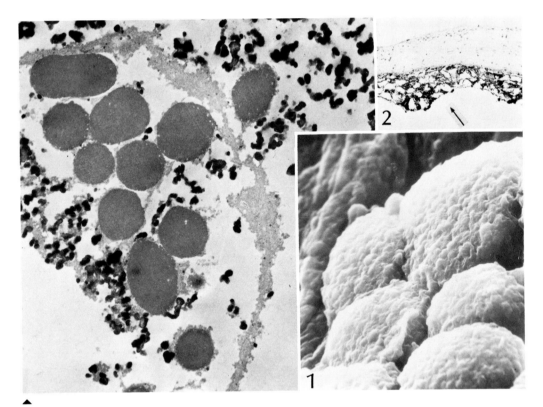

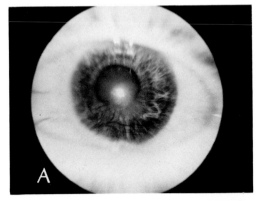

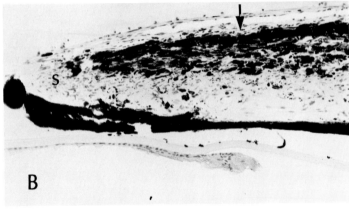

▲
FIG. 15–2. Vacuolation of iris pigment epithelium. **Inset 1** shows swollen posterior layer of iris pigment epithelium from behind as seen by scanning electron microscopy (SEM). **Inset 2** is a section of material seen in **inset 1** to show underlying vacuolation (*arrow*). Larger photograph is transmission electron micrograph of same material stained with TSC. Dark granules of glycogen are now found clumped together due to dehydration required for initial SEM examination. **Main figure,** TSC, ×21,000; **inset 1,** SEM, ×2,900; **inset 2,** post SEM, toluidine blue, ×100.

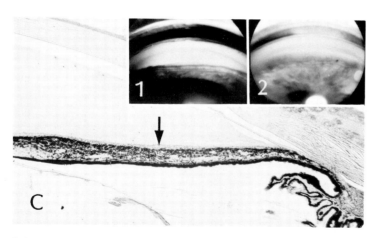

FIG. 15–3. Rubeosis iridis. **A.** Marked rubeosis iridis with large trunk vessel is seen across inferior aspect of iris. **B.** Shrinkage of fibrovascular membrane (*arrow*) causes anterior turning of pupillary pigment epithelium and sphincter muscle (*s*), i.e., ectropion uveae. **C.** Fibrovascular membrane (*arrow*) is present anterior to pigmented anterior border layer of iris. Note peripheral anterior synechia. **Inset 1** shows early anterior chamber rubeosis iridis. Even though angle still open, glaucoma can occur due to mechanical blockage (secondary open angle glaucoma). **Inset 2** shows moderate rubeosis iridis with peripheral anterior synechias causing secondary angle closure glaucoma. **A,** clinical; **B,** H&E, ×100; **C,** H&E, ×21; ◀ **inset 1,** gonioscopy; **inset 2,** gonioscopy.

FIG. 15–4. Neovascularization glaucoma. Rubeosis iridis tends to bleed and lead to hyphema; condition has been called incorrectly hemorrhagic glaucoma. Hemorrhage is not responsible for glaucoma, rubeosis iridis and peripheral anterior synechias (*arrow*) are. Note lacy vacuolation of iris pigment epithelium. H&E, ×75.

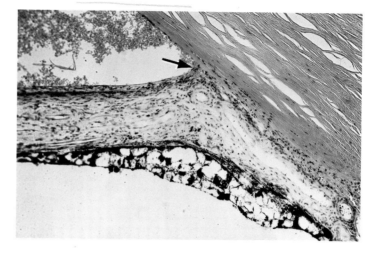

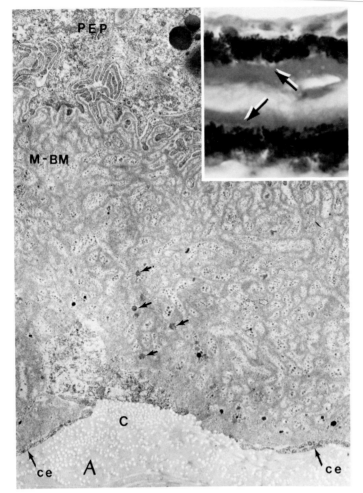

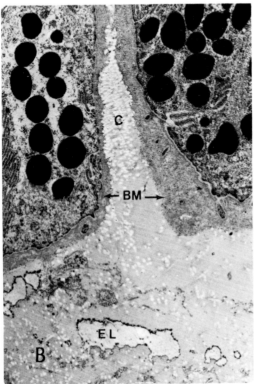

FIG. 15–5. Basement membrane of ciliary pigment epithelium. **A.** Multilaminar external basement membrane (*M-BM*) of ciliary epithelium in region of pars plicata is thickened markedly. Distal edge is demarcated by plane of attenuated non-pigmented uveal cells (*ce*). Numerous small granules or spherules presumably calcific (*arrows*) are present in distal parts of basement membrane. *PEP*, bases of pigment epithelial cells; *C*, collagen. **Inset** shows light microscopic appearance of thickened basement membrane (*arrows*) of pigmented ciliary epithelium. Note marked decrease in number of core capillaries. **B.** Normally thick external basement membrane (*BM*) of ciliary epithelium in region of pars plana from same patient as in **A** is not altered. *C*, collagen; *EL*, elastic lamina. **A,** ×13,200; **inset,** PAS, ×750; **B,** ×9,000 (**A** and **B,** 28-year-old diabetic).

fine neovascularization, which may remain stationary for years. This type of pupillary rubeosis iridis may occur in an eye in which the anterior chamber angle remains open without angle rubeosis also for many years.

III. Early, rubeosis of the anterior chamber angle causes a secondary open angle glaucoma, but then it progresses rapidly to form peripheral anterior synechias and a chronic secondary angle closure glaucoma.

With shrinkage of the fibrovascular tissue on the anterior iris surface, an *ectropion uveae* may develop. The new blood vessels tend to bleed easily, hence the misused and poor term *hemorrhagic glaucoma; neovascularization glaucoma* is the preferred term so as not to confuse the entity with glaucoma secondary to traumatic hemorrhage without rubeosis iridis. Even without the development of rubeosis iridis, there is an increased incidence of chronic simple glaucoma in diabetes.

CILIARY BODY AND CHOROID

BASEMENT MEMBRANE OF CILIARY PIGMENT EPITHELIUM (External Basement Membrane)
(Figs. 15–5 and 15–6)

I. The multilaminar basement membrane of the pigment epithelium is diffusely thickened in the region of the pars plicata.
II. The diffuse thickening of the external basement membrane in diabetics is different from the "spotty" or "patchy" thickening that may be seen in elderly nondiabetics.

BASEMENT MEMBRANE OF CILIARY NONPIGMENTED EPITHELIUM
(Internal Basement Membrane)

The multilaminar basement membrane of the nonpigmented epithelium does not appear affected.

FIBROVASCULAR CORE OF CILIARY PROCESSES
(Fig. 15–5)

I. There is an increase in fibrosis with an obliteration of capillaries within the "core" of the ciliary processes.
II. The capillary basement membrane does not appear thickened significantly in this region.

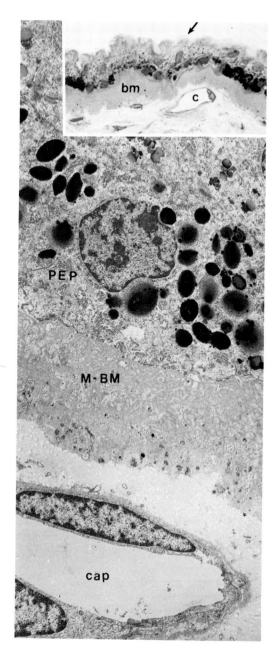

FIG. 15–6. Basement membrane of ciliary pigment epithelium. **Inset** is portion of ciliary process showing thickened basement membrane of pigment epithelium (*bm*). Basement membranes of nonpigmented ciliary epithelium (*arrow*) and of nearby capillary (*c*) are not altered. Electron micrograph from similar region of same material shows that multilaminar basement membrane (*M-BM*) of pigment epithelium (*PEP*) is thickened. There is no significant alteration in thickness of nearby capillary (*cap*) basement membrane. **Main figure,** ×7,500; **inset,** 1.5 μ section, PD, ×395.

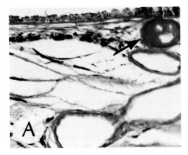

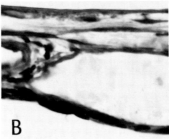

FIG. 15–7. Choroid. **A.** Artery (*arrow*) almost occluded by PAS-positive material. **B.** Choriocapillaris in foveal region shows almost complete occlusion by PAS-positive material. **A,** PAS, ×200; **B,** PAS, ×475.

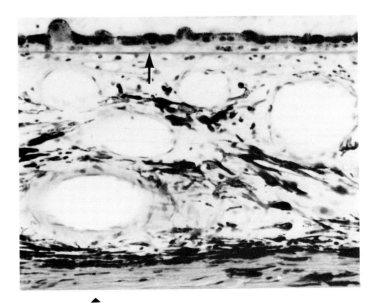

FIG. 15–8. Bruch's membrane (*arrow*) appears thickened. Note early drusen formation by RPE. H&E, ×176.

FIG. 15–9. Normal retinal capillary shows approximately 1:1 pericyte (*p*) to endothelial cell (*e*) ratio. PAS, ×630.

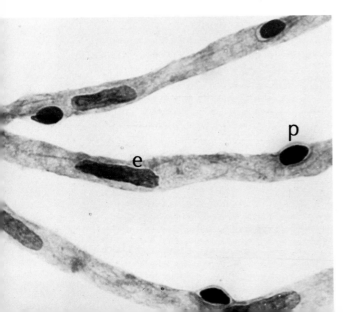

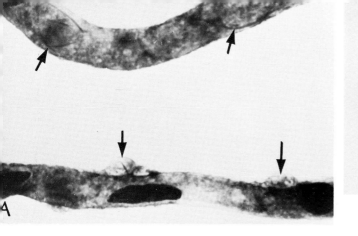

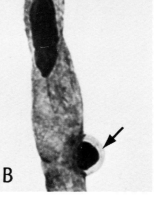

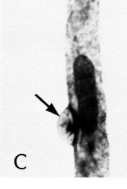

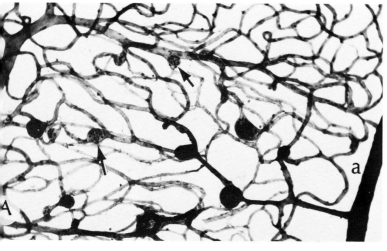

FIG. 15–10. Diabetic retinal capillary. **A.** Basement membrane shell (*arrows*) only evidence remaining to indicate where pericytes had been. **B.** Nondiabetic normal capillary to show basement membrane shell (*arrow*) around pericyte. **C.** Diabetic capillary has only basement membrane shell (*arrow*) with nucleus absent. **A,** PAS, ×630; **B,** PAS, ×850; **C,** PAS, ×630.

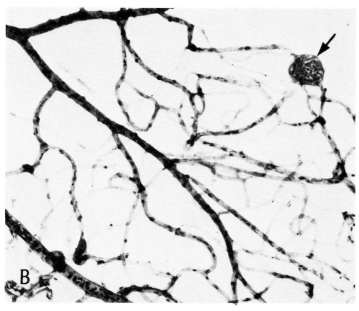

FIG. 15–11. Retinal capillary microaneurysm (RCM). **A.** RCMs occur in random distribution between arteriole (*a*) and venule (*v*). "Young" RCMs are seen as saccular capillary outpouchings with proliferated endothelial cells (*arrows*). "Old" RCMs appear as solid black balls with their lumens obliterated by PAS-positive material. Note darker color of capillaries with thickened basement membranes and arteriolar-venular connections. **B.** Very large RCM (*arrow*) or tiny hemorrhages associated with abnormal vessels probably are responsible for clinically seen RCMs. **A,** PAS, ×40; **B,** PAS, ×115.

ARTERIES AND ARTERIOLES OF CHOROID
(Fig. 15–7)

The onset of arteriosclerosis occurs at a younger age in diabetics than in the general population with a sharp increase in the incidence beyond the fifteenth year of the disease. The change is reflected in atherosclerosis and arteriolarsclerosis of the choroidal vessels.

CHORIOCAPILLARIS AND BRUCH'S MEMBRANE
(Fig. 15–8)

I. PAS-positive material thickens and may partially obliterate the lumen of the choriocapillaris at the posterior pole.
II. The cuticular portion of Bruch's membrane (basement membrane of the retinal pigment epithelium) may become thickened and drusen are common.
III. Because Bruch's membrane is made up in large part by the basement membrane of the retinal pigment epithelium and the adjacent connective tissue layer, it may be thickened.

RETINA

SPECIFIC CONSTELLATION OF VASCULAR FINDINGS
(Clinical "Background" Retinopathy)

I. Loss of capillary pericytes (Figs. 15–9 and 15–10 and part G in Color Plate III)
  A. In the normal retinal capillary the pericyte to endothelial cell ratio is 1:1.
  B. In the diabetic retinal capillary the pericyte to endothelial cell ratio is < 1:1 because of a selective loss of pericytes.
II. Capillary microaneurysms (Figs. 15–11 through 15–14 and parts E and F in Color Plate III)
  A. An increase in the number of retinal capillary microaneurysms can be correlated directly with the loss of pericytes.
  B. There is a random distribution of the microaneurysms across the arteriolar and venular sides of the capillary network.
  C. The microaneurysms start as thin outpouchings (saccular) from the wall of a capillary; then the endothelial cells proliferate and lay down increased amounts of basement membrane. Ultimately all the endothelial cells may disappear. The lumen of the microaneurysm may remain patent or may become occluded by the accumulated basement membrane material.
  D. There are many more microaneurysms present microscopically than seen clinically (unless intravenous fluorescein is used).
  E. Formation of retinal capillary microaneurysms most likely represents a response to an hypoxic environment in the form of either abortive attempts at neovascularization or regressed changes, or both, in a previously proliferating vessel.
III. Thickening of retinal capillary basement membrane (Figs. 15–11 and 15–12)
IV. Arteriolar-venular connections ("shunts") (Figs. 15–11, 15–12 and 15–14)
  A. Arteriolar-venular (A-V) connections (collaterals) are secondary phenomena, i.e., secondary to the surrounding environmental hypoxic stimulus.
  B. The A-V connections have a decreased rate of blood flow.

EXUDATIVE RETINOPATHY

I. "Hard" or "waxy" exudates (Figs. 15–13 and 15–15 through 15–18)
  A. Hard or waxy discrete exudates are collections of serum and glial-neuronal breakdown products located predominantly in the outer plexiform (Henle fiber) layer.
  B. The discrete exudates are removed by macrophages, usually in 4 to 6 months; it may take a year or more if the exudates are confluent.
  C. When they are distributed around the fovea, they form a macular "star."
II. "Soft" or "cotton-wool" spots (see p. 397 in Chap. 11).
  A. They are present most commonly in the early part of the proliferative stage of diabetic retinopathy, especially during a phase of rapid progression.
  B. Microinfarcts of the nerve fiber layer are the cause of the clinically seen cotton-wool spots.
  C. Cytoid bodies are found within the histologic counterpart of the cotton-

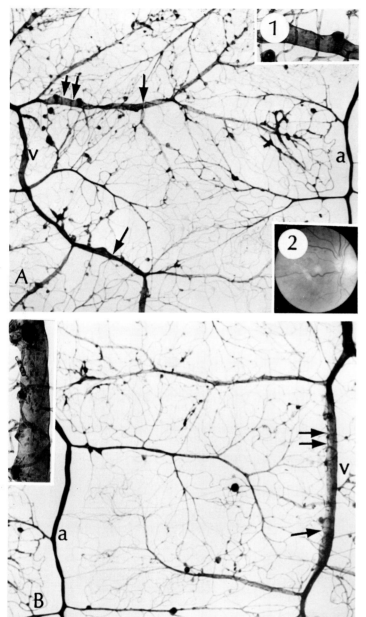

A

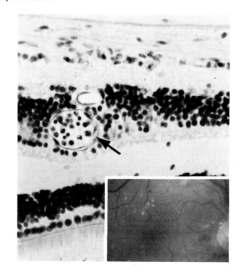

FIG. 15–12. Sausage-shaped venules (*arrows* in **A** and **B**) are due to irregularities in venular walls. Note arteriolar-venular connections and thickened capillary basement membranes (dark-colored capillaries) in **A** and **B**. Retinal capillary microaneurysms tend to arise from cellular (viable) capillaries and cluster around acellular (nonviable) capillaries. Venular walls not only are irregular but also have unusual presence of saccular microaneurysms (**inset 1** in **A** and **inset** in **B** from areas of *double arrows*). a, arteriole; v, venule. **Inset 2** in **A** shows fundus appearance of microaneurysms, cotton-wool spot, irregular venules and intraretinal neovascularization in form of rete mirabile. **A,** PAS, ×16; **inset 1,** PAS, ×40; **inset 2,** fundus; **B,** PAS, ×16; **inset,** PAS, ×54.

FIG. 15–13. Retinal capillary microaneurysm (*arrow*) is characterized by thin wall and presence in capillary area of retina (middle retinal layers) rather than major vessel area (inner retinal layers). **Inset** shows fundus appearance of microaneurysms and hard or waxy exudates. **Main figure,** H&E, ×176; **inset,** fundus.

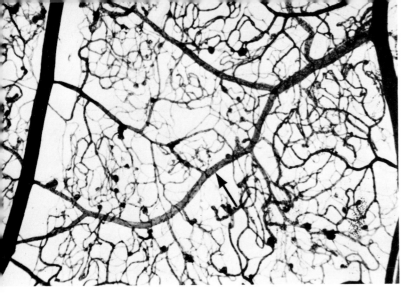

FIG. 15–14. Arteriolar-venular connection (collateral) consists of dilated cellular capillary (*arrow*) in area with increased number of anuclear (apparently nonviable) capillaries. PAS, ×16.

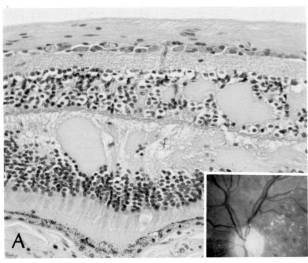

A.

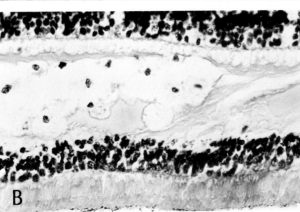

B

FIG. 15–15. Hard or waxy exudates. **A.** Retinal exudates accumulate in outer plexiform (Henle fiber) or in inner nuclear (bipolar cell) layers. Note that here middle limiting membrane separates layers. **Inset** shows fundus appearance of moderate background diabetic retinopathy. **B.** Fat-filled (lipoidal) histiocytes in outer plexiform (Henle fiber) layer of macula. Fat has dissolved out leaving histiocyte nuclei apparently "floating in air." **C.** Massive exudation with foamy histiocytes present in outer plexiform layer. **A,** H&E, ×220; **inset,** fundus; **B,** H&E, ×300; **C,** H&E, ×137.

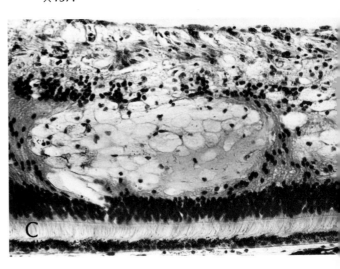

C

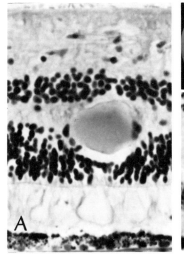

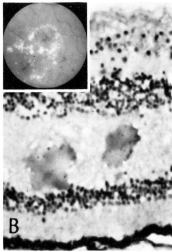

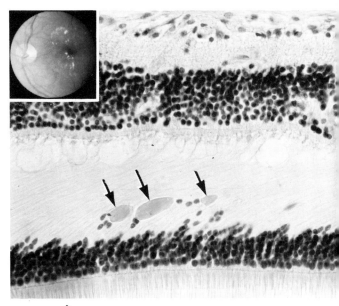

FIG. 15–16. Outer plexiform (hard) exudate (**A**) stains positively for fat (**B**) when special stain is used on frozen section. **Inset** in **B** shows "circinate" or circular type of retinal exudation. **A,** H&E, ×160; **B,** oil red-O, ×160; **inset,** fundus.

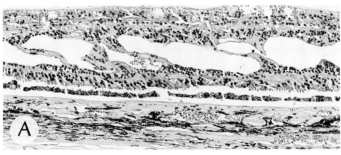

FIG. 15–17. Exudates in Henle nerve fiber layer around fovea (*arrows*) form macular star (**inset**). **Main figure,** H&E, ×250; **inset,** fundus.

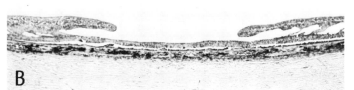

FIG. 15–18. Microcystoid (**A**) or macrocystoid (**B**), i.e., retinoschisis, may occur as result of exudation, usually in macular area. Note hole in inner wall of macular retinoschisis (cyst) in **B. A,** H&E, ×100; **B,** H&E, ×32.

wool spot and are caused by the swollen ends of ruptured axons in the nerve fiber layer in the infarcted area (Figs. 11–14 and 11–15).

D. They generally disappear from view in weeks to months.

III. Microcystoid degeneration of the retinal macula (Fig. 15–18)

A. Exudates may cause pressure atrophy of the retina or enlargement of the intercellular spaces resulting in microcystoid degeneration, especially in the macular area.

B. Microcystoid retinal degeneration may progress to macular retinoschisis ("cyst") and even partial (inner layer of schisis) or complete macular hole formation.

HEMORRHAGIC RETINOPATHY

I. "Dot" and "Blot" hemorrhages (Fig. 15–19)

A. Dot and blot hemorrhages are relatively small hemorrhages located in the inner nuclear layer with spread to the outer plexiform layer of the retina.

B. In three-dimensional view they appear serpiginous.

II. "Splinter" or "flame-shaped" hemorrhages (Fig. 15–20). These are relatively small hemorrhages located in the nerve fiber layer of the retina.

III. Globular hemorrhages (Fig. 15–21). These are caused by the spread of dot and blot hemorrhages within the middle retinal layers.

IV. Confluent hemorrhages (Fig. 15–21). This type of hemorrhage is larger and involves all the retinal layers.

V. Massive hemorrhages (Fig. 15–21). These may break through the internal limiting membrane into the vitreous body or, rarely, into the subretinal space.

VI. Larger hemorrhages, i.e., globular and confluent, may herald the onset of the malignant (proliferative) phase of the disease.

PROLIFERATIVE RETINOPATHY ("Malignant" Stage)
(Figs. 15–12 and 15–22 through 15–27)

I. The proliferative phase of diabetic retinopathy probably is a vascular response to an hypoxic retinal environment.

II. The neovascularization, which is initially intraretinal, generally breaks through the internal limiting membrane and lies between this structure and the vitreous.

Vitreous shrinkage (i.e., detachment) may rip the new vessels, leading to a hemorrhage. If a subvitreal hemorrhage results (the common type of diabetic "vitreous" hemorrhage), it clears rapidly in weeks to a few months. If a hemorrhage into the formed vitreous (vitreous framework) results, it may take many months to years to clear.

III. Pure neovascularization eventually is accompanied by a fibrous component; it is then called *retinitis proliferans*.

Shrinkage of the fibrous component often leads to a retinal detachment, the majority of which are nonrhegmatogenous, i.e., without a retinal hole. Ultimately the whole process of diabetic retinopathy tends to "burn out" and become quiescent.

IV. Less than 40 percent of patients with malignant retinopathy, even if they are

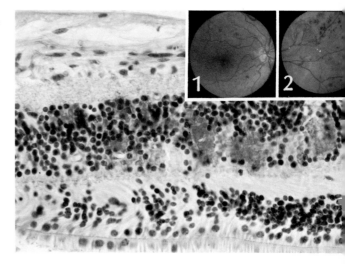

FIG. 15–19. Dot and blot hemorrhages consist of small collections of blood in inner nuclear and outer plexiform layers of retina. **Insets 1** and **2** show fundus appearances of dot and blot hemorrhages. **Main figure,** H&E, ×260; **inset 1,** fundus; **inset 2,** fundus.

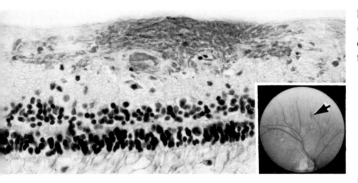

FIG. 15–20. Splinter-shaped hemorrhage (*arrow* in **inset**) consists of small collection of blood in nerve fiber layer of retina. **Main figure,** H&E, ×260; **inset,** fundus.

FIG. 15–21. Large collections of blood have dissected throughout all retinal layers. Pigment (*arrows*) is hemosiderin. **Inset** shows globular, confluent and massive retinal hemorrhages and preretinal fibrosis. **Main figure,** H&E, ×130; **inset,** fundus.

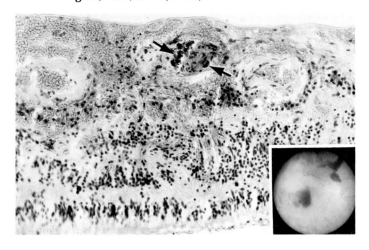

FIG. 15–22. Neovascularization of retina. Note increased number of abnormal intraretinal capillaries (compare to normal capillary shown in Figures 15–9 and 15–10). *a*, arteriole; *v*, venule. PAS, ×100.

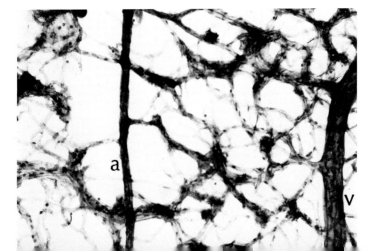

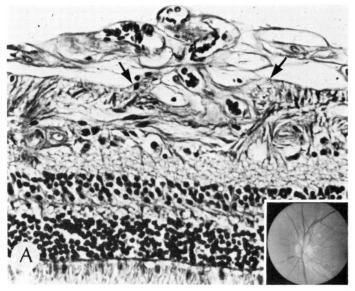

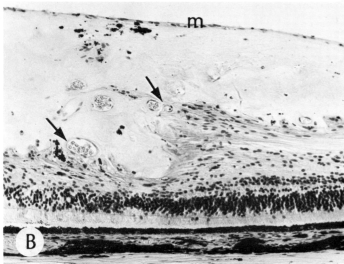

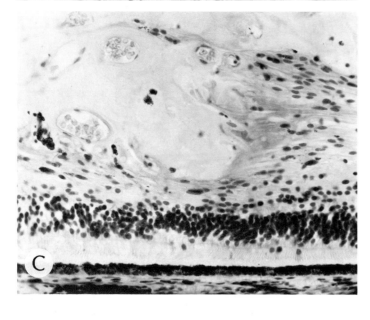

FIG. 15–23. Intraretinal neovascularization. **A.** New vessels are breaking through internal limiting membrane (*arrows*) to reach potential space between retina and vitreous. **Inset** shows extensive neovascularization of retina temporal to optic disc. **B** and **C** show another case with new vessels coming out of retina through internal limiting membrane (*arrows* in **B**) to reach preretinal space. *m*, membrane on posterior surface of vitreous body in **B**. **A**, trichrome, ×160; **inset**, fundus; **B**, H&E, ×130; **C**, H&E, ×200.

Color Plate III. **A–D** all from same case of hyperplasia of nonpigmented ciliary epithelium (see Figure 9–20). **A.** Tumor from anterior chamber stained with periodic acid-Schiff. Cells forming cords or acini are highly positive, while extracellular materials are mildly positive. **B.** Nearby section stained with PAS after treatment with diastase. Intracellular staining (glycogen) is lost. **C.** Extracellular materials stain well with Hale technique for acid mucopolysaccharides. **D.** Extracellular materials fail to stain blue with Hale method for acid mucopolysaccharides after pretreatment of tissue section with hyaluronidase, i.e., they contain hyaluronic acid. **E** and **F**, diabetic retina. **E.** Trypsin digest of retinal periphery. Note marked tortuosity of smallest vessels and multiple capillary aneurysms. Darkly stained vessels with capillary-free zone (above) are arterioles, single multinucleate vessel (below) is venule. **F.** Higher magnification of portion of **E**. Note U-shaped kinking and aneurysmal formations on capillaries and relative loss of pericytes. **G.** Normal capillaries in retinal periphery of nondiabetic. Note symmetry of arrangement, 1:1 ratio of pericyte nuclei to endothelial cell nuclei and lack of aneurysms. **H.** Touton giant cell in juvenile xanthogranuloma. Globules of fat within peripheral portion of cell cytoplasm stain bright red with oil red-O. **A**, PAS, ×115; **B**, diastase-PAS, ×115; **C**, AMP, ×115; **D**, hyaluronidase-AMP, ×115; **E**, PAS, ×100; **F**, PAS, ×700; **G**, PAS, ×700; **H**, frozen section of eyelid, oil red-O, ×320.

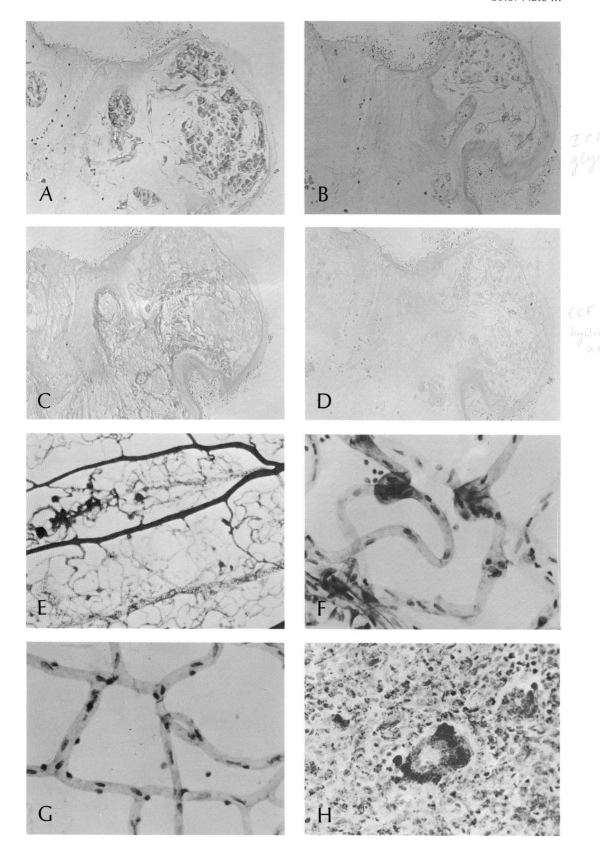

ICF: glycerin

ECF: hyaluronic acid

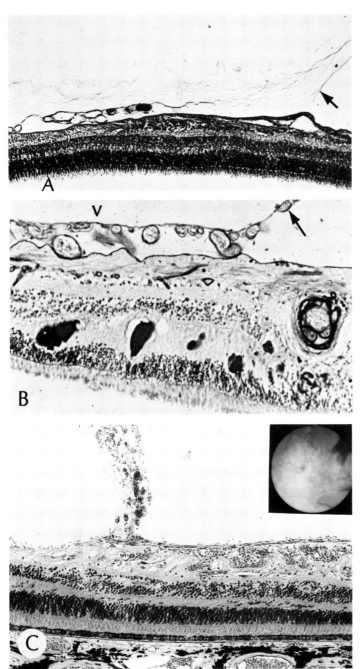

FIG. 15–24. After new vessels leave retina, they may stay in potential space between retina and vitreous (**A**), "climb up" posterior aspect of detached vitreous (*arrow* in **B;** *v,* vitreous) or become ruptured by posteriorly detaching vitreous with resulting hemorrhage (**C**). **Inset** in **C** shows fundus appearance of retinal neovascularization, fibrosis and vitreous hemorrhage. Note early detachment of vitreous (*arrow*) in **A. A,** trichrome, ×54; **B,** PAS, ×160; **C,** H&E, ×100; **inset,** fundus.

not blind, survive 10 years, and less than 25 percent of the diabetic blind survive 10 years.

VITREOUS

VITREOUS DETACHMENT
(Figs. 15–24 through 15–26 and 15–28)

I. Vitreous detachments ("contractures") are very common in diabetics and seem to occur at an earlier age than in non-diabetics.
II. The proliferating fibrovascular tissue from the optic nerve head or retina generally grows between the vitreous and the retina, i.e., along the inner surface of the internal limiting membrane of the retina, along the external surface of a detached vitreous or into Cloquet's canal; almost never does it grow directly into a formed vitreous, i.e., into the vitreous framework.

HEMORRHAGE INTO VITREOUS COMPARTMENT
(Figs. 15–24 and 15–25)

I. A hemorrhage into the subvitreal space is more common than into the vitreous body (see above, p. 578).
II. Organization of the hemorrhage with fibrous overgrowth may occur, usually along the external surface of the detached vitreous.

ASTEROID HYALOSIS

Asteroid hyalosis is an aging change unrelated to diabetes mellitus (see p. 472 in Chap. 12).

OPTIC NERVE

NEOVASCULARIZATION

The optic disc is a site of predilection for neovascularization, which tends to grow out into Cloquet's canal.

ISCHEMIC OPTIC NEUROPATHY

Retrobulbar neuritis, papillitis, papilledema and optic atrophy, all occurring infrequently, may be ischemic manifestations of diabetic micro-

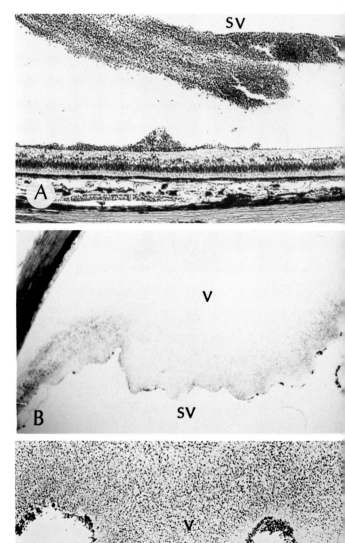

FIG. 15–25. Blood may be suspected of being in vitreous (**A**). **B** and **C** show that vitreous is completely detached and contains some blood, so that blood seen in **A** is in subvitreal (preretinal) area. *v*, vitreous; *sv*, subvitreal area. **A,** H&E, ×40; **B,** H&E, ×16; **C,** H&E, ×40.

angiopathy within the optic papilla in the absence of adequate collateral circulation.

CENTRAL RETINAL VEIN OCCLUSION

See p. 398 in Chapter 11.

582

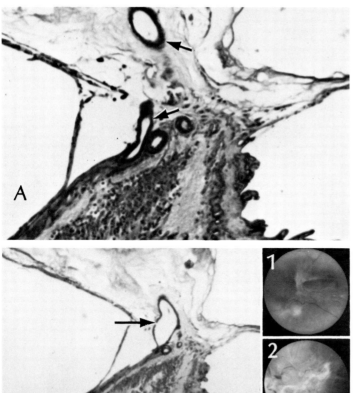

FIG. 15–26. Retinitis proliferans. **A.** Thick fibrovascular band on posterior surface of detached vitreous tents up retina. Note large vessel in band and in retina (*arrows*). These same vessels meet as shown in **B** (*arrow*). **Insets 1** and **2** in **B** show fundus appearances of retinitis proliferans. **A,** PAS, ×160; **B,** PAS, ×44; **inset 1,** fundus; **inset 2,** fundus.

FIG. 15–27. Retinitis proliferans. **A.** Shrinkage of fibrovascular membrane (*fm*) has caused total retinal detachment. **Inset 1** shows fundus with only mild background diabetic retinopathy present. **Inset 2** shows same fundus one year later. Massive fibrovascular-ization arising from area of optic disc is present. **B.** Higher magnification shows thick preretinal fibrovascular membrane (*fm*), which has caused retinal detachment and fixed folds of internal limiting membrane (*arrows*). Intraretinal cystic spaces present in long-standing detachment. **A,** H&E, ×16; **inset 1,** fundus; **inset 2,** fundus; **B,** H&E, ×40.

▼

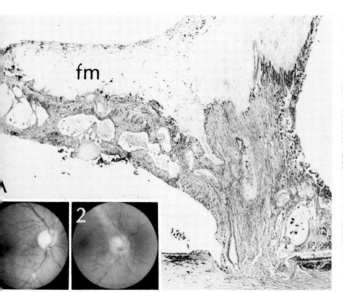

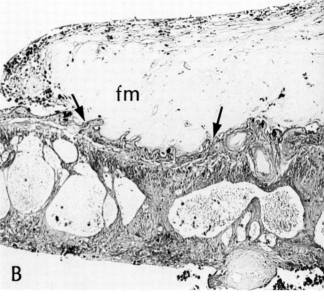

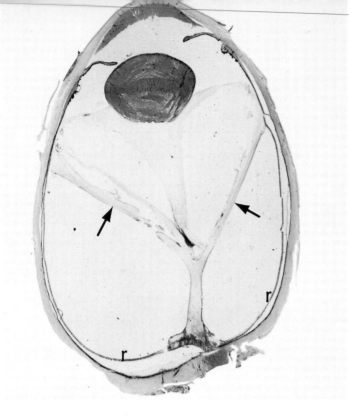

FIG. 15–28. Posterior vitreous detachment is present. *Arrows* show posterior vitreous surface. Vitreous is adherent to area around optic nerve. Note intumescent, cataractous lens and peripheral anterior synechias. *r*, retina. H&E, ×6.

BIBLIOGRAPHY

NATURAL HISTORY

Berkow JW, Shugarman RG, Maumenee AE, Patz A: A retrospective study of blind diabetic patients. J Am Med Assoc 193:867, 1965

Caird FI, Pirie MA, Ramsell TG: Diabetes and the Eye. Oxford, Blackwell, 1969, pp 1–7, 98–100

Danowski TS, Fisher ER, Park EJ, Khurana RC, Nolan S, Stephan T: Capillary basement membranes in muscle in glucose intolerance of the chemical diabetes type. Am J Clin Pathol 61:718, 1974

Kahn HA, Hiller R: Blindness caused by diabetic retinopathy. Am J Ophthalmol 78:58, 1974

Lister J: The Clinical Syndrome of Diabetes Mellitus. London, Lewis, 1959, p 43

Lundbaeb K: Late developments in long-term diabetic vascular disease, *in* Diabetes Mellitus. Edited by K Oberdisse, K Johoke. Stuttgart, Thieme, 1959, p 141

Romani J-D: La microangiopathie du diabète. Étude des relations entre les données de la biopsie cutanée, l'âge du malade, le type et la durée du diabète. Acta Diabetol Lat 9:709, 1972

Sevel D, Bristow JH, Bank S, Marks I, Jackson P: Diabetic retinopathy in chronic pancreatitis. Arch Ophthalmol 86:245, 1971

Vracko R: Basal lamina layering in diabetes mellitus: evidence for accelerated rate of cell death and cell regeneration. Diabetes 23:94, 1974

Vracko R, Benditt EP: Manifestations of diabetes mellitus—their possible relationships to an underlying cell defect. A review. Am J Pathol 75:204, 1974

White P: Childhood diabetes. Diabetes 9:345, 1960

CONJUNCTIVA AND CORNEA

Armaly MF, Baloglon PJ: Diabetes mellitus and the eye. I. Changes in the anterior segment. Arch Ophthalmol 77:485, 1967

Cook DAG: The significance of conjunctival aneurysms in diabetes. XVII Concilium Ophthalmologicum 1954, Acta V, 3. Toronto, University of Toronto Press, 1955, p 1878

English FB, Bell JR, English KP: Conjunctival vascular pathology associated with diabetic lipemia retinalis. Arch Ophthalmol 89:120, 1973

Henkind P, Wise GM: Descemet's wrinkles in diabetes. Am J Ophthalmol 52:371, 1961

LENS

Brown CA, Burman D: Transient cataracts in a diabetic child with hyperosmolar coma. Br J Ophthalmol 57:429, 1973

Yanoff M: Ocular pathology of diabetes mellitus. Am J Ophthalmol 67:21, 1969

IRIS

Armaly MF, Baloglon PJ: Diabetes mellitus and the eye. I. Changes in the anterior segment. Arch Ophthalmol 77:485, 1967

Fine BS, Berkow JW, Helfgott JA: Diabetic lacy vacuolation of iris pigment epithelium. Am J Ophthalmol 69:197, 1970

Madsen PH: Rubeosis of the iris and hemorrhagic glaucoma in patients with proliferative diabetic retinopathy. Br J Ophthalmol 55:368, 1971

Ohrt V: The frequency of rubeosis iridis in diabetic patients. Acta Ophthalmol (Kbh) 49:301, 1971

Yamashita T, Becker B: The basement membrane in the human diabetic eye. Diabetes 10:167, 1961

Yanoff M: Ocular pathology of diabetes mellitus. Am J Ophthalmol 67:21, 1969

Yanoff M, Fine BS, Berkow JW: Diabetic lacy vacuolation of iris pigment epithelium. Am J Ophthalmol 69:201, 1970

CILIARY BODY AND CHOROID

Yamashita T, Becker B: The basement membrane in the human diabetic eye. Diabetes 10:167, 1961

Yanoff M: Ocular pathology of diabetes mellitus. Am J Ophthalmol 67:21, 1969

RETINA

Adnitt PI, Taylor E: Progression of diabetic retinopathy. Lancet 1:652, 1970

Ashton N: Studies of retinal capillaries in relation to diabetic and other retinopathies. Br J Ophthalmol 47:521, 1963

Ashton N: Vascular basement membrane changes in diabetic retinopathy. Brit J Ophthal 58:344, 1974

Ballantyne AJ, Lowenstein A: Diseases of the retina. I. The pathology of diabetic retinopathy. Trans Ophthalmol Soc UK 63:95, 1943

Bloodworth JMB Jr: Diabetic microangiopathy. Diabetes 12:99, 1963

Cogan DG, Toussaint D, Kuwabara T: Retinal vascular patterns. IV. Diabetic retinopathy. Arch Ophthalmol 66:366, 1961

Garner A: Pathology of diabetic retinopathy. Br Med Bull 26:137, 1970

Hutton WL, Snyder WB, Vaiser A, Siperstein MD: Retinal microangiopathy without associated glucose intolerance. Trans Am Acad Ophthalmol Otolaryngol 76:968, 1972

Lundbaek K: Diabetic angiopathy. Acta Diabetol Lat 10:183, 1973

Michaelson IC, Yanko L, Berson D, Irvy M: The reac-

tive phase of diabetic retinopathy and the role of the reticuloendothelial system. Am J Ophthalmol 78:400, 1974

Roth AM, Foos RY: Surface wrinkling retinopathy in eyes enucleated at autopsy. Trans Am Acad Ophthalmol Otolaryngol 75:1047, 1971

Tolentino FI, Lee PF, Schepens CL: Biomicroscopic study of vitreous cavity in diabetic retinopathy. Arch Ophthalmol 75:238, 1966

Werner AV, Larsen HW: Immunohistologic studies in human diabetic and nondiabetic eyes: fluorescent labelling of insulin and insulin antibodies. Acta Ophthalmol (Kbh) 47:937, 1969

Williams DK, Drance SM, Harris GS, Fairclough M: Diabetic cotton-wool spots: evaluation using perimetric and angiographic techniques. Can J Ophthalmol 5:68, 1970

Yanoff M: Diabetic retinopathy. N Engl J Med 274:1344, 1966

Yanoff M: Ocular pathology of diabetes mellitus. Am J Ophthalmol 67:21, 1969

Yanoff M: Histopathogenesis of diabetic retinopathy. Acta Diabetol Lat 9:527, 1972

VITREOUS

Luxenberg M, Sime D: Relationship of asteroid hyalosis to diabetes mellitus and plasma lipid levels. Am J Ophthalmol 67:406, 1969

Tolentino FI, Lee PF, Schepens CL: Biomicroscopic study of vitreous cavity in diabetic retinopathy. Arch Ophthalmol 75:238, 1966

Yanoff M: Ocular pathology of diabetes mellitus. Am J Ophthalmol 67:21, 1969

OPTIC NERVE

Lubow M, Makley TA Jr: Pseudopapilledema of juvenile diabetes mellitus. Arch Ophthalmol 85:417, 1971

Saraux H, Lestradet H, Biais B: La névrite optique du jeune diabétique. Ann Ocul (Paris) 205:35, 1972

Yanko L, Ticko U, Ivry M: Optic nerve involvement in diabetes. Acta Ophthalmol (Kbh) 50:556, 1972

chapter 16

Glaucoma

DEFINITION

Glaucoma is a syndrome caused by a group of different ocular diseases and characterized by an intraocular pressure sufficiently elevated to produce ocular tissue damage, either transient or permanent.

I. Individuals with increased intraocular pressure but without detectable ocular tissue damage or visual functional impairment properly are labelled as individuals with ocular hypertension. The ocular hypertension may be normal for the individual or may lead to ocular tissue damage and hence glaucoma.

II. Glaucoma is *not* an intraocular pressure reading; it is a syndrome.

NORMAL OUTFLOW

HYPERSECRETION

I. Hypersecretion glaucoma is rare and has no antecedent cause.

II. There is a normal outflow facility, and the elevated intraocular pressure is presumed to be due to an increased production of aqueous humor.

III. The glaucoma mainly affects middle-aged women, especially when they have essential hypertension.

IV. Histologically the angle of the anterior chamber shows no abnormalities.

IMPAIRED OUTFLOW

CONGENITAL GLAUCOMA

I. General Information
   A. The incidence of congenital glaucoma ranges from about 1:5000 to 1:10,000 live births.
   B. It is usually inherited as an autosomal recessive but can have an infectious etiology, e.g., rubella.
   C. There is a 60 to 70 percent male predominance.
   D. The disease is bilateral in 64 to 88 percent of cases.
   E. Age of onset:
      1. Present at birth, 40 percent.
      2. Between birth and 6 months, 34 percent.
      3. Between 6 months and 1 year, 12 percent.
      4. Between 1 year and 6 years, 11 percent.
      5. Over 6 years, 2 percent.
      6. No information, 1 percent.

II. Pathogenesis (many theories):
   A. *Barkan's membrane* (mesodermal surface membrane or imperforate innermost uveal sheet) mechanically prevents the aqueous from leaving the eye. There is little convincing histologic proof for this theory.
   B. Congenital absence of Schlemm's canal
      1. Congenital absence of Schlemm's canal is very rare, if it exists at all.
      2. Most often the canal is compressed secondarily and therefore difficult to find histologically.
   C. An *"embryonic"* anterior chamber angle that results from *faulty cleavage* of tissue during embryonic development of the eye prevents the aqueous from leaving the eye. Histologically the angle shows an anterior "insertion" of the iris root, anteriorly displaced ciliary processes, insertion of the ciliary meridional muscles into the trabecular meshwork instead of into (or over) the scleral roll and mesenchymal tissue in the anterior chamber angle (Fig. 16–1).
      1. Many nonglaucoma infant eyes

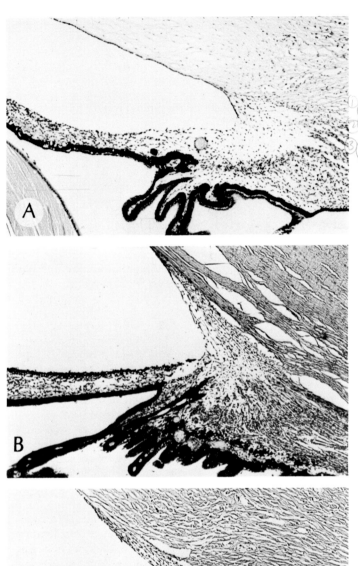

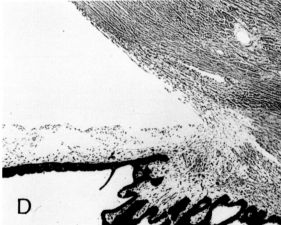

FIG. 16–1. Congenital glaucoma. **A, B** and **C** are from premature infants (**A,** 700 g—died shortly after birth; **B,** 905 g—lived 3½ months; **C,** 1050 g—lived 1 day), none of whom had clinical or histological evidence of glaucoma. Note in all three anterior "insertion" of iris root, anteriorly displaced ciliary processes, continuity of ciliary meridional muscles with uveal trabecular meshwork and mesenchymal tissue in anterior chamber angle. **D.** Eye obtained from 2-year-old child at time of accidental drowning. Bilateral congenital glaucoma well documented; goniotomy and goniopuncture had been performed in another area of eye—pressure well controlled following surgery. Note similarity to non-glaucomatous premature eyes shown in **A, B** and **C. A,** H&E, ×40; **B,** H&E, ×40; **C,** H&E, ×40; **D,** H&E, ×40.

show similar structure of the anterior chamber angle.

2. To be accurate in interpretation of the angle histology, one needs truly meridional sections through the anterior chamber angle. Tangential sectioning makes interpretation difficult. Unfortunately in the usual serial sectioning of the whole eye, because of the continuously curved surface very few sections from the exact center of the embedded tissue are truly meridional.

D. Probably the true cause, or even more likely causes, is not as yet known.

Although due to impaired outflow, the site or sites of the defect may vary from case to case, the major obstruction lying near the entrance to the meshwork, within the meshwork or near the efferent vessels of the drainage angle, or any combination thereof. Thus the question, as in chronic simple (open angle) glaucoma in the adult, may be a quantitative one (see pp. 594–598 in this chapter).

III. Associated diseases and conditions
A. Iris anomalies (see pp. 329–332 in Chap. 9).
1. Hypoplasia of the iris ("aniridia") and iris coloboma may be associated with congenital glaucoma.
2. Axenfeld's anomaly and Rieger's syndrome (see pp. 268–270 in Chap. 8).
B. Peters' anomaly (see p. 265 in Chap. 8).
C. Phakomatoses
1. Sturge-Weber (see pp. 30–32 in Chap. 2).
2. Neurofibromatosis (see pp. 32–35 in Chap. 2).
D. Lowe's syndrome (see p. 360 in Chap. 10).
E. Pierre Robin Syndrome
1. Pierre Robin syndrome consists of hypoplasia of the mandible, glossoptosis, cleft palate and ocular anomalies.
2. The ocular anomalies found in the condition are glaucoma, high myopia, cataract, retinal detachment and microphthalmos.
F. Rubella (see pp. 48–50 in Chap. 2).

IV. Secondary histologic ocular effects in young eyes (less than 10 years of age).
A. Buphthalmos or a large eye is caused by an enlargement, stretching and thinning of the coats of the eye, especially marked in the anterior segment (Figs. 16–2 and 16–3).
B. With enlargement of the eye, including the cornea, a deep anterior chamber results (Figs. 16–2 and 16–3).

These eyes may develop subluxated lenses.

C. Ruptures of Descemet's membrane (*Haag's striae*) may be found in the enlarged corneas (Figs. 16–2 and 16–4), are usually horizontal in the central area and concentric toward the limbus, generally are in the lower half of the

FIG. 16–2. Congenital glaucoma with enlargement, stretching and thinning of cornea and sclera, especially in limbal region (limbal ectasia). Note deep anterior chamber and rupture in Descemet's membrane (*arrow*). Fibrosis of iris root and trabecular meshwork is present. **Inset** shows markedly enlarged corneas in child with bilateral congenital glaucoma. **Main figure,** H&E, ×8; **inset,** clinical.

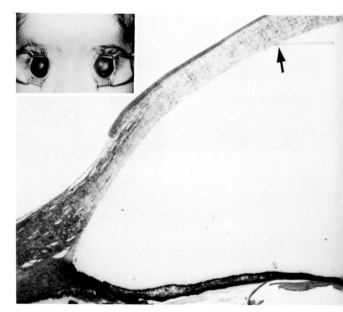

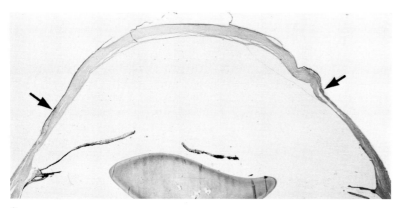

Fig. 16–3. Eye enucleated from 7-year-old girl with congenital glaucoma. Left side shows extreme thinning over limbal and anterior ciliary body (intercalary ectasia), whereas right side shows similar ectatic area lined by iris in form of peripheral anterior synechia (intercalary staphyloma). Iris coloboma due to peripheral iridectomy. Note deep anterior chamber, thinned and enlarged cornea and bullous keratopathy. *Arrows* indicate periphery of Bowman's membrane. H&E, ×10.

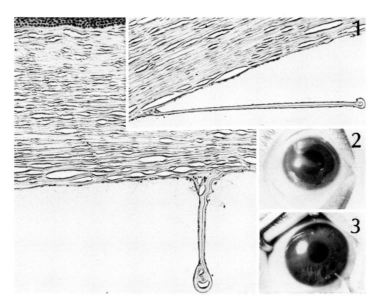

FIG. 16–4. Ruptured end of Descemet's membrane has been healed over so that scroll-like extension of Descemet's membrane hanging into anterior chamber is covered completely by endothelium. Photomicrographic **inset 1** shows higher magnification of rupture in Figure 16–2. Clinical **insets** shows rupture of Descemet's membrane from 10 toward 4 o'clock (**2**) and from 8 toward 2 o'clock (**3**). **Main figure,** H&E, ×54; **inset 1,** H&E, ×40; **inset 2,** clinical; **inset 3,** clinical.

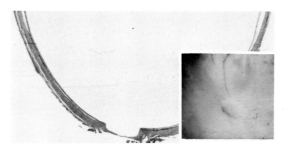

FIG. 16–5. Deep glaucomatous optic nerve-head excavation is present in eye removed from 7-year-old girl with congenital glaucoma (see Figure 16–3). **Inset** shows macroscopic appearance. **Main figure,** H&E, ×5; **inset,** macroscopic.

cornea and frequently are associated with corneal edema.

D. The limbal region becomes stretched and thin with a resultant *limbal ectasia* (Figs. 16–2 and 16–3).

When the limbal ectasia is lined by uvea, e.g., with peripheral anterior synechias, it is called a *limbal staphyloma,* or when extensive and extending posteriorly so as to involve the sclera over the ciliary body, an *intercalary staphyloma* (Fig. 16–3).

E. Fibrosis of the iris root and trabecular meshwork is a late manifestation (Fig. 16–2).

F. Disappearance of Schlemm's canal is also a late result.

G. With continued high intraocular pressure atrophy of the ciliary body, choroid and retina, cupping of the optic disc (Fig. 16–5) and atrophy of the optic nerve result.

PRIMARY GLAUCOMA

I. Closed angle (narrow angle; acute congestive) (Figs. 16–6 and 16–7)

A. Eyes that develop primary angle closure glaucoma have an anatomic predisposition to the condition.

   1. The surface of the peripheral iris is close to the inner surface of the trabecular meshwork, i.e., a narrow or shallow anterior chamber angle.

   2. Small hypermetropic eyes are especially vulnerable.

   3. A normal sized or large lens may be present.

If the lens becomes large enough, e.g., a swollen intumescent lens, it may push the iris diaphragm anteriorly such that an angle closure can result even though the anterior chamber angle was of normal or average width.

B. The trabecular meshwork is normal before an initial attack of acute primary angle closure glaucoma. Following repeated attacks (often at subclinical level) the anterior chamber angle although open may become damaged

(sclerosed or fibrotic) and then may simulate chronic simple (open angle) glaucoma.

C. A sudden rise in intraocular pressure results from the apposition of the peripheral iris to the trabecular meshwork due to the mechanisms of pupillary block.

D. Histology

   1. Segmental iris atrophy

      a. It results from necrosis of the iris stroma secondary to occlusion of its arterial supply due to swelling of the iris root and occlusion of the greater arterial circle of the iris or one or more of its branches.

      b. Segmental iris atrophy usually is seen in the upper half of the iris in a sector configuration.

The atrophy may be extreme resulting in a through and through iris hole, thus curing the condition.

      c. Histologically there is marked atrophy of the stromal layer of the iris and varying degrees of iris pigment epithelial atrophy.

   2. Irregular pupil is due to:

      a. Necrosis of the dilator and sphincter muscle.

      b. Histologically segments or the entire length of dilator muscle is absent. The sphincter muscle shows varying degrees of atrophy.

   3. Glaukomflecken (*cataracta disseminata subcapsularis glaukomatosa*) (Figs. 16–7 and 16–8)

      a. Glaukomflecken probably results from the interference of normal metabolism of the anterior lens cells due to a stagnation of aqueous humor that contains toxic products of necrosis, or from foci of pressure necrosis.

      b. Anterior subcapsular, multiple, tiny, gray-white opacities are seen clinically.

      c. Histologically small areas of epithelial cell necrosis together with tiny adjacent areas of subcap-

FIG. 16–6. Closed angle glaucoma is characterized by "crowded" anterior segment (**inset 1**). Surface of peripheral iris occludes posterior portion of trabecular meshwork. **Inset 2** shows segmental necrosis of iris with absence of dilator muscle and atrophy of stroma. **Main figure,** PAS, ×80; **inset 1,** H&E, ×6; **inset 2,** PAS, ×40.

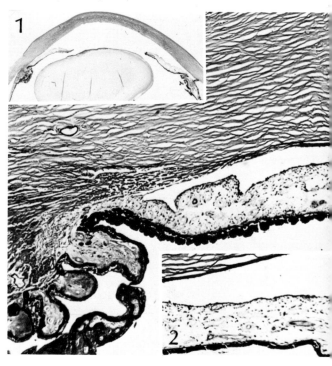

FIG. 16–7. Following acute attack of closed angle glaucoma, iris is necrotic (**A**). **Inset** shows clinical triad of irregular pupil, segmental iris atrophy (only iris from 5 to 9 o'clock relatively normal) and glaukomflecken, i.e., tiny white anterior subcapsular lens opacities. **B.** In this area almost total iris necrosis is present. **A,** H&E, ×101; **inset,** clinical; **B,** H&E, ×101.

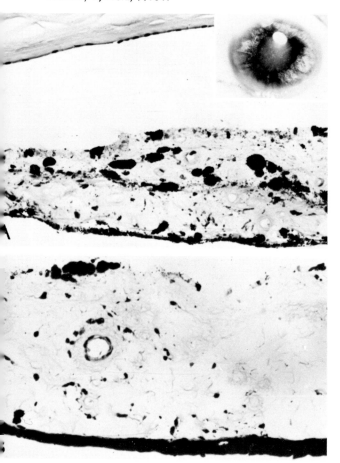

FIG. 16–8. Glaukomflecken is characterized by small areas of lens epithelial necrosis with tiny adjacent areas of subcapsular cortical degeneration. H&E, ×300.

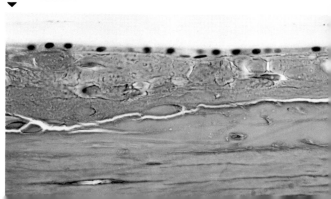

sular cortical degeneration are found.

4. Papilledema
   a. The nerve fibers in the optic nerve are more susceptible to an acute rise in intraocular pressure than are the retinal ganglion cells.
   b. Irreversible visual impairment following an acute attack is due mainly to optic nerve damage.

   The papilledema occurs early and is due probably to a temporary obstruction of the venous return at the nerve head by the increased intraocular pressure. If the associated corneal edema is cleared with glycerol during an acute glaucoma, the papilledema can be seen ophthalmoscopically in almost all cases.

   c. Histology—see p. 489 in Chapter 13.
5. Rubeosis iridis
   a. Rubeosis iridis generally is secondary to a central retinal vein or artery thrombosis caused by the elevated intraocular pressure during the acute attack.
   b. Histologically fibrovascular tissue is found in the anterior chamber angle and on the anterior surface of the iris.

II. Open angle (chronic simple glaucoma) (Figs. 16–9 through 16–11)
A. The angle appears open and normal gonioscopically.
B. The site or sites of resistance to outflow of aqueous humor lie within the structures of the drainage angle of the anterior chamber.

   There is widespread belief that the major site of obstruction lies near to the canal of Schlemm.

C. The condition is almost always bilateral and involves about 1 percent of the adult population.
   1. One eye may develop glaucoma months to years before the fellow eye.
   2. One eye may be more severely affected than the other eye.
D. Heredity
   1. In most cases the condition probably is inherited as an autosomal recessive.
      a. There is a frequent family history of open angle glaucoma.
      b. A high incidence of impaired facility of outflow is found in younger members of families with glaucoma.
E. Histology
   1. Very little is known about the early histology.
   2. Very little meaningful information can be derived from long-standing, "end stage" diseased eyes or from tiny biopsies taken during surgery for control of glaucoma.

   Many reported histologic changes such as "sclerosis" of the trabecular meshwork, compression or absence of Schlemm's canal and decrease in number of macrovacuoles in the endothelial lining of Schlemm's canal are probably "end stage" changes, artifacts or misinterpretations.

   3. "Aging" changes within the trabecular meshwork:
      a. Thickening and alteration in the connective tissue adjacent to Schlemm's canal (i.e., the juxtacanalicular connective tissue) may result in decreased permeability with or without endothelial or associated connective tissue proliferations into Schlemm's canal.
      b. Similar changes may take place in the longitudinal ciliary muscle (e.g., "hyalinization") or in the stroma of the iris root.
      c. Compression or aggregation of the connective tissue cores of the uveal meshwork overlying the youthful scleral roll produces the adult scleral spur.
      d. The changes listed above are mostly irreversible aging changes within the drainage angle of the anterior chamber.

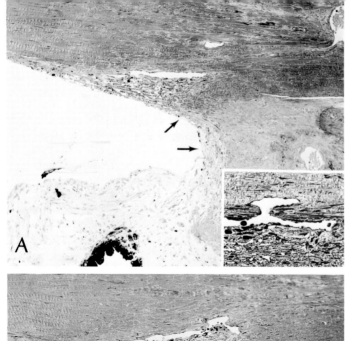

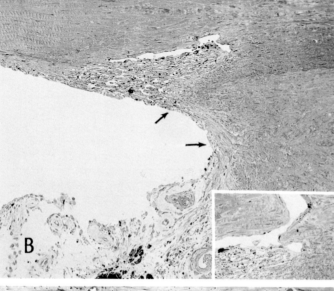

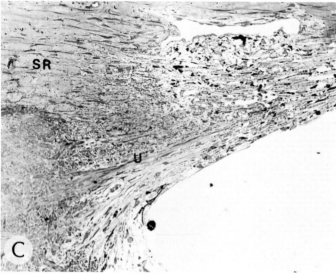

FIG. 16–9. Open angle glaucoma. **A** and **B.** Meridional sections of drainage angle from right (**B**) and left (**A**) eyes of patient with chronic open angle glaucoma. Note compression of uveal meshwork against scleral roll to produce prominent scleral spur in both eyes as well as increased compression of loose tissues in angle recess (*arrows*). **Insets** indicate that continuity is present between canal of Schlemm and openings to at least some of collector channels. **C.** Higher power of another section from left eye to show bipartite nature of scleral spur; scleral roll (*SR*), together with superimposed uveal meshwork (*U*). **A,** 1.5 μ section, PD, ×70; **inset,** 1.5 μ section, PD, ×145; **B,** 1.5 μ section, PD, ×90; **inset,** 1.5 μ section, PD, ×130; **C,** 1.5 μ section, PD, ×180.

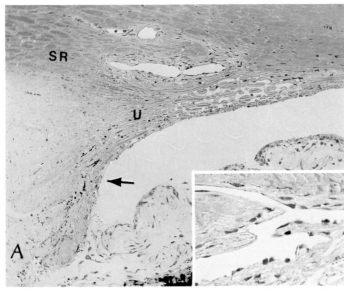

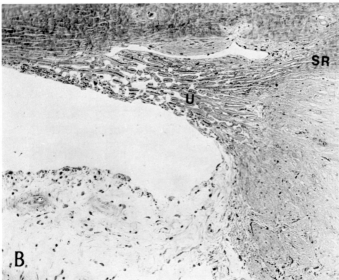

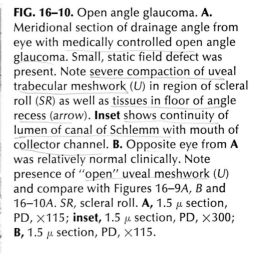

FIG. 16–10. Open angle glaucoma. **A.** Meridional section of drainage angle from eye with medically controlled open angle glaucoma. Small, static field defect was present. Note severe compaction of uveal trabecular meshwork (U) in region of scleral roll (SR) as well as tissues in floor of angle recess (arrow). **Inset** shows continuity of lumen of canal of Schlemm with mouth of collector channel. **B.** Opposite eye from **A** was relatively normal clinically. Note presence of "open" uveal meshwork (U) and compare with Figures 16–9A, B and 16–10A. SR, scleral roll. **A,** 1.5 μ section, PD, ×115; **inset,** 1.5 μ section, PD, ×300; **B,** 1.5 μ section, PD, ×115.

FIG. 16–11. Material from eye with increased intraocular pressure and highly positive water provocative test. Eye was removed because of choroidal malignant melanoma. **Inset 1** shows endothelial cells (e) proliferating across lumen of canal of Schlemm and long cytoplasmic projection (arrow) from endothelial lining of inner wall of canal. Electron micrograph shows endothelial projection to be forming basement membranelike material (arrow) similar to that lying within adjacent juxtacanalicular connective tissue (JCT). Some melanin granules can be seen in extracellular as well as intracellular locations. **Inset 2** shows scarring focally occluding canal of Schlemm. Focal scar is presumably progression of changes observed in **inset 1.** Note that scleralike tissue is absent from scar indicating that this region is not collagenous septum, which normally separates segments of canal of Schlemm. Scarring involves cells of juxtacanalicular connective tissue region and "endothelium" of canal itself. Identical changes also may be observed in same location in older but otherwise normal eyes. **Main figure,** ×6,700; **inset 1,** 1.5 μ section, PD, ×300; **inset 2,** 1.5 μ section, PD, ×450.

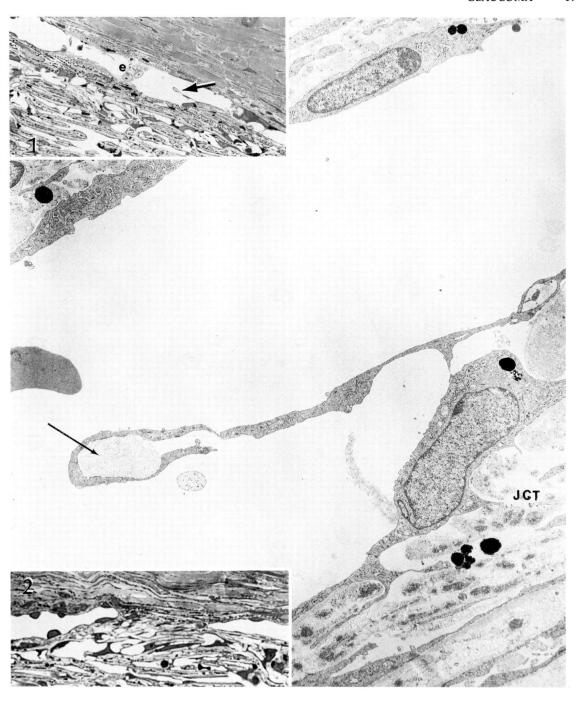

The changes in aggregate can cause diminished aqueous outflow.

Somewhat analogous aging changes occur in the regions of aqueous production, thus diminishing aqueous inflow. Any imbalance between the rate of aqueous obstruction and aqueous secretion will result in either ocular hypertension or hypotension. Histologically such "primary" changes within the drainage angle are detectable when they are localized quantitatively to a specific region.

SECONDARY GLAUCOMA

I. Closed angle is usually due to peripheral anterior synechias.
  A. Chronic primary closed angle glaucoma (Fig. 16–12)
    1. Repeated attacks of primary angle closure glaucoma may give rise to peripheral anterior synechias and secondary angle closure glaucoma. If synechias do not occur, the trabecular damage caused by the repeated attacks can cause a secondary chronic open angle glaucoma.
    2. Histologically peripheral anterior synechias are formed, sometimes with very broad bases.
  B. Phakomorphic
    1. Swelling of the lens may cause peripheral anterior synechias (via pupillary block and iris bombé).
    2. More frequently a swollen lens occurs rapidly and simulates primary closed angle glaucoma.
  C. Subluxated or anterior dislocated lens can cause a pupillary block, which if not broken leads to peripheral anterior synechias and secondary angle closure.
  D. Persistent flat chamber following surgical or nonsurgical trauma may lead to broad-based peripheral anterior synechias, occasionally causing total anterior synechia (see pp. 123–127 in Chap. 5).
  E. Essential iris atrophy (Fig. 16–13)
    1. Essential iris atrophy is usually unilateral, is most often found in women and is of unknown cause. The onset generally is in the third decade.
    2. The initial event is the formation of a peripheral anterior synechia distorting the pupil to that side. The pupil becomes more and more distorted with the development of an ectropion uveae, i.e., exposure of the iris pigment epithelium.
    3. Through-and-through holes develop in the iris opposite to the distorted pupil.
    4. Peripheral anterior synechias increase circumferentially, and an intractable glaucoma develops.
    5. Histologically the iris stroma is atrophic, and in the areas of iris hole formation the stroma and pigment epithelium are absent. Endothelialization of anterior chamber angle with formation of new Descemet's membrane may be present.
  F. Chandler's syndrome
    1. The condition is almost always unilateral.
    2. There is a corneal endothelial dystrophy with a tendency to develop corneal edema at an intraocular pressure not much above normal.
    3. Small peripheral anterior synechias with mild pupillary distortion are found.
    4. There are small areas of iris stromal thinning without through-and-through holes.
    5. The glaucoma is usually mild.
    6. The etiology is unknown.

    Many cases of Chandler's syndrome may very well represent the iris nevus syndrome.

  G. Iris nevus syndrome—see p. 649 in Chapter 17.
  H. Iridoschisis (Fig. 16–14)
    1. The condition mainly starts in the seventh decade of life and is usually bilateral with the sexes equally affected.
    2. The pupil is not displaced and remains reactive.
    3. The anterior iris stromal layers separate widely from the deeper layers.

a. The lower half of the iris most frequently is involved.

b. Initially the loosened stromal fibers remain attached centrally and peripherally so that the delicate middle part of the fibers bow forward into the anterior chamber.

c. Ultimately the fibers break with the free ends floating in the aqueous.

4. Glaucoma develops in about 50 percent of affected eyes; it begins as peripheral anterior synechias develop.

5. Cause

a. The majority seem to be a peculiar type of senile change.

b. It may follow trauma.

c. Rarely it may occur with chronic open angle glaucoma.

I. Anterior uveitis (Fig. 16–15)

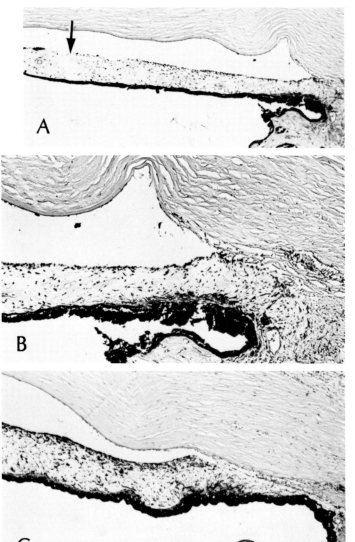

FIG. 16–12. Chronic primary closed angle glaucoma. **A.** Peripheral anterior synechia has formed following repeated closed angle glaucoma attacks. Note segmental atrophy of iris (*arrow*). **B.** Higher magnification shows occlusion and compression of trabecular meshwork. **C.** Another case to illustrate characteristic "bland" (nonfibrovascular) peripheral anterior synechia. **A,** H&E, ×16; **B,** H&E, ×40; **C,** H&E, ×28.

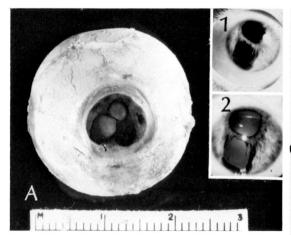

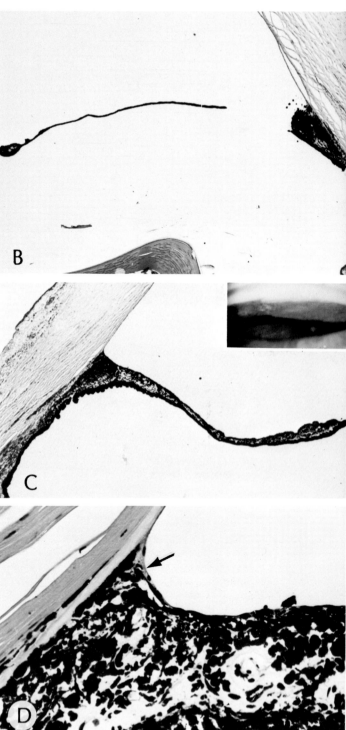

FIG. 16–13. Essential iris atrophy. **A. Insets** show appearance of iris hole with direct light (**1**) and fundus reflex (**2**)—pupil is displaced superiorly toward original synechia. Macroscopic appearance of another case shows hole formation and breaks in stroma. Corneal button removed prior to photography. **B.** Most of iris shows complete atrophy of stroma with only pigment epithelium remaining. Area near iris root demonstrates total atrophy with hole formation. **C.** Opposite iris leaf shows stromal atrophy and peripheral anterior synechia. **Inset** shows gonioscopic appearance of synechia. **D.** Higher magnification of another area demonstrates overgrowth of corneal endothelium over pseudoangle (*arrow*) onto anterior iris with production of new Descemet's membrane. **A**, macroscopic; **inset 1,** clinical; **inset 2,** clinical; **B,** H&E, ×16; **C,** H&E, ×16; **inset,** gonioscopic; **D,** H&E, ×176.

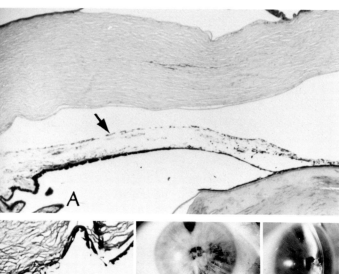

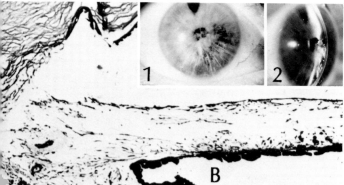

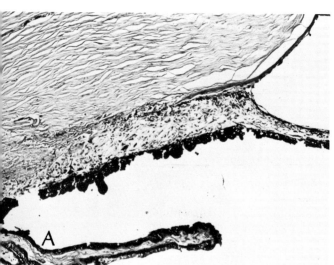

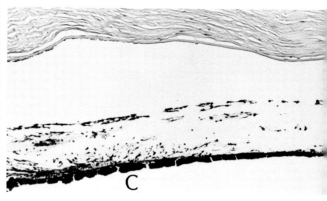

FIG. 16–14. Iridoschisis. **A.** Anterior iris stromal layers (*arrow*) are separated widely from deeper layers. Note bullous keratopathy. **B** and **C.** Anterior stromal layers separated from deeper layers extending from iris root (**B**) toward pupillary iris (**C**). **Insets** in **B** show clinical appearance in another case as viewed directly (**1**) and with slit beam (**2**). **A,** H&E, ×16; **B,** PAS, ×40; **inset 1,** clinical; **inset 2,** slit beam; **C,** H&E, ×40.

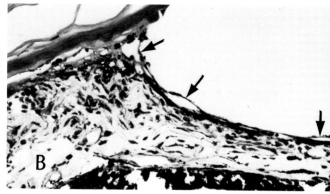

FIG. 16–15. Secondary angle closure glaucoma in congenital syphilis. **A.** Anterior chamber angle is occluded by peripheral anterior synechia. **B.** Higher magnification shows growth of endothelium over pseudoangle onto anterior surface of iris (*arrows*). New, thin Descemet's membrane has been produced by proliferating endothelium. Note Hassall-Henle warts of peripheral Descemet's in **A** and **B.** **A,** PAS, ×40; **B,** PAS, ×136.

Any cause of anterior uveitis, e.g., traumatic, infectious, "allergic" (sympathetic uveitis, phacoanaphylactic endophthalmitis), may result in posterior synechias, iris bombé and then peripheral anterior synechias.

J. Retrolental fibroplasia
   1. The retrolental mass pushes the lens forward and causes "crowding" of the anterior chamber angle.
   2. Angle closure glaucoma may result, sometimes years after the initial damage.

K. Spherophakia (Weill-Marchesani syndrome)—see p. 382 in Chapter 10.

L. Persistent hyperplastic primary vitreous—see p. 698 in Chapter 18.
   1. Swelling of the lens or iris bombé can produce angle closure.
   2. More frequently, repeated hemorrhages result in organization and iridocorneal synechias.

M. Epithelialization or endothelialization (Fig. 16–16) of anterior chamber angle —see pp. 132, 148 in Chapter 5.

N. Neovascularization of anterior surface of iris (Rubeosis iridis) (Fig. 16–17) The many causes include diabetes mellitus, central retinal vein or artery occlusion, branch retinal artery occlusion, diffuse retinal vascular disease, carotid artery ischemia, retinoblastoma, malignant melanoma of uvea (see Table 16–1), long-standing retinal detachment, any chronic retinal disease, penetrating or contusive ocular injuries (see p. 145 in Chap. 5) and Fuchs's heterochromic iridocyclitis (see p. 67 in Chap. 3).

O. Juvenile xanthogranuloma (see pp. 338–339 in Chap. 9).

P. Secondary to uveal malignant melanoma (see Table 16–1) (Fig. 16–18)
   1. Posterior synechias and iris bombé.
      a. A large posterior malignant melanoma and a total retinal detachment combine to displace the iris-lens diaphragm anteriorly, resulting in posterior synechias and iris bombé followed by secondary peripheral anterior synechias.
      b. Similar changes may occur with a large posterior metastatic neoplasm.
   2. Rubeosis iridis.
      a. When rubeosis iridis is associated with a malignant melanoma, the tumor generally is large and posterior.
      b. The rubeosis iridis causes peripheral anterior synechias.
      c. Similar changes may occur with a large posterior metastatic neoplasm.
   3. Diffuse iris malignant melanoma.
      a. A diffuse iris malignant melanoma, or even a diffuse iris

TABLE 16–1.
Histopathologic Mechanisms Producing Secondary Glaucoma in Eyes Containing Uveal Malignant Melanomas*

Mechanism	Underlying cause
Peripheral anterior synechias and angle closure	1. Posterior synechias, iris bombé and peripheral anterior synechias 2. Rubeosis iridis and peripheral anterior synechias 3. Diffuse iris nevus or melanoma and peripheral anterior synechias
Cellular obstruction of aqueous drainage area of an open angle	1. Seeding of neoplasm into anterior chamber angle 2. Ring melanoma with invasion of anterior chamber angle structures 3. Melanin phagocytosis by macrophages with obstruction of anterior chamber angle (melanomalytic glaucoma)

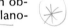

* Modified from Yanoff, 1970.

nevus, may induce peripheral
anterior synechias.
b. The condition may simulate essential iris atrophy or Chandler's
syndrome.

II. Open Angle
A. Secondary to cells or debris in angle
1. Hyphema (see p. 145 in Chap. 5).
2. Uveitis (see p. 74 in Chap. 3).
a. A cyclitis (or iridocyclitis) may
lead to excessive cellular production that clogs up and mechanically obstructs the open angle.

With an anterior uveitis aqueous
inflow is generally decreased so that
glaucoma rarely ensues. Also glaucoma is less likely if the cyclitis is
segmental rather than circumferential and is most unlikely with
a posterior cyclitis or pars planitis.

b. Glaucomatocyclitic crisis (Posner-Schlossman syndrome)
1) The condition mainly occurs
as an unilateral acute rise in
intraocular pressure in people
in their third through fifth
decades; it may be recurrent.
2) Epithelial edema and one or
more keratic precipitates
(tiny and fine at first, but
they may become mutton fat)
are seen clinically.
3) There is little or no reaction
in the aqueous humor and the
angle generally appears normal to gonioscopy.
4) The disease is self-limited and
subsides in from 1 to 3 weeks
without treatment.
5) The cause and histology are
unknown.

Recent evidence suggests
strongly that there is a predilection for glaucomatocyclitic
crises to occur in patients with,
or who will develop, primary
open angle glaucoma.

3. Phacolytic glaucoma (see pp. 378–
380 in Chap. 10).
4. Nondenatured lens material-in-

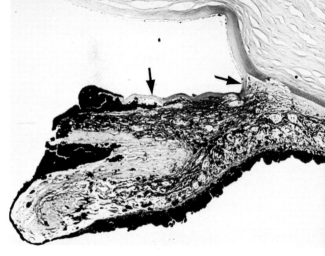

FIG. 16–16. Endothelialization of pseudo-
anterior chamber angle has occurred
following blunt trauma to eye. Anterior
surface of iris is covered by corneal endothelium, which has produced new Descemet's membrane (*arrows*). PAS, ×54.

FIG. 16–17. Rubeosis iridis. **A.** Marked
fibrovascular proliferation has occurred on
anterior iris surface following central retinal
vein occlusion. **Inset** shows clinical appearance of advanced rubeosis iridis in another
case. **B.** Shrinkage of fibrovascular membrane
results in eversion of pupillary iris (pigment
seam and sphincter muscle), i.e., ectropion
uveae. **A,** H&E, ×40; **inset,** clinical; **B,** H&E,
×16.

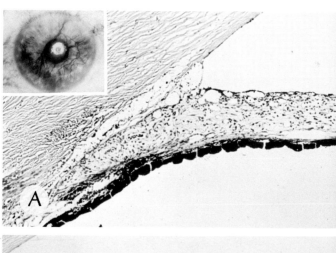

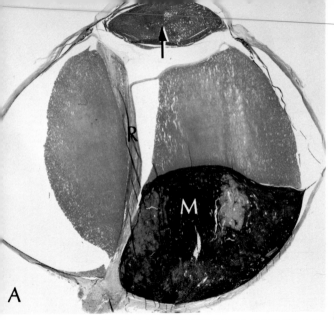

A

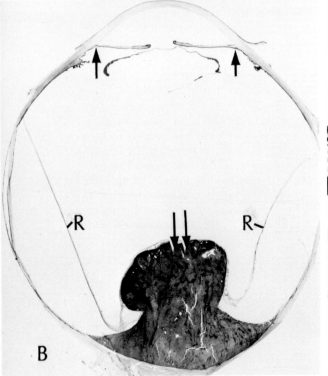

B

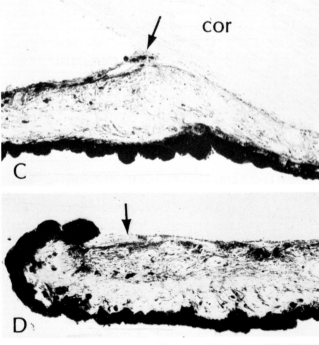

C

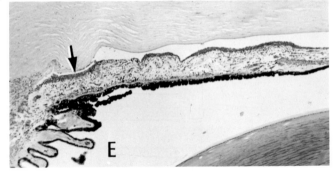

D

E

FIG. 16–18. Closed angle glaucoma secondary to uveal melanomas. **A.** Large melanoma (*M*) and complete retinal detachment (*R*) have displaced lens (*arrow*) anteriorly with resultant posterior and anterior synechias and closed anterior chamber angle. **B, C,** and **D** show large melanoma (*double arrow*), total retinal detachment (*R*) and rubeosis iridis (*single arrows*), with peripheral anterior synechia (**C**) and ectropion uveae (**D**). *cor*, cornea. **E.** Diffuse nevus of anterior iris surface has induced peripheral anterior synechia formation (see Figure 17–38). *Arrow* shows artifactitious cleft between nevus and posterior cornea. **A,** H&E, ×3; **B,** H&E, ×3; **C,** H&E, ×100; **D,** H&E, ×100; **E,** H&E, ×32.

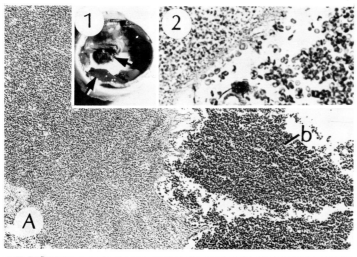

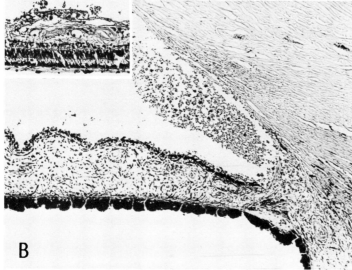

FIG. 16–19. Hemolytic glaucoma. **A.** Fresh blood in subvitreal area (*b*, and *arrows* in **inset 1**) and old blood within vitreous. **Inset 2** shows difference in size between whole erythrocytes in subvitreal area (toward right lower) and fragmented erythrocytes in vitreous (toward left upper). **B.** Fragmented erythrocytes lie both freely and within macrophages in anterior chamber angle. Unless preceded by microincineration, material does not stain positively with Prussian blue reaction for iron. **Inset** shows retinal neovascularization, which was responsible for vitreous hemorrhage. **A,** H&E, ×40; **inset 1,** macroscopic; **inset 2,** H&E, ×176; **B,** H&E, ×40; **inset,** H&E, ×54.

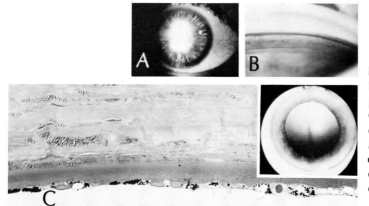

Pigmentary glaucoma

FIG. 16–20. Pigment dispersion syndrome. **A.** Extensive increased iris transillumination present mainly in middle third of iris. **B.** Gonioscopic view to show marked deposition of pigment in anterior chamber angle. **C.** Melanin pigment granules present in corneal endothelial cytoplasm responsible for clinically seen Krukenberg spindle (**inset**). **A,** clinical; **B,** gonioscopy; **C,** 1.5 μ section, PD, ×300; **inset,** clinical.

duced glaucoma generally follows a very recent traumatic rupture of the lens.

   a. Following a needling of a soft cataract the glaucoma, if it develops at all, is seen generally within the first week of needling.

   b. Following penetrating ocular injury (see p. 148 in Chap. 5).

   c. The glaucoma is due to physical occlusion of the open anterior chamber angle by the swollen lens material and is *not* related to phagocytic action.

The ruptured lens may not release its material but may swell resulting in pupillary block and a secondary acute or chronic angle closure glaucoma.

5. Hemolytic glaucoma (Fig. 16–19)

   a. Clinically hemolytic glaucoma presents as an acute open angle glaucoma.

   b. The glaucoma results as a complication of long-standing vitreous hemorrhage due to any cause.

   c. Histologically the anterior chamber angle is obstructed by debris, hemoglobin and macrophages filled mainly with hemoglobin but also containing some hemosiderin.

6. Pigment dispersion syndrome (Pigmentary "glaucoma") (Figs. 16–20 and 16–21)

   a. The pigment dispersion syndrome is found mainly in young adult male myopes.

   b. Depigmentation of the iris epithelium, especially peripherally, results in the clinically observed circumferential foci of increased iris transillumination mainly where the peripheral third of the iris meets the middle third.

A band of increased granular iris pigmentation can be seen directly biomicroscopically overlying the ring of increased retroillumination (best seen in blue irises but also seen fairly easily in brown). The band presumably is due to the

FIG. 16–21. Pigment dispersion syndrome. **A.** ▶ **Inset 1** shows row of depigmented patches on posterior surface of iris, which correspond to translucent patches seen clinically and macroscopically (**inset 2**), to areas of atrophy and distortion (*arrows*) of pigment epithelium seen in scanning electron micrograph and to regions of dilator muscle hyperplasia seen in **inset 3** by thin section light microscopy. *Arrow* in **inset 1** points to heavily pigmented trabecular band in angle. *Arrows* in **inset 3** indicate pigment-filled macrophages. **B. Inset** is transmission electron micrograph (TEM) showing region of atrophy of posterior layer of iris pigment epithelium. Some poorly developed dilator muscle (*MY*) is present in stroma above. *Arrow* shows basement membrane surrounding smooth muscle cell. **Main figure** shows many layers of hyperplastic dilator muscle with complete leiomyomatous differentiation of neuroepithelial cells. Note basement membrane surrounding smooth muscle cells (*arrows*) and presence of typical stromal melanocyte (*ST*) near one of smooth muscle cells (*MY*). **C.** TEM is sample of juxtacanalicular connective tissue and inner endothelial lining of Schlemm's canal. There is some increase in patchy aggregates of basement membrane materials (homogeneous, filamentous and banded varieties; see p. 640 in Chap. 17), which appear within normal limits for age. **Inset 1** is macroscopic photograph of angle of opened eye. *Arrows* point to heavily pigmented band of trabecular meshwork, while *double arrows* indicate band of pigment phagocytosed by peripheral corneal endothelium (clinically called Sampaolesi's line). **Inset 2** shows widespread phagocytosis of neuroepithelial pigment granules by cells of trabecular meshwork. *cs,* canal of Schlemm; *ac,* anterior chamber. **Inset 3** shows edge of iris lesion (*arrow*) and all tissues of nearby drainage angle. Note pigment-filled macrophages in peripheral iris stroma, prominence of muscle spur of Grunert and pigmentation of trabecular meshwork. *cs,* canal of Schlemm. **A,** SEM, ×100; **inset 1,** macroscopic; **inset 2,** macroscopic transilluminated; **inset 3,** 1.5 μ section, PD, ×120; **B,** ×16,000; **inset,** ×16,000; **C,** ×22,000; **inset 1,** macroscopic; **inset 2,** 1.5 μ section, PD, ×485; **inset 3,** 1.5 μ section, PD, ×70.

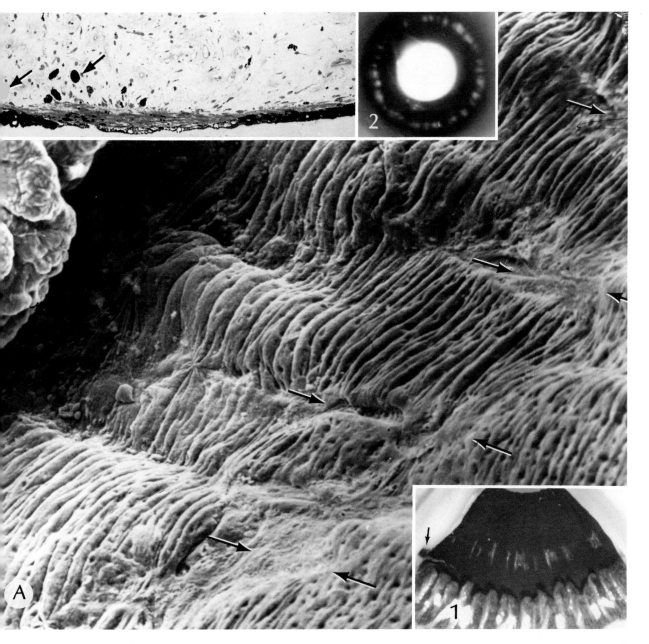

(continued)

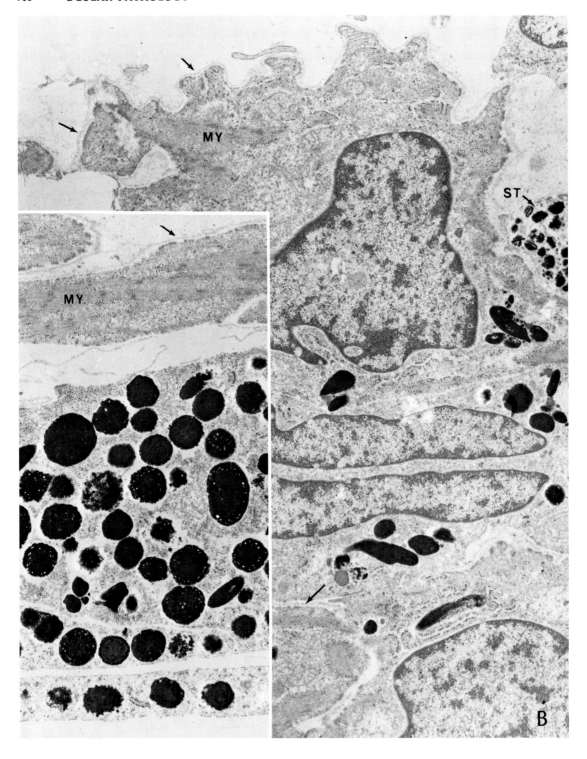

(continued)

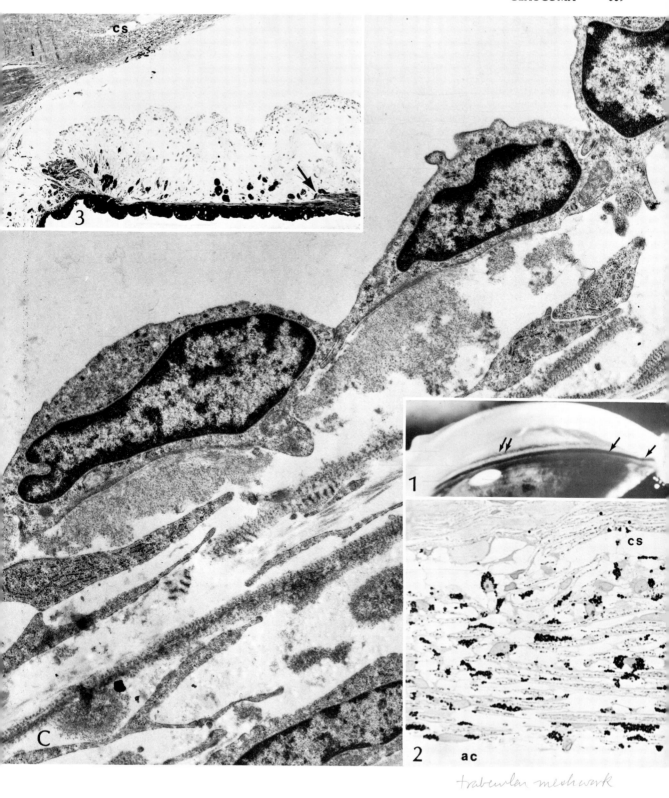

trabecular meshwork

many pigment-filled macrophages in this region of stroma.

c. Iridodonesis may be present.
d. *Krukenberg's spindle* consists of melanin pigment phagocytosed by the central and inferior corneal endothelium in a vertical band.
e. The pigment is deposited on the iris surface, lens and zonules.
f. Marked pigmentation of the trabecular meshwork occurs.
g. The cause is uncertain but the pigmentary changes may be coincidental to, rather than the cause of, the glaucoma.

Glaucoma seems to be present in fewer than 50 percent of cases. Perhaps the relationship of the iris pigment epithelial defect and the glaucoma is a matter of two independent gene loci that are very close together on the same chromosome and tend to be inherited together, but not necessarily so.

h. Histologically the posterior layer of iris pigment epithelium atrophies in foci corresponding to the clinically observed peripheral foci of increased iris transillumination, mainly at the junction of middle and peripheral thirds of the iris.
   1) The dilator muscle is dysplastic in the area and is present in excessive amounts, atrophic or absent. The adjacent iris stroma contains considerable numbers of pigment-filled macrophages.
   2) Melanin granules of neuroepithelial type are widely distributed within the endothelium of the posterior cornea (Krukenberg's spindle) and within the endothelium of the trabecular meshwork.
7. Pseudoexfoliation of lens capsule (see pp. 362–366 in Chap. 10).
8. Secondary to uveal malignant melanomas (see Table 16–1).

a. *Seeded malignant melanoma cells* may mechanically block the anterior chamber angle (Fig. 16–22).
   Similar seeding can occur with metastatic neoplastic cells or juvenile xanthogranuloma cells.
b. *A ring malignant melanoma* may invade directly the anterior chamber angle structures and mechanically block the open angle (Fig. 16–22).

A ring melanoma arises from the root of the iris and anterior ciliary body for 360 degrees. It is not to be confused with a segmental iris or ciliary body melanoma that may seed the anterior chamber angle 360 degrees.

c. *Melanomalytic glaucoma* (Fig. 16–23)
   1) Necrosis (partial or complete) of a ciliary body and iris root malignant melanoma causes the liberation of melanin pigment.
   2) The liberated melanin then induces phagocytosis by macrophages.
   3) The melanin-laden macrophages are carried to the anterior chamber where they cause an obstruction of the open chamber angle.
d. *Epithelialization or endothelialization* of anterior chamber angle (see pp. 132, 148 in Chap. 5).
B. Secondary to damaged outflow channels.
   1. Old uveitis may result in "scarring" of the tissues within the drainage angle (see p. 67 in Chap. 3).
   2. Repeated attacks of acute angle closure glaucoma may cause damage to the trabecular meshwork so that the angle appears open, but the facility of outflow is decreased.
   3. Repeated hyphema may damage the aqueous outflow tissue.
   4. Siderosis or hemosiderosis bulbi. Iron has a "toxic" effect on tissues within the drainage angle and induces "scarring."

FIG. 16–22. Open angle glaucoma secondary to uveal melanomas. **A** and **B** show seeding of iris melanoma onto anterior surface of iris (*arrows*). Melanoma cells also cover angle recess and trabecular meshwork (*double arrow* in **B**). **C.** Ring melanoma involves root of iris and anterior ciliary body 360 degrees with invasion of anterior chamber angle structures. **A,** H&E, ×7; **B,** H&E, ×100; **C,** H&E, ×7.

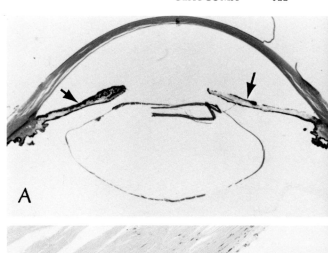

A

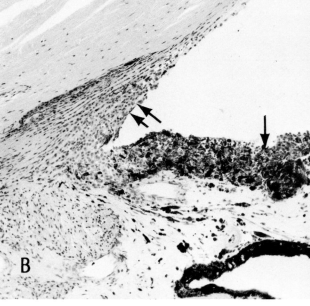

B

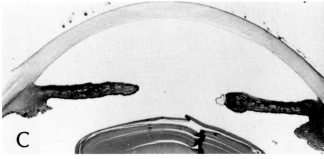

C

5. Trauma
   a. The trauma may have a *direct effect* on the tissues of the drainage angle, inducing scarring (sclerosis) of the trabecular meshwork.
   b. It may cause a *postcontusion deformity* of the anterior chamber angle (see pp. 145–148 in Chap. 5).
6. Cornea guttata (see pp. 308–309 in Chap. 8).
7. Early rubeosis. Before peripheral anterior synechias form, an open anterior chamber angle may be obstructed by an almost transparent, delicate fibrovascular membrane arising from the iris root or anterior face of the ciliary body.

C. Secondary to corneoscleral and extraocular diseases such as interstitial keratitis, orbital venous thrombosis, cavernous sinus thrombosis, carotid cavernous fistula, encircling band following retinal detachment surgery, retrobulbar mass, leukemia and mediastinal syndromes.

D. Unknown mechanisms (generally reversible).
   1. Steroid-induced glaucoma.
   2. α-Chymotrypsin-induced glaucoma.

E. Combinations of the above listed four possibilities.

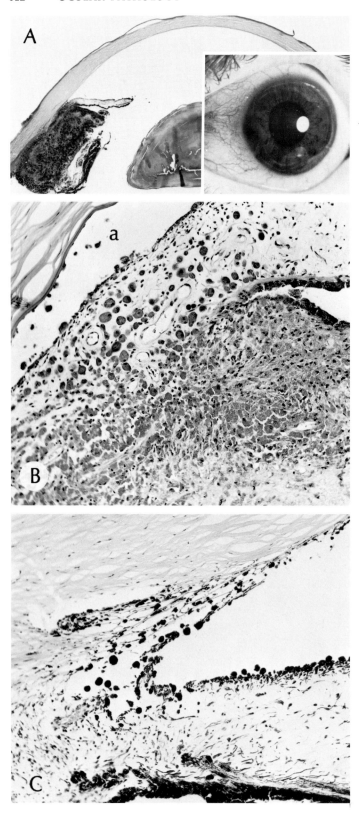

FIG. 16–23. Melanomalytic glaucoma. **A.** Ciliary body melanoma is completely necrotic. **Inset** shows clinical appearance of tumor protruding into anterior chamber angle from 8 to 9 o'clock. **B.** Bleached section shows necrosis of tumor and many pigment-laden macrophages in tumor, iris root and anterior chamber (a). **C.** Anterior chamber angle away from tumor is open but occluded by pigment-laden macrophages. Bleached sections showed cells to be macrophages. **A,** H&E, ×7; **inset,** clinical; **B,** bleached, H&E, ×100; **C,** H&E, ×100.

TISSUE CHANGES CAUSED BY ELEVATED INTRAOCULAR PRESSURE

CORNEAL (Figs. 16–24 and 16–25)

I. Edema of stroma and epithelium.
II. Epithelial bullae.
III. Degenerative subepithelial pannus.

The corneal edema is best seen in its earliest stage in the basal layer of the epithelium. With increased edema the basal layer of cells swell (clinically observed as corneal bedewing), causing a form of microcystoid degeneration. The edema then spreads to overlying (anterior) epithelial cells. Further accentuation of the edema ruptures the cell membranes resulting in macrocysts. At the same time the epithelium is lifted off the underlying Bowman's membrane by intercellular collections of fluid. The overlying epithelium then shows an irregular appearance with areas of atrophy and hypertrophy. With chronic edema fibrous or fibrovascular tissue grows between epithelium and Bowman's membrane forming a pannus. Ultimately the vascular component regresses completely, any inflammatory cells, if having been there, disappear and a relatively acellular scar (a *degenerative pannus*) remains between epithelium and Bowman's membrane.

IV. Atrophy of epithelium and endothelium.

ANTERIOR CHAMBER ANGLE

"Scarring" (sclerosis) of the tissues of the drainage angle.

IRIS

I. Dispersion of pigment onto and from the iris.

Melanin pigment liberated from pigment epithelium or uveal melanocytes generally does not exist "free" on surfaces but is present within cells, e.g., within macrophages in iris or within endothelium on posterior cornea or trabecular meshwork.

II. Fibrosis of stroma.
III. Atrophy or necrosis of stroma dilator muscle and pigment epithelium.
IV. Ectropion uveae (usually secondary to rubeosis iridis*).

CILIARY BODY

I. Fibrosis and hyalinization of the core of fibrovascular tissue in the ciliary processes of the pars plicata.
II. Atrophy of pars plicata.

LENS

Cataract, especially after surgery or after an acute attack of glaucoma, e.g., glaukomflecken with acute closed angle glaucoma.

SCLERA

Ectasia (thinning), or if lined by uvea, staphyloma (Fig. 16–26).

RETINA (Fig. 16–27)

I. Degeneration of inner layers, predominantly nerve fiber and ganglion cell layers.
II. Gliosis, especially with secondary glaucoma.

OPTIC NERVE

I. Atrophy
II. Cupping (Figs. 12–10 and 16–28).
III. Cavernous (*Schnabel's*) optic atrophy consists of cystoid spaces generally posterior to scleral lamina cribrosa. They often are filled with hyaluronic acid (see p. 502 in Chap. 13).

---

* Rubeosis iridis is rare, if it occurs at all, in cases of primary open angle glaucoma that have not had intraocular surgery or retinal vascular occlusion. It may occur rarely in cases of primary closed angle glaucoma, even without intraocular surgery, but with central retinal vein thrombosis.

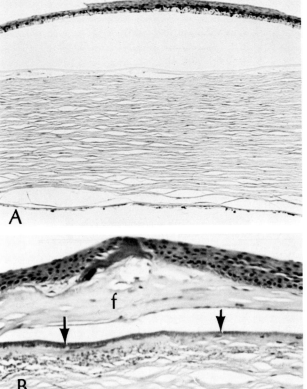

A

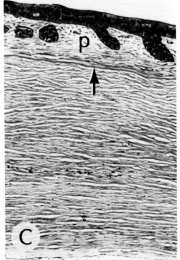

C

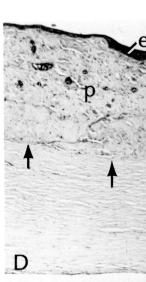

D

FIG. 16–24. Development of degenerative subepithelial pannus. **A.** Longstanding corneal edema leads to bullous keratopathy. Note large bulla and edema of basal epithelium. **B.** Fibrovascular tissue (*f*) grows between epithelium and Bowman's membrane, which here is calcified (*arrows*). **C.** Epithelium has become hyperplastic over degenerative pannus (*p*). Arrow indicates Bowman's membrane. **D.** Ultimately, thick fibrovascular tissue, mostly fibrous, is present as pannus (*p*) between epithelium (*e*) and Bowman's membrane (*arrows*). **A,** H&E, ×54; **B,** H&E, ×101; **C,** trichrome, ×40; **D,** H&E, ×28.

B

FIG. 16–25. Appearance of cornea following diathermy to control painful symptoms of bullous keratopathy. Pannus is present between Bowman's membrane and epithelium. Note scars around diathermy sites. Scars (**inset**) perforate Bowman's membrane. **Main figure,** H&E, ×16; **inset,** H&E, ×40.

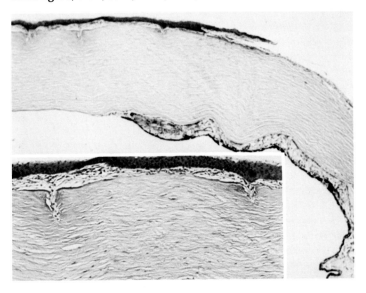

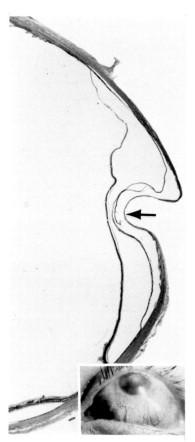

FIG. 16–26. Ectatic (thinned) sclera is redundant (*arrow*) in equatorial area and is lined by underlying choroid, i.e., equatorial staphyloma. **Inset** shows clinical appearance of equatorial staphyloma. **Main figure,** H&E, ×6; **inset,** clinical.

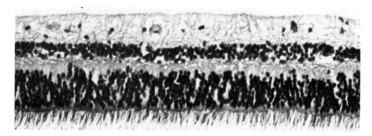

FIG. 16–27. Retina shows atrophy of inner layers, but unlike retina following central retinal artery occlusion, inner layers of retina still are identifiable. H&E, ×100.

FIG. 16–28. Deep excavation of optic nerve-head is present. Optic nerve (*on*) is atrophic and gliotic. **Inset** shows clinical appearance of deep optic cup with shift of blood vessels nasally. **Main figure,** H&E, ×16; **inset,** fundus of left eye.

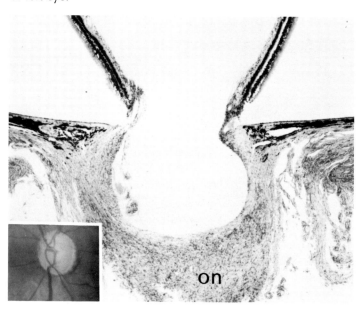

BIBLIOGRAPHY

NORMAL OUTFLOW: HYPERSECRETION

Becker B, Keaky GR, Christensen RE: Hypersecretion glaucoma. Arch Ophthalmol 56:180, 1956

IMPAIRED OUTFLOW: CONGENITAL GLAUCOMA

Anderson DR: Pathology of the glaucomas. Br J Ophthalmol 56:146, 1972

Anderson JR: Hydrophthalmia or Congenital Glaucoma: Its Causes, Treatment and Cure. London, Cambridge Univ Press, 1939

Barkan O: Pathogenesis of congenital glaucoma: gonioscopic and anatomic observations of the anterior chamber in the normal eye and in congenital glaucoma. Am J Ophthalmol 40:1, 1955

Barkan O: Goniotomy for glaucoma associated with nevus flammeus. Am J Ophthalmol 43:545, 1957

Chandler PA, Grant WM: Lectures on Glaucoma. Philadelphia, Lea & Febriger, 1965, pp 296–380

Fine BS, Yanoff M: Ocular Histology: A Text and Atlas. New York, Harper & Row, 1972, pp 214–231

Grant WM, Walton DS: Distinctive gonioscopic findings in glaucoma due to neurofibromatosis. Arch Ophthalmol 79:127, 1968

Kolker AE, Hetherington J Jr: Becker-Shaffer's Diagnosis and Therapy of the Glaucomas. St. Louis, Mosby, 1970, pp. 258–296

Maumenee AE: Further observations on the pathogenesis of congenital glaucoma. Am J Ophthalmol 55:1163, 1963

Merin S, Morin D: Heredity of congenital glaucoma. Br J Ophthalmol 56:414, 1972

Scheie HG: Symposium: congenital glaucoma: diagnosis, clinical course, and treatment other than goniotomy. Trans Am Acad Ophthalmol Otolaryngol 59:309, 1955

Smith JL, Stowe FR: The Pierre Robin syndrome (glossoptosis, micrognathia, cleft palate). A review of 39 cases with emphasis on associated ocular lesions. Pediatrics 27:128, 1961

IMPAIRED OUTFLOW: PRIMARY CLOSED ANGLE

Brini A, Flament J: Cataracta glaucomatosa acuta. Exp Eye Res 16:19, 1973

Chandler PA: Narrow-angle glaucoma. Arch Ophthalmol 47:695, 1952

Christensen L, Irvine AR: Pathogenesis of primary shallow chamber angle closure glaucoma. Arch Ophthalmol 75:490, 1966

Fine BS, Yanoff M: Ocular Histology: A Text and Atlas. New York, Harper & Row, 1972, pp 214–231

Kerman BM, Christensen RE, Foos RY: Angle-closure glaucoma: a clinicopathologic correlation. Am J Ophthalmol 76:887, 1973

Smith ME: Rubeosis iridis and primary angle-closure glaucoma. Int Ophthalmol Clin 11:161, 1971

IMPAIRED OUTFLOW: PRIMARY OPEN ANGLE

Becker B: The genetic problem of chronic simple glaucoma. Ann Ophthalmol 3:351, 1971

Fine BS: Observations on the drainage angle in man and rhesus monkey: a concept of the pathogenesis of chronic simple glaucoma. A light and electron microscopic study. Invest Ophthalmol 3:609, 1964

Fine BS, Yanoff M: Ocular Histology: A Text and Atlas. New York, Harper & Row, 1972, pp 214–231

Fink AI, Felix MD: Schlemm's canal and adjacent structures in glaucomatous patients. Am J Ophthalmol 74:893, 1972

IMPAIRED OUTFLOW: SECONDARY CLOSED ANGLE

Albers EC, Klein BA: Iridoschisis. A clinical and histopathologic study. Am J Ophthalmol 46:794, 1958

Cappin JM: Malignant melanoma and rubeosis iridis. Histopathological and statistical study. Br J Ophthalmol 57:815, 1973

Chandler PA: Atrophy of the stroma of the iris: endothelial dystrophy, corneal edema and glaucoma. Am J Ophthalmol 41:607, 1956

Chandler PA: Choice of treatment in dislocation of lens. Arch Ophthalmol 71:765, 1964

Drysler RM: Central retinal vein occlusion and chronic simple glaucoma. Arch Ophthalmol 73:659, 1965

Garrison LM, Christensen RE, Allen RA: Angle-closure glaucoma from metastatic carcinoma. Am J Ophthalmol 63:503, 1967

Heath P: Essential atrophy of the iris: a histopathologic study. Trans Am Ophthalmol Soc 51:167, 1953

Marchesani O von: Brachydaktylie und angelorene Kugellinse ala Systemerkrankung. Klin Monatsbl Augenheilkd 103:392, 1939

Perraut LE, Zimmerman LE: The occurrence of glaucoma following occlusion of the central retinal artery. Arch Ophthalmol 61:845, 1959

Scheie HG, Yanoff M: Iris nevus (Cogan-Reese) syndrome. Arch Ophthalmol. In press

Yanoff M: Glaucoma mechanisms in ocular malignant melanomas. Am J Ophthalmol 70:898, 1970

Yanoff M: Mechanisms of glaucoma in eyes with uveal malignant melanomas. Int Ophthalmol Clin 12:51, 1972

IMPAIRED OUTFLOW: SECONDARY OPEN ANGLE

Aasved H: Intraocular pressure in eyes with and without fibrillopathia epitheliocapsularis. Acta Ophthalmol (Kbh) 49:601, 1971

Aasved H: The frequency of optic nerve damage and surgical treatment in chronic simple glaucoma and capsular glaucoma. Acta Ophthalmol (Kbh) 49:589, 1971

Bernardino VB, Kim JC, Smith TR: Epithelialization of the anterior chamber after cataract extraction. Arch Ophthalmol 82:742, 1969

Fine BS, Yanoff M, Scheie HG: Pigmentary "glaucoma." A histologic study. Trans Am Acad Ophthalmol Otolaryngol. 78:314, 1974

Hunter WS: Hemolytic glaucoma. Trans Am Acad Ophthalmol Otolaryngol 73:95, 1969

Kass MA, Becker B, Kolker AE: Glaucomatocyclitic crisis and primary open-angle glaucoma. Am J Ophthalmol 75:668, 1973

Kirsch RE: Glaucoma following cataract extraction associated with use of alpha-chymotrypsin. Arch Ophthalmol 72:612, 1964

Layden WE, Shaffer RN: Exfoliation syndrome. Am J Ophthalmol 78:835, 1974

Lichter PR, Schaffer RM: Interstitial keratitis and glaucoma. Am J Ophthalmol 68:241, 1969

Madsen PH: Carotid-cavernous fistulae. A study of 18 cases. Acta Ophthalmol (Kbh) 48:731, 1970

Rich WJ, Radtke ND, Cohan BE: Early ocular hypertension after cataract extraction. Br J Ophthalmol 58:725, 1974

Sugar HS: Pigmentary glaucoma. A 25 year review. Am J Ophthalmol 67:499, 1966

Yanoff M: Glaucoma mechanisms in ocular malignant melanomas. Am J Ophthalmol 70:898, 1970

Yanoff M: Mechanisms of glaucoma in eyes with uveal malignant melanomas. Int Ophthalmol Clin 12:51, 1972

Yanoff M, Scheie HG: Cytology of human lens aspirate and its relationship to phacolytic glaucoma and phacoanaphylactic endophthalmitis. Arch Ophthalmol 80:166, 1968

Yanoff M, Scheie HG: Melanomalytic glaucoma: report of patient. Arch Ophthalmol 84:471, 1970

TISSUE CHANGES CAUSED BY ELEVATED INTRAOCULAR PRESSURE

Albert DM, Gaasterland DE, Caldwell JBH, Howard RO, Zimmerman LE: Bilateral metastatic choroidal melanoma, nevi, and cavernous degeneration. Involvement of the optic nervehead. Arch Ophthalmol 87:39, 1972

Emery JM, Landis D, Paton D, Boniuk M, Craig JM: The lamina cribrosa in normal and glaucomatous human eyes. Trans Am Acad Ophthalmol Otolaryngol 78:290, 1974

Hayreh SS: Optic disc changes in glaucoma. Br J Ophthalmol 56:175, 1972

Lampert PW, Vogel MH, Zimmerman LE: Pathology of the optic nerve in experimental acute glaucoma. Electron microscopic studies. Invest Ophthalmol 7:199, 1968

Schnabel J: Die Entwicklungsgeschichte der glaukomatosen Exkavation. Z Augenheilkd 14:1, 1905

chapter 17

Ocular Melanotic Tumors

OCULAR MELANOCYTES

I. Most authorities agree that dermal, conjunctival and uveal melanocytes are derived from the neural crest. Some authorities, however, dispute this origin. The pigment epithelial melanocytes are derived from neuroepithelium or the layers of the optic cup.

The origin of the pigment epithelium (PE) is not disputed. It is derived from the layers of the optic cup. Unlike the pigment of uveal melanocytes, which is not detectable until late in embryonic life or even until neonatal life, the PE pigment granules can be detected about the fifth week of embryonic life.

II. In histologic sections stained with H&E dermal melanocytes, similar to conjunctival melanocytes, are noted to be solitary dendritic cells with clear cytoplasm (Fig. 17–1).
  A. Silver stains or the dopa reaction demonstrates the cytoplasm.
  B. Uveal melanocytes also are solitary and dendritic, but their cytoplasm contains fine, dustlike, ovoid melanin granules of a size bordering the limits of resolution of the light microscope.
  C. PE cells are neither solitary nor dendritic, but are epithelial and exist as a sheet of cuboidal cells containing large, easily visualized pigment granules.

  The cytoplasm of PE cells contains two basic types of pigment granules: melanin granules, which are large and either ovoid or spherical, and fuscin granules, which generally are spherical. The melanin granules are large and easily seen with light microscopy. Although the fuscin granules also are large, they are relatively nonpigmented and not easily seen with light microscopy.

III. Dermal, conjunctival and uveal melanocytes tend to vary in size, number and melanin content (or ability to make melanin) with racial variation. The normal PE tends to vary little if any in different races and always appears maximally pigmented.

IV. Dermal, conjunctival and uveal melanocytes almost never undergo reactive proliferation under normal circumstances. Neoplastic proliferation, however, does occur.

V. The PE readily undergoes reactive (nonneoplastic) proliferation but rarely becomes neoplastic.

MELANOTIC TUMORS OF EYELIDS

EPHELIS OR FRECKLE — Epidermal

I. An ephelis or freckle is a brown, circumscribed macule normally found only on areas of skin exposed to sunlight.

II. The color is due to increased pigmentation in the basal cell layer of the epidermis. The pigment (melanin) is derived from hyperactive melanocytes that "secrete" their pigment into epidermal basal cells.

III. Melanocytes are *fewer* in number but larger and more functionally active than melanocytes in adjacent, surrounding, paler epidermis.

LENTIGO

I. Lentigo is similar clinically to an ephelis or freckle but is somewhat larger and also may be found on nonexposed skin, usually in older people.

II. In addition to hyperpigmentation of the basal cell layer of epithelium, *increased* numbers of melanocytes are present.

Lentigo maligna (melanotic freckle of Hutchinson) occurs as an acquired pigmented lesion, mostly in adults over 50 years of age. It appears as a brown or black flat lesion primarily on the face, sometimes with involvement of the eyelids and conjunctiva (see Acquired Melanosis in section Melanotic Tumors of Conjunctiva below), enlarging slowly in an irregular manner. About one-third of all lentigo maligna eventuates in malignant melanoma with malignant transformation noted clinically by a thickening or infiltration that becomes elevated into a papule or nodule. Histologically lentigo maligna is indistinguishable from a junctional nevus. An underlying chronic nongranulomatous inflammatory infiltrate is common.

NEVUS*

I. General information
   A. A nevus is a congenital flat or elevated, usually well-circumscribed lesion.

   It may be pigmented early in life or it may not become pigmented until puberty or early adulthood.

   B. The nevus, a hamartomatous tumor, is composed of nevus cells, which are atypical but benign appearing dermal melanocytes.
   C. Five types of nevi:
      1. Junctional.
      2. Intradermal.
      3. Compound.

      A juvenile "melanoma" or spindle-cell nevus is a variety of compound nevus.

      4. Blue.
      5. Congenital oculodermal melanocytosis (nevus of Ota).
II. Junctional nevus (Fig. 17–2)
   A. A junctional nevus generally is flat and well circumscribed and has a uniform brown color.
   B. The nevus cells are located at the

"junction" of the epidermis with the dermis.
   C. The nevus has a low potential for malignancy.
III. Intradermal nevus (Fig. 17–3)
   A. Intradermal nevus generally is elevated, frequently is papillomatous and is the most common type of nevus.
   B. Intradermal nevus or *common mole* has a brown to black color when pigmented. Often, however, it is almost flesh colored.
   C. The nevus cells are entirely in the dermis.
      1. There is a tendency for the cells to become "mature," i.e., smaller, thinner or spindle-shaped and darker as they go deeper into the dermis. This orderly progression in structural change from superficial to deep layers is termed the *normal polarity* of the nevus.
      2. No inflammatory cells are present in or around the nevus unless it is inflamed secondarily.
   D. The nevus may be associated with proliferated Schwann elements, i.e., a *neural nevus*.
   E. This type of nevus probably has no malignant potential.
IV. Compound nevus (Fig. 17–4)
   A. A compound nevus combines junctional and dermal components and usually has a brown color.
   B. The dermal component shows a normal polarity (Fig. 17–5), i.e., cells closest to the epidermis are larger, plumper, rounder and paler than the deeper cells.
   C. The *spindle-cell nevus* (juvenile "melanoma") is a special form of compound nevus that occurs predominantly in children, often as a solitary lesion on the face (Fig. 17–6).
      1. Histologically it superficially resembles a malignant melanoma, but biologically it is benign.
      2. It may contain spindle cells, "epithelioid" cells and single-nucleated and multinucleated giant cells with abundant basophilic cytoplasm.
   D. The compound nevus has a low malignant potential. The malignant mela-

---

* A nevus is any congenital lesion comprised of one of the several types of cells found in the skin. A melanocytic nevus is composed of atypical but benign appearing melanocytes (nevus cells). In this chapter (and elsewhere in the book) the term nevus always refers to the melanocytic nevus.

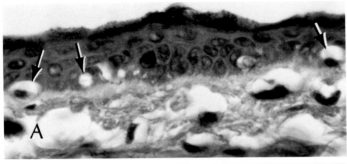

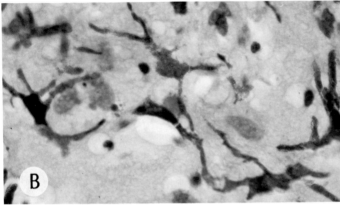

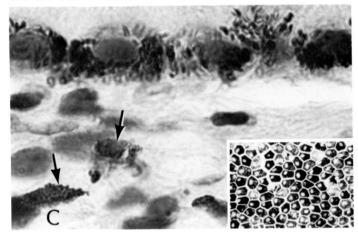

FIG. 17–1. Ocular melanocytes. **A.** Clear cells (*arrows*) in basal epidermal layer represent melanocytes. **B.** Tangential section through choroid shows dendritic configuration of uveal melanocytes. **C.** RPE cells seen in cross-section and in flat preparation (**inset**). Note RPE granules are larger than granules of uveal melanocytes (*arrows*); uveal melanocytes appear spindle-shaped in cross-section. **A,** H&E, ×475; **B,** H&E, ×475; **C,** H&E, ×1,000; **inset,** flat preparation owl monkey RPE, unstained, ×252.

FIG. 17–2. Junctional nevus. Nests of nevus cells (*arrow*) are present at junction of epidermis and dermis. H&E, ×176.

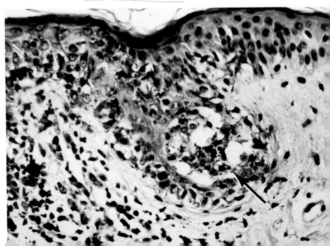

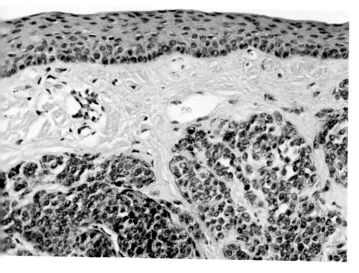

FIG. 17–3. Intradermal nevus. Nests of nevus cells limited to dermis. H&E, ×200.

FIG. 17–4. Compound nevus. **A.** Nevus cells are present at junction of epidermis and dermis and in dermis. **B.** Nevus cells present in junctional and dermal locations. **Inset** from area of *arrow* shows nevus cells in both locations. **A,** H&E, ×101; **B,** H&E, ×40; **inset,** H&E, ×101.

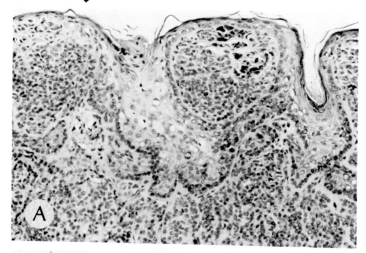

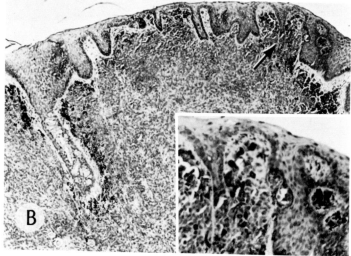

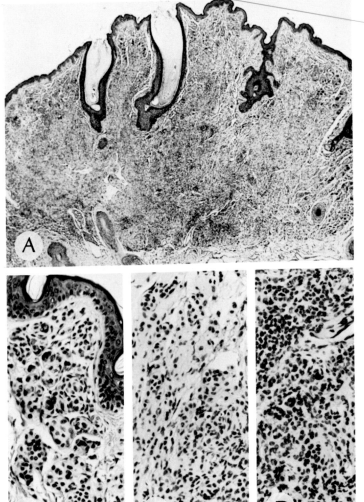

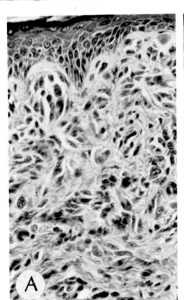

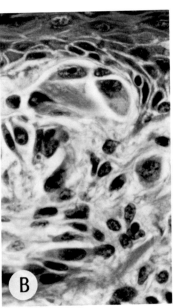

FIG. 17–5. Polarity of nevus. **A.** Papillary nevus. **B.** Plump cells at surface of nevus are larger than cells in middle region (**C**), which are larger than spindle-shaped cells (**D**) toward bottom of lesion. **A,** H&E, ×16; **B,** H&E, ×101; **C,** H&E, ×101; **D,** H&E, ×101.

FIG. 17–6. Spindle-cell nevus (juvenile melanoma). **A.** Spindle-shaped nevus cells predominate. Epithelioid cells and single and multinucleated giant nevus cells are also present. **B.** Higher magnification of another area to show spindle and epithelioid nevus cells. **A,** H&E, ×200; **B,** H&E, ×475.

noma arises from the junctional component.

V. Blue nevus *dermal*,
A. The blue nevus generally is flat and is almost always pigmented from birth; it appears blue to slate gray.
B. Nevus cells are present deep in the dermis in interlacing fasciculi.
  1. The nevus cells in the blue nevus are located deeper than junctional, dermal or compound nevus cells.
  2. The nevus cells are more spindle-shaped, more elongated and contain larger branching processes than other types of nevus cells and more closely resemble uveal nevus cells than do other skin nevus cells.
  3. They may be very cellular, i.e., a *cellular blue nevus* (Fig. 17–7), which has a low malignant potential.
C. Unless the nevus is the cellular type, it has no malignant potential.
VI. Congenital oculodermal melanocytosis (nevus of Ota) (Figs. 17–8 and 17–60)
A. Congenital oculodermal melanocytosis can be considered as a type of blue nevus of the skin around the orbit lids, brow, etc.) associated with an ipsilateral blue nevus of the conjunctiva and a diffuse nevus of the uvea.

The condition is quite common in blacks and orientals but is rare in whites.

B. With diffuse uveal involvement total ipsilateral heterochromia due to a diffuse, maximally pigmented nevus of the uvea is noted, whereas occasionally ipsilateral segmental heterochromia due to segmental ocular involvement is noted.
C. *Congenital dermal melanocytosis* may occur alone or concurrently with orbital melanocytosis, in which case it is called *congenital dermal orbital melanocytosis*, or, as above, it may occur concurrently with ocular melanocytosis, in which case it is called congenital oculodermal melanocytosis.
D. The lesion is potentially malignant only when it occurs in whites.

Malignant melanomas have been reported in the skin, conjunctiva, uvea (most com-

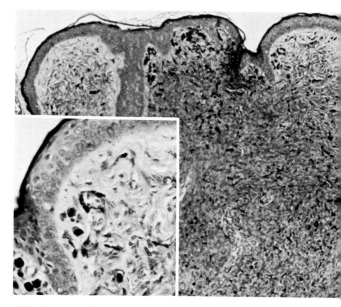

FIG. 17–7. Cellular blue nevus is composed mainly of dendritic-shaped nevus cells, shown with higher magnification in **inset**. **Main figure,** H&E, ×73; **inset,** H&E, ×200.

mon), orbit (rarely) and even in the meninges.

MALIGNANT MELANOMA (Figs. 17–9 and 17–10)

I. Malignant melanoma may arise from a preexisting junctional, compound or, rarely, cellular blue nevus, or it may arise de novo.
II. Skin melanomas are *not* classified according to cell type as are uveal melanomas (see pp. 662–672 in this chapter).*
  A. If the melanoma is limited to the junctional position with invasion of the overlying epithelium, it is classified as a superficial (incipient) malignant melanoma.
  B. If the melanoma invades both epithelium and dermis, it is classified simply as a malignant melanoma.
III. Histology
  A. There is a loss of normal polarity, i.e., the deep cells and superficial cells are indistinguishable.

* On the basis of gross appearance and biologic behavior, melanomas may be divided clinically into superficial spreading melanoma, nodular melanoma and lentigo maligna melanoma.

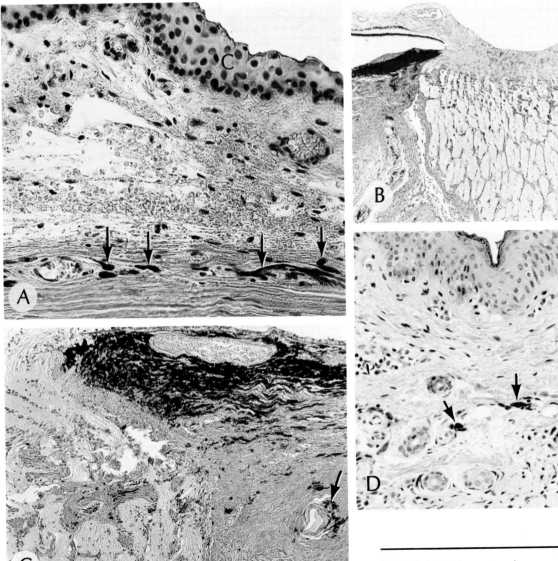

FIG. 17–8. Congenital ocular melanocytosis.
A. Uveal melanocytes (arrows) in episcleral region are responsible for slate blue appearance of conjunctiva. C, conjunctival epithelium. B. Diffuse, maximally pigmented nevus fills choroid. C. Pigmented cells are present in sclera, scleral canal (arrow) and optic nerve septa. D. Dendritic-shaped melanocytes (arrows) are present in dermis of skin in nevus of Ota. A, H&E, ×305; B, H&E, ×18; C, H&E, ×80; D, H&E, ×200.

FIG. 17–9. Malignant melanoma. A. Primary nodular malignant melanoma of skin of back (inset) shows melanoma cells invading epidermis. B. Melanoma has metastasized to skin (inset 2). Metastatic skin melanoma is characterized by clear space between dermal melanoma cells and uninvolved epidermis (shown in lower magnification in inset 1). C and D show fundus appearance (insets) and histology of choroidal metastases to right and left eye, respectively. E. Melanoma cells (emboli) are present in choroidal blood vessels. A, H&E, ×375; inset, clinical; B, H&E, ×750; inset 1, H&E, ×175; inset 2, clinical; C, H&E, ×4; inset, fundus of right eye; D, H&E, ×4; inset, fundus of left eye; E, H&E, ×100.

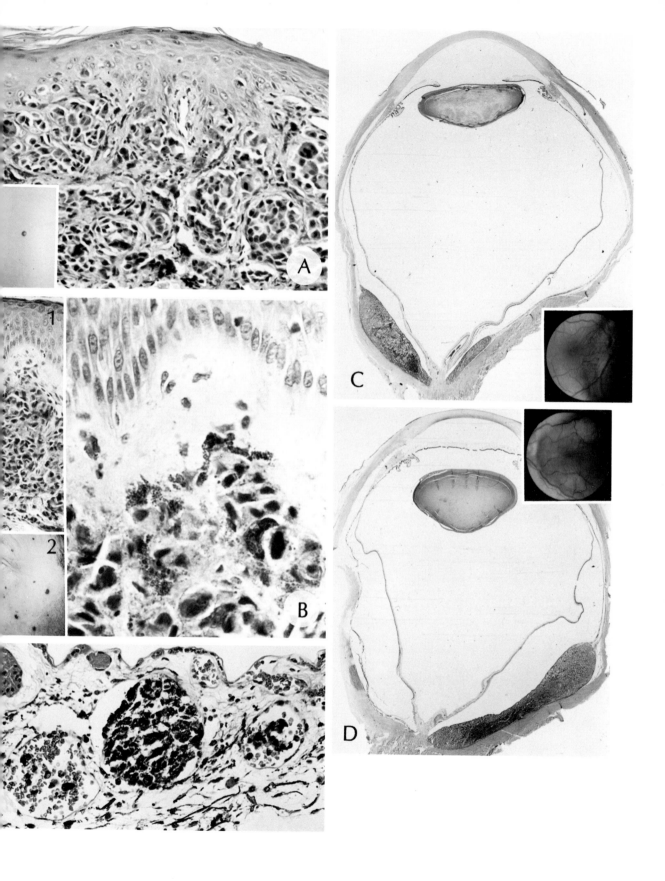

B. There is an invasion of the overlying epithelium.

If this is all that is present, it is called a superficial or incipient malignant melanoma. Pigmentation may or may not be present. If present, it may vary in different parts of the tumor. If not present, the tumor is called an *amelanotic melanoma*.

C. Invasion of the underlying dermis occurs concurrently with or following epithelial invasion.
D. The component cells of the neoplasm are atypical.
  1. There is an increase in the nuclear to cytoplasmic ratio.
  2. Mitotic figures may be present but are frequently absent.
  3. Large, abnormal cells may be present.
E. Frequently the neoplasm has an underlying inflammatory infiltrate of round cells, predominantly lymphocytes.
F. Usually a combination of the above criteria leads to the diagnosis of malignancy rather than any one single criterion.
V. Prognosis
  A. Superficial malignant melanoma, i.e., epithelial invasion but no or only very early dermal invasion has a 75 percent survival rate.
  B. Deep malignant melanoma (majority of melanomas) has a 10 to 39 percent survival rate (variability in survival rates is due to location of tumor and different authors' statistics).

MELANOTIC TUMORS OF CONJUNCTIVA

EPHELIS OR FRECKLE

I. An ephelis or freckle is a brown, patchy, flat lesion with irregular borders.
  A. It may involve the bulbar or palpebral conjunctiva but most frequently involves the bulbar conjunctiva toward the limbus.
  B. The pigmented conjunctiva is movable over the sclera.
  C. The lesion is present at birth.
II. Freckles are common in dark races.

III. The histology consists of an increased pigmentation in the basal cell layer of the conjunctival epithelium with the melanocytes normal or fewer in number.

Histologically the freckle and lentigo are similar, if not identical, to benign acquired melanosis with no junctional activity.

LENTIGO

I. A lentigo is similar to an ephelis or freckle but is somewhat larger in size.
II. Histologically, in addition to the increased pigmentation of the basal cells of the conjunctival epithelium, the melanocytes are increased in number.

NEVUS

I. General information
  A. A nevus is a congenital, flat or elevated, well-circumscribed lesion that may not become pigmented until puberty or early adulthood (especially the junctional, subepithelial and compound types).
  B. The hamartomatous tumor is composed primarily of nevus cells but may also have epithelial elements (see below under compound nevus).
  C. The nevus is the most common conjunctival tumor.
  D. There are five types:
    1. Junctional
    2. Subepithelial (analogous to intradermal nevus of skin).
    3. Compound.

A juvenile "melanoma" or spindle-cell nevus is a variety of compound nevus.

    4. Blue.
    5. Congenital melanocytosis.
      a. Congenital ocular melanocytosis (melanosis oculi).
      b. Congenital oculodermal melanocytosis (nevus of Ota).
II. Junctional nevus (see Table 17–1) (Fig. 17–11)
  A. The junctional nevus is quite similar in appearance to those of the skin.
  B. The nevus moves with the conjunctiva over the sclera.

TABLE 17–1.

Comparison of Conjunctival Nevus, Congenital Ocular Melanocytosis and Primary Acquired Melanosis

	Conjunctival nevus (junctional, subepithelial and compound)	Congenital ocular melanocytosis (melanosis oculi)	Primary acquired melanosis (precancerous and cancerous melanosis)
Onset	Congenital (may not pigment until young adult)	Congenital	Middle age
Structure	Discrete	Diffuse	Diffuse
Color	Brown	Blue or slate gray	Brown
Cysts	May be present (~ 50 percent of time)	None	None
Pigmentation	Variable pigmentation	Always pigmented	Always pigmented
With conjunctival movement	Lesion moves	Lesion does not move	Lesion moves
Growth	Stationary	Stationary	Tends to change
Uvea	Not involved	Heterochromia	Not involved
Skin	Not involved	May be involved (nevus of Ota)	Not involved
Malignant potential	Conjunctival melanoma	Skin or uveal (rarely conjunctival) melanoma	Conjunctival melanoma only

C. The nevus cells appear histologically more "worrisome looking" than those found in skin junctional nevi in that the cells tend to be larger and, unlike in skin, may reach the external surface of the epidermis.

Unlike in the skin the nevus cells are not limited necessarily to the junctional area of the epithelium and subepithelium but may be found within the epithelial layers simulating invasion. Histologically the junctional nevus, when maximally pigmented, is identical to benign acquired melanosis with junctional activity.

D. They have a low malignant potential.

III. Subepithelial nevus (see Table 17–1) (Fig. 17–12)

A. A subepithelial nevus is quite similar to those of the skin and appears flesh colored to brown depending on the degree of pigmentation.

B. The nevus moves with the conjunctiva over the sclera.

C. It is not nearly so common as a junctional or compound nevus.

D. Histologically the cells show normal polarity with smaller, darker, more spindle-shaped cells present in the deeper layers.

E. This type of nevus probably is not potentially malignant.

IV. Compound nevus (see Table 17–1) (Fig. 17–13)

A. A compound nevus is quite similar to those of the skin and appears brown when pigmented.

B. The nevus moves with the conjunctiva over the sclera.

C. Histologically the subepithelial component shows a normal polarity, i.e., the cells closest to the epithelium are plumper, larger, rounder and paler than the deeper cells.

D. The subepithelial hamartomatous component, in addition to the nevus cells, frequently contains epithelial embryonic rests, which may develop into epithelial cysts, i.e., a *cystic nevus* (Fig. 17–14). The epithelial component is present in about 50 percent of conjunctival nevi.

E. Juvenile "melanoma" or spindle-cell nevus

1. The juvenile melanoma is a special form of compound nevus occurring predominantly in children.

2. Histologically it resembles the similar tumor found in the skin.
F. These tumors have a low malignant potential.

At one time these tumors were classified as malignant melanomas. Only in the last few decades has their benign behavior been recognized widely.

V. Blue nevus
   A. The blue nevus is quite similar to those of the skin, appears blue to slate gray in color and is pigmented from birth.
   B. The nevus appears as a diffuse pigmentation that does not move with the conjunctiva over the sclera.
   C. Histologically nevus cells are seen deep in the subepithelial tissue in interlacing fasciculi.
      1. The cells are deeper than the junctional, subepithelial or compound nevus cells.
      2. The nevus cells are more spindle-shaped, elongated and contain larger branching processes than other types of nevus cells.
      3. The nevus may be very cellular, which is called a *cellular blue nevus.*
         a. It appears as a localized blue nodule.
         b. The tumor is potentially malignant but rarely so.
   D. A blue nevus may be difficult to differentiate from other causes of episcleral pigmentation.
   E. Unless it is of the cellular type, it is not potentially malignant.
VI. Congenital melanocytosis (see Table 17–1).
   A. Congenital ocular melanocytosis (melanosis oculi) (Figs. 17–8 and 17–60)
      1. Probably congenital ocular melanocytosis is best considered as a diffuse blue nevus of the conjunctiva.

      It may be a cellular blue nevus but is not always such.

      2. The condition generally is unilateral and mainly present in dark races (blacks and orientals).

3. The lesion has a blue or slate gray color from birth and does not move with the conjunctiva.
4. It is associated with an ipsilateral diffuse uveal nevus that causes heterochromia (the heterochromia at times is subtle, especially in brown-eyed individuals).

Waardenburg's syndrome consists of heterochromia iridis (unilateral or bilateral; segmental or diffuse) usually with a similar (congenital melanocytosis) involvement of the remainder of the uvea; lateral displacement of medial canthi, combined with dystopia of the lacrimal puncta and blepharophimosis; prominent broad root of the nose; growing together of the eyebrows with hypertrichosis of the medial portions; white forelock, a form of partial albinism (early graying of the hair begins soon after puberty); defective pigmentation occurring in any part of the body; and congenital deafness.

5. The involvement may be segmental, i.e., limited to a quadrant (more or less) of the eye.

   When segmental the diffuse uveal nevus generally involves the iris, ciliary body and choroid in the same quadrant (more or less).

6. The condition is potentially malignant when it occurs in whites; a uveal malignant melanoma is the resultant malignancy.

   Rarely the conjunctiva or orbit may be the site of malignancy.

B. Congenital oculodermal melanocytosis (nevus of Ota) (Figs. 17–8 and 17–60)
   1. Congenital oculodermal melanocytosis is a blue nevus of the skin about the orbit (lids, brows, etc.) associated with ipsilateral congenital ocular melanocytosis.
   2. The skin pigmentation generally is prominent but on occasion may be quite subtle.
   3. The condition generally is uni-

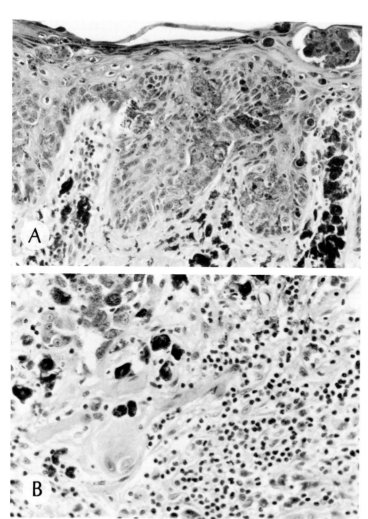

FIG. 17–10. Malignant melanoma. **A.** Melanoma cells are invading epidermis singly and in groups. **B.** Chronic nongranulomatous inflammatory cells underlie melanoma. **A,** H&E, ×200; **B,** H&E, ×275.

FIG. 17–11. Junctional nevus is composed of nest of nevus cells at junction of conjunctival epithelium and subepithelial tissue. H&E, ×340.

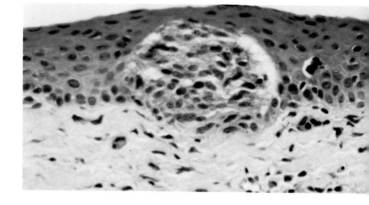

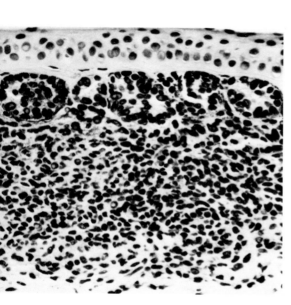

FIG. 17–12. Subepithelial nevus is composed of nests of nevus cells in subepithelial tissue of conjunctiva. H&E, ×176.

(note polarity)

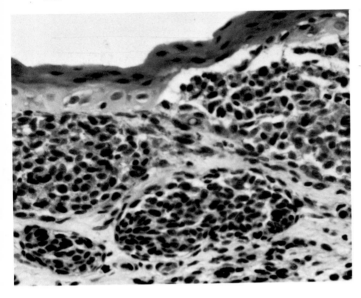

FIG. 17–13. Compound nevus contains nevus cells at junction of conjunctival epithelium and subepithelial tissue and in subepithelial tissue. H&E, ×340.

lateral, occurring mainly in the dark races (blacks and orientals).

4. It is potentially malignant (uveal and skin malignant melanoma; very rarely conjunctival melanoma) when it occurs in whites.

ACQUIRED MELANOSIS

I. Primary acquired melanosis (see Table 17–1)
  A. Clinical characteristics
    1. The melanosis consists of a unilateral, diffuse, brown pigmentation that moves with the conjunctiva over the sclera.

       It is analogous to lentigo maligna of the skin.

    2. The condition has a variable and protracted course.
      a. Rarely it may remain stationary or even recede.
      b. It may remain benign and enlarge slowly over the years.
      c. It may become malignant (about 17 percent), generally 5 to 10 years after onset.
    3. The age of onset is about 40 to 50 years of age.
  B. Classification of unilateral primary acquired melanosis

1. Stage I. Benign acquired melanosis (precancerous melanosis) (Fig. 17–15)
  a. With minimal or no junctional activity:
    1) Hyperpigmentation of the epithelium may be the only finding.
    2) A few clusters of nevus cells may be seen in the junctional position.
  b. With marked junctional activity:
    1) Many nests of nevus cells are seen in the junctional position. Some nests may appear disturbing due to cellular atypia.
    2) Engorged vessels and inflammatory cells are present in the substantia propria.
  c. Without an adequate clinical history it may be impossible to differentiate cytologically from a congenital conjunctival junctional nevus.
2. Stage II. Cancerous acquired melanosis (cancerous melanosis) (Fig. 17–16)
  a. With minimal invasion:
    1) The condition is analogous to superficial or incipient melanoma of skin.
    2) In addition to the cytologic

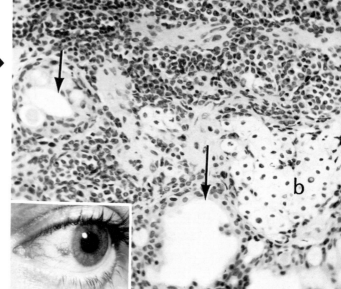

FIG. 17–14. Cystic nevus is compound nevus with hamartomatous, epithelial, cystic structures (*arrows*) admixed with nevus cells in subepithelial tissue. Note collection of balloon cells (*b*) in nevus. **Inset** shows clinical appearance of cystic nevus. **Main figure,** H&E, ×200; **inset,** clinical.

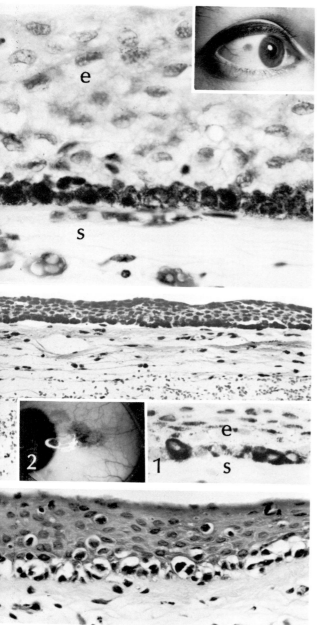

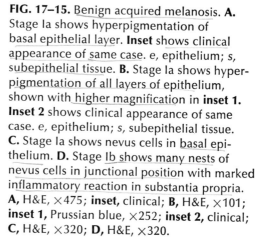

FIG. 17–15. Benign acquired melanosis. **A.** Stage Ia shows hyperpigmentation of basal epithelial layer. **Inset** shows clinical appearance of same case. *e,* epithelium; *s,* subepithelial tissue. **B.** Stage Ia shows hyperpigmentation of all layers of epithelium, shown with higher magnification in **inset 1.** **Inset 2** shows clinical appearance of same case. *e,* epithelium; *s,* subepithelial tissue. **C.** Stage Ia shows nevus cells in basal epithelium. **D.** Stage Ib shows many nests of nevus cells in junctional position with marked inflammatory reaction in substantia propria. **A,** H&E, ×475; **inset,** clinical; **B,** H&E, ×101; **inset 1,** Prussian blue, ×252; **inset 2,** clinical; **C,** H&E, ×320; **D,** H&E, ×320.

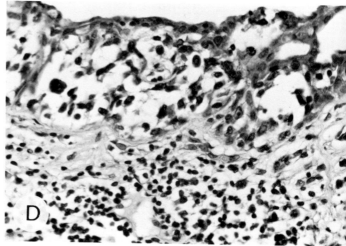

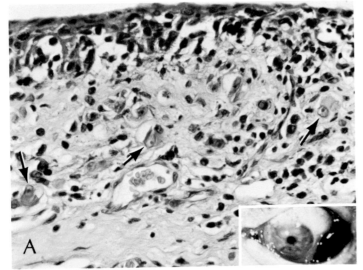

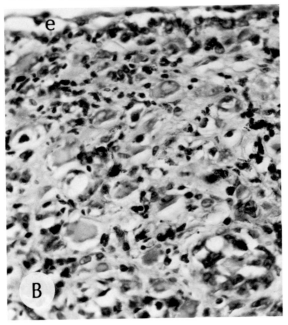

FIG. 17–16. Cancerous acquired melanosis. **A.** Stage IIa shows almost complete replacement of epithelium by atypical nevus cells. Melanoma cells (*arrows*) are present in superficial substantia propria. **Inset** shows clinical appearance of 67-year-old white man who had onset of unilateral conjunctival melanosis 3 years previously; exenteration was performed. **B.** Stage IIb (from same case as shown in **A**) shows frank conjunctival melanoma. e, conjunctival epithelium. **A,** H&E, ×320; **inset,** clinical; **B,** H&E, ×320.

changes as above in Stage I, focal areas of full thickness replacement of epithelium by markedly atypical nevus (melanoma) cells are seen.
3) The substantia propria may be focally and superficially invaded.
4) Mitotic figures may be present.
  b. With marked invasion:
In addition to the cytologic changes as above in Stages I and II, a frankly invasive malignant melanoma is present.
II. Secondary acquired melanosis*
  A. Causes
    1. Radiation.
    2. Metabolic disorders.
      a. Addison's disease.
      b. Pregnancy.
    3. Chemical toxicity.
      a. Arsenic.
      b. Thorazine.
    4. Chronic conjunctival disorders.
      a. Trachoma.
      b. Vernal conjunctivitis.
      c. Keratomalacia.
      d. Xeroderma pigmentosum.
      e. Acanthosis nigricans.

* Modified from Henkind and Friedman, 1971.

MALIGNANT MELANOMA (Figs. 17–17 and 17–18)

I. Primary
  A. Primary conjunctival malignant melanomas arise from junctional① or compound② nevi in 35 to 40 percent of cases, come from acquired melanosis③ in 25 to 30 percent of cases and are de novo④ or indeterminate in 25 to 30 percent of cases. *cellular blue nevus.*
  B. It is rare for a melanoma to arise from congenital ocular melanocytosis.
  C. It is quite rare in black people with only 6 cases reported between 1952 and 1972.
  D. The pathology is quite similar to that seen in malignant melanoma of the eyelids (see pp. 625–628 in this chapter).

The conjunctival melanomas, like the skin melanomas, are *not* classified according to cell type as are uveal melanomas (see pp. 662–672 in this chapter). Most likely the great majority, if not all, of the *"primary malignant melanomas of the cornea"* arise in the limbal conjunctiva and invade the cornea secondarily.

II. Secondary conjunctival malignant melanomas. These tumors may arise from intraocular melanomas or may be metastatic from distant primaries.

Rarely a primary conjunctival malignant melanoma may extend through the anterior scleral canals to invade the eye. The differentiation between a uveal melanoma extending outward into the conjunctiva or a conjunctival melanoma invading inward to the uvea may be difficult.

III. Prognosis
  A. When a conjunctival melanoma arises from a junctional or compound nevus, there is about 20 percent mortality.
  B. When it arises from a primary acquired melanosis, there is about 40 percent mortality.
  C. When it arises de novo or its origin is indeterminate, there is about 40 percent mortality.

LESIONS THAT MAY SIMULATE PRIMARY CONJUNCTIVAL NEVUS OR MALIGNANT MELANOMA*

I. See secondary acquired melanosis, p. 634 in this chapter.
II. See secondary malignant melanoma of conjunctiva, p. 635 in this chapter.
III. Pseudopigmentation
  A. Blue sclera (see p. 314 in Chap. 8).
  B. Ectatic sclera lined by choroid, i.e., *staphyloma*, may simulate a conjunctival melanoma.
  C. Scleromalacia perforans (see p. 317 in Chap. 8).
IV. Endogenous pigmentations
  A. Blood, especially its oxidation product (i.e., *hemosiderin*), may simulate a conjunctival melanoma.
  B. *Bile.* In acute icterus bilirubin is deposited predominantly in the conjunctiva, not in the sclera; with chronic, long-standing icterus the bilirubin, although mainly in the conjunctiva, is also deposited in the sclera.
V. Metabolic disorders
  A. Ochronosis (alkaptonuria) (see p. 315 in Chap. 8).
  B. Gaucher's disease shows conjunctival changes consisting of pigmented, triangular, brown "pinguecula" that contain *Gaucher cells*. They appear in the second decade of life.
VI. Exogenous pigmentations
  A. Epinephrine plaques (see p. 312 in Chap. 8).
  B. Argyrosis (see p. 246 in Chap. 7).
  C. Mascara.
  D. Industrial hazards.
    1. Quinones.
    2. Aniline dyes.
  E. Iron.
  F. Foreign bodies.
VII. Pigment spots of the sclera (Fig. 17–19)
  A. Pigment spots of the sclera are found most commonly with darkly pigmented irises.
  B. They consist of episcleral collections of

* Modified from Henkind and Friedman, 1971.

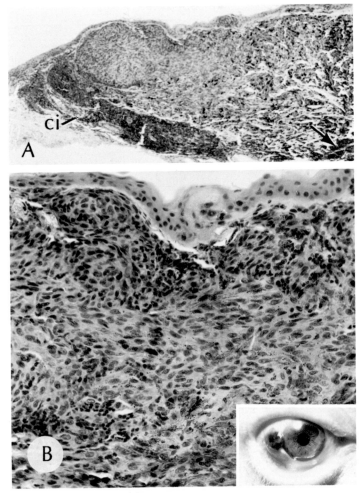

FIG. 17–17. Malignant melanoma. **A.** Conjunctival neoplasm shows underlying chronic inflammation (*ci*) and nests of nevus cells (*arrow*). **B.** Higher magnification shows loss of polarity of atypical nevus cells (melanoma cells). **Inset** shows clinical appearance of tumor (69-year-old man had lesion for at least 30 years; there had been recent growth). **A,** H&E, ×56; **B,** H&E, ×200; **inset,** clinical.

FIG. 17–18. Malignant melanoma. **A.** Large conjunctival neoplasm present. **B.** Higher magnification shows loss of polarity of atypical nevus cells (melanoma cells). **Inset** shows clinical appearance of amelanotic lesion present for many years in 19-year-old woman. Lesion had recently become vascularized. Melanoma recurred following local removal, necessitating exenteration. **A,** H&E, ×16; **B,** H&E, ×69; **inset,** clinical.

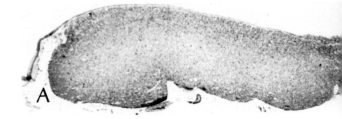

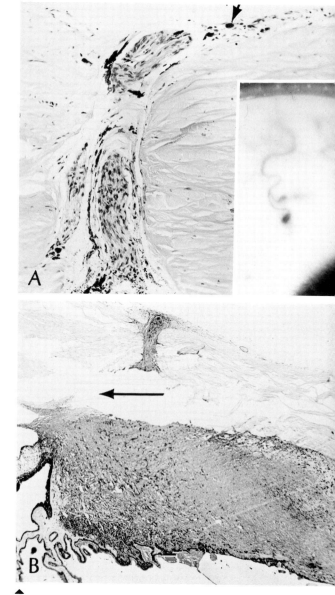

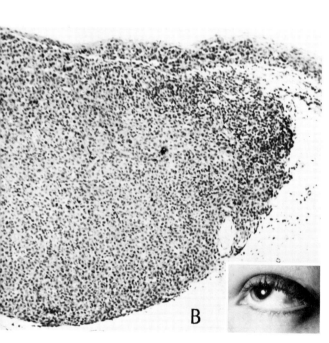

FIG. 17–19. Pigment spot of sclera. **A.** Pigment spot shown in **inset** at site of perforating anterior ciliary vessel is due to presence of pigmented uveal tissue "spilling out" into episclera (*arrow*) from anterior scleral canal. Note intrascleral nerve loop (of Axenfeld) and blood vessels in scleral canal. **B.** Anterior scleral canal may also act as conduit for ciliary body malignant melanoma to reach epibulbar surface. Cleft (*arrow*) is due to sectioning artifact. **A,** H&E, ×125; **inset,** clinical; **B,** H&E, ×72.

uveal melanocytes 3 to 4 mm from the limbus and are always associated with a perforating anterior ciliary vessel, *an intrascleral nerve loop of Axenfeld* or both.

C. Their frequency decreases from superior to inferior to temporal to nasal.

D. The conjunctiva is moveable freely over the pigment spot, and the intrascleral nerve loop remains painful to touch even after local instillation of a topical anesthetic.

MELANOTIC TUMORS OF PIGMENT EPITHELIUM OF IRIS, CILIARY BODY AND RETINA

REACTIVE TUMORS

I. Congenital (Figs. 9–8, 9–9, and 17–20)

A. Proliferation and cyst formation of the iris PE, especially the PE near the iris root, are frequent congenital anomalies.

Although the anomaly is congenital, it may not be noted clinically until adult life.

1. The PE may break off and float freely in the anterior chamber or lodge in the anterior chamber angle. It may be clear and transparent or pigmented.

2. It may simulate a malignant melanoma of the anterior chamber angle or ciliary body.

B. It may result from intrauterine inflammation, trauma, etc.

C. Histologically the PE proliferates in cords, tubes or cystic structures.

II. Drusen (Figs. 17–21 and 17–22)

Most drusen are abnormal basement membrane products of the RPE.

Pigment epithelial cells of the retina, like other ocular epithelia (see cornea, lens and ciliary body), may react to a variety of insults or stimuli by producing abnormal quantities of basement membrane. Although only the variable structure of these abnormal quantities of basement membrane is described, the structure

undoubtedly mirrors the aberrant biochemical activities conducted by the producing cell, e.g., more glycoprotein → more homogeneous basement membrane, more collagen → more filamentous or fibrous basement membrane. The basement membranes so produced are exaggerations of the normal varieties of thin, multilaminar and thick and their variations, which are summarized below.

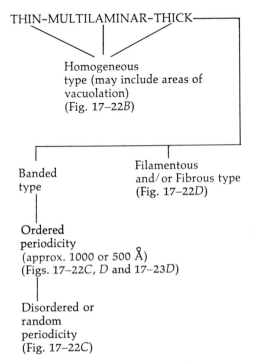

THIN—MULTILAMINAR—THICK

Homogeneous type (may include areas of vacuolation) (Fig. 17–22B)

Banded type

Ordered periodicity (approx. 1000 or 500 Å) (Figs. 17–22C, D and 17–23D)

Disordered or random periodicity (Fig. 17–22C)

Filamentous and/or Fibrous type (Fig. 17–22D)

In contrast to these exaggerations of the normal, the deposition or addition of materials not normally present in basement membranes, e.g., fibrin (Fig. 17–22E), amyloid, or various metals such as silver or copper, would produce more complex pathologic basement membranes.

B. Occasionally they may be observed as collections of exudative material under the RPE from a "leaky" choriocapillaris.

C. Histologically an amorphous, PAS-positive material is present between the RPE and Bruch's membrane. The overlying RPE usually is atrophic, whereas the adjacent RPE frequently is hyperplastic.

III. Pseudoneoplastic proliferations (Color Plate III)

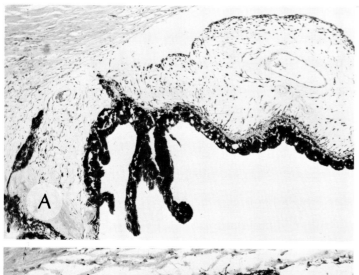

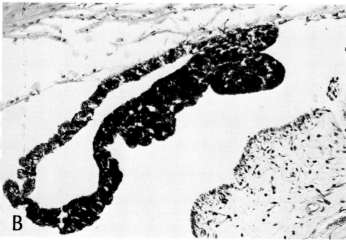

FIG. 17–20. Presumably congenital, papillary, proliferated iris pigment epithelium present at iris root (**A**). Piece probably broke off and became implanted on trabecular meshwork where it grew as pigmented cyst (**B**). Eye was enucleated because of suspected malignant melanoma of anterior chamber angle. **A,** H&E, ×80; **B,** H&E, ×145.

FIG. 17–21. A. Typical druse of moderate size. Pigment epithelium is elevated and somewhat atrophic overlying concretion. **B.** Large druse with probable occlusion of underlying chorio-capillaris. **C, D** and **E** are drusen from same case stained with H&E (**C**), trichrome (**D**) and PAS (**E**). **A,** H&E, ×145; **B,** H&E, ×145; **C,** H&E, ×130; **D,** trichrome, ×40; **E,** PAS, ×40.
▼

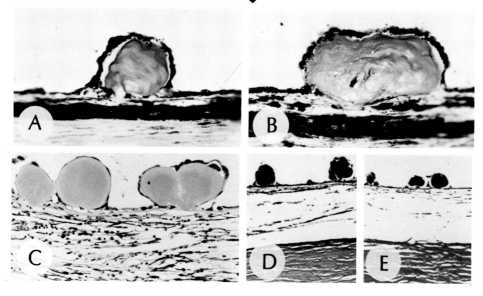

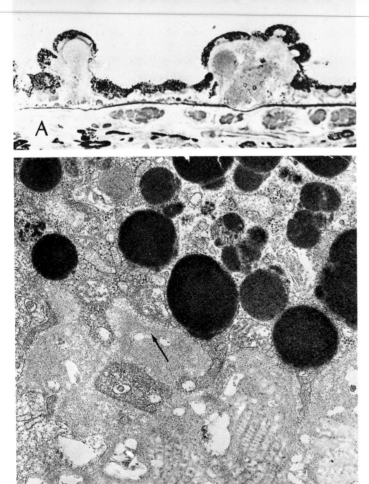

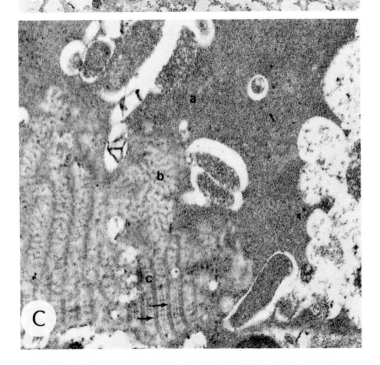

FIG. 17–22. A. Secondary drusen secreted by ▶ pigment epithelium in response to melanoma of choroid. Note attenuation of overlying epithelial cells. Material is PAS-positive in conventional 6 to 8 μ sections. **B.** Production of abnormal quantity of basement membrane (secondary drusen) by reaction of pigment epithelial cell (above) overlying periphery of malignant melanoma. Thin basement membrane (*arrow*) is continuous with large accumulation of similar homogeneous material. Large patch of banded basement membrane with periodicity (*b-bm*) also is present. **C.** Transition of homogeneous basement membrane material (a) through partially ordered region (b) to highly ordered basement membrane (c) with periodicity. Major period is ∼ 1,000 A (*arrows*). **D.** Transition (*arrows*) of thin basement membrane of pigment epithelial cell into larger homogeneous deposit. Second region of basement membrane is clearly filamentous (*f-bm*), while third region has banded basement membrane (*b-bm*) with its characteristic major periodicity of ∼ 1,000 A. **E.** Pigment epithelial cells (*PE*) in placoid formation over choroidal melanoma. Characteristic thin basement membrane is focally thickened by admixture of loose filaments (*arrow*). Masses of fibrin bundles (f, ∼ 200 A periodicity) together with myriad associated random filaments lie beneath and intermix with basement membrane, thus producing more complex pathologic basement membrane. **A,** 1.5 μ section, PD, ×300; **B,** ×7,000; **C,** ×35,000; **D,** ×20,000; **E,** ×20,000.

FIG. 17–23. Juxtapapillary RPE proliferation. ▶ **A.** Nodular proliferation (*arrow*) of RPE, when large, clinically may simulate malignancy. **B.** Higher magnification shows globular accumulations lying between attenuated RPE cells. **C.** Extracellular masses in **B** are PAS-positive. **D.** Electron micrograph shows PAS-positive material to be basement membrane with mixture of banded and vacuolated homogeneous types. Banded type is seen in **inset** at higher magnification. Each stripe is double line with cross-branching at right angles. Banding periodicity is ∼ 1,000 A. **A,** 1.5 μ section, PD, ×150; **B,** 1.5 μ section, PD, ×300; **C,** PAS, ×300; **D,** ×16,000; **inset,** ×51,000.

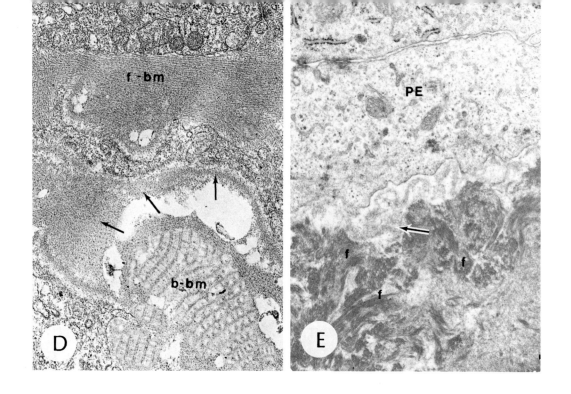

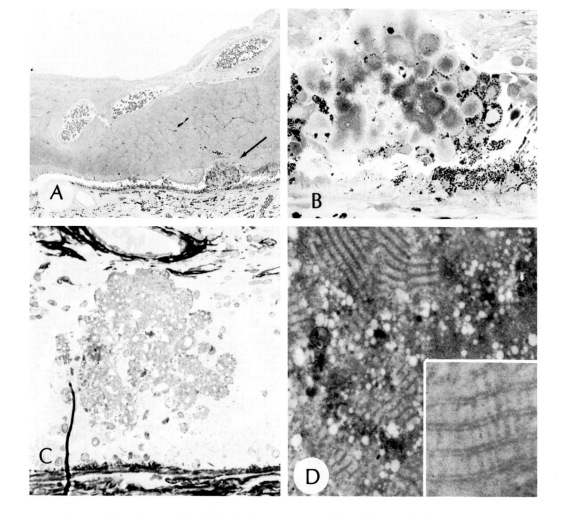

A. Following *miotic therapy* (phospholine iodide for childhood accommodative esotropia), the iris PE may enlarge or proliferate into the pupillary area.

B. Intraretinal (usually from RPE).
1. Juxtapapillary intraretinal pseudo-neoplastic proliferation of the RPE may simulate a neoplasm (Figs. 17–23 and 17–24).
2. It may occur in abiotrophic diseases such as *retinopathia pigmentosa* (Fig. 11–49)

In retinopathia pigmentosa the pigmented cells surrounding the blood vessels appearing as "bone corpuscular" pigmentation of the retina may be pigment-filled macrophages or migrated RPE cells.

3. It may occur in metabolic disorders such as homocystinuria (see p. 380 in Chap. 10); following trauma (see p. 151 in Chap. 5); as a senile change, especially in the region of the macula (see pp. 423–429 in Chap. 11); following ocular inflammation; or in long-standing diabetes.
4. *Ringschwiele* or demarcation line (see p. 462 in Chap. 11).

C. Intravitreal (usually from ciliary PE or RPE but may be from iris PE) (Fig. 17–25).
1. Intravitreal pseudoneoplastic proliferation of the PE is most common following trauma.
2. It may follow purulent endophthalmitis or other ocular inflammations.
3. Histologically, proliferated epithelium, pigmented and nonpigmented, extends out in cords and sheets, generally surrounded by abundant basement membrane material.

IV. Metaplastic
A. Disciform degeneration of the macula (see pp. 423–429 in Chap. 11) represents fibrous metaplasia of the RPE.
B. Bone formation (osseous metaplasia) (Fig. 17–26).
1. It is not certain if the PE undergoes osseous metaplasia or acts as an inducer for surrounding mesenchymal tissue to undergo osseous metaplasia.

2. Intraocular osseous metaplasia is not preceded by cartilage formation.
3. It is common following trauma, long-standing uveitis and endophthalmitis.

NONREACTIVE TUMORS

I. Congenital
A. Glioneuroma (Fig. 17–27)
1. Glioneuromas are rare tumors with only four cases recorded.
2. Histologically the tumor is composed only of brain tissue, containing neurons and glial cells and lacking the embryonic retina, ciliary epithelium and primitive vitreous found in medulloepitheliomas.
B. Medulloepithelioma ("*diktyoma*")— see p. 702 in Chapter 18.
1. Benign medulloepithelioma (Fig. 17–28) is a tumor composed of elements that closely resemble primitive medullary epithelium; it frequently contains structures resembling those derived from the secondary optic cup or optic vesicle, i.e., RPE, ciliary epithelium, vitreous and neuroglia.
2. Malignant tumors (Fig. 17–29) may have elements of the benign type with the addition of tightly packed neuroblastic cells, sometimes showing marked mitotic activity, greatly resembling retinoblastomas.
C. Teratoid medulloepithelioma ("*diktyoma*")
1. Benign teratoid medulloepithelioma (Fig. 17–30) is a tumor having one or more heteroplastic elements (e.g., hyaline cartilage, tissue resembling brain or rhabdomvoblasts) in addition to the medulloepitheliomatous components.
2. Malignant tumors (Fig. 17–31) have sarcomatous changes in one or more elements of the benign type, e.g., rhabdomyosarcoma or chondrosarcoma.
D. Retinal pigment epithelial hypertrophy (benign "melanoma") (Fig. 17–32)
1. Hypertrophy of the RPE clinically is a jet black, flat (or slightly elevated) lesion surrounded by a halo

(due to partial or complete RPE hypopigmentation). It may have drusen of irregular sizes and shapes overlying it.

2. It is a benign, stationary lesion.

3. Histologically the lesion consists of hypertrophy of RPE cells and an increase in size and number of their melanin granules. The surrounding halo is due to atrophy of and/or loss of pigment from the adjacent RPE.

II. Acquired

A. Adenoma (epithelioma) (Figs. 17–33 and 17–34)

1. Adenomas may arise from the pigment epithelium in a solid, papillary or pleomorphic pattern.

2. The cells appear polyhedral in shape and heavily or lightly pigmented. The heavily pigmented cells frequently are vacuolated.

The vacuoles contain a sialomucin that can be digested with neuraminidase (sialidase). These observations together with recent experiments indicating that radioactive fucose is incorporated into the interreceptor matrix show that the pigment epithelium contributes the sialoglycan component to the matrix. The remainder, or greater part, of the matrix is considered to be elaborated by the photoreceptor cells through synthesis within their apical (i.e., inner segment) portions.

3. Histologically the above neoplasm may be difficult to differentiate from simple reactive proliferations of the pigment epithelium.

a. The cells of the adenoma, whether polyhedral or vacuolated, are generally pigmented and are packed together tightly with little or no stroma.

b. Nuclear atypia is common but mitotic figures are rare.

Conversely, the individual cells in pseudoadenomatous hyperplasia tend to be separated by an amorphous basement membranelike material and show little atypia and no mitotic figures.

FIG. 17–24. Intraretinal RPE proliferation. **A.** RPE has proliferated into retina in juxtapapillary area. **B.** Higher magnification to show proliferating pigmented cells (seen with still higher magnification in **inset**). Eye was enucleated because of suspected juxtapapillary malignant melanoma. **A,** H&E, ×16; **B,** H&E, ×40; **inset,** H&E, ×101.

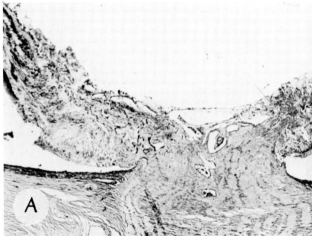

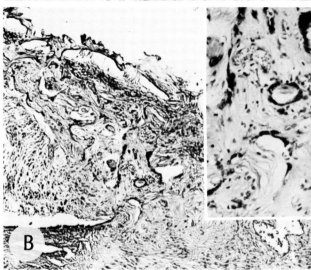

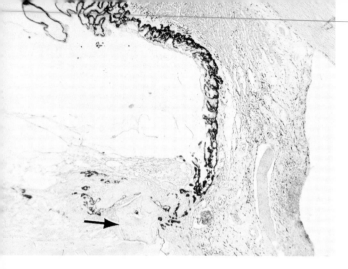

FIG. 17–25. Intravitreal proliferation of pigmented and nonpigmented ciliary epithelium has occurred along with metaplastic bone formation (*arrow*). H&E, ×24.

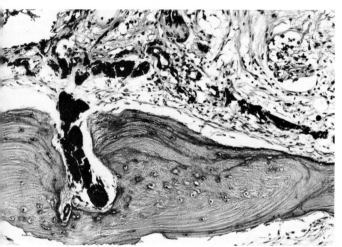

FIG. 17–26. RPE cells are intimately associated with metaplastic bone spicule present in inner rim of choroid. H&E, ×100.

FIG. 17–27. Glioneuroma. **A.** Large tumor present in region of ciliary body is adherent to cataractous displaced lens and extends through scleral dehiscence inferiorly (*arrow*). **B.** Special stain shows presence of bipolar neuron exhibiting long axonal processes. Most neurons in tumor were unipolar. **A,** H&E, ×2.5; **B,** Bodian stain, ×250.

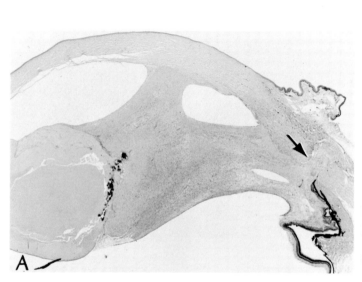

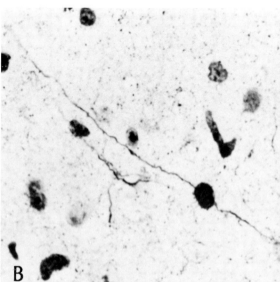

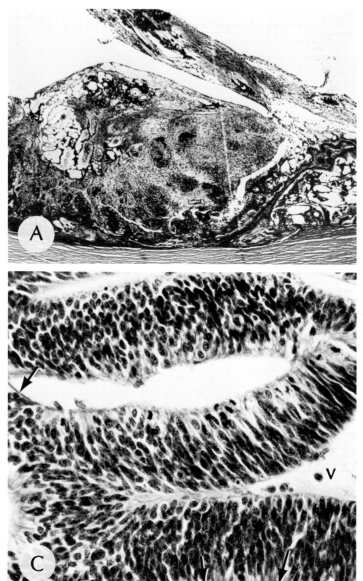

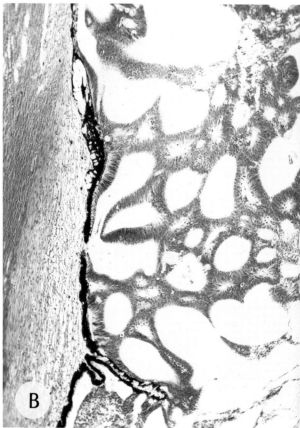

FIG. 17–28. Benign medulloepithelioma. **A.** Ciliary body tumor contains structures that resemble primitive medullary epithelium, ciliary epithelium and vitreous. Note vertical scratch artifact due to defect in microtome knife blade. **B.** Structures resembling medullary epithelium of embryonic ciliary epithelium and retina arise from nonpigmented ciliary epithelium and produce intricate convolutions enclosing lumina of various shapes and sizes. **C.** Multicellular bands are polarized, forming sharply defined structures analogous to external limiting membrane of retina along one surface (*arrow*); less well-defined opposite surface is in contact with primitive vitreous (*v*). **A,** H&E, ×16; **B,** H&E, ×80; **C,** H&E, ×305.

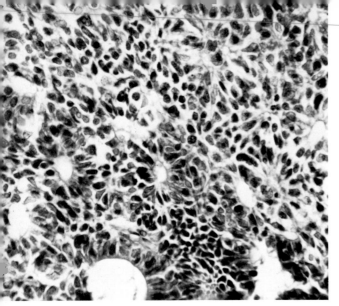

FIG. 17–29. Malignant medulloepithelioma shows atypical cells simulating retino-blastoma cells, many mitotic figures and structures resembling Flexner-Wintersteiner rosettes. H&E, ×380.

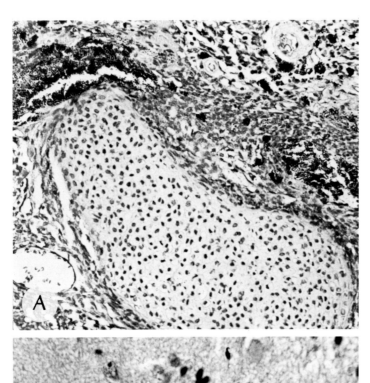

FIG. 17–30. Benign teratoid medulloepithelioma has benign heteroplastic elements such as hyalin cartilage (A) and tissue resembling brain (B). A, H&E, ×130; B, H&E, ×305.

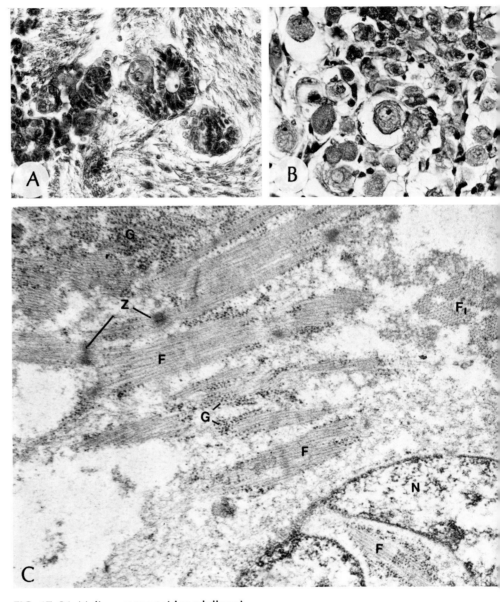

FIG. 17–31. Malignant teratoid medulloepithelioma. A. Neuroepithelial tubules are
present within masses of less well-differentiated (on left) pleomorphic medullary
epithelium. B. Large ganglioform cells
(rhabdomyoblasts) are present among small
undifferentiated cells. C. Electron micrograph
of rhabdomyoblast showing numerous
bundles of cytoplasmic filaments, both thick
and thin, in longitudinal (F) as well as in
cross- (F_1) section; Z bands are present (Z)
as are numerous glycogen particles (G)
scattered about filament bundles. N, infolded
nucleus. A, B and C all from same case. A,
H&E, ×210; B, H&E, ×305; C, ×34,000.

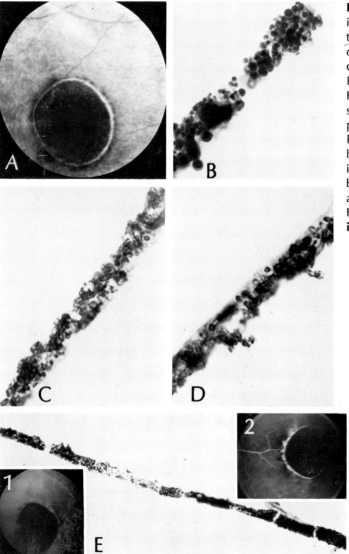

FIG. 17–32. RPE hypertrophy. **A.** Characteristic fundus appearance shows jet black tumor surrounded by halo. **B.** Hypertrophy of RPE cells and melanin granules causes clinical appearance. **C** and **D** show normal RPE anterior and posterior to tumor. **E.** Hypertrophied RPE corresponding to tumor shown on right, depigmented RPE corresponding to halo present in center and normal RPE is on left. **Insets** show fundus appearance before (**1**) and after (**2**) fluorescein. Note increased fluorescence in area of halo and blotting out of background flourescence in area of tumor. **A,** clinical; **B,** H&E, ×990; **C,** H&E, ×990; **D,** H&E, ×990; **E,** H&E, ×305; **inset 1,** fundus; **inset 2,** fluorescein—fundus.

B. Fuchs's adenoma—see p. 347 in Chapter 9.
C. Adenocarcinoma (Fig. 17–35)
   1. Like adenomas adenocarcinomas may have a solid, papillary or pleomorphic pattern.
   2. When the PE becomes malignant, it forms an *incidentally pigmented adenocarcinoma,* not a malignant melanoma.
   3. The neoplasms are relatively benign, generally exhibit only local invasion and metastasize only rarely, if ever.

MELANOTIC TUMORS OF THE UVEA

IRIS

I. Freckle (Fig. 17–36)
   A. An iris freckle is caused by increased pigmentation of anterior border layer melanocytes without increased numbers of melanocytes.

B. There is no discrete mass or nodule.

II. Nevus (Fig. 17–37)

    A. An iris nevus results from an increased number of atypical but benign-appearing melanocytes, i.e., nevus cells, with variable pigmentation.

    B. A discrete mass or nodule is present, frequently on the anterior surface of the iris, i.e., within the anterior border layer of the iris.

    C. There is an increased incidence of iris nevi in eyes of people with neurofibromatosis and with ciliary body or choroidal malignant melanomas.

    D. A diffuse (or rarely segmental) nevus of the iris (and the rest of the uvea) is present in congenital ocular (or oculodermal) melanocytosis.

    E. An acquired diffuse nevus of the iris may be associated with unilateral glaucoma, heterochroma (either eye darker), peripheral anterior synechias, iris nodules, matting and obliteration of the normal iris pattern and occasionally proliferation of endothelium over the anterior iris with the secretion of a new Descemet's membrane. The condition has been called the *iris nevus syndrome* (Fig. 17–38).

        Histologically a diffuse nevus of the anterior surface of the iris is present. Generally peripheral anterior synechias are present between nevus and posterior cornea.

    F. An iris nevus has a low malignant potential.

III. Malignant melanoma (Figs. 17–39 and 17–40)

    A. Iris malignant melanomas constitute approximately 5 to 8 percent of all uveal melanomas.

    B. They usually arise from the anterior border layer tissue of the iris (as do nevi of iris).

    C. Most if not all iris malignant melanomas arise from preexisting nevi of the iris.

    D. Geographic sector distribution of iris malignant melanoma in descending frequency: pupillary zone; entire sector; pupillary and midzone; midzone; periphery; periphery and midzone.

    E. Geographic quadrant distribution of iris malignant melanomas in descending frequency: inferior; temporal; nasal; superior.

    F. Clinically an iris melanoma may present as a discrete mass, a diffuse mass, a heterochromia, a glaucoma (e.g., iris nevus syndrome) or with chronic uveitis.

    G. The tumors may be deeply pigmented, partially pigmented or nonpigmented and frequently show increased vascularity and distortion of the pupil toward the iris quadrant of involvement. An unusual form appearing clinically like "tapioca" has been described.

    H. The vast majority of iris malignant melanomas are composed of spindle cells (see p. 662 in this chapter) and therefore are relatively benign.

        1. They rarely metastasize.

        2. The mortality rate is about 4 to 5 percent.

    I. Differential diagnosis

        1. Anterior *staphyloma*.

        2. Exudative mass in anterior chamber.

            a. Pigmented macrophages in anterior chamber.

            b. *Phacoanaphylactic endophthalmitis.*

            c. *Juvenile xanthogranuloma.*

        3. Corneal or scleral perforation with uveal prolapse.

        4. "Postoperative confusion."

            a. Posterior or anterior chamber epithelial cyst.

                Anterior chamber cysts may also occur "spontaneously" without surgery. The spontaneous "cysts" also have been confused with iris malignant melanomas (Fig. 17–20).

            b. Iridencleisis (unplanned).

        5. Miscellaneous.

            a. *Nodular* thickening and scarring of iris.

            b. *Foreign body* in iris.

            c. *Ectropion uveae.*

            d. *Segmental congenital ocular melanocytosis.*

            e. *Intrairis hemorrhage.*

            f. Other iris tumors, e.g., leiomyoma, metastatic tumors and

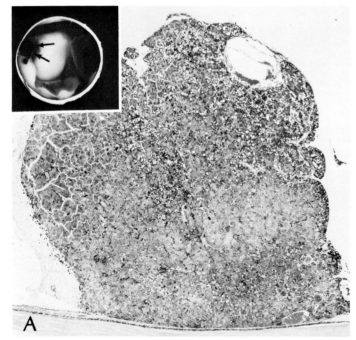

FIG. 17–33. Adenoma. **A.** Solid pattern
in tumor present between equator and ora
serrata (*arrows* in **inset**). Tumor has flat base
and contains vacuolated cells most prominent in inner half. **B.** Tumor consists of light
(containing immature melanosomes) and
dark (containing mature melanosomes) cells.
Cytoplasmic vacuoles are limited mostly to
dark cells. Macrophages are present in loose
cluster within cystoid space (*arrows*). **A,**
H&E, ×28; **inset,** macroscopic; **B,** 1.5 μ
section, PD, ×245.

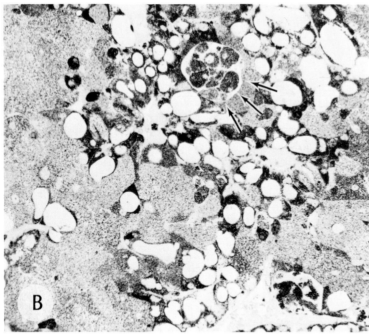

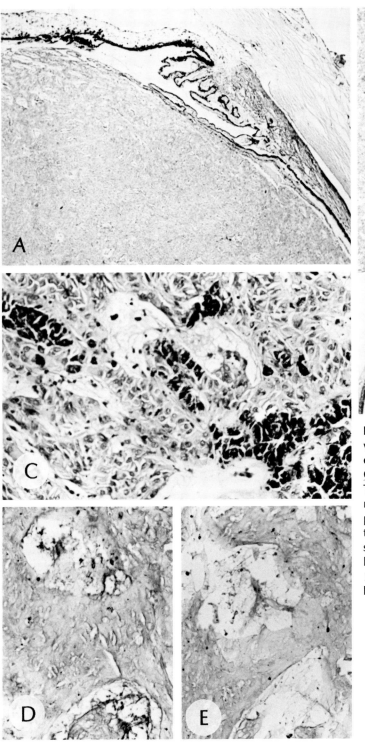

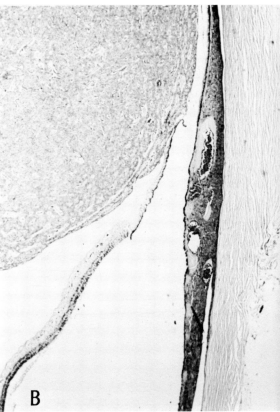

FIG. 17–34. Adenoma. **A.** Large tumor with papillary pattern arises from ciliary epithelium. **B.** Tumor extends to equator. Coincidental choroidal nevus is present. **C.** Tumor is composed of cords of predominantly nonpigmented epithelial cells, but pigmented cells also are present. Spaces in tumor stain positively for acid mucopolysaccharides (**D**) which are digestible with hyaluronidase (**E**). **A,** H&E, ×16; **B,** H&E, ×16; **C,** H&E, ×101; **D,** AMP, ×101; **E,** hyaluronidase—AMP, ×101.

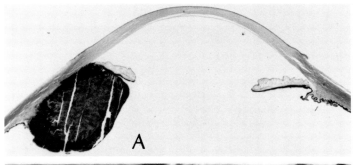

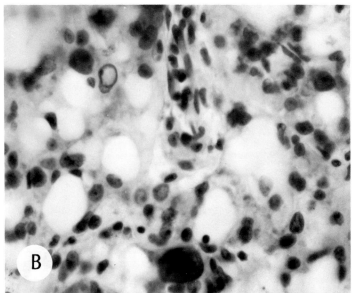

FIG. 17–35. RPE adenocarcinoma. **A.** Heavily pigmented ciliary body tumor has invaded into ciliary muscle, trabecular meshwork and Schlemm's canal. **B.** Bleached section shows considerable nuclear atypia. **A,** H&E, ×7; **B,** bleached, H&E, ×475.

FIG. 17–36. Iris freckle is caused by increased pigmentation of melanocytes of anterior border layer (right two-thirds). **Inset** shows a few iris freckles and one iris nevus at 8 o'clock. **Main figure,** H&E, ×101; **inset,** clinical.

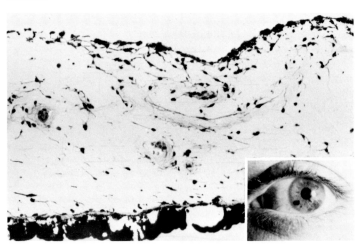

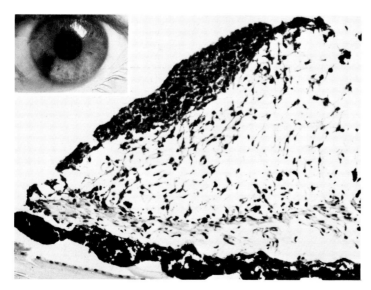

FIG. 17–37. Iris nevus is composed of cluster of nevus cells near pupillary border. **Inset** shows nevus, involving iris root, and present since birth. **Main figure,** H&E, ×101; **inset,** clinical.

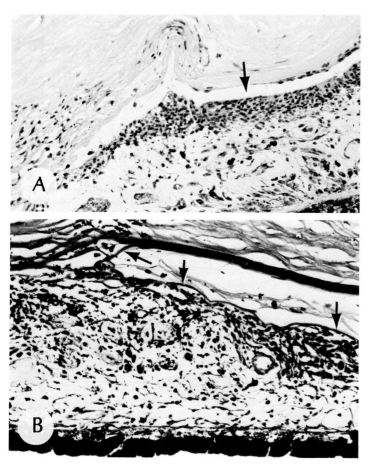

FIG. 17–38. Iris nevus syndrome, i.e., unilateral glaucoma, heterochromia and peripheral anterior synechias, is caused by diffuse nevus of anterior surface of iris (see Figure 16–18*E*). **A.** Nevus in area of peripheral anterior synechia; cleft (*arrow*) is due to fixation artifact. Note posterior extension of Descemet's membrane over trabecular meshwork. **B.** Another case shows diffuse nevus of anterior iris surface and endothelialization of pseudoangle and iris surface (*arrows*). **A,** H&E, ×180; **B,** PAS, ×101.

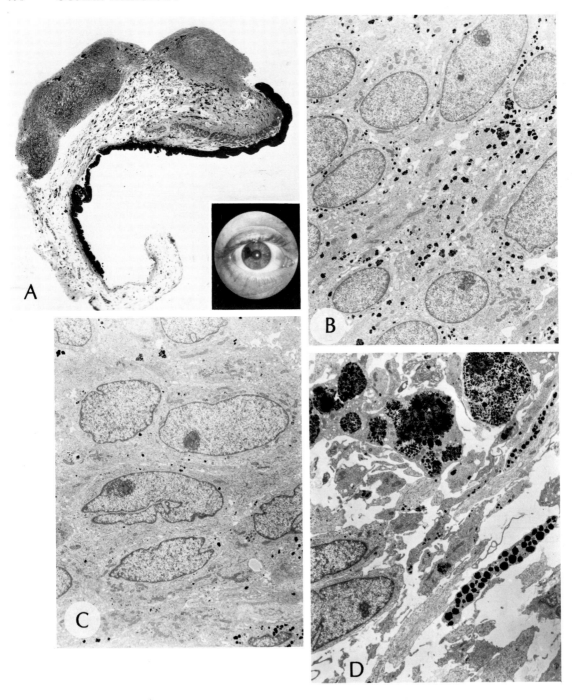

◀ **FIG. 17–39.** Iris melanoma. **A.** Spindle B melanoma of iris is well localized to sector without angle involvement (**inset**). Lobules of tumor involve mostly anterior iris stroma. Some eversion of pupillary pigment epithelium (ectropion uveae) is present. **B.** Electron microscopic sample of pigmented region of tumor in **A.** Cells are mostly spindle-shaped. **C.** Electron microscopic sample of lightly pigmented region of tumor in **A.** Cells are mostly spindle-shaped. Note deep nuclear invaginations in cell near center. This accounts for "line of chromatin" seen by light microscopy in spindle A melanoma cells. **D.** Macrophages (above) are contrasted with normal iris melanocytes (below and to right) by their pigment-filled phagosomes of large and variable sizes. Two spindle-shaped tumor cells are present on left. **A,** 1.5 μ section, PD, ×35; **B,** ×4,000; **C,** ×4,000; **D,** ×4,000.

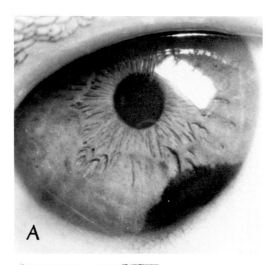

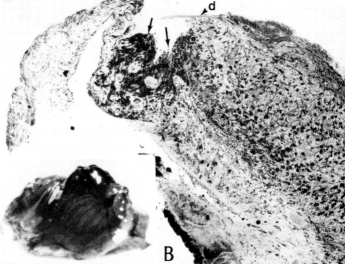

FIG. 17–40. Iris melanoma. **A.** Nevus near iris root had been present at least 7 years. Development of sector cataract led to discovery of ciliary body tumor (**inset in B**). **B.** Light micrograph from iridocyclectomy specimen shows nevus (*arrows*) present at iris root from which arises malignant melanoma, which also invades drainage angle (see fragment of peripheral Descemet's membrane, *d*) and adjacent sclera. **Inset** shows excised specimen. Tumor arises between ciliary crests. Pressure on adjacent lens produced sector cataract. **A,** clinical; **B,** H&E, ×35; **inset,** macroscopic.

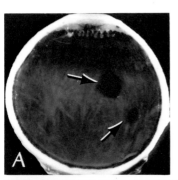

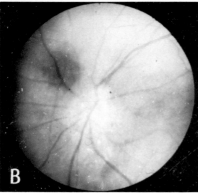

FIG. 17–41. A. Two choroidal nevi (*arrows*) present in eye. **B.** Nevus present just above and nasal to optic disc. **A,** macroscopic; **B,** fundus.

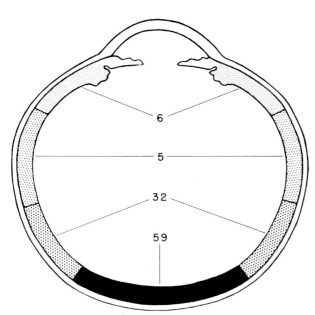

FIG. 17–42. Distribution of 102 nevi in choroid and ciliary body.

ciliary body malignant melanoma.

g. Granulomatous inflammation with Busaca and Koeppe nodules.

CILIARY BODY AND CHOROID

I. Nevus
 A. Incidence
  1. Nevi of the ciliary body and choroid are found in at least 9 to 11 percent of people.
  2. They may be multiple in one eye (Fig. 17–41).
 B. Location (Fig. 17–42)
  1. The majority (59 percent) of nevi are located in the posterior third of the choroid.
  2. The anterior third (5 percent) of the choroid and the ciliary body (6 percent) have almost an equal incidence.
 C. Size and shape (Figs. 17–41 and 17–43 through 17–45)
  1. The diameter of nevi range from about 0.5 mm (0.33 disc diameter [DD]) to 11.0 mm (7 DD) with the majority between 2.5 and 5.5 mm.

2. They generally occupy the entire thickness of the choroid except for the choriocapillaris.
3. Typically nevi are flat, discoid lesions, but 67 percent exceed the thickness of the adjacent choroid.
4. They tend to be relatively avascular.

The relative avascularity of nevi helps to explain their fluorescein fundus picture, which is one of decreased fluorescence. An amelanotic nevus may be detected inadvertently upon examination of a fluorescein angiogram showing a region of persistent choroidal hypofluorescence without the presence of a corresponding pigmented fundus picture. Melanomas, on the other hand, are highly vascular with abnormal vessels, which readily leak fluorescein. Rarely, however, nevi will leak fluorescein and melanomas will not.

 D. Cytology and pigmentation (Figs. 17–46 and 17–47)
  1. Generally nevus cells are plumper than normal melanocytes of the choroid and ciliary body, i.e., they are atypical but benign-appearing melanocytes.
  2. Four types of uveal nevus cells are recognized:
   a. *Plump polyhedral nevus cell*
    1) The plump polyhedral nevus cell is the most common type.
    2) The cell is maximally pigmented.
    3) A nevus made up exclusively of this type of cell is called a melanocytoma.
   b. *Slender spindle nevus cell*
    1) The slender spindle nevus cell is the second most common cell type.
    2) It contains little or no pigment.
    3) The "typical" nevus contains a majority of plump polyhedral cells with some slender spindle nevus cells either admixed or collected together within the nevus, closest to the sclera.
   c. *Plump fusiform and dendritic*

nevus cells are less pigmented than plump polyhedral nevus cells but more so than slender spindle nevus cells.

d. *Balloon cells*
   1) Balloon cells are large cells with abundant foamy cytoplasm.
   2) Similar cells are found occasionally in cutaneous nevi.

3. Congenital ocular (or oculodermal) melanocytosis is a diffuse nevus of the uvea. Rarely it may have a segmental distribution (see p. 625 in this chapter).

This pigment-cell disorder involves skin, conjunctival and uveal melanocytes but not the RPE.

E. Effects of nevus on neighboring tissues
   1. Nevi frequently narrow the overlying choriocapillaris and rarely may completely obliterate it (Fig. 17–48).
   2. They may cause overlying retinal changes, which are usually minimal.
      a. Slight degeneration or proliferation (Figs. 17–48 and 17–50) of pigment epithelium may occur.
      b. Rarely they cause definite disturbances of rod and cone or outer nuclear layer (Fig. 17–49).
      c. More frequently they induce overlying *drusen* formation (Fig. 17–50).
      d. Central serous retinopathy may occur rarely.
F. There is an increased incidence of uveal nevi in eyes that contain uveal melanomas.

II. Malignant melanoma
   A. General information:
      1. The median age is 55 years (it is rare in children but even a congenital case has occurred).
      2. There is a slight preponderance of melanomas in men.
      3. Whites more frequently have intraocular melanomas than blacks in a ratio of 15:1.*

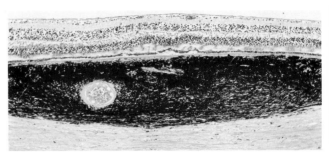

FIG. 17–43. Typical placoid nevus of choroid shows bulging toward retina and sclera. Intensity of pigment characteristically decreases from inner to outer layers. There is a tendency of nevus to spare choriocapillaris. H&E, ×50.

4. Uveal melanomas are slightly more prevalant in individuals with blue irises than in those with brown irises.
5. Bilaterality or multifocal origin is extremely rare.
6. Heredity is not an important factor.
7. The incidence of uveal melanomas in an adult white clinic population is about 0.02 to 0.06 percent.
8. For sites of malignant melanoma within the eye, see Table 17–2.

B. Clinical presentation
   1. A mass found on routine examination or found after a complaint of blurred vision probably is the most frequent clinical presentation (Fig. 17–51).

Orange pigment accumulation over choroidal tumors (Fig. 17–77) is a helpful clinical distinguishing feature between nevi and melanomas. Any lesion resembling a nevus but demonstrating the orange pigment should be strongly suspected of being melanoma.

---

* The often quoted statistic of 150:1 is an absolute figure not corrected for the racial ratio (10:1 whites to blacks) in the United States.

TABLE 17–2.
Site of Malignant Melanomas within the Eye*

Location	Anterior[†]	Equatorial	Posterior	Anterior-posterior[‡]	Total
Superior	3		3	2	8
Inferior	2		2	1	5
Temporal	2	1	9	5	17 ⎫
Inferotemporal	5	3	2		10 ⎪ 51
Superotemporal	2		12	1	15 ⎬
Macula			9		9 ⎭
Nasal	3	2	7	3	15 ⎫
Inferonasal	1		3	1	5 ⎬ 31
Superonasal	5		4	2	11 ⎭
Peripapillary			2		2
Whole eye				3	3
Totals	23	6	53	18	100

* From Yanoff and Zimmerman, Cancer 20:493, 1967.
† Includes ciliary body and choroid anterior to equator; does not include iris.
‡ Diffuse or large neoplasms extending from ciliary body or ora serrata to posterior choroid.

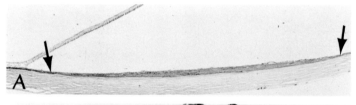

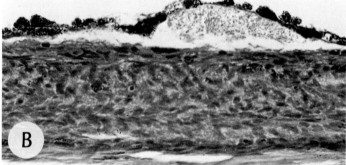

FIG. 17–44. Choroidal nevus. **A.** Nevus measures about 8 mm in diameter; *arrows* indicate extent of nevus. **B.** Higher magnification shows druse overlying relatively amelanotic nevus. **A,** H&E, ×45; **B,** H&E, ×305.

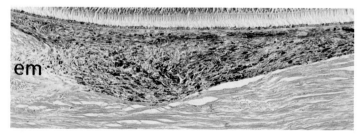

FIG. 17–45. Choroidal nevus extends into sclera adjacent to emissary canal (*em*). H&E, ×70.

bleached
polyhedral cell

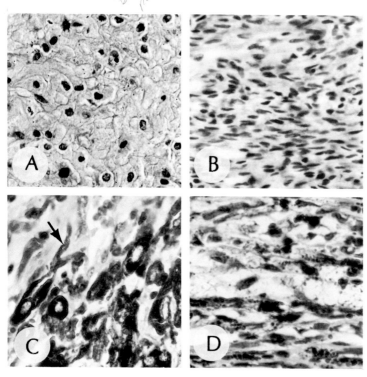

FIG. 17–46. Cell types in nevus. **A.** Plump polyhedral nevus cells. Nuclei are rather small and uniform. Abundance of cytoplasm is striking after pigment is bleached out. **B.** Slender spindle-shaped nevus cells. **C.** Plump fusiform and plump dendritic nevus cells. Note dendritic projections (*arrow*) of heavily pigmented cytoplasm and large nuclei. **D.** Balloon cells are present above slender spindle-shaped nevus cells. **A,** bleached, H&E, ×300; **B,** H&E, ×395; **C,** H&E, ×440; **D,** H&E, ×600.

FIG. 17–47. Nevus of choroid. Cells contain moderate pigmentation, are of moderate plumpness and appear dendritic. ×8,400.

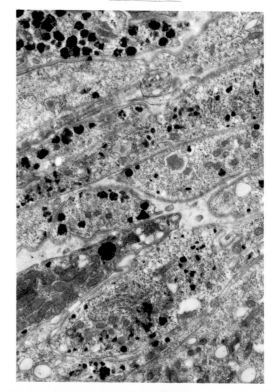

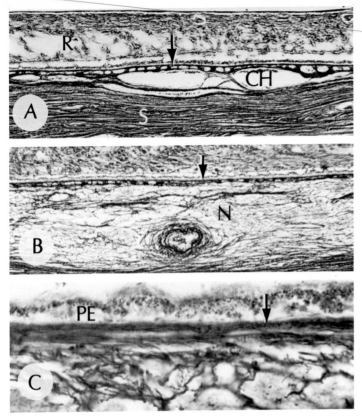

FIG. 17–48. Effects of choroidal nevus on overlying choriocapillaris. **A.** Normal chorio-capillaris (*arrow*) near nevus shown in **B.** and **C.** *R*, retina; *CH*, choroid; *S*, sclera. **B.** Narrowing and partial obliteration of chorio-capillaris (*arrow*) over nevus (*N*). **C.** Almost complete obliteration of choriocapillaris (*arrow*). Also note slight degenerative changes of overlying pigment epithelium (*PE*). **A,** Wilder reticulum, ×120; **B,** Wilder reticulum, ×120; **C,** Wilder reticulum, ×705.

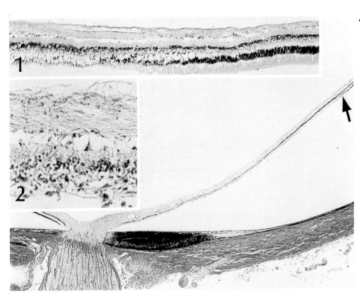

◀ **FIG. 17–49.** Effects of choroidal nevus on overlying retina. Juxtapapillary nevus with marked degeneration of overlying retina. Transitional area between normal retinal and degenerated retina (*arrow*) shown at higher magnification in **inset 1.** Degenerated retina shown at higher magnification in **inset 2.** Retinal changes caused patient to have absolute scotoma, rare with nevus. **Main figure,** H&E, ×10; **inset 1,** H&E, ×55; **inset 2,** H&E, ×140.

FIG. 17–50. Secondary drusen present over nevus. **A.** Nevus produces slight thickening of choroid. **B.** Proliferative and degenerative changes are present in RPE. Druse (*D*) overlies nevus composed here of slender spindle cells. **A,** H&E, ×50; **B,** H&E, ×395.

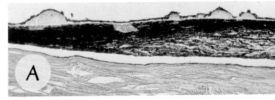

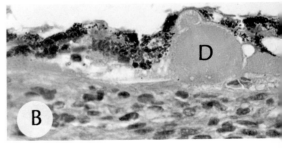

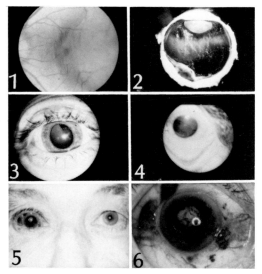

FIG. 17–51. Clinical presentation. **1** and **2** from same patient who presented clinically with blurred vision. Patients in **3** and **4** presented clinically with inferior temporal and superior scotomas, respectively. Patient shown in **5** and **6** presented with cataract, heterochromia and intraocular melanoma extending into episclera anteriorly. **1**, fundus; **2**, macroscopic; **3**, clinical; **4**, clinical; **5**, clinical, both eyes; **6**, clinical, right eye.

FIG. 17–52. Episcleral tumor (*arrow* in **inset 1**) was first clinical sign in ciliary body melanoma (*arrows* in **insets 2** and **3**). Melanoma has invaded Schlemm's canal (*sp*) and has reached episcleral region (*ep*). **Main figure,** H&E, ×37; **inset 1,** clinical; **inset 2,** fundus reflex; **inset 3,** macroscopic. ▼

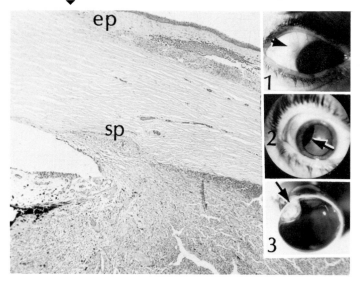

FIG. 17–53. Serous fluid present under macular retina (*arrow*) with peripheral choroidal melanoma. Patient presented with blurred vision due to central serouslike retinopathy. H&E, ×32.

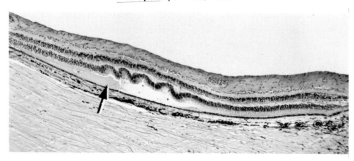

2. Episcleral vascular injection may occur over a ciliary body malignant melanoma.

Some of these patients have been treated for chronic conjunctivitis until the melanoma was discovered with adequate ophthalmoscopy.

3. Decreased intraocular pressure may occur with a ciliary body malignant melanoma.
4. The patient may present with an episcleral extension of a uveal malignant melanoma (Fig. 17–52) that may simulate a conjunctival lesion.
5. Vitreous hemorrhage (see p. 675 in this chapter).
6. Central serous retinopathy (Fig. 17–53) may accompany a peripheral uveal malignant melanoma.

Fluorescein angiography may reveal identical findings to those seen in cystic macula following cataract extraction, hypotony or uveitis.

7. Ocular inflammation may occur (Fig. 17–54), but it is less common than with retinoblastoma (see p. 693 in Chap. 18).
8. Glaucoma (see pp. 602, 610 in Chap. 16).
9. Opaque media (see p. 676 in this chapter).
10. The uveal melanoma may originate in or invade the iris and produce a heterochromia (Fig. 17–51).
11. Metastases usually are a late manifestation of uveal melanomas, whereas frequently they are an early manifestation of skin melanomas.

C. Histogenesis (many theories):
1. *Mesodermal* theory is that the tumor arises from mesodermal elements in the uvea, hence the name *melanosarcoma.*
2. Retinal pigment epithelial theory is that the melanoma arises from the retinal pigment epithelium.
3. Neural theory is that the melanoma arises from Schwann cells associ-

ated with the ciliary nerves (Fig. 17–55).
4. Nevoid theory is that the melanoma arises from a preexisting nevus.

Most evidence points to the nevoid theory of histogenesis, i.e., *the vast majority of uveal malignant melanomas arise from preexisting nevi* (Figs. 17–56 through 17–60).

D. Callender classification and prognosis (Fig. 17–61) (specifically for ciliary body and choroidal malignant melanomas; also may be applied to iris but *not* to conjunctival or skin malignant melanomas).
1. Spindle A (Fig. 17–62)
   a. Spindle A is the second rarest type of melanoma (5 percent) and is made up of cohesive cells with small spindle-shaped nuclei with a central dark stripe (caused by a nuclear fold) but no distinct nucleoli; the cytoplasm is indistinct without easily identifiable cell borders.

   [handwritten margin: cohesive nuclear fold; I: 5%; Suv. 92%]

   The dark stripe is quite helpful in classification when present, but it does not always occur.

   b. Mitotic figures are extremely rare.
   c. The survival rate is approximately 92 percent.*
2. Spindle B and fascicular (Figs. 17–63 through 17–65)
   a. Spindle B is common (39 percent) and is made up of cohesive cells with prominent spindle-shaped nuclei with distinct nucleoli; the cytoplasm is indistinct without easily identifiable cell borders.

   [handwritten margin: cohesive palisades nucleoli; I: 39%; S: 75%]

   b. In about 6 percent of spindle B cell malignant melanomas the spindle-shaped cells form a palisaded arrangement called a *fascicular pattern,* but the cell type in this arrangement remains spindle B.
   c. Mitotic figures are rare.
   d. The survival rate is approximately 75 percent.*

---

* Fifteen-year actuarial survival rates based on a study of 2652 cases by type of cell (Paul et al, 1962).

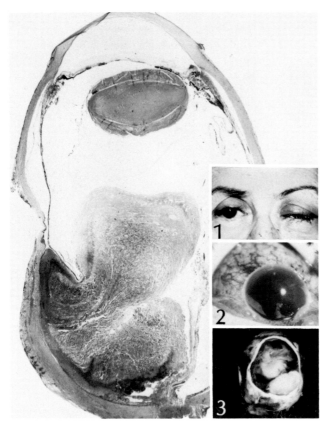

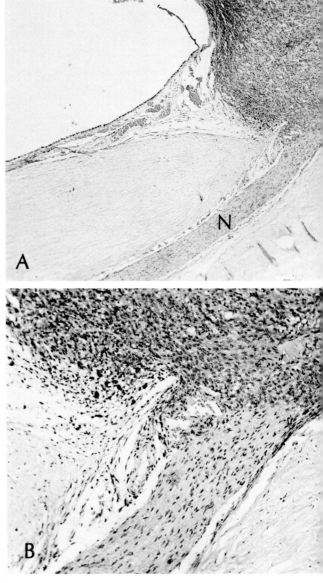

FIG. 17–54. Patient presented (**insets 1** and **2**) with signs and symptoms of acute endophthalmitis. Completely necrotic choroidal melanoma (**inset 3**) and anterior segment necrosis are present. **Main figure,** H&E, ×5; **inset 1,** clinical, both eyes; **inset 2,** clinical, left eye; **inset 3,** macroscopic.

FIG. 17–55. Neural theory of histogenesis of uveal melanoma. **A.** Long posterior ciliary nerve (*N*) enters choroidal melanoma. **B.** Higher magnification to show reactive proliferation of Schwann cells, which may simulate de novo melanoma cells. **A,** H&E, ×32; **B,** H&E, ×100.

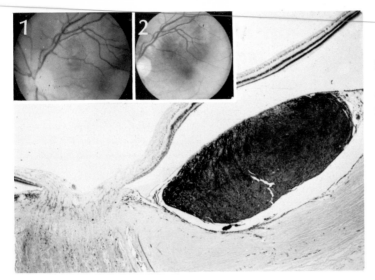

FIG. 17–56. Nevus noted in fundus (**inset 1**). Rapid growth occurred almost 4 years later (**inset 2**), and eye was enucleated. Heavily pigmented melanoma is present in posterior pole. **Main figure,** H&E, ×8; **inset 1,** fundus; **inset 2,** fundus.

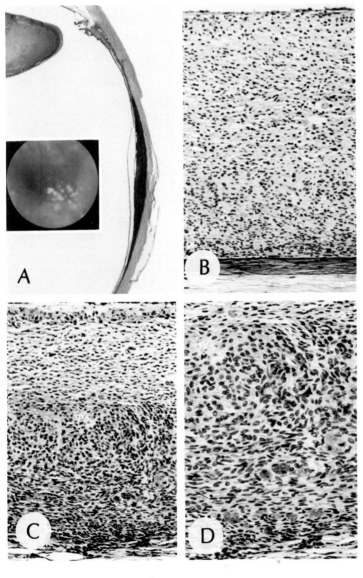

FIG. 17–57. A. Large, heavily pigmented lesion with overlying drusen (**inset**) present in pars plana and anterior choroid. Bleached serial sections show nevus cells throughout most of tumor, as seen in **B. C** shows one of very few areas that may be considered melanoma of low-grade malignancy (spindle A). **D** shows questionable malignant area at higher magnification. **A,** H&E, ×6; **inset,** fundus; **B,** bleached, H&E, ×69; **C,** bleached, H&E, ×69; **D,** H&E, ×101.

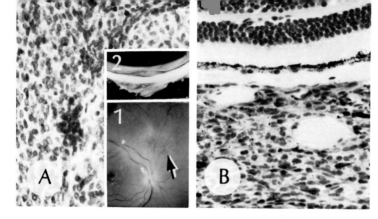

FIG. 17–58. A. Nevus (arrow in inset 1) noted above optic disc some years before. Sudden growth necessitated enucleation (inset 2). Histology shows spindle B type of pattern in this area. B. Most of tumor, however, is composed of nevus cells. A, H&E, ×176; inset 1, macroscopic; inset 2, macroscopic cross-section; B, H&E, ×176.

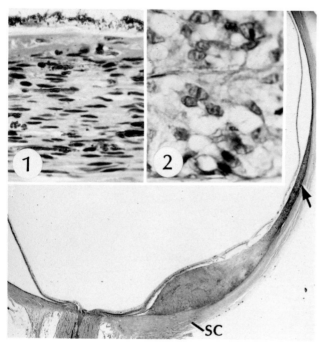

FIG. 17–59. Melanoma arising from nevus. Melanoma, which has invaded scleral canal (sc), has long, tapering (arrow) end. Inset 1 shows higher magnification from area near arrow. Cells are indistinguishable from those observed in choroidal nevi. Inset 2 shows melanoma cells invading scleral canal. Main figure, H&E, ×9; inset 1, H&E, ×500; inset 2, H&E, ×550.

FIG. 17–60. Melanoma arising in diffuse uveal nevus, i.e., congenital ocular melano-cytosis. Uveal tissue is thickened and hyper-pigmented. Note mushroom-shaped, heavily pigmented melanoma posteriorly. Inset 1 shows nevus cells in base of melanoma. Inset 2 shows obviously malignant cells from area above nevus cells. Main figure, H&E, ×8.5; inset 1, bleached, H&E, ×600; inset 2, bleached, H&E, ×600.

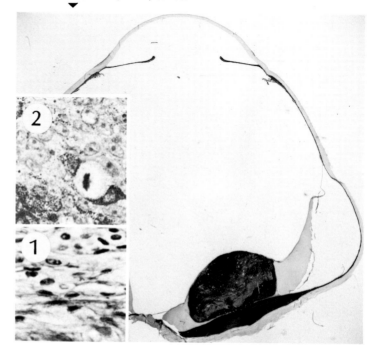

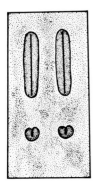

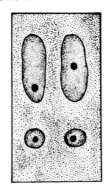

Spindle A   Spindle B

chromatin stripe (nuclear fold)

nucleoli

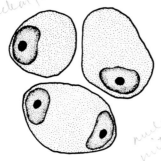

nucleoli mitosis

Epithelioid

FIG. 17–61. Spindle A and spindle B cells are cohesive cells that contain spindle-shaped nuclei with very ill-defined cell borders so that nuclei superficially appear to be in syncytium. Spindle B nuclei are larger and plumper than spindle A nuclei and contain prominent nucleoli rather than nuclear folds ("chromatin stripe"). Epithelioid cells are noncohesive cells that have distinct cell borders and large oval nuclei with prominent nucleoli.

FIG. 17–62. Spindle A melanoma. **A.** Stripe due to infolding of nuclear membrane best noted when nuclei cut in cross-section (*arrows*). Inset shows typical dark stripe parallel to long axis of nuclei. **B.** Spindle A cells are seen along long axis and in cross-section. **A,** 1.5 μ section, toluidine blue, $\times$530; **inset,** H&E, $\times$630; **B,** H&E, $\times$630.

▼

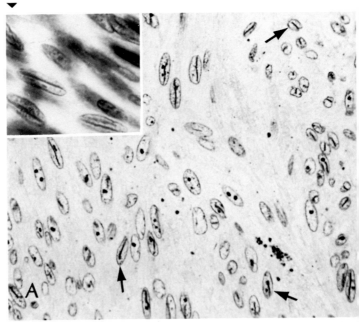

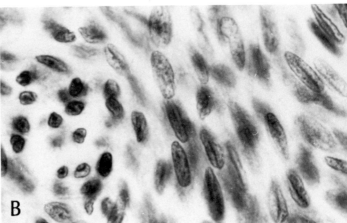

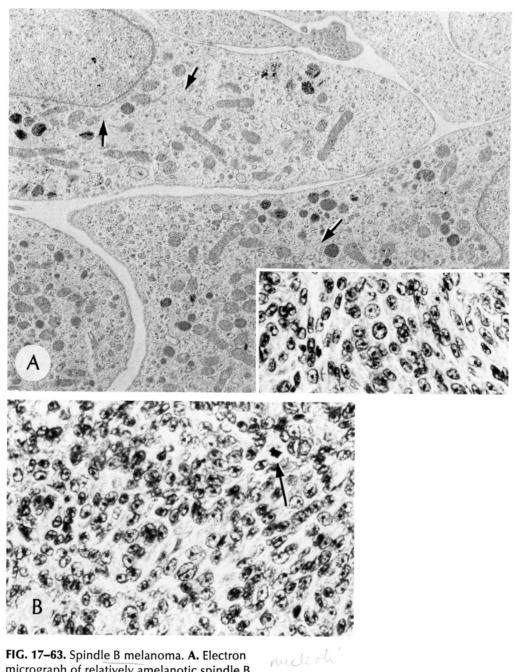

FIG. 17–63. Spindle B melanoma. **A.** Electron micrograph of relatively amelanotic spindle B melanoma. Intracytoplasmic filaments (*arrows*) are present, and mitochondria are elongated and partially oriented along long axis of cell. Melanosomes are all immature. **Inset** shows spindle B cells. **B.** Spindle B cells are identified by their prominent nucleoli. Note mitotic figure (*arrow*). **A,** ×13,000; **inset,** H&E, ×252; **B,** H&E, ×252.

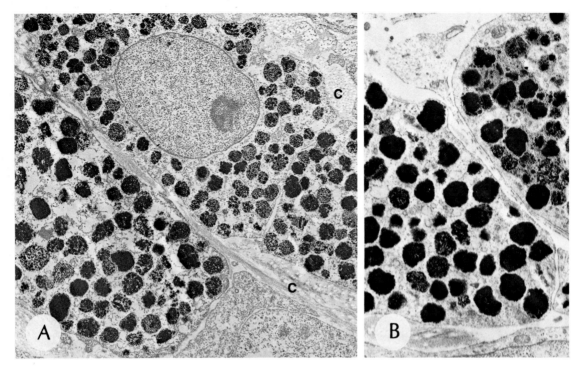

FIG. 17–64. Spindle B melanoma cells. **A.** Many late stage, immature melanosomes are present in cytoplasm. Collagen (i.e., reticulin) of thick and thin diameters (c) is present between cells. **B.** Note macrophage-containing melanin granules of all sizes within phagosomes on right and relatively normal choroidal melanocyte on left. **A,** ×9,000; **B,** ×13,200.

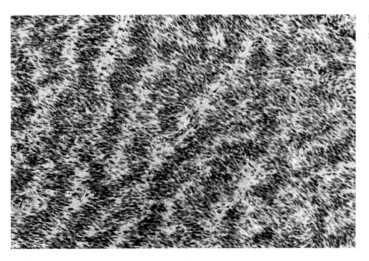

FIG. 17–65. Fascicular pattern formed by spindle B melanoma cells. H&E, ×100.

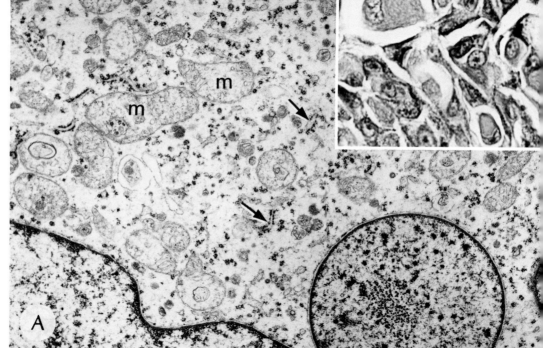

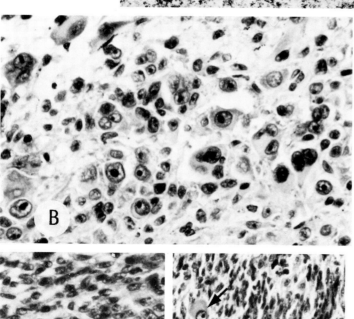

FIG. 17–66. Epithelioid cells. **A.** Cell shows large, watery cytoplasm, lack of cytoplasmic filaments and loose (nonaligned) arrangement of cell organelles (e.g., *m*, mitochondria). There is widespread dispersion of ribosomal clusters (polysomes), while some remain attached to fragments of endoplasmic reticulum (*arrows*). **Inset** is light micrograph to show tendency of cells to separate, i.e., loss of cohesiveness. **B.** Light micrograph shows epithelioid cells recognized by their large oval nuclei with prominent nucleoli and abundant cytoplasm with clearly defined cell borders. Compare to size of spindle B cells in Figure 17–63*B* at same magnification. **A,** ×19,500; **inset,** H&E, ×750; **B,** H&E, ×252.

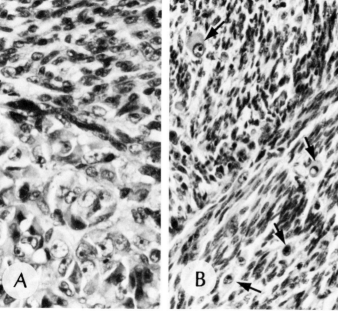

FIG. 17–67. Mixed cell melanoma. **A.** Clusters of epithelioid cells (bottom half) are juxtaposed against clusters of spindle B cells (upper half). **B.** Individual epithelioid cells (*arrows*) may be scattered among spindle B cells. **A,** H&E, ×252; **B,** H&E, ×136.

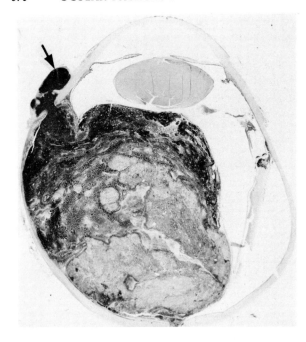

FIG. 17–68. Necrotic melanoma fills most of globe and has extended into epibulbar region at limbus (*arrow*). H&E, ×3.

FIG. 17–69. Necrotic and degenerative ▶ changes in melanoma. **A.** Vacuoles with lipoidal content still intact in vesicles on left. *m,* almost mature melanosome. Lipoidal degeneration of cells of melanoma is seen clearly in thin section in **inset 1.** Electron micrograph shown in **inset 2** shows vacuoles within melanoma cells. **B.** Necrotic material on right is filled with cell debris, pigment-filled macrophages (both melanin and material of hemoglobin origin) as well as clefts of cholesterol crystals. Area of viable tumor cells on left is infiltrated heavily with plasma cells, especially near necrotic border. Some calcium is present within necrotic region (best seen with alizarin stain). **C.** Electron micrograph shows space of dissolved-out cholesterol crystal within mass of necrotic cellular debris. **A.** ×20,000; **inset 1,** 1.5 μ section, PD, ×440; **inset 2,** ×6,000; **B,** H&E, ×35; **C,** ×20,000.

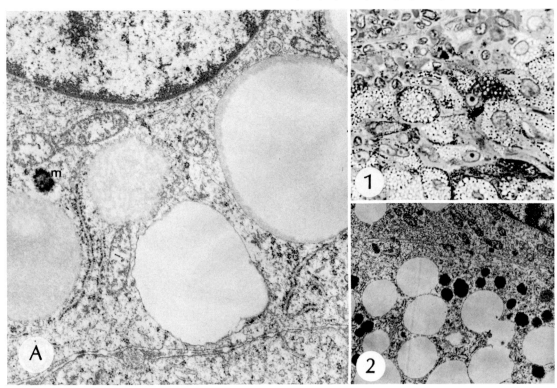

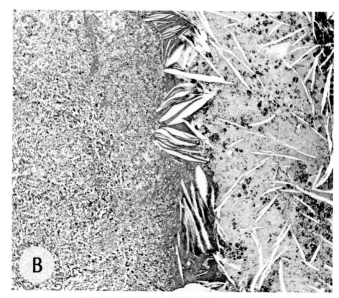

B

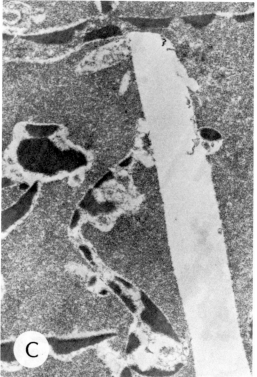

C

FIG. 17–70. Size, shape and pigmentation of tumor. **1–3** show ciliary body tumors. **4** and **5** are same case. Tumors may be deeply melanotic (**5**), amelanotic (**1–3** and **6**), or show gradations of pigmentation (**7–9**). **1**, macroscopic; **2**, macroscopic; **3**, macroscopic; **4**, fundus; **5**, macroscopic; **6**, macroscopic; **7**, macroscopic; **8**, macroscopic; **9**, macroscopic.

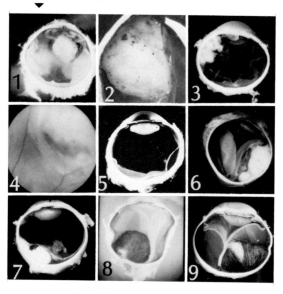

3. Epithelioid (Fig. 17–66)
   a. Epithelioid is the rarest type (3 percent) and is made up of non-cohesive cells with large, round nuclei with prominent nucleoli (frequently pink) and abundant eosinophilic cytoplasm with distinct cell borders.
   b. Mitotic figures are common.
   c. The survival rate is approximately 28 percent.*
4. Mixed (Fig. 17–67)
   a. Mixed cell is the commonest type (45 percent) and consists of a neoplasm showing both a significant spindle-cell component (usually spindle cell B) mixed with a significant epithelioid component (*not* a mixture of spindle A and spindle B cells, but of spindle cells *and* epithelioid cells).
   b. The survival rate is approximately 41 percent.*

* Fifteen-year actuarial survival rates based on a study of 2652 cases by type of cell (Paul et al, 1962).

5. Necrotic (Figs. 17–68 and 17–69)
    a. Necrotic is an uncommon type (7 percent) and consists of a tumor so necrotic that the cell type can not be identified.

    Necrosis may lead to large cystic spaces in the tumor or a large accumulation of eosinophilic debris sometimes containing clefts of cholesterol crystals.

    b. Necrosis of tumor may be due to an autoimmune mechanism as may be evidenced by the presence of a large population of plasma cells.
    c. The survival rate is approximately 41 percent.*
6. Simplified classification
    a. A little under 50 percent of ciliary body and choroidal malignant melanomas are of the spindle-cell variety with an excellent prognosis, i.e., about 73 percent survive.*
    b. A little over 50 percent are of the nonspindle-cell variety (epithelioid, mixed or necrotic) with a poor prognosis, i.e., about 35 percent survive.
E. Other classifications and prognosis
    1. Wilder's stain for reticulin
    In general, heavily fibered malignant melanomas have a better prognosis than lightly fibered ones, but this is not a very reliable criterion.
    2. Degree of pigmentation (Fig. 17–70)
        a. In general, lightly pigmented tumors have a better prognosis than heavily pigmented ones, but this is not a very reliable criterion.
        b. The pigmentation may vary greatly from cell to cell, from region to region and from tumor to tumor.
            1) Unless serial sections are made, one may see only the pigmented part of the tumor or the nonpigmented (amelanotic) part of the tumor.

2) Some tumors are completely amelanotic,* others are maximally pigmented and others show variable pigmentation.
3. Size of tumor (Fig. 17–70)
    a. Malignant melanomas under 1.0 cm³ (approximately 6 DD × 6 DD × 6 DD or smaller clinically) have a very favorable prognosis.

    Of this group of small tumors 69 percent are of the spindle-cell types.

    b. Malignant melanomas over 1.0 cm³ (10 × 10 × 10 mm) have a poor prognosis.

    Of this group of large tumors 57 percent are of the nonspindle-cell types. The poor prognosis in the large tumor group reflects the preponderance of epithelioid cell-containing melanomas.

    c. For practical clinical purposes a solid uveal tumor *under 6 DD in greatest diameter* has a favorable prognosis with a survival rate of of about 73 percent.
F. Associated findings†
    1. Invasion of *Bruch's membrane* occurs in about 63 percent of tumors (Fig. 17–71).
        a. When Bruch's membrane is intact, the tumor generally has an *oval shape.*
        b. With invasion and rupture of Bruch's membrane the tumor takes on a *mushroom shape.*
        c. When ruptured the elastic Bruch's membrane acts as a tourniquet around the base of the tumor such that:
            1) Arterial blood can be pumped easily into the mushroom head, but the venous return is obstructed, thereby leading to

---

* By electron microscopy some poorly formed, immature melanosomes can be found with considerable frequency, even in tumor cells considered completely amelanotic by light microscopy.

† Unpublished data from the 100 consecutive uveal malignant melanomas reported by Yanoff and Zimmerman, 1967.

* Fifteen-year actuarial survival rates based on a study of 2652 cases by type of cell (Paul et al, 1962).

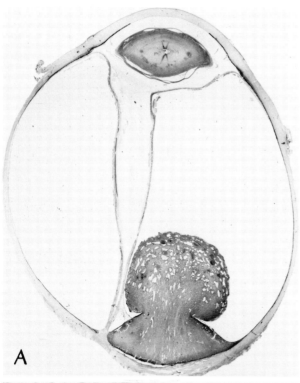

A

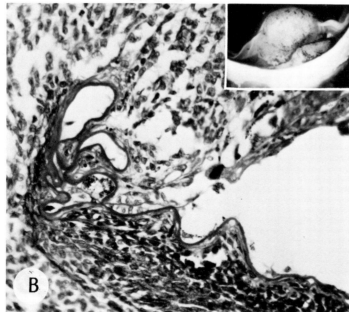

B

FIG. 17–71. **A.** Mushroom shape of melanoma caused by rupture through Bruch's membrane. Note vascular engorgement in head of mushroom and total retinal detachment. **B.** Higher magnification shows curled, ruptured end of Bruch's membrane. **Inset** shows gross appearance of mushroom-shaped melanoma. **A,** H&E, ×4; **B,** H&E, ×340; **inset,** macroscopic.

FIG. 17–72. Melanoma extends into scleral canal (*arrows*). H&E, ×32.

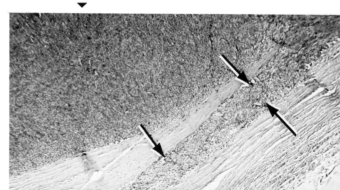

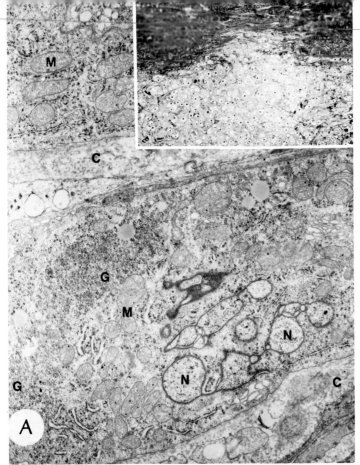

FIG. 17–73. A. Melanoma of choroid invading directly into collagenous lamellas of sclera is seen in **inset.** Electron micrograph of malignant cells within sclera shows that cells contain large quantities of glycogen (*G*), possess large, unoriented mitochondria (*M*) and have bizarre segmentation and infolding of nuclei (*N*). *C*, scleral collagen. **B. Inset** shows that tumor cells from uveal malignant melanoma have been transported by aqueous currents to reach uveal meshwork of anterior chamber drainage angle. Although by light microscopy pigment-bearing cells may be interpreted as macrophages, electron microscopy indicates clearly that cell is producing melanin. Note also area of lipoidal degeneration (*L*). *Tr*, uveal trabecular meshwork. **A,** ×10,500; **inset,** 1.5 μ section, PD, ×130; **B,** ×16,500; **inset,** 1.5 μ section, PD, ×750.

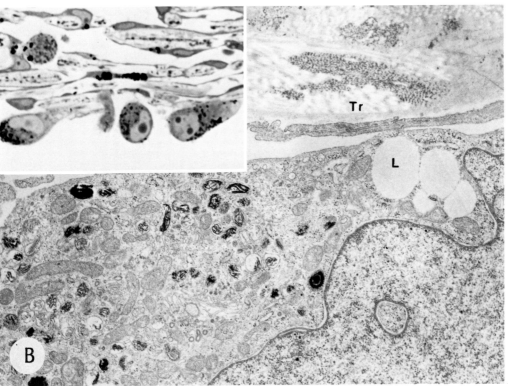

FIG. 17–74. Melanoma arising from juxta-papillary choroid has massively invaded optic nerve, meninges and surrounding orbit. Note retinal detachment. H&E, ×3.

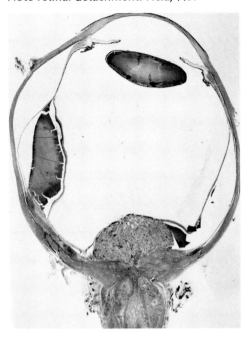

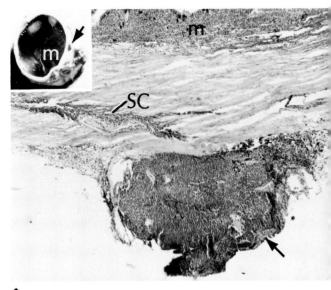

FIG. 17–76. Extraocular extension of melanoma (*arrow*) is present. Note melanoma in scleral canal (*SC*). **Inset** shows macroscopic appearance of same eye. *Arrow* shows extraocular extension. *m*, melanoma. **Main figure,** H&E, ×39; **inset,** macroscopic.

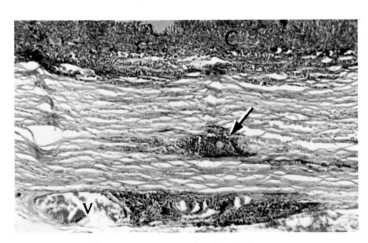

FIG. 17–75. Melanoma is present in choroid (*C*), scleral canal (*arrow*) and vortex vein (*v*). H&E, ×57.

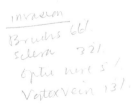

dilated, tortuous venous channels.

2) The vascular abnormalities account for prolonged fluorescein staining.

3) The dilated, thin veins also may lead to intravitreal hemorrhage.

2. Invasion of the scleral canals (Figs. 17–59 and 17–72) occurs in about 32 percent of tumors, thus providing one route by which the tumor gains access to the orbit.

3. Invasion of scleral tissue occurs directly (Fig. 17–73) in about 15 percent of tumors.

4. Invasion of the optic nerve (Fig. 17–74) occurs in about 5 percent of tumors (not nearly as important as invasion of the optic nerve with retinoblastoma—see p. 693 in Chap. 18).

5. Invasion of the vortex veins (Fig. 17–75) occurs in about 13 percent of tumors.

a. One should take sections of the vortex veins routinely for histology on all enucleated globes suspected of harboring an intraocular tumor.

b. Vortex vein invasion carries an extremely unfavorable prognosis.

6. A retinal detachment (Figs. 17–70, 17–71 and 17–74) is present in about 90 percent of cases, but in about 80 percent of these the detachment is localized rather than total.

7. Extraocular extensions (Fig. 17–76) occurs in about 13 percent of tumors.

a. With extraocular extension there is an orbital recurrence rate of 18 percent as compared to 0.7 percent without detectable extraocular extension.

b. If the extraocular portion of the tumor is incised or transected (rather than small and/or well-encapsulated) at the time of enucleation or if it is nonencapsulated, there is an orbital recurrence rate of 50 percent.

c. Frequently discovery of an orbital recurrence precedes the discovery of a metastasis.

Because frequently the orbital recurrence precedes the metastasis, exenteration may be the treatment of choice when there is significant extraocular extension.

8. Reaction of overlying pigment epithelium

a. Secondary drusen (Fig. 17–22).

b. Orange pigment overlying choroidal melanomas is seen clinically in about 47 percent of cases (Fig. 17–77).

Histologically the appearance results from aggregates of RPE cells and lipofuscin-containing macrophages overlying the melanoma.

lipofuscin macrophages

With fluorescein the region of the orange pigment is hypofluorescent.

c. Placoid or adenomatous (see Fig. 11–45) proliferations (Fig. 17–78) frequently are accompanied by degenerative changes in the overlying retina.

G. Unsuspected malignant melanomas

1. Approximately 12 percent of histologically proven ciliary body and choroid malignant melanomas are unsuspected preoperatively.

2. Majority are in glaucoma eyes with *opaque media.*

a. Clinical diagnosis in one series of unsuspected malignant melanomas*:

1) Absolute glaucoma, 50 percent.

2) Secondary glaucoma, 17 percent.

3) Hemorrhagic glaucoma, 8 percent.

4) Retinal detachment, 17 percent.

5) Blind painful eye, 8 percent.

Many of these eyes have a total retinal detachment. Clinically a patient with a retinal detachment plus glaucoma, especially with no previous history of glaucoma and no glaucoma in the other eye, should be considered to have a uveal malignant melanoma until proven otherwise.

H. Unsuspected malignant melanomas Approximately 4 percent of eyes with opaque media enucleated from white patients blind for at least 6 months harbor a malignant melanoma.

This does not mean that 4 percent of in vivo blind eyes with opaque media harbor a malignant melanoma, because the statistics are derived from a study done on already enucleated eyes. The eyes were obviously enucleated for some reason. Therefore, if a blind eye with opaque media becomes clinically symptomatic,

* Unpublished data from the 12 percent of unsuspected malignant melanomas out of the 100 consecutive uveal malignant melanomas reported by Yanoff and Zimmerman, 1967.

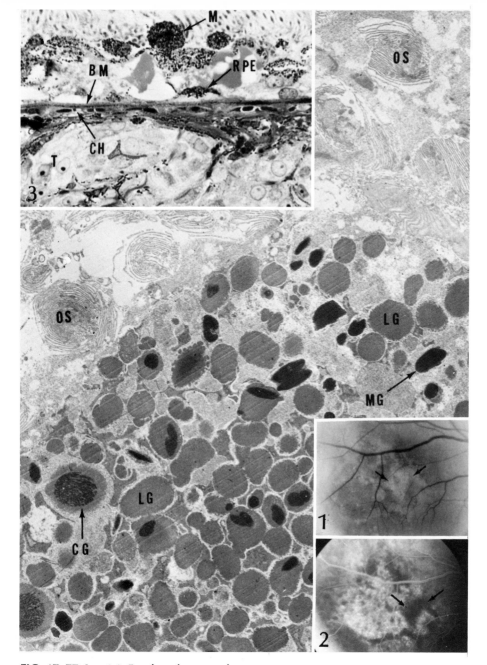

FIG. 17–77. Inset 1. Fundus photograph.
Orange-colored material is present overlying
tumor along *arrows*. Compare with region of
hypofluorescence (*arrows*) as seen in **inset 2.**
Inset 3 shows proliferating pigment epithelium (*RPE*) and associated macrophages
(*M*) overlying tumor (*T*). Macrophages are
migrating into outer layers of neural retina.
BM, Bruch's membrane; *CH,* choriocapillaris.
Electron micrograph shows myriad lipofuscin
granules (*LG*) within pigment-laden macrophage. *OS,* photoreceptor outer segments;
MG, melanin granules; *CG,* compound
granule. **Main figure,** ×11,800; **inset 1,**
fundus; **inset 2,** fundus, fluorescein; **inset 3,**
1.5 μ section, toluidine blue, ×530.

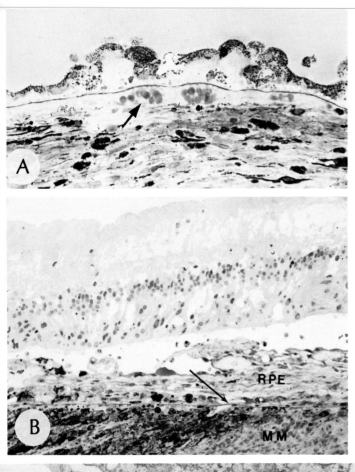

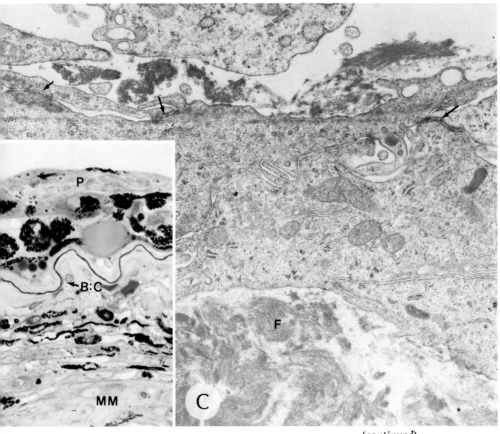

FIG. 17–78. RPE reaction over choroidal melanoma. **A.** Mild RPE cell reaction. Choriocapillaris (*arrow*) is patent. **B.** Plaque of hypopigmented, proliferating, spindle-shaped RPE cells. Underlying choriocapillaris almost obliterated by melanoma (*MM*), and layer of rods and cones is lost. *Arrow* indicates plane of Bruch's membrane. **C. Inset.** Plaque (*P*) of proliferating pigment epithelium overlying choroidal melanoma. *B:C*, Bruch's membrane and choriocapillaris; *MM*, melanoma cells. Electron micrograph shows some of relatively amelanotic proliferated pigment epithelium. Note dense attachments (*arrows*) lying in single plane reminiscent of normal pigment epithelium. Periodicity of finely filamentous extracellular material here indicates that it is fibrin (*F*). **D.** Schematic drawing illustrates flattened papillary growth pattern that may be seen (see Figure 11–45D). Heavy line represents basement membrane, which lines bases of cells. **E.** Retina (*R*) overlying choroidal melanoma (*ME*) shows microcystoid degeneration and widespread loss of photoreceptor layer with adhesion of neural retina to altered RPE. **A,** 1.5 μ section, toluidine blue, ×265; **B,** 1.5 μ section, toluidine blue, ×130; **C,** ×20,000; **inset,** 1.5 μ section, PD, ×395; **E,** H&E, ×50.

(*continued*)

(*continued*)

Neural retina

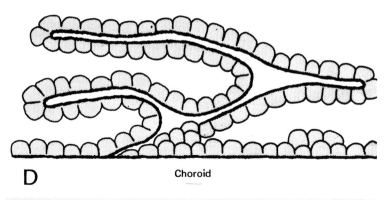

D   Choroid

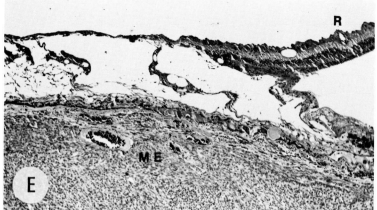

E

the diagnosis of a malignant melanoma should be considered and an enucleation performed. Ultrasonography may be quite helpful in this situation.

I. Differential diagnosis of uveal malignant melanomas
   1. Hemorrhages: choroidal, subpigment epithelial, retinal or subretinal and vitreous.
   2. Cysts: congenital, retinoschisis, solitary and parasitic.
   3. Serous detachment: retinal and choroidal.
   4. Tumors: hemangioma, nevus, metastatic carcinoma, lymphoma, and lesions of pigment epithelium.
   5. Ultrasonography, fluorescein angiography, transillumination and ^{32}P-uptake study are helpful diagnostic methods in determining the correct diagnosis.

J. Primary uveal malignant melanoma

may occur along with another systemic primary tumor.

MELANOTIC TUMORS OF THE OPTIC DISC

MELANOCYTOMA (magnocellular nevus of the nerve head) (Fig. 17–79)

I. A melanocytoma is a nevus composed entirely of maximally pigmented plump polyhedral nevus cells.

In addition to the optic disc, melanocytomas (nevi) may be found in any part of the uvea.

II. Usually they are present at the inferior temporal aspect of the optic disc in patients with "dark" fundi.
   A. Usually the tumor fills less than half the optic disc, but rarely it may fill the

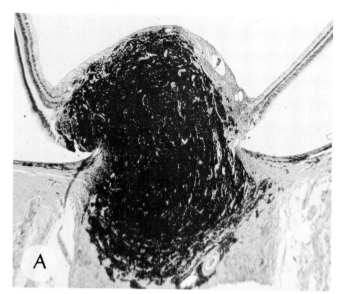

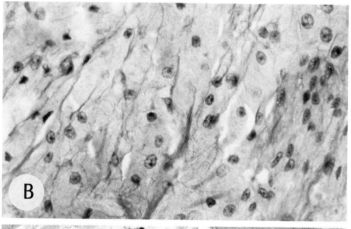

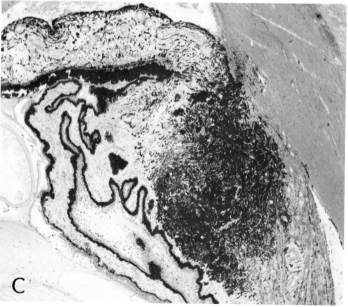

whole disc and may even "spill out" into the adjacent choroid and retina.

    B. It may extend into the vitreous to an "alarming" degree, either directly or as a dispersion of pigment.

III. Whereas the uveal malignant melanoma ratio of white to black is 15:1, the melanocytoma of optic disc ratio of white to black is 0.1:1.0.*

Even when a melanocytoma is present in whites, it generally is seen in patients who have dark fundi. The melanocytoma frequently invades directly into the retina for a short distance and clinically is seen to end in the retina with feathered edges.

IV. It is a benign lesion but probably has the same very low malignant potential of any nevus, and when it occurs in a white individual, it has a higher potential for malignant change than in a black individual.

MALIGNANT MELANOMA

I. Primary malignant melanomas of the optic disc are exceedingly rare, if they occur at all.

II. Most malignant melanomas thought to be primary in the nerve head actually are primary in the juxtapapillary choroid with secondary invasion of the optic disc.

III. About 5 percent of choroidal malignant melanomas invade the optic disc and nerve (Fig. 17–74).

BIBLIOGRAPHY

MELANOTIC TUMORS OF EYELIDS

Allen AC, Spitz S: Clinicopathologic correlation of melanocarcinomas. Cancer 6:1, 1953

Brown EE: Lentigines: their possible significance. Arch Dermatol Syph 47:804, 1943

Clark WH, From L, Bernardino EA, Mihm MC: The histogenesis and biologic behavior of primary human malignant melanomas of the skin. Cancer Res 29:705, 1969

Dorsey CS, Montgomery H: Blue nevus and its distinction from Mongolean spot and the nevus of Ota. J Invest Dermatol 22:225, 1954

Fine BS, Yanoff M: Ocular Histology: A Text and Atlas. New York, Harper & Row, 1972, pp 51–55, 168, 169, 180–186

Fitzpatrik TB, Seiji M, McGugan AD: Melanin pigmentation. N Engl J Med 265:328, 374, 430, 1961

Goldberg M: Waarbenburg's syndrome with fundus and other abnormalities. Arch Ophthalmol 76:797, 1966

Lund HZ, Kraus JM: Melanotic Tumors of the Skin, in Atlas of Tumor Pathology, Section I, Fascicle 3. Washington, D.C., Armed Forces Institute of Pathology, 1962

Schrader WA, Helwig EB: Balloon cell nevi. Cancer 20:1502, 1967

Waardenburg PJ: A new syndrome combining developmental anomalies of the eyelids, eyebrows and nose root, with pigmentary defects of the iris and head hair, and with congenital deafness. Am J Hum Genet 3:195, 1951

MELANOTIC TUMORS OF CONJUNCTIVA

Dhermy P, Barry R: Naevus naevo-cellulaire à cellules ballonnisantes de la conjonctive. A propos de trois nouveaux cas. Arch Ophtalmol (Paris) 34:303, 1974

Elsas FJ, Green WR, Ryan SJ: Benign pigmented tumors arising in acquired conjunctival melanosis. Am J Ophthalmol 78:229, 1974

Gow JA, Spencer WH: Intraocular extension of an epibulbar malignant melanoma. Arch Ophthalmol 90:57, 1973

Henkind P, Friedman AH: External ocular pigmentation. Int Ophthalmol Clin 11:87, 1971

Jay B: Naevi and melanomata of the conjunctiva. Br J Ophthalmol 49:169, 1965

Kielar RA: Limbal melanoma in a Negro. Arch Ophthalmol 87:392, 1972

Pfaffenbach DD, Green WR, Maumenee AE: Balloon cell nevus of the conjunctiva. Arch Ophthalmol 87:192, 1972

Reese AB: Precancerous and cancerous melanosis. Am J Ophthalmol 61:1272, 1966

Welsh NH, Jhavery Y: Malignant melanoma of the cornea in an African patient. Am J Ophthalmol 72:796, 1971

Yanoff M: Pigment spots of the sclera. Arch Ophthalmol 81:151, 1969

Yanoff M, Scheie HG: Argyrosis of conjunctiva and lacrimal sac. Arch Ophthalmol 71:57, 1964

Yanoff M, Zimmerman LE: Histogenesis of malignant melanomas of the uvea. III. The relationship of congenital ocular melanocytosis and neurofibromatosis to uveal melanomas. Arch Ophthalmol 77:331, 1967

Zimmerman LE: Criteria for management of melanosis: in correspondence: Arch Ophthalmol 76:307, 1966

MELANOTIC TUMORS OF PIGMENT EPITHELIUM OF IRIS, CILIARY BODY AND RETINA

Farkas TG, Krill AE, Sylvester VM, Archer D: Familial and secondary drusen: histologic and functional correlations. Trans Am Acad Ophthalmol Otolaryngol 75:333, 1971

---

* The often quoted 1:1 statistic for melanocytomas is not corrected for the racial ratio in the United States and probably should be 0.1:1.0.

Farkas TG, Sylvester V, Archer D: The ultrastructure of drusen. Am J Ophthalmol 71:1196, 1971

Farkas TG, Sylvester V, Archer D, Altona M: The histochemistry of drusen. Am J Ophthalmol 71:1207, 1971

Fine BS: Free floating pigmented cyst in the anterior chamber. A clinicopathologic report. Am J Ophthalmol 67:493, 1969

Fine BS, Yanoff M: Ocular Histology: A Text and Atlas. New York, Harper & Row, 1972, pp 154, 189, 190, 225, 226

Font RL, Zimmerman LE, Fine BS: Adenoma of the retinal pigment epithelium: histochemical and electron microscopic observations. Am J Ophthalmol 73:544, 1972

Frayer WC: Reactivity of the retinal pigment epithelium: an experimental and histopathologic study. Trans Am Ophthalmol Soc 64:586, 1966

Frayer WC: Neoplasms and related lesions of the retinal pigment epithelium. Int Ophthalmol Clin 12:63, 1972

Garner A: Tumors of the retinal pigment epithelium. Br J Ophthalmol 54:715, 1970

Green WR, Iliff WJ, Trotter RR: Malignant teratoid medulloepithelioma of the optic nerve. Arch Ophthalmol 91:451, 1974

Kurz GH, Zimmerman LE: Vagaries of the retinal pigment epithelium. Int Ophthalmol Clin 2:441, 1962

Manz HJ, Rosen DA, Macklin RD, Willis WE: Neuroectodermal tumor of anterior lip of the optic cup. Glioneuroma transitional to teratoid medullo-epithelioma. Arch Ophthalmol 89:382, 1973

Mullaney J: Primary malignant medullopithelioma of the retinal stalk. Am J Ophthalmol 77:499, 1974

Spencer WH, Jesberg DO: Glioneuroma (choristomatous malformation of the optic cup margin). A report of two cases. Arch Ophthalmol 89:387, 1973

Streeten BW, McGraw JL: Tumor of the ciliary pigment epithelium. Am J Ophthalmol 74:420, 1972

Swan KC: Iris pigment nodules complicating miotic therapy. Am J Ophthalmol 37:886, 1954

Tso MOM, Albert DM: Pathological condition of the retinal pigment epithelium. Neoplasms and nodular nonneoplastic lesions. Arch Ophthalmol 88:27, 1972

Vogel MH, Zimmerman LE, Gass JDM: Proliferation of the juxtapapillary retinal pigment epithelium simulating malignant melanoma. Doc Ophthalmol 26:461, 1969

Wallow IHL, Tso MOM: Proliferation of the retinal pigment epithelium over malignant choroidal tumors—a light and electron microscopic study. Am J Ophthalmol 73:914, 1972

Wolter JR: Proliferating pigment epithelium—producing a simple organoid structure in the subretinal space of a human eye. Arch Ophthalmol 77:651, 1967

Yanoff M, Zimmerman LE: Pseudomelanoma of anterior chamber caused by implantation of iris pigment epithelium. Arch Ophthalmol 74:302, 1965

Zimmerman LE: Melanocytes, melanocytic nevi and melanocytomas. Invest Ophthalmol 4:11, 1965

Zimmerman LE: Verhoeff's "terato-neuroma": a critical reappraisal in light of new observations and current concepts of embryonic tumors. Am J Ophthalmol 72:1039, 1971

Zimmerman LE, Font RL, Anderson SR: Rhabdomyosarcomatous differentiation in malignant intraocular medulloepitheliomas. Cancer 30:817, 1972

MELANOTIC TUMORS OF THE UVEA: IRIS

Ferry AP: Lesions mistaken for malignant melanomas of the iris. Arch Ophthalmol 74:9, 1965

Fine BS, Yanoff M: Ocular Histology: A Text and Atlas. New York, Harper & Row, 1972, pp 168–185

Iwamoto T, Reese AB, Mund ML: Tapioca melanoma of the iris. 2. Electron microscopy of the melanoma cells compared with normal iris melanocytes. Am J Ophthalmol 74:851, 1972

Reese AB, Mund ML, Iwamoto T: Tapioca melanoma of the iris. I. Clinical and light microscopy studies. Am J Ophthalmol 74:840, 1972

Rones B, Zimmerman LE: The prognosis of primary tumors of the iris treated by iridectomy. Arch Ophthalmol 60:193, 1958

Scheie HG, Yanoff M: Iris nevus (Cogan-Reese) syndrome. Arch Ophthalmol. In press

Yanoff M, Zimmerman LE: Pseudomelanoma of anterior chamber caused by implantation of iris pigment epithelium. Arch Ophthalmol 74:302, 1965

Zimmerman LE: Clinical pathology of iris tumors. Am J Clin Pathol 39:214, 1963

MELANOTIC TUMORS OF THE UVEA: CILIARY BODY AND CHOROID

Bierring F, Jensen OA: Electron microscopy of melanomas of the human uveal tract: the ultrastructure of four malignant melanomas of the mixed-cell type. Acta Ophthalmol (Kbh) 42:665, 1964

Callender GR: Malignant melanotic tumors of the eye: a study of histologic types in 111 cases. Trans Am Acad Ophthalmol Otolaryngol 36:131, 1931

Char DH, Hollinshead A, Cogan DG, Ballintine EJ, Hogan MJ, Herberman RB: Cutaneous delayed hypersensitivity reaction to soluble melanoma antigen. N Engl J Med 291:274, 1974

Cogan DG, Kuwabara T: Tumors of the ciliary body. Int Ophthalmol Clin 11:27, 1971

Federman JL, Lewis MG, Clark WH, Egerer I, Sarin LK: Tumor-associated antibodies in the serum of ocular melanoma patients. Trans Am Acad Ophthalmol Otolaryngol 78:784, 1974

Ferry AP: Lesions mistaken for malignant melanoma of posterior uvea. Arch Ophthalmol 72:463, 1964

Fine BS, Yanoff M: Ocular Histology: A Text and Atlas. New York, Harper & Row, 1972, pp 185–211

Flocks M, Gerende JH, Zimmerman LE: The size and shape of malignant melanomas of the choroid and ciliary body in relation to prognosis and histologic characteristics. Trans Am Acad Ophthalmol Otolaryngol 59:740, 1955

Font RL, Spaulding AG, Zimmerman LE: Diffuse

malignant melanoma of the uveal tract: a clinicopathologic report of 54 cases. Trans Am Acad Ophthalmol Otolaryngol 72:877, 1968

Font RL, Zimmerman LE, Armaly MF: The nature of the orange pigment over a choroidal melanoma—histochemical and electron microscopic observations. Arch Ophthalmol 91:359, 1974

Hale PN, Allen RA, Straatsma BR: Benign melanomas (nevi) of the choroid and ciliary body. Arch Ophthalmol 74:532, 1965

Henkind P, Roth MS: Breast carcinoma and concurrent uveal melanoma. Am J Ophthalmol 71:198, 1971

Iwamoto T, Jones IS, Howard GM: Ultrastructural comparison of spindle A, spindle B, and epithelioid-type cells in uveal malignant melanoma. Invest Ophthalmol 11:873, 1972

Jensen OA: Malignant melanomas of the uvea in Denmark. Acta Ophthalmol (Kbh) [Suppl 75] p. 1, 1963

Kroll AJ, Kuwabara T: Electron microscopy of uveal melanoma—a comparison of spindle and epithelioid cells. Arch Ophthalmol 73:378, 1965

Litricin O: Unsuspected uveal melanomas. Am J Ophthalmol 76:734, 1974

Makley TA, Teed RW: Unsuspected intraocular tumors. Arch Ophthalmol 60:475, 1958

Naumann G: Pigmentierete Naevi der Aderhaut und des Ciliarkörpers. Adv Ophthalmol 23:187, 1970

Naumann GOH, Hellner K, Naumann LR: Pigmented nevi of the choroid. Clinical study of secondary changes in the overlying tissues. Trans Am Acad Ophthalmol Otolaryngol 75:110, 1971

Naumann G, Yanoff M, Zimmerman LE: Histogenesis of malignant melanomas of the uvea. I. Histopathologic characteristics of nevi of the choroid and ciliary body. Arch Ophthalmol 76:784, 1966

Naumann G, Zimmerman LE, Yanoff M: Visual field defect associated with choroidal nevus. Am J Ophthalmol 62:914, 1966

Newsom WA, Hood CI, Horwitz JA, Fine SL, Sewell JH: Cystoid macular edema: histopathologic and angiographic correlations. A clinicopathologic case report. Trans Am Acad Ophthalmol Otolaryngol 76:1005, 1972

Paul EV, Parnell BL, Fraker M: Prognosis of malignant melanomas of the choroid and ciliary body. Int Ophthalmol Clin 2:387, 1962

Rahi AHS: Autoimmune reactions in uveal melanoma. Br J Ophthalmol 55:793, 1971

Riley FC: Balloon cell melanoma of the choroid. Arch Ophthalmol 92:131, 1974

Scheie HG, Yanoff M: Pseudomelanoma of ciliary body, report of a patient. Arch Ophthalmol 77:81, 1967

Shields JA, Zimmerman LE: Lesions simulating malignant melanoma of the posterior uvea. Arch Ophthalmol 89:466, 1973

Smith LT, Irvine AR: Diagnostic significance of orange pigment accumulation over choroidal tumors. Am J Ophthalmol 76:212, 1973

Starr HJ, Zimmerman LE: Extrascleral extension and orbital recurrence of malignant melanomas of the choroid and ciliary body. Int Ophthalmol Clin 2:369, 1962

Tasman W: Familial intraocular melanoma. Trans Am Acad Ophthalmol Otolaryngol 74:955, 1970

Wallow IHL, Tso MOM: Proliferation of the retinal pigment epithelium over malignant choroidal tumors—a light and electron microscopic study. Am J Ophthalmol 73:914, 1972

Yanoff M: Glaucoma mechanisms in ocular malignant melanomas. Am J Ophthalmol 70:898, 1970

Yanoff M: Mechanisms of glaucoma in eyes with uveal malignant melanomas. Int Ophthalmol Clin 12:51, 1972

Yanoff M, Scheie HG: Melanomalytic glaucoma: report of patient. Arch Ophthalmol 84:471, 1970

Yanoff M, Zimmerman LE: Histogenesis of malignant melanomas of the uvea. II. Relationship of uveal nevi to malignant melanomas. Cancer 20:493, 1967

Yanoff M, Zimmerman LE: Histogenesis of malignant melanomas of uvea. III. The relationship of congenital ocular melanocytosis and neurofibromatosis to uveal melanomas. Arch Ophthalmol 77:331, 1967

Zimmerman LE: Problems in the diagnosis of malignant melanomas of the choroid and ciliary body. Am J Ophthalmol 75:917, 1973

MELANOTIC TUMORS OF THE OPTIC DISC

Wiznia RA, Price J: Recovery of vision in association with a melanocytoma of the optic disc. Am J Ophthalmol 78:236, 1974

Zimmerman LE: Melanocytes, melanocytic nevi and melanocytomas. Invest Ophthalmol 4:11, 1965

chapter 18

Retinoblastoma and Pseudoglioma

RETINOBLASTOMA

HISTORICAL ASPECTS

I. Early Period
   A. Petrus Pawius of Leiden in 1597 probably was the first to describe the entity that we now recognize as retinoblastoma.
   B. In 1767 a very accurate description of bilateral retinoblastoma was given by Hayes of London.

II. Nineteenth Century
   A. James Wardrop of Edinburgh clearly established retinoblastoma as an entity in 1809.
   B. Virchow called the tumor *glioma of the retina* in 1864 in the belief that the tumor arose from glial cells.
   C. In 1891 Flexner and in 1897 Wintersteiner described the rosettes that are frequently found in the tumor. They believed that the tumor arose from precursor cells of the neuroepithelium, i.e., photoreceptors, and called it a *neuroepithelioma*.

III. Twentieth Century
   A. HL Hilgartner was the first to treat retinoblastoma with x ray.
   B. Verhoeff suggested the term retinoblastoma, which was adopted by the American Ophthalmological Society in 1926. Verhoeff believed that the tumor was composed of embryonic retinal cells.
   C. Moore, Stallard and Milner were the first to destroy retinoblastoma with implanted radon seeds.
   D. Gillette and Bodenstein in 1946 pointed out the potential usefulness of triethylene melamine, and in 1953 Kupfer was the first to treat retinoblastoma with nitrogen mustard.
   E. Tso, Fine and Zimmerman demonstrated the presence of photoreceptor differentiation (*fleurettes*) in retinoblastomas in 1970.

GENERAL INFORMATION

I. Retinoblastoma, along with leukemia and neuroblastoma, is one of the most common childhood malignancies and is the most common childhood intraocular neoplasm.
II. It is third to uveal malignant melanoma and metastatic carcinoma as the most common intraocular malignancy in humans.
III. The frequency is approximately 1 in 15,000 to 34,000 live births with a trend toward a higher incidence than presently found.
IV. There is no significant race or sex predilection.
V. Bilaterality occurs in 20 to 35 percent of all cases.
VI. The eye is normal in size at birth but later may become phthisical or buphthalmic.
VII. Age at time of initial diagnosis:
   A. Average age is 13 months with 89 percent diagnosed before 3 years of age.
   B. It is rare after 7 years of age but has been reported in patients past 50 years of age.
VIII. Children with retinoblastoma may have other abnormalities such as the D-deletion (13q−) syndrome, XXX chromosomal abnormality, 21 trisomy, the Pierre Robin syndrome or hereditary congenital cataracts.
IX. Retinoblastoma is the only known cancer in humans inherited through a *dominant autosomal gene*.

HEREDITY*

I. Familial cases
   A. About 6 percent of all retinoblastoma

* An alternative theory to the purely genetic mode of inheritance is one stating that retinoblastoma is not primarily the direct expression of a gene action but

cases are inherited through a dominant autosomal gene with incomplete penetrance (50 to 85 percent).

B. About 50 percent of the cases are bilateral.

II. Sporadic cases

A. About 94 percent of all retinoblastomas develop by mutation (sporadic cases).

The mutation rate is about 2×10^{-5} (1 in 36,000 births) with 25 percent representing a genetic mutation capable of transmitting the retinoblastoma to their offspring as an irregular autosomal dominant. The remaining 75 percent represent a somatic mutation incapable of transmitting the tumor.

genetic

somatic

B. About 30 percent of the cases are bilateral.

III. Genetic counselling

A. Healthy parents with one affected child run about a 6 percent risk of producing more affected children.

B. If two or more siblings are affected, there is a 50 percent risk that each additional child will be affected.

C. A retinoblastoma survivor with the hereditary type has a 50 percent chance of producing affected children.

D. A sporadically affected person has a 12.5 percent chance of producing affected children.

E. Phenotypically normal children of an affected parent may be genetically abnormal.

HISTOLOGY

I. The basic cell type is the radiosensitive, *undifferentiated retinoblastoma cell* (Fig. 18–1).

II. Rosettes are of two types:

A. *Flexner-Wintersteiner rosettes* (Fig. 18–2) are the characteristic rosette of

---

rather the result of some oncogenic factor in the environment, a factor to which retinal cells might become particularly vulnerable as a consequence of an abnormal dominant gene. The oncogenic factor presumably is a virus. The finding of RNA-directed DNA-polymerase type activity in retinoblastomas is circumstantial evidence that a virus is involved in the histogenesis of retinoblastomas.

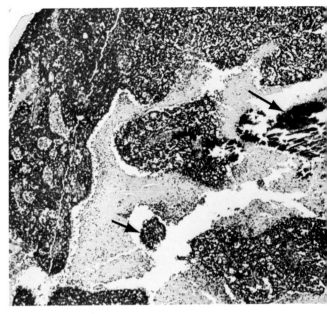

FIG. 18–1. Retinoblastoma is composed of undifferentiated, tightly packed cells with large hyperchromic nuclei and scant cytoplasm. No stroma is present. Areas of necrosis (pale areas) and calcification (*arrows*) are characteristic. H&E, ×40.

has a ... % chance of having the potentiality to produce affected children

→ but 25%

retinoblastoma, but they are not always present. In these rosettes the cells line up around an apparently empty central lumen. Special stains show that the lumen contains a hyaluronidase-resistant acid mucopolysaccharide.

B. *Homer-Wright rosettes* are found in medulloblastomas and neuroblastomas in addition to being seen occasionally in retinoblastomas. In these rosettes the cells line up around an area containing cobweblike material but no acid mucopolysaccharides.

III. Pseudorosette. This is a very poor and confusing term that is often used to refer to arrangements within the tumor that on cursory examination may resemble the above rosettes. These structures are formed by:

A. Viable tumor cells clustering around blood vessels from which they derive their nourishment.

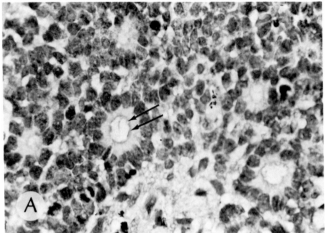

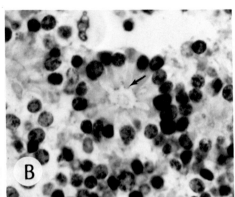

FIG. 18–2. Flexner-Wintersteiner rosettes. **A.** Cuboidal tumor cells with nuclei toward bases are arranged around central lumen. Delicate limiting membrane (*arrows*) can be seen at apexes of cells surrounding lumen. **B.** Delicate limiting membrane consists of interrupted series of small densities (*arrow*). **A,** H&E, ×440; **B,** 1.5 μ section, toluidine blue, ×615.

B. Small foci of necrotic cells between larger masses of viable tumor cells.

C. Incompletely formed Flexner-Wintersteiner or Homer-Wright rosettes.

IV. Fleurettes (Fig. 18–3). These are flowerlike groupings of tumor cells within the retinoblastoma that clearly show evidence of differentiation into photoreceptor elements.

A. Fleurettes may be absent, may be present in small nodules or rarely may be present as the only cells in the tumor, i.e., differentiation of the entire tumor into photoreceptorlike elements.

B. Regions of photoreceptor differentiation generally lack evidence of either necrosis or calcification.

The increased differentiation suggests improved prognosis but also suggests radio resistance.

V. Other histologic features

A. Necrosis is present in most tumors (Figs. 18–4 and 18–5).

Total necrosis may lead to spontaneous and complete regression, a rare occurrence. With complete regression the eye sometimes retains useful vision. The regression or necrosis of the retinoblastoma may be due to a cytotoxic effect of lymphocytes against the retinoblastoma cells.

B. Calcification is a frequent and important diagnostic feature, which may be

FIG. 18–3. Fleurettes. **A.** Retinoblastoma with ▶ photoreceptor differentiation is shown. *Arrows* indicate pale eosinophilic cellular regions of differentiation. **Inset** shows fundus appearance of completely differentiated retinoblastoma. **B.** Note flowerlike arrangement, i.e., fleurette (*double arrow*), of cells undergoing photoreceptor differentiation (as illustrated in **C**). Other regions (*arrows*) have photoreceptor differentiation with less pronounced fleurette arrangement. **C.** Electron micrograph shows photoreceptor inner segments resembling those of cone cells radiating from attachment girdle (*arrows*) of external limiting membrane of zonulae adherentes. *M,* mitochondria. **A,** H&E, ×8; **inset,** fundus; **B,** 1.5 μ section, PD, ×575; **C,** ×5,500.

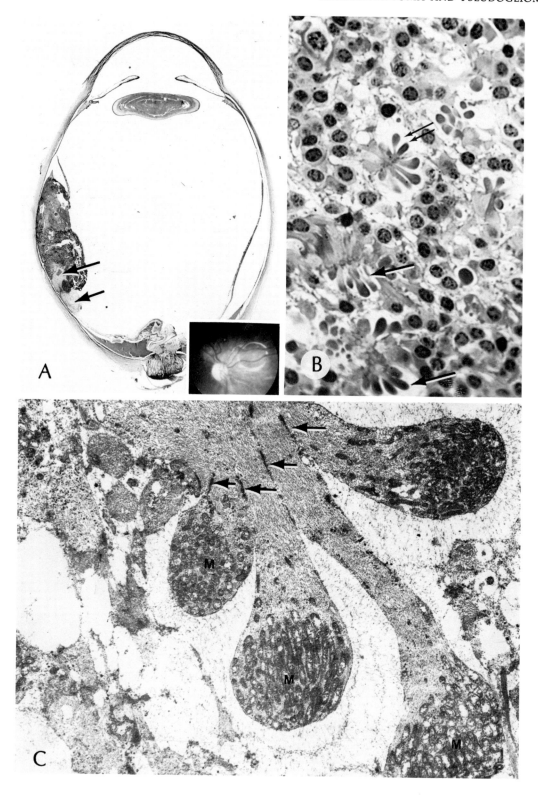

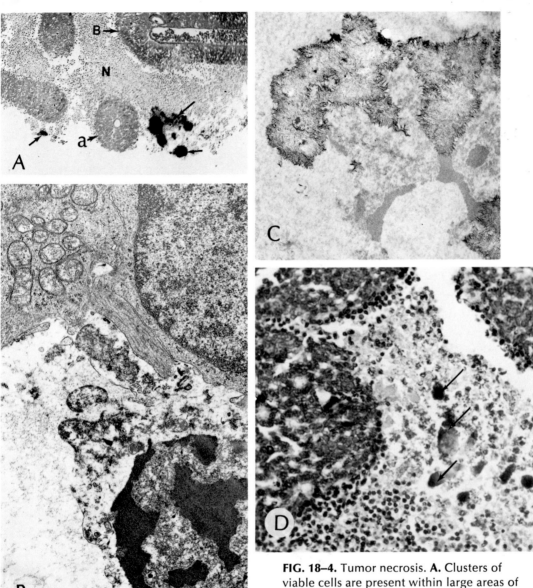

FIG. 18–4. Tumor necrosis. **A.** Clusters of viable cells are present within large areas of necrosis (*N*). Viable cells (*a*) clustering about small lumen or about blood vessel (*B*) may resemble superficially rosettes and hence sometimes are called pseudorosettes, a poor term. Dark areas (*arrows*) are areas of calcification. **B.** Electron micrograph of transition between viable cells (above) and necrotic cells (below). Note clumping of nuclear chromatin and focal densification of cytoplasmic components in necrotic cell. **C.** Calcification, in form of myriad spicules, is occurring in debris of necrotic cell. **D.** Calcification is present here in region of cell necrosis (*arrows,* basophilic region with H&E). Rosettes are plentiful in region of viable cells on left. **A,** alizarin red, ×60; **B,** ×16,000; **C,** ×16,000; **D,** H&E, ×305.

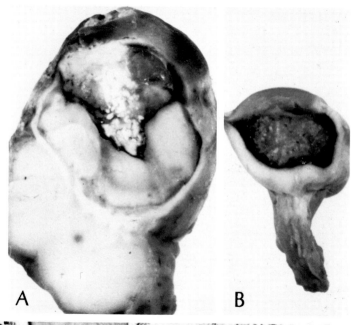

A

B

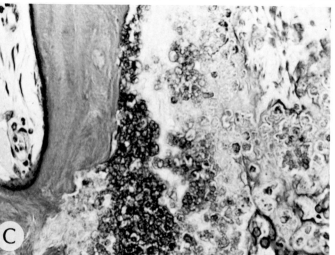

C

FIG. 18–5. Necrosis and spontaneous regression of retinoblastoma. **A** and **B.** Bilateral retinoblastoma with enlargement of one eye (**A**) and phthisis bulbi of other (**B**). **C.** Retinoblastoma cells are fossilized. Ossification is present. **A** and **B,** macroscopic; **C,** H&E, ×300.

FIG. 18–6. Exophytic retinoblastoma is characterized by tumor growing predominantly toward subretinal space. Note multifocal growth of retinoblastoma. **Inset 1** shows macroscopic appearance of tumor. **Inset 2** shows clinical appearance of another exophytic retinoblastoma presenting with bullous retinal detachment. **Main figure,** H&E, ×4; **inset 1,** macroscopic; **inset 2,** clinical.

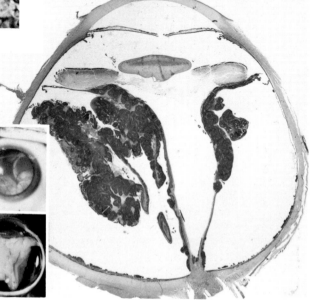

2

1

detected clinically. It is present mainly in areas of necrosis.

C. Basophilic areas around blood vessels and also lying freely within the tumor may represent deoxyribonucleic acid (DNA) deposition.

D. About 1.5 percent of cases have a diffuse, infiltrating type of tumor without a discrete retinal mass. This type of tumor occurs in a slightly older age group than the usual type, tends not to be bilateral and frequently is accompanied by a simulated hypopyon.

GROWTH PATTERN

I. Multifocal growth (Fig. 18–6), i.e., spontaneous development from more than one region of the same retina, is seen frequently within an eye.

II. Bilateral involvement (Fig. 18–5) is a reflection of multifocal retinal involvement affecting both eyes.

III. Endophytic retinoblastoma (Fig. 18–7). This tumor grows predominantly toward the vitreous and the retina is not detached.

IV. Exophytic retinoblastoma (Fig. 18–6). This grows predominantly toward the subretinal space and detaches the retina. Most retinoblastomas have both endophytic and exophytic components.

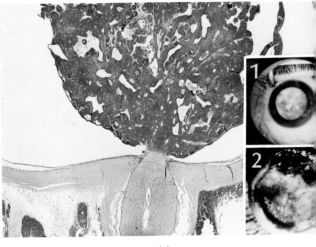

FIG. 18–7. Endophytic retinoblastoma. Retinoblastoma involving almost all of retina on either side of optic nerve head. Growth is mostly inward (endophytum). Although nerve head is involved, there has been no invasion of optic nerve proper. **Insets** show clinical (**1**) and macroscopic (**2**) appearance of endophytic retinoblastoma of another case. Note resemblance of tumor in clinical picture to brain tissue. **Main figure,** H&E, ×6; **inset 1,** clinical; **inset 2,** macroscopic.

MODE OF EXTENSION

I. Local spread
   A. Anteriorly by seeding into the vitreous and aqueous (Fig. 18–8).

   Aqueous seeding may simulate an hypopyon. Deposits may appear on the iris and in the anterior chamber angle and produce a secondary open angle glaucoma.

   B. Posteriorly (Figs. 18–9 and 18–10) by direct extension into the subretinal space, invasion into the choroid where the tumor may gain access to the systemic circulation or spread into the optic nerve where the cells may gain access to the subarachnoid space by passage alongside the central retinal vessels within the nerve to their exit across the subarachnoid space.

II. Extraocular extension
   A. Orbit (Fig. 18–10).
   B. Brain.

III. Metastases. Metastatic spread is assumed to have occurred when examination reveals that the choroid (massively) or the cut end of the optic nerve is invaded by tumor cells.

PROGNOSIS

I. The prognosis for life is much improved in recent years due to earlier diagnosis and improved methods of treatment. Bilateral cases have the same general fatality rate as unilateral cases.

II. Histologic correlation
   A. Cellular differentiation
      1. An individual who has a tumor with abundant Flexner-Wintersteiner rosettes has about a sixfold better prognosis than one with a tumor with no rosettes.
      2. A tumor composed entirely of fleurettes is believed to augur a

better prognosis than one with no fleurettes and probably better than a tumor with abundant Flexner-Wintersteiner rosettes but with no fleurettes.

B. With slight choroidal invasion the mortality rate is around 25 percent; with massive invasion the mortality rate is around 65 percent.

C. Optic nerve involvement:
1. With no invasion the mortality rate is around 8 percent.
2. With invasion to the lamina cribrosa the mortality rate is around 15 percent.
3. With invasion posteriorly beyond the lamina cribrosa the mortality rate is around 44 percent.
4. With invasion to the line of transection or to the posterior point of exit of the central retinal vessels from the optic nerve, the mortality rate is around 65 percent.

D. The presence of rubeosis iridis is a poor prognostic sign.

E. The clinical prognosis is determined by the location and size of the tumor.

CLINICAL FEATURES

I. Early lesions may present with visual difficulties, strabismus or may be completely asymptomatic, as with small fundus lesions found on routine eye examination.

II. Moderate lesions may present as:
A. Leukokoria, i.e., "cat's eye reflex" (Figs. 18–7 and 18–9A).
B. Inflammation with hypopyon, uveitis, endophthalmitis or panophthalmitis (Fig. 18–8). *Suspect any unusual childhood eye inflammation as being retinoblastoma.*
C. Rubeosis iridis (Fig. 18–11) with a hyphema or chronic secondary angle closure glaucoma.

The glaucoma may lead to symptoms of photophobia. With glaucoma of prolonged duration buphthalmos may develop. Not only glaucoma but also hyphema may result from the rubeosis iridis. Spontaneous hyphema in a child should always alert one to suspect retinoblastoma (along with juvenile xanthogranuloma).

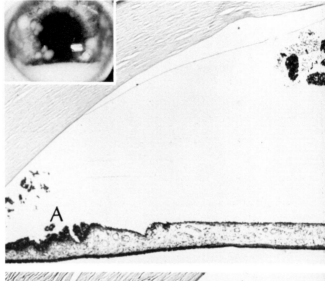

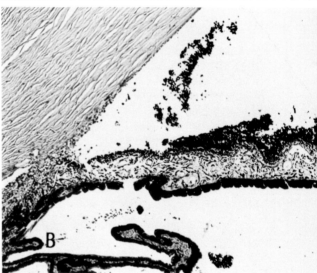

FIG. 18–8. Retinoblastoma is present freely in anterior chamber and on anterior surface of iris (**A**). **Inset** shows clinical appearance of retinoblastoma hypopyon and clumps of cells in aqueous and on iris surface. **B.** Tumor present in anterior chamber angle simulated clinical hypopyon. **A,** H&E, ×16; **inset,** clinical; **B,** H&E, ×40.

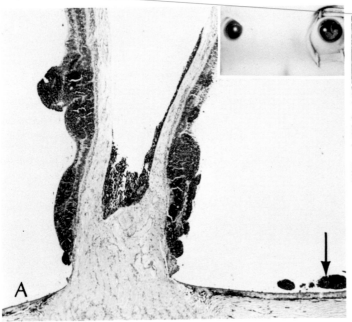

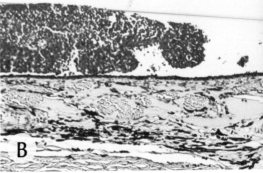

FIG. 18–9. Posterior seeding of retinoblastoma. **A.** Seeding is present on internal and external surfaces of detached retina and in subretinal space (*arrow*). **Inset** shows exophytic retinoblastoma of left eye presenting as bullous retinal detachment. **B.** Retinoblastoma has seeded onto RPE. **A,** H&E, ×16; **inset,** clinical; **B,** H&E, ×69.

FIG. 18–10. Retinoblastoma has massively invaded choroid (c), subarachnoid space around optic nerve (o) and orbit (*arrows*). *L*, lens; *s*, sclera. **Inset** shows macroscopic appearance. **Main figure,** H&E, ×4; **inset,** macroscopic.
▼

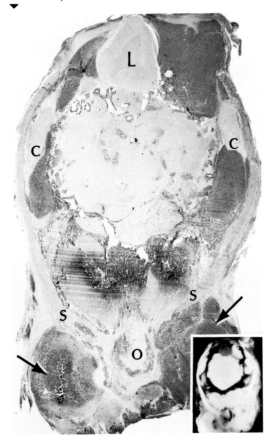

FIG. 18–11. Rubeosis iridis, peripheral anterior synechia and ectropion uveae are present in eye with retinoblastoma. Glaucoma along with photophobia and steamy cornea were present. H&E, ×28.

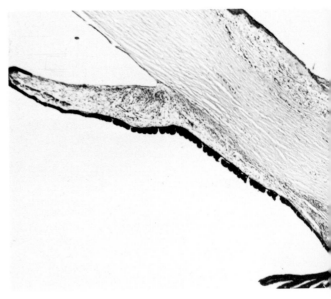

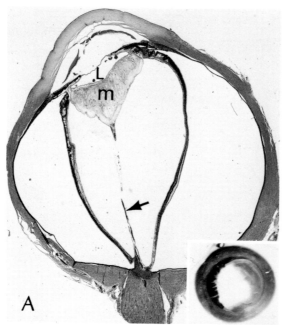

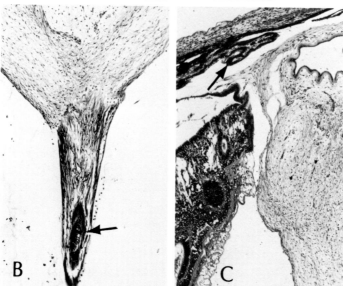

FIG. 18–12. PHPV. **A.** Abundant mesenchymal fibrovascular tissue (*m*) is present just behind posterior lens capsule. Note persistent hyaloid vasculature (*arrow*). *L,* lens. **Inset** shows characteristic clinical appearance with posterior lens opacity and inward drawing of ciliary processes from 7 to 12 o'clock. **B.** Higher magnification to show mesenchymal tissue and blood-filled hyaloid vessel (*arrow*) at posterior aspect. **C.** Ciliary processes (*arrow*) and retina are drawn into retro-lental mass. **A,** H&E, ×5; **inset,** clinical; **B,** H&E, ×55; **C,** H&E, ×55.

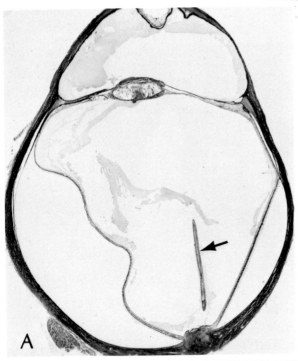

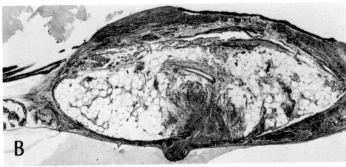

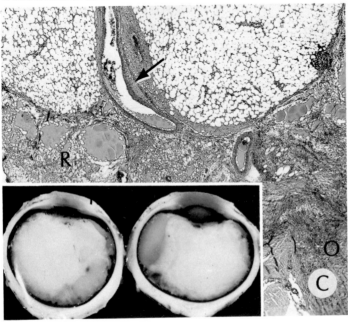

FIG. 18–13. PHPV. **A.** Unusual association of PHPV with intralenticular adipose tissue. Note persistence of hyaloid vessel (*arrow*). **B.** Higher magnification to show replacement of lens by adipose tissue. **C.** Posterior segment of eye with PHPV shown in **inset** demonstrates that vitreous compartment has been replaced by adipose tissue. Retina (*R*) is edematous, gliosed and disorganized. Note prominent hyaloid vessel (*arrow*). O, optic nerve. **A,** H&E, ×4.5; **B,** H&E, ×28; **C,** H&E, ×23; **inset,** macroscopic.

FIG. 18–14. Retinopathy of prematurity in 3½-month-old baby girl (905 g at birth). **A** and **B** show right and left eyes, respectively, with nasal retina pulled over optic nerve head. **Insets** show analogous fundus changes. **C.** Proliferating endothelial cells (*arrow* and shown in higher magnification in **D**) have not reached ora serrata (*double arrow*) in nasal periphery. **E.** Vessels have migrated out of retina into vitreous compartment, formed fibrous component (retinitis proliferans) and with shrinkage have caused retinal detachment. **Inset** shows clinical appearance of bilateral retinal detachment in patient with retinopathy of prematurity. **A,** H&E, ×16; **inset,** clinical, right eye; **B,** H&E, ×21; **inset,** clinical, left eye; **C,** H&E, ×40; **D,** H&E, ×101; **E,** H&E, ×16; **inset,** clinical.

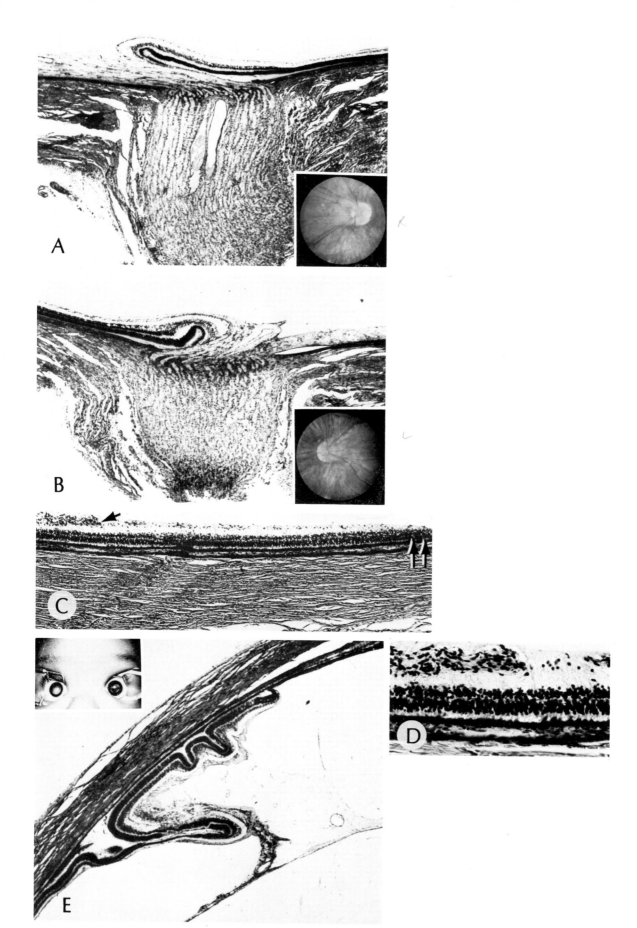

D. Phthisis bulbi (Fig. 18–5B).
III. Advanced lesions may present with proptosis, distant metastases or both.

PSEUDOGLIOMA (Pseudo retinoblastoma)

GENERAL INFORMATION

I. Terminology
   A. The term pseudoglioma was introduced by Collins in 1892 to designate a heterogeneous group of pathologic entities that may be confused clinically with retinoblastomas.
   B. The term pseudoretinoblastoma is a preferred term but has not yet gained wide acceptance.
II. The clinical presentation of pseudoglioma is similar to retinoblastoma, and it may present with *leukokoria,* i.e., large whitish retrolental mass, or with a small endophytic or exophytic tumor.

LEUKOKORIA

I. Persistent hyperplastic primary vitreous (PHPV) (Figs. 18–12 and 18–13)
   A. PHPV is a congenital, unilateral condition that is recognizable at birth; it can be bilateral but rarely so.
   B. It is unrelated to prematurity.
   C. PHPV exists within a microphthalmic eye with a shallow anterior chamber.
   D. Long ciliary processes may be seen around the periphery of a smaller than normal lens.
   E. A lens capsule dehiscence usually is present posteriorly, and occasionally the lens is cataractous.
   F. The condition is a result of persistence of the primary vitreous and hyaloid vasculature system from the embryo.

   Preretinal glial nodules may occur with PHPV. The preretinal nodules are thought to represent neuroectodermal proliferations.

II. Retinal dysplasia (Figs. 2–12 and 11–2) p.392
   A. Retinal dysplasia is congenital, usually bilateral and recognizable at birth but is unrelated to prematurity.
   B. Retinal dysplasia is accompanied by a

microphthalmic eye with a shallow anterior chamber. Frequently it is associated with systemic anomalies as part of trisomy 13–15 (see p. 39 in Chap. 2). It may be unilateral, and then generally it is not associated with systemic anomalies and trisomy 13–15.
   C. Histologically tubular and rosettelike formations form the dysplastic retina with four general types of rosettes recognized:
      1. Three-layer rosettes that have the appearance of mature retina that has been thrown into folds secondarily.
      2. Two-layer rosettes in which the innermost layer resembles a photoreceptor cell layer with an external limiting membrane and a relatively large lumen usually containing several undifferentiated cells. Surrounding this is a more peripheral layer of bipolarlike cells or poorly differentiated cells.
      3. One-layer rosettes with a single layer of moderately well-differentiated neural cells, usually several cells in thickness, having an external limiting membranelike structure and surrounding a lumen. Within the lumen larger undifferentiated cells usually are observed.
      4. Primitive unilayer rosettes in which a single layer of undifferentiated retinal cells surround a lumen or are arranged in a circle with a tangle of fibrils seen centrally.
III. Retinopathy of prematurity (retrolental fibroplasia) (Fig. 18–14)
   A. Retinopathy of prematurity is bilateral and not present at birth.

   A number of cases of "congenital retrolental fibroplasia" have been reported. The term retrolental fibroplasia probably should be reserved for the clinicopathologic entity as described below and not used as a purely histologic diagnosis.

   B. It occurs in premature infants with a history of oxygen therapy.

   The retinal vessels must be immature to be affected by increased oxygen tension.

If the baby is premature but the retinal vessels are mature, oxygen therapy will not cause retinopathy of prematurity; conversely, oxygen therapy in a full-term baby with immature retinal vessels may cause retinopathy of prematurity.

C. The eyes are normal in size at birth but may become microphthalmic and may develop shallow anterior chambers.

D. Ciliary processes may be seen in the periphery of the retrolental mass.

E. Histology:
1. Early, the retinal capillary endothelium proliferates into whorls within the peripheral retina.
2. The young vessels break through the internal limiting membrane and grow into the subvitreal space.
3. A fibrous component develops, and with shrinkage, a retinal detachment takes place.
4. The macula and posterior retinal vessels are displaced temporally.
5. The earliest retinal changes are seen in the periphery of the temporal retina. (The retinal changes are not necessarily progressive and may cease at any stage.)
6. There is a tendency to hemorrhage.
7. Glaucoma, generally a chronic secondary angle closure type, may occur in later years.

IV. Toxocara endophthalmitis (see pp. 93–94 in Chap. 4) (Figs. 4–25 and 4–26)
A. Toxocara endophthalmitis is a unilateral ocular condition in an otherwise healthy child, generally 3 to 12 years old.

B. The involved eye is quiet and asymptomatic. The only complaint is one of decreased vision.

C. Toxocara canis is the responsible parasite; it migrates to the eye in the larval stage.

D. Histologically a localized eosinophilic granulomatous inflammatory reaction occurs around the dead worm.

The nematode tends to have a peripheral retinal location, although on occasion the macula may be the only site of involvement.

V. Coats's disease (Figs. 18–15 and 18–16)
A. Coats's disease is a unilateral condition (rarely bilateral) that generally affects children between 18 months and 18 years; the peak incidence is found toward the end of the first decade.

B. Two-thirds of the cases occur in boys.

C. Telangiectatic retinal vessels, probably Leber's miliary aneurysms, leak fluid resulting in the exudative, bullous retinal detachment called Coats's disease.

D. Histologically telangiectatic retinal vessels, an eosinophilic transudate predominantly in the outer retinal layers and a rich subretinal exudate containing foamy macrophages and the "slits" of cholesterol crystals are characteristic.

VI. Norrie's disease (Fig. 18–17)

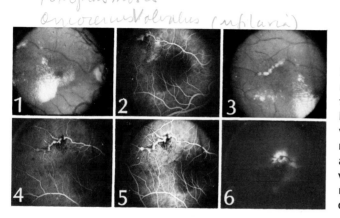

FIG. 18–15. Coats's disease in 16-year-old man. 1 and 2 demonstrate fundus and fluorescein appearance of posterior pole. Note foveomacular exudation and abnormal vessel at 11 o'clock. 3. Fundus shows abnormal vessel with typical light bulb appearance. 4, 5 and 6 show early, arteriolar-venular and 30-minute fluorescein phases, respectively. 1, clinical; 2, fluorescein; 3, clinical; 4, 5 and 6, fluorescein.

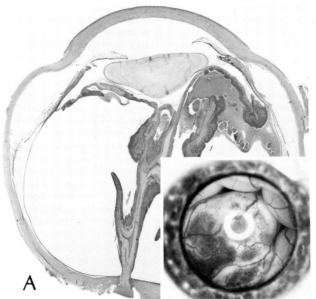

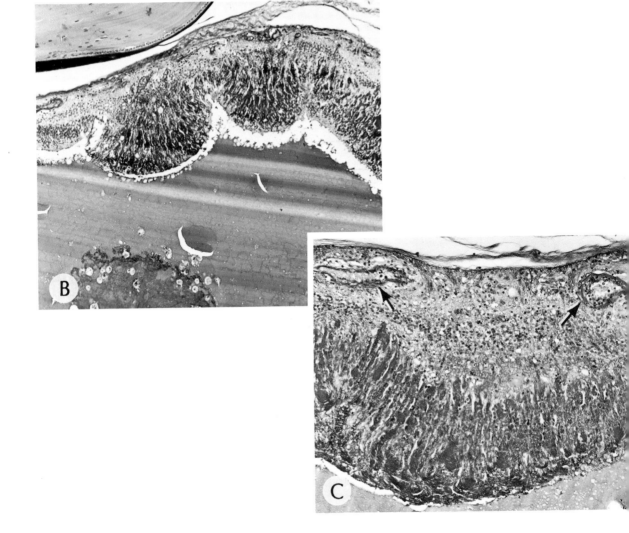

FIG. 18–16. Coats's disease in 2-year-old boy whose eye had been enucleated with clinical diagnosis of retinoblastoma. **A.** Retina is detached completely. **Inset** shows clinical appearance. Note telangiectatic vessels on surface of exudatively detached retina. **B.** Exudate in subretinal space contains foamy macrophages. PAS-positive exudate in degenerating outer retinal layers and telangiectatic blood vessels in inner retinal layers are present. **C.** PAS-positive exudate and foamy macrophages spread out degenerating outer retinal layers. Note telangiectatic blood vessels (*arrows*). **A,** H&E, ×3; **inset,** clinical; **B,** PAS, ×68; **C,** PAS, ×100.

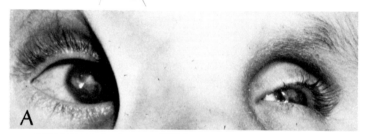

inverse epicanthal fold.

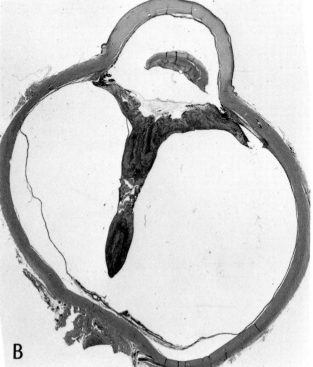

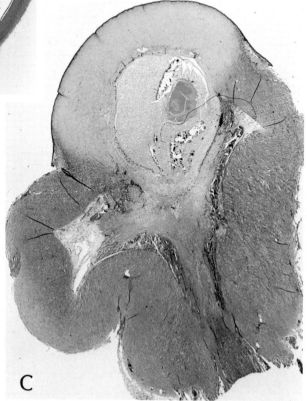

FIG. 18–17. Norrie's disease. **A.** Clinical appearance showing leukokoria of both eyes. **B** and **C** show histology of right (**B**) and left (**C**) eyes. Findings are nonspecific. **A,** clinical; **B,** H&E, ×6; **C,** H&E, ×6.

A. Norrie's disease is a bilateral condition that starts in early childhood.

B. It is characterized by deafness, mental retardation and pseudoglioma and has a sex-linked recessive inheritance pattern.

C. The ocular histology is nonspecific with a hemorrhagic retinal detachment and retinal necrosis common.

VII. Incontinentia pigmenti (Block-Sulzberger syndrome) (Fig. 18–18)

A. Incontinentia pigmenti has its onset in infancy with dermal, central nervous system, ocular and dental involvement.

B. The dermal lesions can be divided into three stages:
1. An initial papular rash.
2. A verrucous pigmented stage.
3. A pigmented nonelevated stage.

C. The central nervous system involvement consists of deformities of calvarium, convulsions, paresis and mental retardation.

D. The ocular changes consist of strabismus, nystagmus, blue sclera, myopia and pseudoglioma.

E. Dental abnormalities usually are present.

F. Hereditary as well as infectious theories of etiology have been proposed.

G. The ocular histology is nonspecific with retinal detachment, intraocular hemorrhage and retinal necrosis common.

Fluorescein study has shown changes consistent with an initial obliterative endarteritis starting peripherally and proceeding centrally. The arterioles ultimately become occluded.

VIII. Massive retinal fibrosis

A. Massive retinal fibrosis is due to organization of a massive retinal hemorrhage in the newborn.

B. Organization, fibrosis and contracture may simulate growth of a retinoblastoma.

IX. Metastatic retinitis (see Chap. 11)

X. Congenital nonattachment of retina (see Chap. 11) (Fig. 10–3)

XI. Secondary retinal detachment (see Chap. 11)

XII. Juvenile retinoschisis (Fig. 11–48)

XIII. Embryonal medulloepithelioma (diktyoma) (Figs. 17–28 and 17–29) (see p. 642 in Chap. 17)

A. Embryonal medulloepithelioma is a unilateral ocular tumor and is usually observed at birth because of a peculiar pupillary reflex.

B. It arises from the ciliary epithelium as a well-circumscribed mass, or it may infiltrate the area around the lens.

Rarely the tumor can arise from the optic nerve in the region of the optic disc.

C. Glaucoma may be the presenting sign.

D. Heteroplastic elements may be present and then it is termed a *teratoid medulloepithelioma* (Figs. 17–30 and 17–31).

Cartilage is present in 20 percent of cases. The tumor may contain rhabdomyoblasts (large benign globular cells superficially resembling ganglion cells).

E. Histologically the tumor consists of poorly differentiated neuroectodermal tissue, which in places resembles embryonic retina. The cells frequently are arranged in a double layer, forming tubes with the innermost layer secreting hyaluronic acid ("vitreous").

XIV. Congenital cataract may be confused with a retinoblastoma because of the leukokoria.

XV. Coloboma of Choroid

DISCRETE RETINAL OR CHORIORETINAL LESIONS

I. Small endophytic tumors
A. Retinal Hamartomas.
1. Tuberous sclerosis (see Chap. 2).
2. Neurofibromatosis (see Chap. 2).
B. Myelinated (medullated) nerve fibers (Fig. 11–5)
C. Coloboma of choroid (see pp. 329–332 in Chap. 9).
D. Retinochoroiditis is especially easy to confuse with retinoblastoma when deposits of white exudates are present on the retina.

II. Small exophytic tumors
A. Coats's disease may occur as a localized posterior lesion.

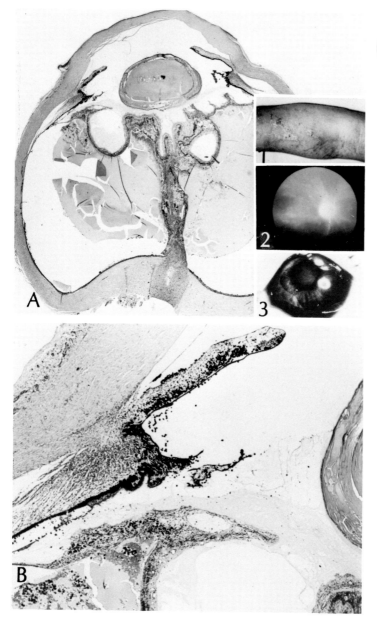

FIG. 18–18. Incontinentia pigmenti. **A.** Cataract, retinal detachment and intraocular necrosis (see **B**) are present. **Insets 1** and **2** from another case to demonstrate both verrucous and nonelevated pigmented dermal lesions (**1**) and obliterative endarteritis of retinal vessels coming off optic disc (**2**); fluorescein showed nonperfusion of retinal blood vessels beyond four disc diameters from optic disc. **Inset 3** shows another case with leukokoria. **B.** Higher magnification illustrates necrosis of iris, ciliary body and peripheral retina. **A,** H&E, ×7; **inset 1,** clinical of arm; **inset 2,** fundus; **inset 3,** clinical; **B,** H&E, ×16.

B. Larval (*Toxocara canis*) granulomas may present with posterior locations, especially in the macula.

C. Choroiditis or acute exudative retinitis with subretinal exudate.

D. Von Hippel-Lindau angiomatosis (see p. 30 in Chap. 2).

E. Proliferative lesions of retinal pigment epithelium (see pp. 638–642 in Chap. 17).

BIBLIOGRAPHY

RETINOBLASTOMA

Historical Aspects

Dunphy EB: The story of retinoblastoma. Trans Am Acad Ophthalmol Otolaryngol 68:249, 1964

Ts'o MOM, Fine BS, Zimmerman LE: The nature of retinoblastoma. II. An electron microscopic study. Am J Ophthalmol 69:350, 1970

Ts'o MOM, Zimmerman LE, Fine BS: The nature of

retinoblastoma. I. Photoreceptor differentiation. Am J Ophthalmol 69:339, 1970

General Information

Albert DM, Reid TW: RNA-directed DNA-polymerase activity in retinoblastoma: report of its presence and possible significance. Trans Am Acad Ophthalmol Otolaryngol 77:630, 1974

Dunphy EB: The story of retinoblastoma. Trans Am Acad Ophthalmol Otolaryngol 68:249, 1964

Ellsworth RM: The practical management of retinoblastoma. Trans Am Ophthalmol Soc 67:462, 1969

Francois J, Matton-Van Leuven MT: Recent data on the heredity of retinoblastoma, in Ocular and Adnexal Tumors. Edited by M Boniuk. St. Louis, Mosby, 1964, pp 123–141

Friendly DS, Parks MM: Concurrence of hereditary congenital cataracts and hereditary retinoblastoma. Arch Ophthalmol 84:525, 1970

Grace E, Drennan J, Colver D, Gordon RR: The 13q— deletion syndrome. J Med Genet 8:351, 1971

Howard RO, Breg WR, Albert DM, Lesser RL: Retinoblastoma and chromosome abnormality. Partial deletion of the long arm of chromosome 13. Arch Ophthalmol 92:490, 1974

Jensen RD, Miller RW: Retinoblastoma: epidemiologic characteristics. N Engl J Med 285:307, 1971

Leelawong N, Regan CDJ: Retinoblastoma: a review of ten years. Am J Ophthalmol 66:1050, 1968

Makley TA: Retinoblastoma in a 52-year-old man. Arch Ophthalmol 69:325, 1963

O'Grady RB, Rothstein TB, Romano PE: D-group deletion syndromes and retinoblastoma. Am J Ophthalmol 77:40, 1974

Ramírez LC, deBuen S: Clinical and pathologic findings in 100 retinoblastoma patients. J Pediatr Ophthalmol 10:12, 1973

Reese AB: Retinoblastoma: past, present and future (editorial). Arch Ophthalmol 77:293, 1967

Schappert-Kimmijser J, Hemmes GC, Nijland R: The heredity of retinoblastomas. Ophthalmologica 151:197, 1966

Stafford W, Zimmerman LE: Retinoblastoma. In preparation

Heredity

Albert DM, Rabson AS: The role of viruses in the pathogenesis of ocular tumors. Int Ophthalmol Clin 12:195, 1972

Albert DM, Reid TW: RNA-directed DNA-polymerase activity in retinoblastoma: report of its presence and possible significance. Trans Am Acad Ophthalmol Otolaryngol 77:630, 1973

Char DH, Ellsworth R, Rabson AS, Albert DM, Herberman RB: Cell-mediated immunity to a retinoblastoma tissue culture line in patients with retinoblastoma. Am J Ophthalmol 78:5, 1974

Char DH, Herberman RB: Cutaneous delayed hypersensitivity responses of patients with retinoblastoma to standard recall antigens and crude membrane extracts of retinoblastoma tissue culture cells. Am J Ophthalmol 78:40, 1974

Falls HF, Neel JV: Genetics of retinoblastoma. Arch Ophthalmol 46:367, 1951

Jensen RD, Miller RW: Retinoblastoma: epidemiologic characteristics. N Engl J Med 285:307, 1971

Knudson AG: Mutation and cancer: statistical study of retinoblastoma. Proc Natl Acad Sci USA 68:820, 1971

Morgan SS, Bair HL: Hereditary retinoblastoma: report of a family with retinoblastoma occurring in three successive generations. Am J Ophthalmol 65:43, 1968

Pruett R, Atkins L: Chromosome studies in patients with retinoblastoma. Arch Ophthalmol 82:177, 1969

Reese AB: Retinoblastoma: past, present and future (editorial). Arch Ophthalmol 77:293, 1967

Schappert-Kimmijser J, Hemmes GD, Nijland R: The heredity of retinoblastomas. Ophthalmologica 151:197, 1966

Zimmerman LE: Changing concepts concerning the pathogenesis of infectious diseases. Am J Ophthalmol 69:947, 1970

Histology

Bernardino V Jr, Salceda SR: DNA precipitation (in correspondence). Arch Ophthalmol 84:547, 1970

Bill AH: Immune aspects of neuroblastoma: current information. Am J Surg 122:142, 1971

Boniuk M, Zimmerman LE: Spontaneous regression of retinoblastoma. Int Ophthalmol Clin 2:525, 1962

Hogan MJ, Zimmerman LE (eds): Ophthalmic Pathology. An Atlas and Text (2nd ed). Philadelphia, Saunders, 1962, p 519

Morgan G: Diffuse infiltrating retinoblastoma. Br J Ophthalmol 55:600, 1971

Morris WE, LaPiana FG: Spontaneous regression of bilateral multifocal retinoblastoma with preservation of normal visual acuity. Ann Ophthalmol 6:1192, 1974

Mullaney J: Retinoblastomas with DNA precipitation. Arch Ophthalmol 82:454, 1969

Ramírez LC, deBuen S: Clinical and pathologic findings in 100 retinoblastoma patients. J Pediatr Ophthalmol 10:12, 1973

Sevel D, Röhm GF, Sealy R: Clinical significance of the fleurette in retinoblastoma. Br J Ophthal 58:687, 1974

Ts'o MOM, Fine BS, Zimmerman LE: The nature of retinoblastoma. II. An electron microscopic study. Am J Ophthalmol 69:350, 1970

Ts'o MOM, Zimmerman LE, Fine BS: The nature of retinoblastoma. I. Photoreceptor differentiation. Am J Ophthalmol 69:339, 1970

Ts'o MOM, Fine BS, Zimmerman LE: The Flexner-Wintersteiner rosettes in retinoblastoma. Arch Pathol 88:664, 1969

Wallow IHL, Fine BS, Tso MOM: Morphologic changes in photoreceptor outer segments following photic injury. A comparative study. Ophthalmol Res 5:10, 1973

Zimmerman LE, Fine BS: Production of hyaluronic acid by cysts and tumors of the ciliary body. Arch Ophthalmol 72:365, 1964

Growth Pattern

Dunphy EB: The story of retinoblastoma. Trans Am Acad Ophthalmol Otolaryngol 68:249, 1964

Herm RL, Heath P: A study of retinoblastoma. Am J Ophthalmol 41:22, 1956

Leelawong N, Regan CDJ: Retinoblastoma: a review of ten years. Am J Ophthalmol 66:1050, 1968

Parkhill EM, Benedict WL: Gliomas of the retina: a histopathologic study. Am J Ophthalmol 24:1354, 1941

Stafford W, Zimmerman LE: Retinoblastoma. In preparation

Mode of Extension

Carbajal UM: Metastasis in retinoblastoma. Am J Ophthalmol 48:47, 1959

Dunphy EB: The story of retinoblastoma. Trans Am Acad Ophthalmol Otolaryngol 68:249, 1964

Herm RL, Heath P: A study of retinoblastoma. Am J Ophthalmol 41:22, 1956

Leelawong N, Regan CDJ: Retinoblastoma: a review of ten years. Am J Ophthalmol 66:1050, 1968

Parkhill EM, Benedict WL: Gliomas of the retina: a histopathologic study. Am J Ophthalmol 24:1354, 1941

Stafford W, Zimmerman LE: Retinoblastoma. In preparation

Prognosis

Boniuk M: Discussion of "Retinoblastoma," in Ocular and Adnexal Tumors. Edited by M Boniuk. St. Louis, Mosby, 1964, pp 197–200

Carbajal UM: Metastasis in retinoblastoma. Am J Ophthalmol 48:47, 1959

Dunphy EB: The story of retinoblastoma. Trans Am Acad Ophthalmol Otolaryngol 68:249, 1964

Ellsworth RM: Treatment of retinoblastoma. Am J Ophthalmol 66:49, 1968

Herm RL, Heath P: A study of retinoblastoma. Am J Ophthalmol 41:22, 1956

Leelawong N, Regan CDJ: Retinoblastoma: a review of ten years. Am J Ophthalmol 66:1050, 1968

Parkhill EM, Benedict WL: Gliomas of the retina: a histopathologic study. Am J Ophthalmol 24:1354, 1941

Stafford W, Zimmerman LE: Retinoblastoma. In Preparation

Ts'o MOM, Zimmerman LE, Fine BS, Ellsworth RM: A cause of radioresistance in retinoblastoma: photoreceptor differentiation. Trans Am Acad Ophthalmol Otolaryngol 74:959, 1970

Clinical Features

Binder PS: Unusual manifestations of retinoblastoma. Am J Ophthalmol 77:674, 1974

Boniuk M, Zimmerman LE: Spontaneous regression of retinoblastoma. Int Ophthalmol Clin 2:525, 1962

Brockhurst RJ, Donaldson DD: Spontaneous resolution of probable retinoblastoma. Arch Ophthalmol 84:388, 1970

Dunphy EB: The story of retinoblastoma. Trans Am Acad Ophthalmol Otolaryngol 68:249, 1964

Herm RL, Heath P: A study of retinoblastoma: a review of ten years. Am J Ophthalmol 41:22, 1956

Leelawong N, Regan CDJ: Retinoblastoma: a review of ten years. Am J Ophthalmol 66:1050, 1968

Stafford WR, Yanoff M, Parnell BL: Retinoblastoma initially misdiagnosed as primary ocular inflammations. Arch Ophthalmol 82:771, 1969

Stafford W, Zimmerman LE: Retinoblastoma. In preparation

Walton DS, Grant WM: Retinoblastoma and iris neovascularization. Am J Ophthalmol 65:598, 1968

PSEUDOGLIOMA

General Information

Kogan L, Boniuk M: Causes for enucleation in childhood with special reference to pseudoglioma and unsuspected retinoblastoma. Int Ophthalmol Clin 2:507, 1962

Yanoff M: Pseudogliomas: differential diagnosis of retinoblastoma. Ophthalmol Dig 34:9, 1972

Leukokoria: Persistent Hyperplastic Primary Vitreous

Blodi FC: Preretinal glial nodules in persistence and hyperplasia of primary vitreous. Arch Ophthalmol 87:531, 1972

Font RL, Yanoff M, Zimmerman LE: Intraocular adipose tissue and persistent hyperplastic primary vitreous. Arch Ophthalmol 82:43, 1969

Leukokoria: Retinal Dysplasia

Hoepner J, Yanoff M: Spectrum of ocular abnormalities in trisomy 13–15. Am J Ophthalmol 74:729, 1972

Hunter WS, Zimmerman LE: Unilateral retinal dysplasia. Arch Ophthalmol 74:23, 1965

Lahav M, Albert DM: Clinical and histopathologic classification of retinal dysplasia. Am J Ophthalmol 75:648, 1973

Silverstein AM, Osburn BI, Pendergast RA: The pathogenesis of retinal dysplasia. Am J Ophthalmol 72:13, 1971

Leukokoria: Retinopathy of Prematurity

Flower RW, Patz A: Oxygen studies in retrolental fibroplasia. IX. The effects of elevated arterial oxygen tension on retinal vascular dynamics in the kitten. Arch Ophthalmol 85:197, 1971

Kalina RE, Forrest GL: Proliferative retrolental fibroplasia in infant retinal vessels. Am J Ophthalmol 76:811, 1973

Karlsberg RC, Green WR, Patz A: Congenital retrolental fibroplasia. Arch Ophthalmol 89:122, 1973

Stefani FH, Heidi E: Non-oxygen induced retinitis proliferans and retinal detachment in full-term infants. Br J Ophthalmol 58:490, 1974

Tasman W: Vitreoretinal changes in cicatricial retrolental fibroplasia. Trans Am Ophthalmol Soc 68:548, 1970

Tyner GS, Frayer WC: Clinical and autopsy findings in early retrolental fibroplasia. Arch Pathol 46:647, 1951

Leukokoria: Toxocara Endophthalmitis

Brown DH: Ocular *Toxocara canis.* J Pediatr Ophthalmol 7:182, 1970

Wallace GD: Sarcocystis in mice inoculated with toxoplasma-like oocysts from cat feces. Science 180:1375, 1973

Wilder HC: Nematode endophthalmitis. Trans Am Acad Ophthalmol Otolaryngol 54:99, 1950

Wilkinson CP, Welch RB: Intraocular toxocara. Am J Ophthalmol 71:921, 1971

Leukokoria: Coats's Disease

Archer DB: Leber's miliary aneurysms. Ophthalmol Dig 33:8, 1971

Ergerer I, Tasman W, Tomer TL: Coats' disease. Arch Ophthalmol 92:109, 1974

Farkas TG, Potts AM, Boone C: Some pathologic and biochemical aspects of Coats' disease. Am J Ophthalmol 75:289, 1973

Meythaler H: Zur pathologischen Anatomie der Retinitis exsudativa externa. Klin Monatsbl Augenheilkd 156:644, 1970

Reese AB: Telangiectasis of the retina and Coats' disease. Am J Ophthalmol 42:1, 1956

Tripathi R, Ashton N: Electron microscopical study of Coats' disease. Br J Ophthalmol 55:289, 1971

Leukokoria: Norrie's Disease

Apple DJ, Fishman GA, Goldberg MF: Ocular histopathology of Norrie's disease. Am J Ophthalmol 78:196, 1974

Brini A, Sacrez P, Levy JP: Maladie de Norrie. Ann Ocul (Paris) 205:1, 1972

Fradkin AH: Norrie's disease: congenital progressive oculo-acoustico-cerebral degeneration. Am J Ophthalmol 72:947, 1971

Holmes LB: Norrie's disease—an X-linked syndrome of retinal malformation, mental retardation and deafness. N Engl J Med 284:367, 1971

Townes PL, Roca PD: Norrie's disease (hereditary oculo-acoustic-cerebral degeneration). Report of a United States family. Am J Ophthalmol 76:797, 1973

Leukokoria: Incontinentia Pigmenti

Benedikt O, Ehalt H: Familiär auftretendes Bloch-Sulzberger-Syndrom (Incontinentia pigmenti) mit Augenbeteiligung. Klin Monatsbl Augenheilkd 157:652, 1970

McCrary JA, Smith JL: Conjunctival and retinal incontinentia pigmenti. Arch Ophthalmol 79:417, 1968

Leukokoria: Massive Retinal Fibrosis

Reese AB: Massive retinal fibrosis in children. Am J Ophthalmol 19:576, 1936

Leukokoria: Embryonal Medulloepithelioma

Anderson SR: Medulloepithelioma of the retina. Int Ophthalmol Clin 2:483, 1962

Apt L, Heller MD, Moskovitz M, Foos RY: Dictyoma (embryonal medulloepithelioma): recent review and case report. J Pediatr Ophthalmol 10:30, 1973

Green WR, Iliff WJ, Trotter RR: Malignant teratoid medulloepithelioma of the optic nerve. Arch Ophthalmol 91:451, 1974

Mullaney J: Primary malignant medulloepithelioma of the retinal stalk. Am J Ophthalmol 77:499, 1974

Zimmerman LE: Verhoeff's "terato-neuroma." A critical reappraisal in light of new observations and current concepts of embryonic tumors. Am J Ophthalmol 72:1039, 1971

Appendix

CHAPTER 1

Fig. 1–1. **Main figure,** SEI 73-166; **inset,** SEI 73-167.
Fig. 1–2. **A,** SEI 73-249; **B,** SEI 73-250.
Fig. 1–3. **Upper left,** SEI 73-171; **lower left,** SEI 73-175.
Fig. 1–4. **Inset,** AFIP Neg. 66-504; rabbit.
Fig. 1–5. **Main figure,** SEI 73-176.
Fig. 1–6. **Main figure,** SEI 73-330; **inset 1,** SEI 73-332; **inset 2,** SEI 73-331.
Fig. 1–7. SEI 73-169.
Fig. 1–8. **Main figure,** SEI 73-168.
Fig. 1–9. **Main figure,** SEI 73-170; **inset 1,** SEI 73-170; **inset 2,** SEI 73-300.
FIG. 1–10. SEI 73-137.
Fig. 1–11. SEI 73-172.
Fig. 1–12. **Inset,** AFIP Neg. 70-4565; **B,** SEI 73-183.
Fig. 1–13. **Main figure,** SEI 73-178; **inset,** SEI 73-179.
Fig. 1–14. SEI 73-3.
Fig. 1–15. **Main figure,** SEI 73-177; **inset,** SEI 73-333.
Fig. 1–16. **Main figure,** SEI 73-336; **inset,** SEI 73-335.
Fig. 1–17. **Inset,** SEI 73-18.
Fig. 1–18. **Inset,** SEI 73-46.
Fig. 1–19. **B,** SEI 73-45; **inset 1,** SEI 73-47; **inset 2,** SEI 73-46; **inset 3,** SEI 73-173; **inset 4,** SEI 73-49; **inset 5,** SEI 73-49.
Fig. 1–20. **A,** SEI 73-18; **B,** SEI 73-696. Courtesy of Dr. J. D. M. Gass.
Fig. 1–21. SEI 73-289.
Fig. 1–22. SEI 73-136.
Fig. 1–23. AFIP Neg. 64-1140. From Zimmerman LE; Trans Am Acad Ophthalmol Otolaryngol 69:412, 1965.
Fig. 1–24. **A,** SEI 73-50; **B,** SEI 73-161; **C,** SEI 73-72.
Fig. 1–25. **Main figure,** SEI 73-184; **inset 1,** SEI 73-496; **inset 2,** SEI 73-4.
Fig. 1–26. **Main figure,** AFIP Neg. 58-13252. From Fine BS, Zimmerman LE: Am J Ophthalmol 48:151, 1959.
Fig. 1–30. **Main figure,** SEI 73-456; **inset,** SEI 73-457.
Fig. 1–31. SEI 73-443.
Fig. 1–32. SEI 73-30.
Fig. 1–33. SEI 73-471.
Fig. 1–34. SEI 73-531.
Fig. 1–35. SEI 73-731.
Fig. 1–36. SEI 73-286.
Fig. 1–37. SEI 73-283.
Fig. 1–38. **A,** SEI 73-252; **B,** SEI 73-253.
Fig. 1–39. **A,** SEI 73-459; **B,** SEI 73-460.
Fig. 1–40. **Main figure,** SEI 73-469; **inset,** SEI 73-409.

CHAPTER 2

Fig. 2–1. **Main figure,** SEI 73-207; **inset 1,** SEI 73-209; **inset 2,** SEI 73-479. **Main figure** and **inset 1** courtesy of Dr. D. H. Nicholson.
Fig. 2–2. **A,** SEI 73-883; **B,** SEI 73-187; **inset 1,** SEI 73-382; **insets 2** and **3,** SEI 73-478. **A,** from Tasman W: Retinal Diseases in Children. New York, Harper and Row, 1971, p. 72. **B** and **inset 1** courtesy of Dr. R. Cordero-Moreno.
Fig. 2–3. **Main figure,** SEI 73-244; **inset,** SEI 73-245.
Fig. 2–4. **Main figure,** SEI 73-216; **inset 1,** SEI 73-123; **inset 2,** SEI 73-122. **Inset 1** courtesy of Dr. H. G. Scheie.
Fig. 2–5. **Main figure,** SEI 73-242; **inset,** SEI 73-106.
Fig. 2–6. **A,** SEI 73-243; **inset,** SEI 73-113. **B,** SEI 73-191; **inset,** SEI 73-247. Courtesy of Dr. L. Calkins.
Fig. 2–7. **Main figure,** SEI 73-267; **inset 1,** SEI 73-268; **inset 2,** SEI 73-115.
Fig. 2–8. SEI 73-497.
Fig. 2–9. SEI 73-882. From Archer DB, et al.: Am J Ophthalmol 75:224, 1973.
Fig. 2–10. SEI 73-392.
Fig. 2–11. SEI 73-392.
Fig. 2–12. **Main figure,** SEI 73-387; **inset,** SEI 73-399.
Fig. 2–13. **Main figure,** Derm No. 9777-10; **inset,** Derm No. 9777. From Hoepner J, Yanoff M: Am J Ophthalmol 74:729, 1972.
Fig. 2–14. Derm No. 9777-20. From Hoepner J, Yanoff M: Am J Ophthalmol 74:729, 1972.
Fig. 2–15. **A,** Derm No. 9777; **B,** Derm No. 9777. From Hoepner J, Yanoff M: Am J Ophthalmol 74:729, 1972.
Fig. 2–16. **Main figure,** Derm No. 9777-14; **inset,** Derm No. 9777-9. From Hoepner J, Yanoff M: Am J Ophthalmol 74:729, 1972.
Fig. 2–17. From Rodrigues MM, et al.: Am J Ophthalmol 76:265, 1973.
Fig. 2–18. **Main figure,** SEI 73-274; **inset,** SEI 73-477. Courtesy of Dr. W. C. Frayer.
Fig. 2–19. **Main figure,** SEI 73-198; **inset,** SEI 73-200. Courtesy of Dr. W. C. Frayer.
Fig. 2–20. **A,** Derm No. 9001; **B,** SEI 73-394. From Yanoff M, et al.: Am J Ophthalmol 70:391, 1970.
Fig. 2–21. **Main figure,** Derm No. 8926-24; **inset 1,** SEI 73-400; **inset 2,** Derm No. 8926-22. From Yanoff M, et al.: Am J Ophthalmol 70:391, 1970.
Fig. 2–22. **Main figure,** Derm No. 8926-19; **inset,** Derm No. 8926-20. From Yanoff M, et al.: Am J Ophthalmol 70:391, 1970.
Fig. 2–23. **Main figure,** SEI 73-476; **inset,** SEI 73-579. Modified from Cameron JD, et al.: Am J Ophthalmol 78:852, 1974.
Fig. 2–24. **Main figure,** SEI 73-213; **inset 1,** SEI 73-185; **inset 2,** SEI 73-255. From Cameron JD, et al.: Am J Ophthalmol 78:852, 1974.
Fig. 2–25. **Inset 1,** SEI 73-395; **inset 2,** SEI 73-396; **inset 3,** SEI 73-397; **inset 4,** SEI 73-398. From Yanoff M, Rorke LB: Am J Ophthalmol 75:1036, 1973.
Fig. 2–26. **Main figure,** Derm No. 7786-3; **inset 2,** SEI 73-633. **Main figure** and **inset 1** from Yanoff M, et al.: Trans Am Acad Ophthalmol Otolaryngol 72:896, 1968. **Inset 2** courtesy of Dr. H. G. Scheie.

Fig. 2–27. **Main figure,** Derm No. 7786-8; **inset,** SEI 73-631. **Main figure** from Yanoff M, et al.: Trans Am Acad Ophthalmol Otolaryngol 72:896, 1968. **Inset** courtesy of Dr. H. G. Scheie.

Fig. 2–28. Derm No. 7786-9. From Yanoff M, et al.: Trans Am Acad Ophthalmol Otolaryngol 72:896, 1968.

Fig. 2–29. **Main figure,** Derm No. 8852; **inset 1,** Derm No. 8852-3; **inset 2,** Derm No. 8852-3; **inset 3,** Derm No. 8852-2. From Yanoff M: *In* Retinal Diseases in Children. New York, Harper & Row, 1971, pp 223–232.

Fig. 2–30. **Main figure,** Derm No. 8852-6; **inset 1,** Derm No. 7786; **inset 2,** SEI 73-637. **Main figure** and **inset 1** from Yanoff M: *In* Retinal Diseases in Children. New York, Harper & Row, 1971, pp 223–232.

Fig. 2–31. AFIP Neg. 65-4111. From Zimmerman LE, Font RL: J Am Med Assoc 196:684, 1966.

Fig. 2–32. **A,** SEI 73-378; **B,** SEI 73-345; **C,** SEI 73-346. **A** from Bogdanoff B, et al.: Am J Dis Child 123:145, 1972.

Fig. 2–33. **Main figure,** SEI 73-188; **inset 1,** SEI 73-275; **inset 2,** SEI 73-131. Courtesy of Dr. A. P. Ferry.

Fig. 2–34. **A,** AFIP Neg. 65-3904; **B,** AFIP Neg. 65-3910; **C,** AFIP Neg. 65-3910. From Zimmerman LE, Font RL: J Am Med Assoc 196:684, 1966.

CHAPTER 3

Fig. 3–1. **A,** SEI 73-149; **B,** SEI 73-150.

Fig. 3–3. **A,** SEI 73-487; **B,** SEI 73-486.

Fig. 3–4. SEI 73-223.

Fig. 3–5. **Main figure,** SEI 73-379.

Fig. 3–6. **Main figure,** SEI 73-344; **inset 1,** SEI 73-343; **inset 2,** SEI 73-341; **inset 3,** SEI 73-342. Courtesy of Dr. W. R. Green. Case reported by Green WR, Koo BS: Survey Ophthalmol 12:324, 1967.

Fig. 3–7. **Main figure,** SEI 73-484; **inset 1,** SEI 73-551; **inset 2,** SEI 73-485.

Fig. 3–8. **Main figure,** SEI 73-204; **inset 1,** SEI 73-262; **inset 2,** SEI 73-296.

Fig. 3–9. **Main figure,** Derm No. 8926-9. Case reported by Nelson DA, et al.: Arch Ophthalmol 84:613, 1970.

Fig. 3–10. **Inset 1,** SEI 73-412; **inset 2,** SEI 73-413. Modified from Nelson DA, et al.: Arch Ophthalmol 84:613, 1970.

Fig. 3–11. **Inset 1,** SEI 73-410; **Inset 3,** SEI 73-404. **Main figure** and **insets 1** and **2** modified from Nelson DA, et al.: Arch Ophthalmol 84:613, 1970.

Fig. 3–12. **Bottom,** AFIP Neg. 72-1523. Modified from Font RL, et al.: Arch Pathol 96:168, 1973.

Fig. 3–13. **A,** SEI 73-838; **inset,** SEI 73-130. **B,** SEI 73-836. **C,** SEI 73-836. From Perry H, et al.: Arch Ophthalmol. In press.

Fig. 3–14. From Perry H, et al.: Arch Ophthalmol. In press.

Fig. 3–15. **Main figure,** SEI 73-521; **inset,** SEI 73-522.

Fig. 3–16. SEI 73-519.

Fig. 3–17. SEI 73-729.

Fig. 3–18. **A,** SEI 73-90; **inset 1,** SEI 73-92; **B,** SEI 73-1; **C,** SEI 73-2. From Winslow RL, et al.: Arch Ophthalmol 92:33, 1974.

Fig. 3–19. **A,** SEI 73-450; **inset,** SEI 73-617; **B,** SEI 73-451.

Fig. 3–20. SEI 73-518.

Fig. 3–21. **Main figure,** SEI 73-263; **inset 1,** SEI 73-133; **inset 2,** SEI 73-264.

Fig. 3–22. **Main figure,** SEI 73-445; **inset,** SEI 73-444.

Fig. 3–33. SEI 73-447.

Fig. 3–24. From Perry H, et al.: Arch Ophthalmol. In press.

Fig. 3–25. **Main figure,** SEI 73-206; **inset 1,** SEI 73-193; **inset 2,** SEI 73-205.

Fig. 3–26. **A,** SEI 73-194; **B,** SEI 73-196; **inset,** SEI 73-495; **C,** SEI 73-197.

CHAPTER 4

Fig. 4–1. **Main figure,** SEI 73-854; **inset,** SEI 77-884. From Kay ML, et al.: Am J Ophthalmol 78:90, 1974.

Fig. 4–2. **A,** SEI 73-51; **B,** SEI 73-56; **C,** SEI 73-54.

Fig. 4–3. **Main figure,** SEI 73-7; **inset 1,** SEI 73-298; **inset 2,** SEI 73-50; **inset 3,** SEI 73-55. **Inset 1** courtesy of Dr. H. G. Scheie.

Fig. 4–4. **A,** SEI 73-163; **inset 1,** SEI 73-315; **inset 2,** SEI 73-316; **B,** SEI 73-162. **Insets 1** and **2** courtesy of Dr. H. G. Scheie.

Fig. 4–5. **A,** SEI 73-9; **B,** SEI 73-19; **inset,** SEI 73-69; **C,** SEI 73-71.

Fig. 4–6. **Main figure,** SEI 73-14; **inset 1,** SEI 73-70; **inset 2,** SEI 73-317.

Fig. 4–7. **A,** SEI 73-299; **B, inset 1,** SEI 73-461; **inset 2,** SEI 73-464; **inset 3,** SEI 73-462; **inset 4,** SEI 73-302; **inset 5,** SEI 73-301.

Fig. 4–8. **Main figure,** SEI 73-189; **inset 1,** SEI 73-287; **inset 2,** SEI 73-286. Courtesy of Dr. Francisco Contreras.

Fig. 4–9. **Main figure,** SEI 73-10; **inset,** SEI 73-571.

Fig. 4–10. **Main figure,** SEI 73-513; **inset,** SEI 73-572. Courtesy of Dr. A. Steinberg.

Fig. 4–11. **A,** SEI 73-192; **inset,** SEI 73-124; **B,** SEI 73-290; **C,** SEI 73-281. **A** and **B** courtesy of Dr. P. Henkind.

Fig. 4–12. **Main figure,** SEI 73-27; **inset 1,** SEI 73-280; **inset 2,** SEI 73-279. Courtesy of Dr. M. O. M. Tso.

Fig. 4–13. **Main figure,** SEI 74-540; **inset,** SEI 74-541.

Fig. 4–14. **A,** SEI 73-270; **B,** SEI 73-269. Courtesy of Dr. R. S. Smith.

Fig. 4–15. **Main figure,** SEI 73-235; **inset 1,** SEI 73-323; **inset 2,** SEI 73-266; **inset 3,** SEI 73-324; **inset 4,** SEI 73-501; **inset 5,** SEI 73-500.

Fig. 4–16. **Main figure,** SEI 73-502; **inset,** SEI 73-499.

Fig. 4–17. **Main figure,** SEI 73-564; **inset,** SEI 73-566. Courtesy of Dr. A. Steinberg.

Fig. 4–18. **Main figure,** SEI 73-186; **inset,** SEI 73-134. Courtesy of Dr. H. Rodman.

Fig. 4–19. **A,** SEI 73-258; **inset,** SEI 73-322. **B,** SEI 73-260; **inset,** SEI 73-261. Courtesy of Dr. A. Bunyor.

Fig. 4–20. **Main figure,** SEI 73-1056; **inset,** SEI 73-851.

Fig. 4–21. SEI 73-251. Courtesy of Dr. G. Klintworth.

Fig. 4–22. **Main figure,** SEI 73-229; **inset 1,** SEI 73-420; **inset 2,** SEI 73-233.

Fig. 4–23. **Main figure,** SEI 73-573; **inset,** SEI 73-574.

Fig. 4–24. **A,** SEI 74-656; **inset,** SEI 74-618; **B,** SEI 74-567; **C,** SEI 74-568.

Fig. 4–25. **Main figure,** SEI 73-190; **inset 1,** SEI 73-314; **inset 2,** SEI 73-114. **Main figure** and **inset 1** courtesy of Dr. M. Rodrigues.

Fig. 4–26. **Main figure,** SEI 73-785; **inset 1,** 73-424; **inset 2,** SEI 73-407.

Fig. 4–27. **1,** SEI 74-410; **2,** SEI 74-411; **3,** SEI 74-412; **4,** SEI 74-413; **5,** SEI 74-415; **6,** SEI 74-416; **7,** SEI 74-405; **8,** SEI 74-406; **9,** SEI 74-407.

Fig. 4–28. **Main figure,** SEI 73-295; **inset 1,** SEI 73-326; **inset 2,** SEI 73-325; **inset 3,** SEI 73-293. **Main figure** and **inset 3** courtesy of Dr. M. J. Reeh.

Fig. 4–29. **Main figure,** SEI 73-543; **inset 1,** SEI 73-292;

inset 2, SEI 73-291; inset 3, SEI 73-291. Courtesy of Dr. M. J. Reeh.

Fig. 4–30. Main figure, SEI 74-531; inset 1, SEI 74-387; inset 2, SEI 74-388.

Fig. 4–31. A, SEI 73-562; B, SEI 73-563.

Fig. 4–32. Main figure, AFIP Neg. 69-720; inset 1, AFIP Neg. 69-723; inset 2, AFIP Neg. 69-719. Courtesy of Dr. R. L. Font.

Fig. 4–33. Main figure, SEI 73-541; inset, SEI 73-542. Courtesy of Dr. J. Butcher.

Fig. 4–34. A, SEI 73-536; inset, SEI 73-627. B, SEI 73-537; inset 1, SEI 73-539; inset 2, SEI 73-540; inset 3, SEI 73-540; inset 4, SEI 73-538; inset 5, SEI 73-538. Courtesy of Dr. G. de Venecia. Case reported by de Venecia G, et al.: Arch Ophthalmol 86:44, 1971.

Fig. 4–35. From Wyhinny GJ, et al.: Am J Ophthalmol 76:773, 1973.

Fig. 4–36. A, AFIP Neg. 65-7056; B, SEI 73-385; inset, SEI 74-424; C, SEI 73-339. A from Naumann G, et al.: Am J Ophthalmol 65:533, 1968. B and C courtesy of Dr. R. L. Font.

Fig. 4–37. Main figure, SEI 73-160; inset 1, SEI 73-632; inset 2, SEI 73-628.

Fig. 4–38. A, SEI 73-695; inset, SEI 73-304. B, SEI 73-694; inset, SEI 73-303. Courtesy of Dr. J. D. M. Gass. Case reported by Gass JDM, Olson CL: Trans Am Acad Ophthalmol Otolaryngol 77:739, 1973.

Fig. 4–39. A, SEI 74-234; B, SEI 73-692. A from Laties AM, Scheie HG: Am J Ophthalmol 74:60, 1972. B courtesy of Dr. J. D. M. Gass. Case reported by Gass JDM, Olson CL: Trans Am Acad Ophthalmol Otolaryngol 77:739, 1973.

Fig. 4–40. A, SEI 73-544; B, SEI 74-213; C, SEI 74-210; D, SEI 74-212. A courtesy of Dr. I. W. McLean.

Fig. 4–41. AFIP Neg. 64-5340. From Zimmerman LE: *In* The Cornea World Congress. Washington, DC, Butterworths, 1965, p 30.

Fig. 4–42. A, B and C, AFIP Neg. 56-20159. Case reported by Fine BS, Gilligan JH: Am J Ophthalmol 43:433, 1957.

CHAPTER 5

Fig. 5–1. A, upper, SEI 73-490; lower left, SEI 73-489; lower right, SEI 73-488. B, inset 1, AFIP Neg. 74-11278. Courtesy of Drs. D. MacKeen and B. Fine, unpublished observations.

Fig. 5–2. A, AFIP Neg. 64-4603; B, AFIP Neg. 73-12174. B courtesy of Dr. D. Barsky.

Fig. 5–3. SEI 73-438.

Fig. 5–4. SEI 73-774.

Fig. 5–5. SEI 73-835.

Fig. 5–6. SEI 73-549.

Fig. 5–7. SEI 73-775.

Fig. 5–8. Main figure, SEI 73-719; inset, SEI 73-720.

Fig. 5–9. Main figure, SEI 73-1062; inset 1, SEI 73-899; inset 2, SEI 73-901.

Fig. 5–10. SEI 73-664.

Fig. 5–11. SEI 73-640.

Fig. 5–12. AFIP Neg. 72-13861.

Fig. 5–13. A, SEI 73-963; B, SEI 73-770.

Fig. 5–14. SEI 73-721.

Fig. 5–15. SEI 73-638.

Fig. 5–16. SEI 73-650.

Fig. 5–17. Main figure, SEI 73-649; inset, SEI 73-13.

Fig. 5–18. SEI 73-964.

Fig. 5–19. A, SEI 74-528; inset, SEI 74-565; B, SEI 73-645.

Fig. 5–20. Main figure, SEI 73-778; inset 1, SEI 73-589; inset 2, SEI 73-772.

Fig. 5–21. Main figure, SEI 73-717; inset, SEI 73-718.

Fig. 5–22. Main figure, Derm No. 7915-3; inset 1, SEI 73-595; inset 2, SEI 73-596; inset 3, SEI 73-597. Main figure from Yanoff M, Scheie HG: Arch Ophthalmol 80:166, 1968.

Fig. 5–23. A, SEI 73-446; B, SEI 73-724.

Fig. 5–24. A, SEI 73-781; B, SEI 73-797; inset, SEI 73-594.

Fig. 5–25. Main figure, SEI 73-734; inset, SEI 73-699.

Fig. 5–26. SEI 73-195.

Fig. 5–27. Main figure, SEI 73-670; inset 1, SEI 73-997; inset 2, SEI 73-998.

Fig. 5–28. Main figure, SEI 73-671; inset 1, SEI 73-581; inset 2, SEI 73-580.

Fig. 5–29. A, SEI 73-646; B, SEI 73-806.

Fig. 5–30. A, SEI 73-606; B, SEI 73-607.

Fig. 5–31. Main figure, SEI 73-763; insets 1 and 2, SEI 73-603; inset 3, SEI 73-602. Insets 1, 2 and 3 courtesy of Dr. G. Naumann.

Fig. 5–32. SEI 73-702.

Fig. 5–33. A, SEI 73-522; B, SEI 73-522; C, SEI 73-872.

Fig. 5–34. Main figure, SEI 73-783; inset, SEI 73-598.

Fig. 5–35. A, AFIP Neg. 64-5361-1; B, AFIP Neg. 63-5278; C, AFIP Neg. 63-5281; D, AFIP Neg. 63-5280; E, AFIP Neg. 63-5279.

Fig. 5–36. Main figure, SEI 73-527; inset 1, SEI 73-582; inset 2, SEI 73-795.

Fig. 5–37. A, SEI 73-800; B, SEI 73-802.

Fig. 5–38. SEI 73-796.

Fig. 5–39. A, SEI 73-587; B, SEI 73-788; C, SEI 73-788; D, SEI 73-666; E, SEI 73-665; F, SEI 73-848; inset, SEI 73-849.

Fig. 5–40. SEI 73-700.

Fig. 5–41. Main figure, SEI 73-707; inset 1, SEI 73-585; inset 2, SEI 73-608; inset 3, SEI 73-586; inset 4, SEI 73-708.

Fig. 5–42. A, AFIP Neg. 71-7378; B, AFIP Neg. 71-7377.

Fig. 5–43. A, SEI 73-789; B, SEI 73-701.

Fig. 5–44. SEI 73-612. Courtesy of Dr. H. G. Scheie.

Fig. 5–45. Main figure, AFIP Neg. 61-1028; inset 1, SEI 73-623; inset 2, SEI 73-624. Main figure modified from Fine BS: Lab Invest 11 (pt. 2):1161, 1962.

Fig. 5–46. A, SEI 73-714; inset, SEI 73-622. B, SEI 73-715; inset, SEI 73-715.

Fig. 5–47. Main figure, SEI 73-661; inset 1, SEI 73-578; inset 2, SEI 73-590; inset 3, SEI 73-599.

Fig. 5–48. Main figure, SEI 73-791; inset 1, SEI 73-760; inset 2, SEI 73-761.

Fig. 5–49. Main figure, SEI 73-662; inset, SEI 73-801.

Fig. 5–50. Main figure, SEI 73-1063; inset, SEI 74-429.

Fig. 5–51. A, SEI 73-952; inset 1, SEI 73-609; inset 2, SEI 73-610; inset 3, SEI 73-503; B, SEI 73-1049; C, SEI 73-1048; D, SEI 73-1047.

Fig. 5–52. From Eagle RC, et al.: Am J Ophthalmol 75:426, 1973.

Fig. 5–53. Main figure, SEI 73-712; inset, SEI 73-611.

Fig. 5–54. A, SEI 74-153; inset, SEI 74-39; B, SEI 74-152.

Fig. 5–55. SEI 73-967.

Fig. 5–56. SEI 73-954.

Fig. 5–57. Main figure, SEI 73-732; **inset 1,** SEI 73-723; **inset 2,** SEI 73-373; **inset 3,** SEI 73-372; **inset 4,** SEI 73-371. Insets 2, 3 and 4 courtesy of Dr. G. Naumann.

Fig. 5–58. Main figure, SEI 73-787; **inset 1,** SEI 73-604; **inset 2,** SEI 73-605.

Fig. 5–59. Main figure, SEI 73-383; **inset,** SEI 73-374. Inset courtesy of Dr. G. Naumann.

Fig. 5–60. **A,** SEI 73-382; **B,** SEI 73-381.

Fig. 5–61. **A,** SEI 73-642; **B,** SEI 73-659.

Fig. 5–62. SEI 73-968.

Fig. 5–63. **A,** SEI 73-639; **B,** SEI 73-811.

Fig. 5–64. Main figure, SEI 73-810; **inset,** SEI 73-377.

Fig. 5–65. Main figure, SEI 74-367; **inset,** SEI 73-126.

Fig. 5–66. SEI 73-474.

Fig. 5–67. Main figure, SEI 73-798; **inset 1,** SEI 73-405; **inset 2,** SEI 73-583; **inset 3,** SEI 73-982.

Fig. 5–68. Main figure, SEI 73-782; **inset 1,** SEI 73-971; **inset 2,** SEI 73-366. Inset 2 courtesy of Dr. G. Naumann.

Fig. 5–69. Main figure, SEI 73-804; **inset 1,** SEI 73-363; **inset 2,** SEI 73-973.

Fig. 5–70. SEI 73-805.

Fig. 5–71. **A,** SEI 73-1050; **inset 1,** SEI 73-320; **inset 2,** SEI 74-228; **inset 3,** SEI 74-229; **B,** SEI 73-1051; **inset,** SEI 73-319. From Eagle RC, Yanoff M: Albrecht v Graefes Arch klin exp Ophthal 193:121, 1975.

Fig. 5–72. **A,** SEI 74-555; **B,** SEI 74-557.

Fig. 5–73. Main figure, SEI 73-765; **inset 1,** SEI 73-365; **inset 2,** SEI 73-427.

Fig. 5–74. **A,** SEI 73-644; **B,** SEI 73-759.

Fig. 5–75. SEI 73-673.

Fig. 5–76. **A,** SEI 73-654; **B,** SEI 73-780.

Fig. 5–78. **A,** SEI 73-777; **inset,** SEI 73-364. **B,** SEI 73-194; **inset,** SEI 73-370.

Fig. 5–80. SEI 73-641.

Fig. 5–81. SEI 73-663.

Fig. 5–82. Main figure, SEI 73-776; **inset 1,** SEI 73-1002; **inset 2,** SEI 73-1003.

Fig. 5–83. Main figure, SEI 73-784; **inset,** SEI 73-674.

Fig. 5–84. Courtesy of Dr. F. La Piana.

Fig. 5–85. Main figure, SEI 73-803; **inset,** SEI 73-368.

Fig. 5–86. Main figure, AFIP Neg. 65-1401; **inset 1,** AFIP Neg. 65-1398; **inset 2,** AFIP Neg. 65-1399. All from Johnson FB, Zimmerman LE: Am J Ophthalmol 44:533, 1965.

Fig. 5–87 **A,** SEI 73-762; **inset,** SEI 73-813. **B,** AFIP Neg. 61-6823; **inset,** AFIP Neg. 61-6824. **B** from Fine BS: Lab Invest 11 (pt. 2):1161, 1962.

Fig. 5–88. Main figure, SEI 73-491; **inset 1,** SEI 73-425; **inset 2,** SEI 73-426.

Fig. 5–89. Main figure, SEI 73-769; **inset 1,** SEI 73-369; **inset 2,** SEI 73-790.

Fig. 5–90. Main figure, SEI 73-768; **inset,** SEI 73-809.

Fig. 5–91. AFIP Neg. 71-10250.

Fig. 5–92. From Blodi FC: Int Ophthalmol Clin 11:1, 1971.

Fig. 5–93. From Hanna CH, Fraunfelder FT: Arch Ophthalmol 87:184, 1972.

Fig. 5–95. Courtesy of Dr. S. Hirsch.

Fig. 5–96. **C,** AFIP Neg. 73-2758.

Fig. 5–97. **A,** AFIP Neg. 68-8713-1; **B,** AFIP Neg. 68-8713-2. **A** and **B** courtesy of Dr. J. W. Berkow. **C** from Curtin TL, Boyden DG: Am J Ophthalmol 65:188, 1968.

Fig. 5–98. **Inset 1,** AFIP Neg. 64-3945. **A** from Fine BS in Mc Pherson A (ed): New York, Harper & Row, 1968, p 16. **Inset 1** and **B** from Fine BS, Geeraets WJ: Acta Ophthalmol 43:684, 1965.

Fig. 5–99. **B,** AFIP Neg. 66-3316. **B** from Fine BS, et al.: Am J Ophthalmol 64:209, 1967.

CHAPTER 6

Fig. 6–2. Main figure, SEI 73-141; **inset,** SEI 73-142.

Fig. 6–3. SEI 73-433.

Fig. 6–4. **A,** SEI 73-925; **B,** AFIP Neg. 73-2198.

Fig. 6–5. SEI 73-1076.

Fig. 6–6. SEI 73-80.

Fig. 6–8. SEI 73-454.

Fig. 6–9. SEI 73-532.

Fig. 6–10. SEI 74-184.

Fig. 6–11. **A,** SEI 74-117; **B,** SEI 74-116.

Fig. 6–12. Main figure, SEI 73-878; **inset,** SEI 74-452. Courtesy of Dr. D. M. Kozart and Dr. J. A. Katowitz.

Fig. 6–13. **A,** SEI 74-236; **inset 1,** SEI 74-235; **inset 2,** SEI 74-237; **B,** SEI 74-238; **inset,** SEI 74-239. Modified from Katowitz JA, et al.: Arch Ophthalmol 91:208, 1974.

Fig. 6–14. Main figure, SEI 73-1017; **inset,** SEI 74-104. Courtesy of Dr. F. C. Riley.

Fig. 6–15. **A,** SEI 74-109; **B,** SEI 74-110.

Fig. 6–16. Main figure, SEI 73-455; **inset,** SEI 74-61.

Fig. 6–17. SEI 74-123.

Fig. 6–18. Main figure, SEI 74-122; **inset 1,** SEI 74-50; **inset 2,** SEI 74-101.

Fig. 6–19. **A,** SEI 73-956; **B,** SEI 73-893; **inset 1,** SEI 73-889; **inset 2,** SEI 74-94.

Fig. 6–20. **A,** SEI 73-908; **inset 1,** SEI 74-93; **inset 2,** SEI 73-907; **B,** SEI 73-1046; **inset 3,** SEI 74-48; **inset 4,** SEI 74-49.

Fig. 6–21. Main figure, SEI 73-891; **inset,** SEI 73-892.

Fig. 6–22. **A,** SEI 73-1079, **inset,** SEI 74-36; **B,** SEI 73-1080.

Fig. 6–23. **A,** SEI 73-1038; **inset 1,** SEI 74-62; **inset 2,** SEI 74-96; **B,** SEI 73-1014; **inset,** SEI 73-1013.

Fig. 6–24. Main figure, SEI 74-185; **inset 1,** SEI 74-186; **inset 2,** SEI 74-35. Main figure and inset 1 courtesy of Dr. J. Butcher.

Fig. 6–25. Main figure, SEI 74-188; **inset,** SEI 74-187.

Fig. 6–26. **A,** SEI 73-732; **inset 1,** SEI 74-614; **inset 2,** SEI 74-612; **inset 3,** SEI 74-610; **B;** SEI 73-576; **C,** SEI 73-577. From Katowitz JA, et al.: In preparation.

Fig. 6–27. Main figure, SEI 74-526; **inset,** SEI 74-539. Courtesy of Dr. J. Butcher.

Fig. 6–28. **A,** SEI 74-245; **inset,** SEI 74-244. **B,** SEI 74-242; **inset,** SEI 74-243. Courtesy of Dr. L. B. Rorke.

Fig. 6–29. **A,** SEI 74-202; **B,** SEI 74-205; **C,** SEI 74-206. Case reported by Frayer WC: Arch Ophthalmol 64:58, 1960.

Fig. 6–30. **A,** SEI 74-197; **B,** SEI 74-198. Courtesy of Dr. J. Butcher.

Fig. 6–31. Main figure, SEI 74-190; **inset 1,** SEI 74-442; **inset 2,** SEI 74-441.

Fig. 6–32. **A,** SEI 73-912; **inset,** SEI 74-99. **B,** SEI 73-911; **inset,** SEI 74-67.

Fig. 6–33. Main figure, SEI 73-923; **inset,** SEI 73-924.

Fig. 6–34. Main figure, SEI 73-1022; **inset 1,** SEI 74-47; **inset 2,** SEI 73-1023. Courtesy of Dr. J. R. Duke.

Fig. 6–35. **B,** SEI 74-569; **C,** Derm No. 7017-1. **B** from and **C** modified from Frayer WC, et al.: Trans Am Ophthalmol Soc 66:233, 1968.

Fig. 6–36. Main figure, SEI 73-894; **inset,** SEI 73-895.

Fig. 6–37. SEI 73-520.

Fig. 6–38. SEI 73-896.

Fig. 6–39. **A,** SEI 73-951; **inset,** SEI 73-902. **B,** SEI 73-

903; inset, SEI 73-904. **C,** SEI 73-905; inset, SEI 73-906.

Fig. 6–40.   Main figure, SEI 73-1081; inset, SEI 74-54.

Fig. 6–42.   SEI 73-926.

Fig. 6–43.   A, SEI 73-958; inset, SEI 74-74; **B,** SEI 73-927.

Fig. 6–44.   Main figure, SEI 73-79; inset, SEI 73-82.

Fig. 6–45.   Main figure, SEI 73-914; inset 1, SEI 74-55; inset 2, SEI 73-915.

Fig. 6–46.   Main figure, SEI 74-114; inset, SEI 74-113.

Fig. 6–47.   A, SEI 74-16; inset, SEI 74-106; **B,** SEI 73-1041; **C,** SEI 73-1042; **D,** SEI 73-1046. **A, B** and **C** courtesy of Dr. J. Ramírez Macías.

Fig. 6–48.   A, SEI 73-959; **B,** SEI 73-932; **C,** SEI 73-933.

Fig. 6–49.   A, SEI 74-128; inset 1, SEI 74-63; inset 2, SEI 74-58; **B,** SEI 73-936; **C,** SEI 74-127.

Fig. 6–50.   A, SEI 73-559; inset 1, SEI 73-560; **B,** SEI 73-937; inset 2, SEI 73-938; inset 3, SEI 73-938; **C,** SEI 73-934; inset 4, SEI 74-98; inset 5, SEI 74-102; **D,** SEI 73-935.

Fig. 6–51.   Main figure, SEI 73-1077; inset 1, SEI 74-70; inset 2, SEI 73-1078.

Fig. 6–52.   Main figure, SEI 74-145; inset 1, SEI 74-146; inset 2, SEI 74-46.

Fig. 6–53.   SEI 74-183.

Fig. 6–54.   A, SEI 74-111; **B,** SEI 74-112.

Fig. 6–55.   A, SEI 73-917; **B,** SEI 73-918.

Fig. 6–56.   A, SEI 74-191; **B,** SEI 74-192.

Fig. 6–57.   Main figure, SEI 74-195; inset, SEI 74-196.

Fig. 6–58.   A, Derm No. 5218-1; inset, SEI 74-43; **B,** Derm No. 5218-3; **C,** Derm No. 5218-2. Modified from Scheie HG, et al.: Arch Ophthalmol 72:800, 1964.

Fig. 6–60.   A, SEI 74-151; inset, SEI 74-64; **B,** SEI 74-150; **C,** SEI 74-147; **D,** SEI 74-148.

Fig. 6–61.   Main figure, SEI 73-1017; inset, SEI 74-227. Courtesy of Dr. C. J. Lee.

Fig. 6–62.   A, SEI 73-960; inset, SEI 73-834; **B,** SEI 74-107; **C,** SEI 74-108.

Fig. 6–63.   A, SEI 73-957; **B,** SEI 73-920.

Fig. 6–64.   SEI 74-133.

Fig. 6–65.   A, SEI 74-193; **B,** SEI 74-194.

Fig. 6–66.   A, SEI 73-439; **B,** SEI 73-440.

Fig. 6–67.   A, SEI 74-137; inset, SEI 74-138; **B,** SEI 74-139; **C,** SEI 74-140.

Fig. 6–68.   A, SEI 73-909; **B,** SEI 73-910.

Fig. 6–69.   Main figure, SEI 74-141; inset, SEI 74-142.

Fig. 6–70.   A, AFIP Neg. 71-9109; **B,** AFIP Neg. 71-9100. From Ryan SJ, Font RL: Am J Ophthalmol 76:73, 1973.

Fig. 6–71.   A, AFIP Neg. 71-9114; **B,** AFIP Neg. 71-9115. From Ryan SJ, Font RL: Am J Ophthalmol 76:73, 1973.

Fig. 6–72.   A, AFIP Neg. 71-9104; **B,** AFIP Neg. 71-9102. From Ryan SJ, Font RL: Am J Ophthalmol 76:73, 1973.

CHAPTER 7

Fig. 7–1.   SEI 73-1071.

Fig. 7–2.   Main figure, SEI 74-129; inset 1, SEI 73-375; inset 2, SEI 73-376.

Fig. 7–3.   Main figure, SEI 73-877; inset, SEI 73-634.

Fig. 7–4.   A, AFIP Neg. 64-3754; **B,** AFIP Neg. 74-3755.

Fig. 7–5.   Main figure, SEI 73-1040; inset 1, SEI 74-103; inset 2, SEI 73-1039. Courtesy of Dr. F. M. Polack.

Fig. 7–6.   A, SEI 73-824; **B,** SEI 73-713.

Fig. 7–7.   A, SEI 73-822; inset 1, SEI 73-629; inset 2, SEI 73-821; **B,** SEI 73-820; inset 3, SEI 73-630; inset 4, SEI 73-819.

Fig. 7–8.   Main figure, SEI 73-818; inset, SEI 73-626.

Fig. 7–9.   Main figure, SEI 73-825; inset, SEI 73-826.

Fig. 7–10.   A, SEI 73-1030; inset 1, SEI 74-45; inset 2, SEI 74-66; **B,** SEI 73-1029. Courtesy of Dr. S. L. Biggs.

Fig. 7–11.   From Wang S-P, Grayston JT: Am J Ophthalmol 63:1133, 1967.

Fig. 7–12.   A, SEI 73-1067; inset, SEI 73-819; **B,** SEI 73-881.

Fig. 7–13.   A, SEI 73-740; inset, SEI 73-741; **B,** SEI 73-739.

Fig. 7–14.   Main figure, SEI 73-1060; inset, SEI 74-43. Modified from Scheie HG, et al.: Arch Ophthalmol 72:800, 1964.

Fig. 7–15.   A, Derm No. 4941-1; inset, SEI 74-71; **B,** Derm No. 4941-2. **A** and **B** modified from Yanoff M, Scheie HG: Arch Ophthalmol 72:57, 1964.

Fig. 7–16.   Main figure, SEI 73-342; inset, SEI 74-41.

Fig. 7–17.   Inset, SEI 74-59. **Main figure** from Ostler HB, et al.: Trans Am Acad Ophthalmol Otolaryngol 74:1254, 1970. **Inset** courtesy of Dr. J. A. Katowitz.

Fig. 7–18.   SEI 74-546.

Fig. 7–19.   A, SEI 73-1052; **B,** SEI 73-1053; **C,** SEI 73-1054.

Fig. 7–20.   A, SEI 73-735; inset, SEI 73-737; **B,** SEI 73-738; **C,** SEI 74-130.

Fig. 7–21.   Main figure, SEI 74-626; inset, SEI 74-401; **B,** SEI 74-624.

Fig. 7–22.   A, SEI 74-56; **B,** SEI 74-136; **C,** SEI 74-51; **D,** SEI 73-1070.

Fig. 7–23.   A, SEI 73-1072; inset 1, SEI 74-52; inset 2, SEI 74-53; **B,** SEI 73-1075. All modified from Yanoff M: Arch Ophthalmol 79:291, 1968.

Fig. 7–24.   A, SEI 74-69; **B,** SEI 73-77.

Fig. 7–25.   Main figure, SEI 73-879; inset, SEI 73-880.

Fig. 7–26.   A, SEI 73-815; **B,** SEI 73-816.

Fig. 7–27.   A, SEI 73-754; inset, SEI 74-392; **B,** SEI 73-755; **C,** SEI 73-753.

Fig. 7–28.   A, SEI 73-792; **B,** SEI 73-747; **C,** SEI 73-751; **D,** SEI 73-749; **E,** SEI 73-750; **F,** SEI 73-752.

Fig. 7–29.   Main figure, SEI 73-950; inset 1, SEI 73-885; inset 2, SEI 73-876. Courtesy of Dr. C. J. Lee.

Fig. 7–30.   A, SEI 73-843; **B,** SEI 73-844; **C,** SEI 73-846; **D,** SEI 73-847.

CHAPTER 8

Fig. 8–1.   A, SEI 74-427; **B,** SEI 74-428; **C,** SEI 74-390; **D,** SEI 74-447. **B** Courtesy of Dr. J. A. Katowitz.

Fig. 8–2.   AFIP Neg. 67-4579. Experimental lesion in rabbit.

Fig. 8–3.   Main figure, SEI 73-509; inset, SEI 74-422. **Inset** courtesy of Dr. H. G. Scheie.

Fig. 8–4.   AFIP Neg. 73-12175. Courtesy of Dr. D. Barsky.

Fig. 8–5.   SEI 73-437.

Fig. 8–6.   A, SEI 74-553; **B,** SEI 73-875; inset, SEI 74-443.

Fig. 8–7.   A, SEI 74-8; inset, SEI 74-451; **B,** SEI 74-34.

Fig. 8–8.   A, SEI 74-231; **B,** SEI 74-233; inset 1, SEI 74-90; inset 2, SEI 74-89; inset 3, SEI 74-86. Modified from Scheie HG, Yanoff M: Arch Ophthalmol 87:525, 1972.

Fig. 8–9.   A, AFIP Neg. 73-6965; **B,** AFIP Neg. 73-6969.

Fig. 8–10.   SEI 74-347.

Fig. 8–11.   A, SEI 73-955; **B,** SEI 73-855; **C,** SEI 73-857. Courtesy of Dr. R. Cordero-Moreno.

Fig. 8–12. **A,** SEI 73-953; **B,** SEI 73-862; **C,** SEI 73-861.

Fig. 8–13. **A,** SEI 74-13; **inset 1,** SEI 74-83; **inset 2,** SEI 74-82; **B,** SEI 74-118; **C,** SEI 74-119; **D,** SEI 74-120.

Fig. 8–14. **A,** SEI 74-240; **B,** SEI 74-241; **C,** SEI 73-868; **inset 1,** SEI 74-455; **inset 2,** SEI 74-404. **A** and **B** courtesy of Dr. J. A. Katowitz. **Insets 1** and **2** courtesy of Dr. H. G. Scheie.

Fig. 8–15. **Main figure,** SEI 73-1065; **inset 1,** SEI 74-450; **inset 2,** SEI 73-1066; **inset 3,** SEI 73-1066. **Inset 1** courtesy of Dr. J. A. Katowitz.

Fig. 8–16. **Left eye,** SEI 73-636; **Right eye,** SEI 73-635.

Fig. 8–17. **Main figure,** SEI 73-512; **inset,** SEI 74-423.

Fig. 8–18. SEI 73-794.

Fig. 8–19. **A,** Derm No. 9601-2; **inset,** Derm No. 9601-3. **B,** Derm No. 9601-1; **inset,** Derm No. 9601-4. Case reported by Scheie HG, et al.: Ann Ophthalmol 3:697, 1971.

Fig. 8–20. **A,** SEI 74-11; **inset,** SEI 74-396; **B,** SEI 73-730. **Inset** courtesy of Dr. D. M. Kozart.

Fig. 8–21. **A,** SEI 73-609; **B,** SEI 73-593; **C,** SEI 74-14. **A** courtesy of Dr. H. G. Scheie.

Fig. 8–22. **Main figure,** SEI 74-131; **inset,** SEI 74-426.

Fig. 8–23. **A,** AFIP Neg. 69-9833. **B** and **C** from Font RL: Arch Ophthalmol 90:382, 1973.

Fig. 8–24. **A,** SEI 73-356; **inset 1,** SEI 73-359; **inset 2,** SEI 74-448; **B,** SEI 74-547; **inset,** SEI 74-532. **Inset 2** courtesy of Dr. H. G. Scheie.

Fig. 8–25. **A,** AFIP Neg. 73-10965; **B,** AFIP Neg. 73-10966; **C,** AFIP Neg. 73-10963; **D,** AFIP Neg. 73-10967; **E,** AFIP Acc. 831164; **F,** AFIP Acc. 831164. **A** through **D** modified from Zimmerman LE: Survey Ophthalmol 8:1, 1963. **E** and **F** from Fine BS: *In* The Cornea. Washington, DC, Butterworths, 1965.

Fig. 8–26. **Main figure,** SEI 73-863; **inset,** SEI 74-454.

Fig. 8–27. **A,** SEI 73-353; **inset,** SEI 74-60; **B,** SEI 74-354.

Fig. 8–28. **Inset 1,** SEI 74-57. **Main figure** and **inset 2** from Levine RA, Robb MF: Arch Ophthalmol 86:525, 1971.

Fig. 8–29. SEI 73-866.

Fig. 8–30. **A,** AFIP Neg. 58-662. **B,** SEI 73-792; **inset,** SEI 73-996. **Inset,** AFIP Neg. 72-12849.

Fig. 8–31. **A,** SEI 73-744; **inset,** SEI 73-625; **B,** SEI 73-745.

Fig. 8–32. **A,** SEI 73-864; **inset,** SEI 73-865; **B,** SEI 73-705; **C,** SEI 73-841; **D,** SEI 73-840; **inset,** SEI 73-842.

Fig. 8–33. **A,** SEI 74-224; **B,** SEI 74-225; **C,** SEI 74-226. Courtesy of Dr. P. R. Laibson.

Fig. 8–34. **Main figure,** SEI 73-874; **inset 1,** SEI 73-308; **inset 2,** SEI 73-307; **inset 3,** SEI 73-618; **inset 4,** SEI 73-309.

Fig. 8–35. **C,** AFIP Neg. 72-9776; **D,** AFIP Neg. 72-8866-6. **A** from Fine BS, et al.: Am J Ophthalmol 66:1, 1968. **B** from Berkow JW, et al.: Am J Ophthalmol 66:812, 1968.

Fig. 8–36. **Inset 1,** AFIP Neg. 71-6349; **inset 2,** AFIP Neg. 72-1568-2. Modified from Brownstein S, et al.: Am J Ophthalmol 75:799, 1973.

Fig. 8–37. **A,** SEI 74-174; **inset,** SEI 74-434; **B,** SEI 74-175; **C,** SEI 74-176. **Inset** courtesy of Dr. H. G. Scheie.

Fig. 8–38. **C,** AFIP Neg. 72-17316; **D,** AFIP Neg. 72-13708; **inset,** AFIP Neg. 72-12978. **C** from and **D** modified from Fine BS, et al.: Am J Ophthalmol 78:12, 1974.

Fig. 8–39. **A,** AFIP Neg. 64-6590; **B,** AFIP Neg. 64-7088; **C,** AFIP Neg. 64-7089. From Stafford WL, Fine BS: Arch Ophthalmol 75:53, 1966.

Fig. 8–40. **Inset 2,** AFIP Neg. 73-10956; **inset 3,** AFIP Neg. 73-10955.

Fig. 8–42. **A,** AFIP Neg. 72-13250. From Rodrigues MM, et al.: Am J Ophthalmol. 92:475, 1974.

Fig. 8–43. **B,** AFIP Neg. 73-1168. From Rodrigues MM, et al.: Am J Ophthalmol. 92: 475, 1974.

Fig. 8–44. **A,** AFIP Neg. 73-1171. From Rodrigues MM, et al.: Am J Ophthalmol. 92:475, 1974.

Fig. 8–45. **A, inset 1,** AFIP Neg. 70-4869; **B, inset 1,** AFIP Neg. 75-2233; **inset 2,** AFIP Neg. 75-2232. Case reported by Font RL, Fine BS: Am J Ophthalmol 73:419, 1972.

Fig. 8–46. **Inset in A,** AFIP Neg. 73-4217. **Inset in B,** AFIP Neg. 73-4216. **C,** AFIP Neg. 67-144; **inset 1,** SEI 74-431; **inset 2,** AFIP Neg. 66-6698. **A** modified from Griffith DG, Fine BS: Am J Ophthalmol 63:1659, 1967. **Inset 1** courtesy of Dr. P. R. Laibson.

Fig. 8–47. **Inset in B,** AFIP Neg. 70-8873. From Brownstein S, et al.: Am J Ophthalmol. 77:701, 1974.

Fig. 8–48. **A,** AFIP Neg. 73-11039; **B,** AFIP Neg. 73-11041; **inset,** AFIP Neg. 64-565.

Fig. 8–49. **Inset 1 in A,** AFIP Neg. 71-9575; **inset 2 in A,** AFIP Neg. 61-9578. **Inset 1 in B,** AFIP Neg. 61-9576.

Fig. 8–50. **Inset,** AFIP Neg. 64-3522.

Fig. 8–51. **A,** SEI 74-657. **A, C** and **D** from Kenyon KR, Maumenee AE: Invest Ophthalmol 7:475, 1968. **Inset 1** modified from Kenyon KR, Maumenee AE: Am J Ophthalmol 76:419, 1973.

Fig. 8–52. From Kenyon KR, et al.: Am J Ophthalmol 73:718, 1972.

Fig. 8–53. From Frazier PD, Wong VG: Arch Ophthalmol 80:87, 1968.

Fig. 8–54. **A,** AFIP Neg. 65-4495; **B,** AFIP Neg. 65-4496; **C,** AFIP Neg. 65-12185; **inset,** AFIP Neg. 65-13104; **D,** SEI 74-302; **E,** SEI 74-303. **A, B** and **C** modified from McTigue JW: Trans Am Ophthalmol Soc 65:591, 1967.

Fig. 8–55. **A, inset 1,** AFIP Neg. 74-12991; **C,** AFIP Neg. 67-145; **D,** AFIP Neg. 71-9595. **C** from McTigue JW: Trans Am Ophthalmol Soc 65:591, 1967.

Fig. 8–56. **A,** SEI 73-869; **inset,** SEI 73-870; **B,** SEI 73-966.

Fig. 8–57. AFIP Neg. 74-1652-1. From Gass JDM: Arch Ophthalmol 71:348, 1964.

Fig. 8–58. SEI 73-138.

Fig. 8–59. AFIP Neg. 74-1293-3.

Fig. 8–60. AFIP Neg. 74-1293-2. Modified from Gass JDM: Arch Ophthalmol 71:348, 1964.

Fig. 8–61. **B,** AFIP Neg. 73-2582; **C,** AFIP Neg. 73-2583. From Tso MOM, et al.: Am J Ophthalmol 79:479, 1975.

Fig. 8–62. **Main figure,** SEI 74-173; **inset 1,** SEI 74-394; **inset 2,** SEI 74-393. **Insets 1** and **2** courtesy of Dr. J. A. Katowitz.

Fig. 8–63. **A,** AFIP Neg. 61-1065; **B,** AFIP Neg. 64-552. From Ferry AP, Zimmerman LE: Am J Ophthalmol 58:205, 1964.

Fig. 8–64. **A,** SEI 74-309; **inset,** SEI 74-473; **B,** SEI 74-311. Courtesy of Dr. W. R. Green.

Fig. 8–65. **A,** SEI 73-1024; **inset,** SEI 74-44. **B,** SEI 73-1025; **inset,** SEI 73-1026. All courtesy of Dr. W. M. Townsend.

Fig. 8–66. **Main figure,** SEI 74-207; **inset,** SEI 74-80.

Fig. 8–67. **Main figure,** SEI 73-545; **inset,** SEI 74-472. **Main figure** courtesy of Dr. I. W. McLean.

Fig. 8–68. SEI 74-527.

Fig. 8–69. **A,** SEI 74-201; **B,** SEI 74-204; **inset,** SEI 74-

471. **A** and **B** from case reported by Frayer WC: Arch Ophthalmol 64:58, 1960.

Fig. 8–70. **A**, SEI 74-211; **B**, SEI 74-208; **inset**, SEI 74-209.

Fig. 8–71. Courtesy of Dr. A. P. Ferry. Case reported by Ferry AP, Hein HF: Am J Ophthalmol 70:764, 1970.

CHAPTER 9

Fig. 9–1. **A**, SEI 74-252; **inset 1**, SEI 74-463; **inset 2**, SEI 74-462; **B**, SEI 74-253.

Fig. 9–2. **A**, SEI 74-249; **B**, SEI 74-251; **C**, SEI 74-250.

Fig. 9–3. **Main figure**, SEI 74-305; **inset**, SEI 74-306. Courtesy of Dr. L. Christensen.

Fig. 9–4. **A**, SEI 73-812; **inset**, SEI 74-84; **B**, SEI 74-121; **inset 1**, SEI 74-397; **inset 2**, SEI 74-475.

Fig. 9–5. **1**, SEI 74-421; **2**, SEI 74-420; **3**, SEI 74-419; **4**, SEI 74-418; **5**, SEI 74-417; **6**, SEI 74-469; **7**, SEI 74-458; **8**, SEI 74-459; **9**, SEI 74-461.

Fig. 9–6. SEI 73-210.

Fig. 9–7. **A**, Derm No. 9527-5; **inset 1**, SEI 74-87; **inset 2**, SEI 74-88; **B**, Derm No. 9527-6; **C**, SEI 73-1085. From Scheie HG, Yanoff M: Arch Ophthalmol 87:525, 1972.

Fig. 9–8. **Inset 2**, AFIP Neg. 67-11210.

Fig. 9–10. **A**, AFIP Neg. 63-6910; **B**, AFIP Neg. 69-5607; **1**, SEI 74-439; **2**, SEI 74-474; **3**, SEI 74-437; **4**, SEI 74-436. **1, 3** and **4** courtesy of Dr. D. M. Kozart.

Fig. 9–11. **A**, SEI 74-584; **inset**, AFIP Neg. 62-4608; **B**, SEI 74-586; **C**, SEI 74-587. **Inset** from Zimmerman LE, Fine BS: Arch Ophthalmol 72:365, 1964.

Fig. 9–12. From Johnson BL, Storey JD: Arch Ophthalmol 84:166, 1970.

Fig. 9–13. **Main figure**, SEI 74-163; **inset**, SEI 74-162. Courtesy of Dr. J. B. Crawford.

Fig. 9–14. **Main figure**, SEI 74-596; **inset 1**, SEI 74-617; **inset 2**, SEI 74-615; **inset 3**, SEI 74-598. **Insets 1** and **2** courtesy of Dr. H. G. Scheie.

Fig. 9–15. **A**, SEI 74-15; **inset 1**, SEI 73-312; **inset 2**, SEI 73-313; **inset 3**, SEI 73-310; **B**, SEI 74-166; **inset 4**, SEI 74-167; **inset 5**, SEI 74-165. **Inset 1** courtesy of Dr. H. G. Scheie. **Inset 3** courtesy of Dr. G. Naumann.

Fig. 9–16. **A**, SEI 73-349; **inset**, SEI 73-350; **B**, SEI 73-347; **C**, SEI 73-348.

Fig. 9–17. **A**, SEI 73-941; **inset**, SEI 73-942; **inset 1**, SEI 74-321; **inset 2**, SEI 74-323; **C**, SEI 73-962; **D**, SEI 73-214. Case in **D** reported by Cameron JD, Yanoff M, Frayer WC: Am J Ophthalmol 78:852, 1974.

Fig. 9–18. From Ferry AP, et al.: Arch Ophthalmol 88:39, 1972.

Fig. 9–19. **A**, SEI 74-159; **B**, SEI 74-158. Courtesy of Dr. W. S. Hunter.

Fig. 9–21. **Main figure**, SEI 73-943; **inset**, SEI 74-468.

Fig. 9–22. **A**, AFIP Neg. 67-11603; **inset 1**, AFIP Neg. 67-11611; **inset 2**, AFIP Neg. 68-2837; **B**, AFIP Neg. 68-592. **A** modified from, **B** same case as and **C** from Meyer SL, et al.: Am J Ophthalmol 66:1061, 1968.

Fig. 9–23. **A**, SEI 73-391; **B**, SEI 73-361.

Fig. 9–24. **A**, SEI 74-622; **B**, SEI 74-600; **C**, SEI 74-602; **D**, SEI 74-604; **E**, SEI 74-606. Case to be reported by Dr. E. K. Rahn.

Fig. 9–25. **A**, SEI 73-667; **inset**, SEI 74-359; **B**, SEI 74-366; **C**, SEI 74-359; **D**, SEI 74-361; **E**, SEI 74-364. Case to be reported by Dr. E. K. Rahn.

Fig. 9–26. **A**, SEI 74-9; **B**, SEI 74-160; **C**, SEI 74-161. Courtesy of Dr. R. B. O'Grady. Case reported by Ryan SJ, et al.: Trans Am Acad Ophthalmol Otolaryngol 76:652, 1972.

Fig. 9–27. **A**, SEI 74-621; **inset 1**, SEI 73-986; **inset 2**, SEI 73-987; **B**, SEI 74-582; **C**, SEI 74-583.

Fig. 9–28. **Main figure**, SEI 73-778; **inset**, SEI 73-773.

Fig. 9–29. **Main figure**, SEI 74-580; **inset**, SEI 74-620.

CHAPTER 10

Fig. 10–1. SEI 74-85.

Fig. 10–2. **Main figure**, SEI 73-553; **inset 1**, SEI 73-327; **inset 2**, SEI 74-395.

Fig. 10–3. SEI 73-159.

Fig. 10–4. Derm No. 9374. From Hoepner J, Yanoff M: J Ped Ophthalmol 8:107, 1971.

Fig. 10–5. **A**, SEI 73-388; **B**, SEI 73-389; **inset 1**, AFIP Neg. 72-11902; **inset 2**, AFIP Neg. 72-9783. **A** and **B** courtesy of Dr. D. B. Schaffer. **C** from and **D** modified from Yanoff M, et al.: Am J Ophthalmol 76:363, 1973.

Fig. 10–6. **A**, SEI 73-234; **B**, SEI 73-503; **C**, SEI 73-505; **D**, SEI 73-504; **E**, SEI 73-386. Courtesy of Dr. V. T. Curtin.

Fig. 10–7. SEI 73-38.

Fig. 10–8. SEI 73-37.

Fig. 10–9. From Burde RM, et al.: Arch Ophthalmol 82:651, 1969.

Fig. 10–10. **Inset**, AFIP Neg. 74-3371.

Fig. 10–11. **B**, SEI 73-985; **C**, SEI 74-346. **B** courtesy of Dr. H. G. Scheie. **C** courtesy of Dr. G. Naumann.

Fig. 10–12. **A**, SEI 73-352; **B**, SEI 73-73; **inset**, AFIP Neg. 72-6760.

Fig. 10–13. **A**, SEI 73-517; **B**, AFIP Neg. 72-2762.

Fig. 10–15. **A**, SEI 73-23; **B**, SEI 73-24; **C**, SEI 73-29; **inset**, AFIP Neg. 74-4876.

Fig. 10–16. **Main figure**, SEI 73-31; **inset 1**, SEI 73-367; **inset 2**, SEI 73-119.

Fig. 10–17. SEI 73-25.

Fig. 10–18. **A**, SEI 73-26; **inset**, SEI 73-121; **B**, SEI 73-27; **C**, SEI 73-28; **inset**, SEI 73-125.

Fig. 10–19. **A**, SEI 74-68; **B**, SEI 73-39; **C**, SEI 73-524.

Fig. 10–20. From Eagle RC, et al.: Am J Ophthalmol 75:426, 1973.

Fig. 10–22. **Main figure**, SEI 73-36; **inset**, SEI 73-129.

Fig. 10–23. SEI 73-355.

Fig. 10–25. **Main figure**, SEI 73-15; **inset**, SEI 73-117.

Fig. 10–26. **Main figure**, SEI 73-354; **inset**, SEI 73-600.

Fig. 10–27. **Main figure**, SEI 73-40; **inset 1**, SEI 73-110; **inset 2**, SEI 73-109.

Fig. 10–28. **A**, SEI 73-236; **B**, AFIP Neg. 67-4974. **B** from Font RL, et al.: Arch Ophthalmol 82:43, 1969.

Fig. 10–29. **A**, SEI 73-11; **B**, SEI 73-523.

Fig. 10–30. **A**, SEI 73-1001; **B**, SEI 73-1000.

Fig. 10–31. **Main figure**, SEI 73-12; **inset**, SEI 73-108.

Fig. 10–34. **Main figure**, SEI 73-782; **inset**, SEI 73-651.

Fig. 10–35. **A**, SEI 73-65; **inset 1**, SEI 73-104; **inset 2**, SEI 73-3; **B**, SEI 73-67. **Inset 1**, courtesy of Dr. T. R. Thorp.

Fig. 10–36. **Inset 1**, AFIP Neg. 71-2795; **inset 3**, AFIP Neg. 71-9587. From Ramsey MS, et al.: Am J Ophthalmol 74:377, 1972.

Fig. 10–37. **A**, AFIP Neg. 71-4880-1; **B**, AFIP Neg. 70-8860. From Ramsey MS, et al.: Am J Ophthalmol 74:377, 1972.

Fig. 10–38. **B**, AFIP Neg. 71-11407; **C**, AFIP Neg. 71-11408; **D**, AFIP Neg. 72-3729-1. From Ramsey MS, et al.: Am J Ophthalmol 76:102, 1973.

Fig. 10–39. Main figure, AFIP Neg. 72-3729-8; **inset,** AFIP Neg. 72-907. From Ramsey MS, et al.: Am J Ophthalmol 76:102, 1973.

Fig. 10–40. Inset, AFIP Neg. 72-2764.

CHAPTER 11

Fig. 11–1. Inset, SEI 73-994. **A–D** from Shields JA, Tso MOM: Arch Ophthalmol (Grouped Pigmentation), in press. Copyright American Medical Association.

Fig. 11–2. From Lahav M, et al.: Am J Ophthalmol 75:648, 1973.

Fig. 11–3. Main figure, SEI 74-310; **inset,** SEI 74-81.

Fig. 11–4. SEI 74-341.

Fig. 11–5. A, AFIP Neg. 72-10790; B, AFIP Neg. 72-10791; C, Right, SEI 74-900; left, SEI 74-901.

Fig. 11–6. Main figure, SEI 74-328; **inset,** SEI 74-329.

Fig. 11–7. A, AFIP Neg. 69-10044-7; B, AFIP Neg. 70-7275. Modified from Brownstein S, et al.: Arch Ophthalmol 90:49, 1973.

Fig. 11–8. A, SEI 74-492; B, SEI 74-493. Courtesy of Dr. W. R. Green. Case reported by Michelson PE, et al.: Arch Ophthalmol 86:274, 1971.

Fig. 11–9. A, SEI 74-368; B, SEI 74-369.

Fig. 11–10. A, AFIP Neg. 72-12099; B, SEI 74-1090; inset 1, SEI 74-1088; inset 2, SEI 74-1097. A from Eagle RC, et al.: Arch Ophthalmol. 92:28, 1974.

Fig. 11–11. A, SEI 74-488; inset, SEI 74-399; B, SEI 74-516; C, SEI 74-518; D, SEI 74-519.

Fig. 11–12. A, SEI 74-824. B, SEI 74-634. C, SEI 74-648; inset, SEI 74-1014. D, SEI 74-650; inset, SEI 74-1013. Case to be reported by Cameron JD, et al.

Fig. 11–13. A, SEI 74-674; B, SEI 74-675; C, SEI 74-678; D, SEI 74-676.

Fig. 11–14. A, AFIP Neg. 73-10953; B, AFIP Neg. 73-10952.

Fig. 11–15. From Kroll AJ: Arch Ophthalmol 79:453, 1968.

Fig. 11–16. A, SEI 74-478; B, SEI 74-325; inset, SEI 74-843; C, SEI 74-324; D, SEI 74-681; E, SEI 74-679. B–E same eye from patient with polycythemia vera.

Fig. 11–17. AFIP Neg. 61-3075.

Fig. 11–18. Main figure, SEI 74-506; inset 1, SEI 74-903; inset 2, SEI 74-845.

Fig. 11–19. SEI 74-566.

Fig. 11–20. Main figure, SEI 74-559; inset, SEI 74-560.

Fig. 11–21. A, SEI 74-562; B, SEI 74-561.

Fig. 11–22. SEI 74-563.

Fig. 11–23. A, AFIP Neg. 67-1691; B, AFIP Neg. 67-143, C, AFIP Neg. 61-3074; D, AFIP Neg. 66-505.

Fig. 11–24. A and B courtesy of Dr. B. W. Streeten.

Fig. 11–25. A, SEI 74-5; B, SEI 74-4; inset 1, SEI 74-884; inset 2, SEI 74-885; C, SEI 74-3; D, SEI 74-1. All from Eagle RC, et al.: Arch Ophthalmol 92:28, 1974.

Fig. 11–26. AFIP Neg. 58-13199-3. From Fine BS: Lab Invest 11 (pt. 2):1161, 1962.

Fig. 11–27. SEI 74-314.

Fig. 11–28. AFIP Neg. 65-2836.

Fig. 11–29. A, SEI 73-688; B, SEI 73-689.

Fig. 11–30. A, AFIP Neg. 61-3948; B, AFIP Neg. 61-3946. C from Yanoff M, Tsou K-C: Am J Ophthalmol 60:311, 1965.

Fig. 11–32. A, AFIP Neg. 63-2326; B, AFIP Neg. 63-2325; C, SEI 74-312. C courtesy of Dr. R. Y. Foos.

Fig. 11–33. AFIP Neg. 61-3945. From Fine BS: *In* New and Controversial Aspects of Retinal Detachment.

Edited by A McPherson. New York, Harper & Row, 1968.

Fig. 11–34. A, AFIP Neg. 63-2323; B, SEI 74-738; C, SEI 74-737.

Fig. 11–35. A, AFIP Neg. 73-3704. A courtesy of Dr. M. O. M. Tso.

Fig. 11–36. A, SEI 74-370; inset 1, SEI 74-470; inset 2, SEI 74-400; B, SEI 74-371.

Fig. 11–37. SEI 74-664.

Fig. 11–38. A, AFIP Neg. 64-5771; B, SEI 74-661; C, SEI 74-660.

Fig. 11–40. A, SEI 73-886; B, SEI 73-887; C, SEI 73-888.

Fig. 11–41. A, SEI 74-833; B, SEI 74-839; C, SEI 74-521.

Fig. 11–42. From Gass JDM: Am J Ophthalmol 63:573, 1967.

Fig. 11–43. A, SEI 74-760; inset, SEI 74-761; B, SEI 74-759. Courtesy of Dr. D. G. Cogan.

Fig. 11–44. A, SEI 74-545; B, SEI 74-524; C, SEI 74-491; D, SEI 74-481. A, B and C courtesy of Dr. W. C. Frayer. Case depicted in A, B and C reported by Frayer WC: Arch Ophthalmol 53:82, 1955.

Fig. 11–45. A, AFIP Neg. 61-10840-1; B, AFIP Neg. 73-12393; C, AFIP Neg. 73-12392; D, AFIP Neg. 73-12390.

Fig. 11–46. From Klintworth GK, et al.: Arch Ophthalmol 90:45, 1973.

Fig. 11–47. Inset A, AFIP Neg. 70-11112. From Ramsey MS, Fine BS: Am J Ophthalmol 73:229, 1972.

Fig. 11–48. A, AFIP Neg. 66-9564; inset, Derm No. 7228. B, AFIP Neg. 66-9570. C, AFIP Neg. 66-9567. D, SEI 74-667. E, SEI 74-668; inset, SEI 74-898. F, SEI 74-669. G, SEI 74-671; inset, SEI 74-897. H, SEI 74-672; inset, SEI 74-896. I, AFIP Neg. 66-9563; inset, SEI 74-905. Modified from Yanoff M, et al.: Arch Ophthalmol 79:49, 1968.

Fig. 11–49. A, SEI 74-376; B, SEI 74-379; C, SEI 74-373; D, SEI 74-372; inset, SEI 74-841; E, SEI 74-572; F, SEI 74-577; G, SEI 74-574; H, SEI 74-575; I, SEI 74-374, J, SEI 74-576.

Fig. 11–50. A, SEI 74-348; inset 1, SEI 73-619; inset 2, SEI 73-620; B, SEI 74-350.

Fig. 11–51. A, SEI 74-662; inset, SEI 73-128. B, SEI 74-663; inset, SEI 73-995. Histology courtesy of Dr. D. G. Cogan.

Fig. 11–52. A, SEI 74-332; inset, SEI 74-457; B, SEI 74-335; C, SEI 74-498; D, SEI 74-497.

Fig. 11–53. A, AFIP Neg. 74-6726; B, AFIP Neg. 74-6722; F, AFIP Neg. 67-11221; G, AFIP Neg. 68-5139.

Fig. 11–54. From Robb RM, Kuwabara T: Invest Ophthalmol 12:366, 1973.

Fig. 11–55. A, AFIP Neg. 64-5265; B, AFIP Neg. 64-5279; C, AFIP Neg. 64-5278. From Yanoff M, Schwarz GA: Trans Am Acad Ophthalmol Otolaryngol 69:701, 1965.

Fig. 11–56. SEI 74-682.

Fig. 11–57. A, SEI 74-315; inset, SEI 74-320; B, AFIP Neg. 71-9580.

Fig. 11–58. Courtesy of Dr. R. Machemer.

Fig. 11–59. SEI 74-517.

Fig. 11–60. A, AFIP Neg. 65-3113; B, AFIP Neg. 70-6718; C, AFIP Neg. 70-6719; D, AFIP Neg. 70-6143; E, AFIP Neg. 70-6312; F, AFIP Neg. 70-6294; G, AFIP Neg. 70-6146; H, AFIP Neg. 70-6305. From Yanoff M, et al.: Int Ophthalmol Clin 11:211, 1971.

Fig. 11–61. Inset 1, AFIP Neg. 65-230; inset 2, AFIP Neg. 65-7007.

Fig. 11–62. A, SEI 74-479; B, SEI 74-480.

Fig. 11–63. **A,** SEI 74-338; **inset,** SEI 73-592. **B,** SEI 74-773; **inset,** SEI 74-830.
Fig. 11–64. SEI 74-339.
Fig. 11–65. SEI 74-772.
Fig. 11–66. **A,** SEI 74-10; **B,** SEI 74-126.
Fig. 11–67. **C,** AFIP Neg. 74-6718; **inset in D,** AFIP Neg. 74-6721; **inset in E,** AFIP Neg. 74-6723. All modified from Streeten BW: Am J Ophthalmol 74:1201, 1972.
Fig. 11–68. **A,** AFIP Neg. 62-6119; **B,** AFIP Neg. 62-6741; **C,** AFIP Neg. 62-6737; **D,** AFIP Neg. 63-23. From Meyer E, Kurz GH: Arch Ophthalmol 70:640, 1963.
Fig. 11–69. **Main figure,** SEI 74-564; **inset,** SEI 73-615.
Fig. 11–70. **Main figure,** SEI 74-489; **inset,** SEI 73-616.
Fig. 11–71. SEI 74-327.
Fig. 11–72. **A,** SEI 74-340; **B,** SEI 74-342; **inset,** SEI 73-613.
Fig. 11–73. **A,** SEI 73-147; **B,** SEI 73-146.

CHAPTER 12

Fig. 12–1. AFIP Neg. 73-10959.
Fig. 12–2. **A,** SEI 74-889; **B,** SEI 74-888; **C,** SEI 74-658.
Fig. 12–3. **Main figure,** SEI 74-724; **inset,** AFIP Neg. 71-7272-2.
Fig. 12–4. AFIP Neg. 61-6384.
Fig. 12–5. **A,** AFIP Neg. 70-4564; **inset,** AFIP Neg. 70-4565.
Fig. 12–6. **A,** SEI 74-867; **B,** SEI 74-910. **B** courtesy of Dr. H. G. Scheie.
Fig. 12–7. **A,** AFIP Neg. 53-10592; **B, AFIP** Neg. 59-3208; **C,** AFIP Neg. 59-3208. **A-C** from Rodman HI, et al.: Arch Ophthalmol 66:552, 1961, **D** from March W, et al.: Invest Ophthalmol 13:701, 1974.
Fig. 12–8. **Main figure,** SEI 74-725; **inset,** SEI 72-229.
Fig. 12–9. SEI 74-831.
Fig. 12–10. SEI 74-734.
Fig. 12–11. SEI 74-1034.
Fig. 12–12. **A,** SEI 74-530; **B,** SEI 74-343.
Fig. 12–13. **A,** SEI 73-1031; **B,** SEI 73-1032; **C,** SEI 73-1033; **D,** SEI 73-1034. **A–D** and **inset** courtesy of Dr. J. D. M. Gass.
Fig. 12–14. AFIP Neg. 74-4881.
Fig. 12–15. **A,** AFIP Neg. 74-4882; **B,** AFIP Neg. 74-4883.
Fig. 12–16. AFIP Neg. 67-143.
Fig. 12–17. Derm No. 8107. From Yanoff M: Am J Ophthalmol 67:21, 1969.

CHAPTER 13

Fig. 13–1. **A,** SEI 74-692; **B,** SEI 74-689. Case reported by Yanoff M, Rorke LB: Am J Ophthalmol 75:1036, 1973.
Fig. 13–2. **Main figure,** AFIP Neg. 62-2328; **inset 2,** AFIP Neg. 54-26330. **Main figure** from Ferry AP: Arch Ophthalmol 70:346, 1963. **Inset** 2 modified from Grear JN: Arch Ophthalmol 28:467, 1942 and from Hogan MJ, Zimmerman LE (eds): Ophthalmic Pathology: An Atlas and Textbook (2nd ed). Philadelphia, Saunders, 1962.
Fig. 13–3. **A,** AFIP Neg. 67-183-3; **B,** AFIP Neg. 68-3044; **C,** AFIP Neg. 67-5196. From Willis R, et al.: Arch Ophthalmol 88:139, 1972.
Fig. 13–4. **A,** SEI 73-434; **inset,** SEI 74-857; **B,** SEI 73-436; **C,** SEI 73-435.
Fig. 13–5. **A,** SEI 74-727; **inset,** SEI 74-893; **B,** SEI 74-728.

Fig. 13–6. SEI 73-68.
Fig. 13–7. SEI 74-726.
Fig. 13–8. AFIP Neg. 73-6971.
Fig. 13–9. SEI 73-546. Courtesy of Dr. S. Brownstein. Case reported by Brownstein S, Jannotta FS: Can J Ophthalmol 9:372, 1974.
Fig. 13–10. **A,** SEI 73-1057; **B,** SEI 73-1059; **inset,** SEI 73-1058. Courtesy of Dr. T. R. Hedges, Jr.
Fig. 13–11. From Henkind P, et al.: Am J Ophthalmol 69:78, 1970.
Fig. 13–12. **A,** SEI 74-1037; **B,** SEI 74-1038; **C,** SEI 74-1039; **D,** SEI 74-1036; **E,** SEI 74-1040. Courtesy of Dr. L. B. Rorke.
Fig. 13–13. **A,** SEI 74-950; **B,** SEI 74-947; **C,** SEI 74-951; **D,** SEI 74-952. Courtesy of Dr. L. B. Rorke.
Fig. 13–14. **A,** SEI 74-380; **B,** SEI 74-386; **C,** SEI 74-382.
Fig. 13–15. **A,** SEI 74-1030; **B,** SEI 74-1033. Courtesy of Dr. L. B. Rorke.
Fig. 13–16. **A,** SEI 74-987; **B,** SEI 74-954; **C,** SEI 74-955. Courtesy of Dr. L. B. Rorke.
Fig. 13–17. **A,** SEI 74-825; **B,** SEI 74-696; **C,** SEI 74-697; **D,** SEI 74-1017.
Fig. 13–18. **A,** Derm No. 7310. **A** to **E** from Rahn EK, et al.: Am J Ophthalmol 66:1143, 1968.
Fig. 13–19. **A,** SEI 74-731; **B,** SEI 74-730; **inset,** SEI 74-859.
Fig. 13–20. **A,** SEI 74-1018; **B,** SEI 74-1019; **C,** SEI 74-477; **D,** SEI 74-476.
Fig. 13–21. **A,** SEI 74-345; **B,** SEI 74-222; **C,** SEI 74-223; **D,** SEI 74-221; **E,** SEI 74-220; **F,** SEI 74-219; **G,** SEI 74-218; **H,** SEI 74-214; **inset,** SEI 74-216.
Fig. 13–22. **A,** AFIP Neg. 70-5810; **B,** AFIP Neg. 71-4680; **C,** AFIP Neg. 70-5823; **D,** AFIP Neg. 71-4678; **E,** AFIP Neg. 71-4675. From Karp LA, et al.: Arch Ophthalmol 91:24, 1974.
Fig. 13–23. SEI 74-285.
Fig. 13–24. **A,** SEI 74-808; **inset,** SEI 73-423; **B,** SEI 74-807; **C,** SEI 74-809; **inset,** SEI 74-858.
Fig. 13–25. **A,** SEI 73-683; **B,** SEI 73-682.
Fig. 13–26. **A,** SEI 73-143; **B,** AFIP Neg. 67-4573.
Fig. 13–27. SEI 73-139.
Fig. 13–28. **A,** AFIP Neg. 65-1302. From Zimmerman LE, Fine BS: Arch Ophthalmol 74:394, 1965.

CHAPTER 14

Fig. 14–1. Derm No. 8926-23. From Yanoff M, et al.: Am J Ophthalmol 70:391, 1970.
Fig. 14–2. **A,** SEI 74-619; **B,** SEI 74-284.
Fig. 14–3. **Main figure,** SEI 74-172; **inset,** SEI 74-912.
Fig. 14–4. **A,** SEI 73-220; **B,** SEI 73-221; **C,** SEI 73-222. All courtesy of Dr. H. Ring.
Fig. 14–5. SEI 74-551.
Fig. 14–6. **A,** AFIP Neg. 65-7170-B; **B,** AFIP Neg. 65-7175-B; **C,** AFIP Neg. 65-7169-B. From Font RL, et al.: Am J Clin Pathol 48:365, 1967.
Fig. 14–7. **Main figure,** SEI 73-340. Case reported by Streeten BW, et al.: Am J Ophthalmol 77:750, 1974.
Fig. 14–8. **A, C** and **D** from Kroll AJ, Kuwabara T: Arch Ophthalmol 76:244, 1966. **B** courtesy of Dr. A. J. Kroll.
Fig. 14–9. **A,** AFIP Neg. 64-6604; **B,** AFIP Neg. 64-6605; **C,** AFIP Neg. 64-6606. From Yanoff M: Med Ann DC 34:319, 1965.
Fig. 14–10. **A,** SEI 74-247; **B,** SEI 74-248. Courtesy of Dr. L. B. Rorke.

Fig. 14–11. **1,** SEI 74-878; **2,** SEI 74-877; **3,** SEI 74-876; **4,** SEI 74-875.

Fig. 14–12. SEI 74-510.

Fig. 14–13. **A,** AFIP Neg. 64-831; **B,** AFIP Neg. 64-830; **C,** AFIP Neg. 64-990; **D,** AFIP Neg. 64-5061; **E,** AFIP Neg. 61-3169. From Ferry AP: Survey Ophthalmol 10:434, 1965.

Fig. 14–14. **A,** SEI 74-687; **inset 1,** SEI 74-78; **inset 2,** SEI 74-75; **B,** SEI 74-688.

Fig. 14–15. **Main figure,** SEI 73-208; **inset,** SEI 73-208. Courtesy of Dr. D. H. Nicholson.

Fig. 14–16. **A,** SEI 74-280; **B,** SEI 74-281.

Fig. 14–17. **A,** SEI 73-961; **inset,** SEI 74-895; **B,** SEI 73-1082.

Fig. 14–18. **Main figure,** SEI 73-928; **inset 1,** SEI 74-37; **inset 2,** SEI 74-38. **Insets 1** and **2** courtesy of Dr. H. G. Scheie.

Fig. 14–19. **Main figure,** SEI 74-144; **inset,** SEI 74-79.

Fig. 14–20. **A,** SEI 74-788; **B,** SEI 74-780.

Fig. 14–21. **A,** SEI 74-932; **B,** SEI 74-934. Courtesy of Dr. H. T. Enterline.

Fig. 14–22. **A,** SEI 73-1035; **B,** SEI 73-1037. Courtesy of Dr. J. B. Crawford.

Fig. 14–23. SEI 74-815. Courtesy of Dr. J. Myers.

Fig. 14–24. **D,** SEI 74-941; **E,** SEI 74-942. **A** and **C** from Enterline HT, et al.: Cancer 13:932, 1960. **B** courtesy of Dr. H. T. Enterline. **D** and **E** courtesy of Dr. A. J. Steinberg.

Fig. 14–25. **A,** AFIP Neg. 65-2047; **B,** AFIP Neg. 65-1492; **C,** AFIP Neg. 65-1497; **D,** AFIP Neg. 65-1491. From Font RL, Zimmerman LE: Arch Ophthalmol 75:475, 1966.

Fig. 14–26. **A,** SEI 74-282; **B,** SEI 74-283.

Fig. 14–27. **A,** SEI 74-784; **inset,** SEI 74-923; **B,** SEI 74-787; **C,** SEI 74-786.

Fig. 14–28. **A,** Derm No. 6482-5; **inset 1,** SEI 74-913; **inset 2,** SEI 74-914; **B,** Derm No. 6482-9; **C,** Derm No. 6482-4; **D,** Derm No. 6482-11. **A–D** from Yanoff M, Scheie HG: Cancer 19:1711, 1966.

Fig. 14–29. **A,** SEI 74-549; **B,** SEI 74-550; **C,** SEI 74-552.

Fig. 14–30. SEI 74-533.

Fig. 14–31. **A,** SEI 74-756; **inset,** SEI 74-95; **inset 1,** SEI 74-408; **inset 2,** SEI 74-409; **C,** SEI 74-982.

Fig. 14–32. **Main figure,** AFIP Neg. 61-3782; **inset,** SEI 74-983. **Main figure** from Porterfield JF, Zimmerman LE: Virchows Arch [Pathol Anat] 335:329, 1962.

Fig. 14–33. From Kroll AJ, et al.: Invest Ophthalmol 2:523, 1963.

Fig. 14–34. **A,** SEI 74-1054; **B,** SEI 74-1053; **C,** SEI 74-1058; **D,** SEI 74-1061.

Fig. 14–35. **A,** SEI 74-762; **B,** SEI 74-763. Courtesy of Dr. J. D. M. Gass.

Fig. 14–36. **A,** SEI 74-508; **B,** SEI 74-509. Courtesy of Dr. J. R. Wolter.

Fig. 14–37. SEI 73-217.

Fig. 14–38. **A,** SEI 74-289; **B,** SEI 74-288; **C,** SEI 74-30.

Fig. 14–39. **A,** SEI 74-1041; **inset,** SEI 74-1043; **B,** SEI 74-1045; **C,** SEI 74-1049.

Fig. 14–40. **A,** SEI 74-929; **B,** SEI 74-931; **C,** SEI 74-930. Courtesy of Dr. H. T. Enterline.

Fig. 14–41. **A,** SEI 74-514; **inset 1,** SEI 74-915; **inset 2,** SEI 74-890; **B,** SEI 74-512; **C,** SEI 74-513; **D,** SEI 74-515; **E,** AFIP Neg. 73-12397; **F,** AFIP Neg. 73-12398; **G,** AFIP Neg. 73-12399.

Fig. 14–42. **A,** AFIP Neg. 61-5871; **B,** AFIP Neg. 61-5844. From Zimmerman LE, et al.: Int Ophthalmol Clin 2:337, 1962.

Fig. 14–43. **A,** SEI 74-275; **B,** SEI 74-276; **C,** SEI 74-277; **D,** SEI 74-279.

Fig. 14–44. **A,** SEI 73-151; **inset,** SEI 74-403; **B,** SEI 73-152.

Fig. 14–45. **Main figure,** SEI 74-154; **inset,** SEI 74-155. Courtesy of Dr. W. R. Lee.

Fig. 14–46. **A,** SEI 74-7; **B,** SEI 74-156. Courtesy of Dr. L. E. Zimmerman. Case illustrated by Hogan MJ, Zimmerman LE (eds): Ophthalmic Pathology: An Atlas and Textbook. Philadelphia, Saunders, 1962.

Fig. 14–47. **A,** SEI 74-1029; **inset,** SEI 73-305; **B,** SEI 74-750; **C,** SEI 74-713; **D,** SEI 74-1027.

Fig. 14–48. **1,** SEI 74-464; **2,** SEI 74-465; **3,** SEI 74-466; **4,** SEI 74-467; **5,** SEI 74-1028; **6,** SEI 74-1025.

Fig. 14–49. **A,** Derm No. 8674-1; **inset,** SEI 74-919; **B,** Derm No. 8674-4. From Yanoff M, et al.: Ophthalmol Res 1:245, 1970.

Fig. 14–50. **A,** SEI 74-748; **inset 1,** SEI 74-832; **inset 2,** SEI 74-838; **B,** SEI 74-750.

Fig. 14–51. **Inset,** SEI 74-837. From Yanoff M, Scheie HG: Survey Ophthalmol 12:133, 1967.

Fig. 14–52. **A,** SEI 74-751; **B,** SEI 74-753; **C,** SEI 74-755; **D,** SEI 74-754.

Fig. 14–53. **A,** SEI 74-769; **B,** SEI 74-767; **C,** SEI 74-768; **D,** SEI 74-771. Courtesy of Dr. T. R. Hedges and Dr. J. P. Decker.

Fig. 14–54. **A,** AFIP Neg. 68-7157-5; **B,** AFIP Neg. 69-4179; **C,** AFIP Neg. 69-4178. From Karp LA, et al.: Arch Ophthalmol 85:295, 1971.

Fig. 14–55. **A,** SEI 74-792; **inset 1,** SEI 74-922; **inset 2,** SEI 74-892; **B,** SEI 74-791; **C,** SEI 74-793. Case reported by Brooks HW, et al.: Arch Otolaryngol 100:304, 1974.

Fig. 14–56. **A,** SEI 74-1000; **inset,** SEI 74-977; **B,** SEI 74-1001. Courtesy of Dr. S. J. Ryan.

CHAPTER 15

Fig. 15–1. **A,** AFIP Neg. 69-2110; **B,** AFIP Neg. 69-3732-1. **A** modified from Fine BS, et al.: Arch Ophthalmol 69:197, 1970. **B** and **C** modified from Yanoff M, et al.: Arch Ophthalmol 69:201, 1970.

Fig. 15–2. **Inset 2,** AFIP Neg. 70-11415.

Fig. 15–3. **A,** SEI 74-844; **B,** Derm No. 8194-1; **C,** Derm No. 8107–10; **inset 1,** SEI 74-921; **inset 2,** SEI 74-920. **B** and **C** from Yanoff M: Am J Ophthalmol 67:21, 1969. **Insets 1** and **2** courtesy of Dr. H. G. Scheie.

Fig. 15–6. **Inset,** AFIP Neg. 71-7387.

Fig. 15–7. **A,** Derm No. 8194-2; **B,** Derm No. 8194-3. From Yanoff M: Am J Ophthalmol 67:21, 1969.

Fig. 15–8. SEI 74-716.

Fig. 15–9. SEI 74-718.

Fig. 15–10. **A,** SEI 74-719; **B,** SEI 74-717; **C,** SEI 74-720.

Fig. 15–11. **B,** SEI 74-989.

Fig. 15–12. **A,** SEI 74-503; **inset 1,** SEI 74-504; **inset 2,** SEI 74-869; **B,** SEI 74-502; **inset,** SEI 74-505.

Fig. 15–13. **Main figure,** SEI 74-722; **inset,** SEI 74-873.

Fig. 15–15. **A,** AFIP Neg. 65-6483; **inset,** SEI 74-872; **B,** AFIP Neg. 64-5767; **C,** SEI 74-816.

Fig. 15–16. **A,** Derm No. 8107; **B,** Derm No. 8107; **inset,** SEI 74-864. From Yanoff M: Am J Ophthalmol 67:21, 1969.

Fig. 15–17. **Inset,** SEI 73-419.

Fig. 15–18. B, SEI 74-1004.

Fig. 15–19. Main figure, Derm No. 8107-3; **inset 1,** SEI 73-421; **inset 2,** SEI 74-871. **Main figure** from Yanoff M: Am J Ophthalmol 67:21, 1969.

Fig. 15–20. Main figure, Derm No. 8107-4; **inset,** SEI 74-874. **Main figure** from Yanoff M: Am J Ophthalmol 67:21, 1969.

Fig. 15–21. Main figure, Derm No. 8107-5; **inset,** SEI 74-865. **Main figure** from Yanoff M: Am J Ophthalmol 67:21, 1969.

Fig. 15–23. A, SEI 74-994; **inset,** SEI 74-870; **B,** SEI 74-990; **C,** SEI 74-991. **A** courtesy of Dr. S. de Buen. **B** and **C** from Yanoff M: Am J Ophthalmol 67:21, 1969.

Fig. 15–24. A, SEI 74-723; **B,** SEI 74-993; **inset,** SEI 74-866. **A** and **B** courtesy of Dr. S. de Buen.

Fig. 15–25. A, SEI 74-814; **B,** SEI 74-978; **C,** SEI 74-979.

Fig. 15–26. A, Derm No. 8107; **B,** Derm No. 8107; **inset 1,** SEI 74-883; **inset 2,** SEI 74-868. **B** from Yanoff M: Am J Ophthalmol 67:21, 1969.

Fig. 15–27. A, SEI 74-985; **inset 1,** SEI 74-882; **inset 2,** SEI 74-881; **B,** SEI 74-986.

**Fig. 15–28. Derm No. 8194-5. Modified from Yanoff M: Am J Ophthalmol 67:21, 1969.

CHAPTER 16

Fig. 16–1. A, SEI 74-799; **B,** SEI 74-733; **C,** SEI 74-800; **D,** SEI 74-801.

Fig. 16–2. Main figure, SEI 74-806; **inset,** SEI 74-829. **Inset** courtesy of Dr. H. G. Scheie.

**Fig. 16–3. SEI 74-529.

Fig. 16–4. Main figure, SEI 74-804; **inset 1,** SEI 74-803; **inset 2,** SEI 74-828; **inset 3,** SEI 74-827.

Fig. 16–5. Main figure, SEI 74-12; **inset,** SEI 74-77.

Fig. 16–6. Main figure, SEI 73-87; **inset 1,** SEI 73-88; **inset 2,** SEI 73-87.

Fig. 16–7. A, SEI 73-432; **inset,** SEI 74-826; **B,** SEI 73-431.

**Fig. 16–8. AFIP Neg. 74-4880.

Fig. 16–9. A, AFIP Neg. 65-13106; **inset,** AFIP Neg. 67-6959; **B,** AFIP Neg. 65-6480; **inset,** AFIP Neg. 65-6482; **C,** AFIP Neg. 67-6972. Courtesy of Dr. A. E. Maumenee.

Fig. 16–10. A, AFIP Neg. 64-2273; **inset,** AFIP Neg. 64-2665; **B,** AFIP Neg. 64-2274. Courtesy of Dr. L. C. Moss.

Fig. 16–11. Inset 1, AFIP Neg. 73-962; **inset 2,** AFIP Neg. 73-1179. Courtesy of Dr. H. G. Scheie.

Fig. 16–12. A, SEI 73-429; **B,** SEI 73-430; **C,** SEI 73-672.

Fig. 16–13. A, AFIP Neg. 58-952-1; **inset 1,** SEI 74-907; **inset 2,** SEI 74-906; **B,** SEI 74-998; **C,** SEI 74-999; **inset,** SEI 74-908; **D,** SEI 74-997. **Insets 1** and **2** in **A** courtesy of Dr. H. G. Scheie. **Inset** in **C** courtesy of Dr. G. Naumann.

Fig. 16–14. A, SEI 73-679; **B,** SEI 73-681; **inset 1,** SEI 74-909; **inset 2,** SEI 74-899; **C,** SEI 73-680. **Insets 1** and **2** courtesy of Dr. G. Naumann.

Fig. 16–15. A, SEI 74-1003; **B,** SEI 74-1002.

**Fig. 16–16. SEI 73-969.

Fig. 16–17. A, SEI 73-441; **inset,** SEI 74-904; **B,** SEI 73-442.

Fig. 16–18. A, Derm No. 8926-25; **B,** Derm No. 9001-3; **C,** Derm No. 8926-15; **D,** Derm No. 8926-17; **E,** Derm No. 9113-2. From Yanoff M: Am J Ophthalmol 70:898, 1970.

Fig. 16–19. A, SEI 74-797; **inset 1,** SEI 74-917; **inset 2,** SEI 74-798; **B,** SEI 74-795; **inset,** SEI 74-794.

Fig. 16–20. A, SEI 74-880; **B,** SEI 74-846; **C,** AFIP Neg. 74-3370; **inset,** SEI 74-73. **A** courtesy of Dr. H. G. Scheie.

Fig. 16–21. Inset 3 in **A,** AFIP Neg. 73-2588; **inset 2** in **C,** AFIP Neg. 73-3712; **inset 3** in **C,** AFIP Neg. 73-5134. All except **main figure** in **C** from Fine BS, et al.: Trans Am Acad Opthalmol Otolaryngol 78:314, 1974.

Fig. 16–22. A, Derm No. 8926-26; **B,** Derm No. 8926-12; **C,** Derm No. 8926-28. From Yanoff M: Am J Ophthalmol 70:898, 1970.

Fig. 16–23. A, Derm No. 8926–29; **inset,** SEI 74-694; **B,** Derm No. 8926-17; **C,** Derm No. 8926-18. From Yanoff M, Scheie HG: Arch Ophthalmol 84:471, 1970.

Fig. 16–24. A, SEI 73-521; **B,** SEI 73-873; **C,** SEI 73-965; **D,** SEI 73-871.

Fig. 16–25. Main figure, SEI 73-757; **inset,** SEI 73-758.

Fig. 16–26. Main figure, SEI 74-732; **inset,** SEI 74-847.

**Fig. 16–27. SEI 73-472.

Fig. 16–28. Main figure, SEI 73-470; **inset,** SEI 73-403.

CHAPTER 17

Fig. 17–1. A, Derm No. 9778-44; **B,** Derm No. 9778-42; **C,** SEI 73-182; **inset,** SEI 74-918.

**Fig. 17–2. SEI 74-705.

**Fig. 17–3. Derm No. 9778-34.

Fig. 17–4. A, SEI 73-224; **B,** SEI 74-703; **inset,** SEI 74-704.

Fig. 17–5. A, SEI 74-628; **B,** SEI 74-629; **C,** SEI 74-630; **D,** SEI 74-631.

Fig. 17–6. A, Derm No. 9778-36; **B,** Derm No. 9778-39.

Fig. 17–7. Main figure, Derm No. 9778-27; **inset,** Derm No. 9778-28.

Fig. 17–8. A, AFIP Neg. 57-17020; **B,** AFIP Neg. 59-6074; **C,** AFIP Neg. 57-8750; **D,** Derm No. 9778-33. **A–C** from Zimmerman LE: Invest Ophthalmol 4:11, 1965. **D** courtesy of Dr. S. de Buen.

Fig. 17–9. A, SEI 73-60; **inset,** SEI 73-240; **B,** SEI 73-58; **inset 1,** SEI 73-57; **inset 2,** SEI 73-239; **C,** SEI 73-5; **inset,** SEI 73-238; **D,** SEI 73-6; **inset,** SEI 73-237; **E,** SEI 73-43. Case to be reported by R. C. Lanciano, Jr. and S. Bresalier.

Fig. 17–10. A, Derm No. 9778-37; **B,** Derm No. 9778-38.

**Fig. 17–11. Derm No. 9778-45.

**Fig. 17–12. SEI 74-695.

**Fig. 17–13. Derm No. 9778-46.

Fig. 17–14. Main figure, Derm No. 9778-30; **inset,** SEI 73-989.

Fig. 17–15. A, Derm No. 9778-32; **inset,** SEI 73-991; **B,** SEI 73-823; **inset 1,** SEI 73-756; **inset 2,** SEI 73-992; **C,** Derm No. 9778-53; **D,** Derm No. 9778-54.

Fig. 17–16. A, Derm No. 9778-55; **inset,** SEI 74-821; **B,** Derm No. 9778-56.

Fig. 17–17. A, Derm No. 9778-10; **B,** Derm No. 9778-18; **inset,** SEI 73-990. **Inset** courtesy of Dr. H. G. Scheie.

Fig. 17–18. A, SEI 74-683; **B,** SEI 74-684; **inset,** SEI 73-993. **Inset** courtesy of Dr. H. G. Scheie.

Fig. 17–19. A, Derm No. 8057-6; **inset,** Derm No. 8058; **B,** Derm No. 8057-5. **Inset** and **B** from Yanoff M: Arch Ophthalmol 81:151, 1969.

Fig. 17–20. A, AFIP Neg. 64-6619; **B,** AFIP Neg. 64-6615. From Yanoff M, Zimmerman LE: Arch Ophthalmol 74:302, 1965.

Fig. 17–21. A, AFIP Neg. 64-5769; **B,** AFIP Neg. 64-5770; **C,** Derm No. 9778-19; **D,** SEI 73-687; **E,** SEI 73-686.

Fig. 17–22. A, AFIP Neg. 74-3368.

Fig. 17–23.   A, AFIP Neg. 66-1282; **B,** AFIP Neg. 68-5140; **C,** AFIP Neg. 68-5141.

Fig. 17–24.   A, SEI 74-709; **B,** SEI 74-710; **inset,** SEI 74-711. Courtesy of Dr. E. Howes. Case reported by Vogel MH, et al.: Doc Ophthalmol 26:461, 1969.

Fig. 17–25.   Derm No. 9778-5.

Fig. 17–26.   SEI 73-17.

Fig. 17–27.   A, SEI 74-693. From Spencer WH, Jesbury DO: Arch Ophthalmol 89: 387, 1973.

Fig. 17–28.   A, SEI 74-1023; **B,** AFIP Neg. 70-9499; **C,** AFIP Neg. 70-8362. **A** courtesy of Dr. J. S. McGavic. **B** and **C** from Zimmerman LE: Am J Ophthalmol 72:1039, 1971.

Fig. 17–29. AFIP Neg. 70-8781. From Zimmerman LE: Am J Ophthalmol 72:1039, 1971.

Fig. 17–30.   A, SEI 73-61; **B,** AFIP Neg. 70-8775. **A** courtesy of Dr. B. W. Streeten. **B** from Zimmerman LE: Am J Ophthalmol 72:1039, 1971.

Fig. 17–31.   A, AFIP Neg. 71-6850; **B,** AFIP Neg. 69-9903. **A** and **B** from and **C** modified from Zimmerman LE, et al.: Cancer 30:817, 1972.

Fig. 17–32.   A, AFIP Neg. 61-5908-2; **B,** AFIP Neg. 61-3087; **C,** AFIP Neg. 61-3087; **D,** AFIP Neg. 61-3086; **E,** AFIP Neg. 61-6691; **inset 1,** SEI 73-983; **inset 2,** SEI 73-984. **A–C** from Kurz GH, Zimmerman LE: Int Ophthalmol Clin 2:441, 1962. **Insets 1** and **2** courtesy of Mr. T. H. Tomer.

Fig. 17–33.   A, AFIP Neg. 70-7096; **B,** AFIP Neg. 70-7091. From Font RL, et al.: Am J Ophthalmol 73:544, 1972.

Fig. 17–34.   A, SEI 73-945; **B,** SEI 73-946; **C,** SEI 73-947; **D,** SEI 73-948; **E,** SEI 73-949.

Fig. 17–35.   A, Derm No. 8926-27; **B,** Derm No. 9778-48.

Fig. 17–36.   Main figure, SEI 73-704; **inset,** SEI 73-1004.

Fig. 17–37.   Main figure, SEI 73-703.

Fig. 17–38.   A, Derm No. 9113-1; **B,** SEI 74-26. Modified from Scheie HG, Yanoff M: Arch Ophthalmol. In press.

Fig. 17–39.   A, AFIP Neg. 71-7379.

Fig. 17–40.   B, AFIP Neg. 73-6964.

Fig. 17–41.   AFIP Neg. 65-7044. From Naumann G, et al.: Arch Ophthalmol 76:784, 1966.

Fig. 17–42.   A, AFIP Neg. 65-2263-1; **B,** SEI 74-891. **A** from Naumann G, et al.: Arch Ophthalmol 76:784, 1966.

Fig. 17–43.   AFIP Neg. 65-2608. From Naumann G, et al.: Arch Ophthalmol 76:784, 1966.

Fig. 17–44.   A, AFIP Neg. 65-6910; **B,** AFIP Neg. 65-3151. From Naumann G, et al.: Arch Ophthalmol 76:784, 1966.

Fig. 17–45.   AFIP Neg. 65-6914. From Naumann G, et al.: Arch Ophthalmol 76:784, 1966.

Fig. 17–46.   A, AFIP Neg. 63-2245; **B,** AFIP Neg. 65-3980; **C,** AFIP Neg. 65-2610; **D,** AFIP Neg. 65-443. **A–C** from Naumann G, et al.: Arch Ophthalmol 76:784, 1966. **D** from Yanoff M, Zimmerman LE: Cancer 20:493, 1967.

Fig. 17–48.   A, AFIP Neg. 65-3148; **B,** AFIP Neg. 65-3149; **C,** AFIP Neg. 65-3159. From Naumann G, et al.: Arch Ophthalmol 76:784, 1966.

Fig. 17–49.   Main figure, AFIP Neg. 65-5944; **inset 1,** AFIP Neg. 65-3158; **inset 2,** AFIP Neg. 65-3158. From Naumann G, et al.: Am J Ophthalmol 62:914, 1966.

Fig. 17–50.   A, AFIP Neg. 65-6912; **B,** AFIP Neg. 65-3145. From Naumann G, et al.: Arch Ophthalmol 76:784, 1966.

Fig. 17–51.   1, SEI 73-978; **2,** SEI 74-855; **3,** SEI 73-1008; **4,** SEI 73-1006; **5,** SEI 73-1011; **6,** SEI 73-1012.

Fig. 17–52.   Main figure, Derm No. 9778-8; **inset 1,** SEI 73-1009; **inset 2,** SEI 73-1010; **inset 3,** SEI 73-999.

Fig. 17–53.   Derm No. 9778-20.

Fig. 17–54.   Main figure, SEI 74-735; **inset 1,** SEI 74-449; **inset 2,** SEI 74-72; **inset 3,** SEI 74-854.

Fig. 17–55.   A, Derm No. 9778-12; **B,** Derm No. 9778-13.

Fig. 17–56.   Main figure, SEI 74-746; **inset 1,** SEI 73-979; **inset 2,** SEI 73-980.

Fig. 17–57.   A, SEI 74-739; **inset,** SEI 73-977; **B,** SEI 74-743; **C,** SEI 74-742; **D,** SEI 74-745.

Fig. 17–58.   A, SEI 74-686; **inset 1,** SEI 73-417; **inset 2,** SEI 73-418; **B,** SEI 74-685.

Fig. 17–59.   Main figure, AFIP Neg. 62-2240; **inset 1,** AFIP Neg. 65-2241; **inset 2,** AFIP Neg. 65-2244.

Fig. 17–60.   Main figure, AFIP Neg. 65-3386; **inset 1,** AFIP Neg. 65-3382; **inset 2,** AFIP Neg. 65-3383.

Fig. 17–62.   A, AFIP Neg. 73-11443; **inset,** SEI 74-1011; **B,** SEI 74-1010.

Fig. 17–63.   Inset, SEI 74-1008; **B,** SEI 74-1007.

Fig. 17–65.   Derm No. 9778-57.

Fig. 17–66.   Inset, SEI 73-35; **B,** SEI 74-1005.

Fig. 17–67.   A, SEI 74-486; **B,** SEI 74-487.

Fig. 17–68.   AFIP Neg. 65-966. From Yanoff M, Zimmerman LE: Cancer 20:493, 1967.

Fig. 17–69.   Inset 1, AFIP Neg. 72-12985; **B,** AFIP Neg. 72-12987.

Fig. 17–70.   1, SEI 74-849; **2,** SEI 74-230; **3,** SEI 74-850; **4,** SEI 73-976; **5,** SEI 73-116; **6,** SEI 74-848; **7,** SEI 74-851; **8,** SEI 74-856; **9,** SEI 74-852.

Fig. 17–71.   A, SEI 74-736; **B,** Derm No. 9778-47; **inset,** SEI 74-853.

Fig. 17–72.   Derm No. 9778-22.

Fig. 17–73.   Inset in A, AFIP Neg. 73-1172; **inset in B,** AFIP Neg. 73-964.

Fig. 17–74.   AFIP Neg. 65-968. From Yanoff M, Zimmerman LE: Cancer 20:493, 1967.

Fig. 17–75.   Derm No. 9778-21.

Fig. 17–76.   Main figure, Derm No. 9778-23; **inset,** SEI 73-1007.

Fig. 17–77.   Inset 3, AFIP Neg. 72-12745. Modified from Font RL, et al.: Arch Ophthalmol 91:359, 1974.

Fig. 17–78.   A, AFIP Neg. 73-11445; **B,** AFIP Neg. 70-10435; **inset,** AFIP Neg. 71-7385; **E,** AFIP Neg. 73-11450. **B** and **D** from Wallow IHL, Tso MOM: Am J Ophthalmol 73:914, 1972.

Fig. 17–79.   A, Derm No. 9778-4; **B,** SEI 74-1021; **C,** AFIP Neg. 65-3155. **A** and **B** courtesy of Dr. P. J. G. Maris. **C** from Naumann G, et al.: Arch Ophthalmol 76:784, 1966.

CHAPTER 18

Fig. 18–1.   SEI 73-284.

Fig. 18–2.   A, AFIP Neg. 69-3354; **B,** AFIP Neg. 69-3351. From Tso MOM, et al.: Arch Pathol 88:664, 1969.

Fig. 18–3.   A, AFIP Neg. 68-7851; **inset,** SEI 74-916; **B,** AFIP Neg. 68-9466. **Inset** courtesy of Dr. D. B. Schaffer. **C** modified from Tso MOM, et al.: Am J Ophthalmol 69:339, 350, 1970.

Fig. 18–4.   A, AFIP Neg. 72-9777; **D,** AFIP Neg. 65-239.

Fig. 18–5.   A and **B,** AFIP Neg. 53-5706; **C,** AFIP Neg. 61-3515. From Boniuk M, Zimmerman LE: Int Ophthalmol Clin 2:525, 1962. **A** and **B** modified from Hogan MJ, Zimmerman LE (eds): Ophthalmic Pathology. An Atlas and Text (2nd ed). Philadelphia, Saunders, 1962.

Fig. 18–6.   **Main figure,** SEI 73-779; **inset 1,** SEI 74-834; **inset 2,** SEI 73-415.

Fig. 18–7.   **Main figure,** AFIP Neg. 65-240; **inset 1,** SEI 73-416; **inset 2,** SEI 74-818.

Fig. 18–8.   **A,** SEI 73-678; **inset,** SEI 74-925; **B,** SEI 74-1012. **Inset** courtesy of Dr. G. Naumann.

Fig. 18–9.   **A,** SEI 73-675; **inset,** SEI 74-817; **B,** SEI 73-677.

Fig. 18–10.   **Main figure,** SEI 74-534; **inset,** SEI 74-607.

Fig. 18–11.   SEI 74-1016.

Fig. 18–12.   **A,** AFIP Neg. 73-12379; **inset,** SEI 74-836; **B,** AFIP Neg. 73-12380; **C,** AFIP Neg. 73-12381. **Inset** courtesy of Dr. H. G. Scheie.

Fig. 18–13.   **A,** AFIP Neg. 67-5562; **B,** AFIP Neg. 67-4974; **C,** AFIP Neg. 67-10893; **inset,** AFIP Neg. 67-4770-1. From Font RL, et al.: Arch Ophthalmol 82:43, 1969.

Fig. 18–14.   **A,** SEI 74-774; **inset,** SEI 74-924; **B,** SEI 74-775; **inset,** SEI 74-927; **C,** SEI 74-779; **D,** SEI 74-780; **E,** SEI 74-776; **inset** SEI 74-835. Case shown in **A–E** reported by Tyner GS, Frayer WC: Arch Pathol 46:647, 1951. **Inset** in **E** courtesy of Dr. D. B. Schaffer.

Fig. 18–15.   **1,** SEI 74-887; **3,** SEI 74-886. **2** and **4–6** courtesy of Dr. A. J. Kroll.

Fig. 18–16.   **A,** SEI 73-3; **inset,** SEI 73-401; **B,** SEI 73-63; **C,** SEI 73-64.

Fig. 18–17.   From Townes PL, Roca PD: Am J Ophthalmol 76:797, 1973.

Fig. 18–18.   **A,** SEI 74-535; **inset 1,** SEI 74-911; **inset 2,** SEI 74-926; **inset 3,** SEI 74-819; **B,** SEI 74-254. **Inset 3** courtesy of Dr. E. K. Rahn.

Color Plate I.   **A,** AFIP Neg. 74-3375; **B,** AFIP Neg. 74-3376; **C,** AFIP Neg. 74-3380; **D,** AFIP Neg. 74-3381; **E,** AFIP Neg. 74-3379; **F,** AFIP Neg. 74-3374; **G,** AFIP Neg. 74-3378; **H,** AFIP Neg. 74-3377; **I,** AFIP Neg. 74-3383.

Color Plate II.   **A,** AFIP Neg. 66-6694; **B,** AFIP Neg. 66-6695; **C,** AFIP Neg. 66-6696; **D,** AFIP Neg. 71-9576; **E,** AFIP Neg. 71-9577; **F,** AFIP Neg. 63-4651; **G,** AFIP Neg. 63-4653; **H,** AFIP Neg. 61-2802.

Color Plate III.   **A,** AFIP Neg. 68-10005; **B,** AFIP Neg. 68-9997; **C,** AFIP Neg. 68-10004; **D,** AFIP Neg. 68-10000. **H** from Zimmerman LE: Trans Am Acad Ophthalmol Otolaryngol 69:412, 1965.

Index

[Handwritten annotations:]

Stains
PAS : hyalin, basem. membr.
          glycogen,
Orcein , ? : Elastic
Weigert |
Perl : iron
Ziehl-Nielsen : acidfast
                        leprosy(?)

Collagen   (?)
    width   240 A° (X-section) P.300
    periodic(640 A° (?)
    hydroxy proline }
    hydroxy lysine   } tropocollagen
            glycogen |

Amyloid :
    Metachromasia
    Dichroism
    Birefringence
    fine fibrillar pattern .

P. 89   India ink }
             muci carmin } : fungi
             Gomori
             PAS

P.91   Gridley for hyphae

2.670 alizarin stain : Ca

P. 294   Mason-Trichrome stain : collagen→
                                              blue

P.294   Congo-Red : Amyloid [fibrillar
                    P.478   (2M)
                                            birefring.
                                            dichroism
                                            polychromasia

P.294   Colloidal-iron : acid mucopolysacch.
                                              → blue
P.302 Alcean Blue }

P.580 : Diastase digests glycogen
          hyaluronidase " hyaluronic acid
          Elastase   ↓ Elastin

P.580 : Hale technic : for acid mucopoly-
                                        saccharide

P.580   oil-red-O : for fat
       celloidin (?)(H)

Cover and text designed by
Maria S. Karkucinski

Composition in linotype, Palatino, by
American Book–Stratford Press, Inc.
Photo-lithography by Murray Printing Co.

Harper and Row, Publishers

75 76 77 78 79 80 10 9 8 7 6 5 4 3 2 1

Neovascularization
rec List p. 602

Congen. glaucoma

1. aniridia, Axenfeld's Rieger
2. Peters
3. Phakomatoses
   Sturge-Weber
   Neurofibromatosis
4. Lowe's syndrome
5. Pierre-Robin
6. Rubella

Cataract — cat

Cornea — corn

glaucoma — glee club

iris — flower

Lowe's Syndrome : Sex linked rec. (♂)
congen. cat + glaucoma
+ renal (NH₃) ∴ acidosis

Miller's "

p.702 Norrie's " : deafness
mental b
Hem. retinal detachment (pseudoglioma)
sex-linked recessive

Blue Sclera: E.D.
Paget
Osteog. imperfecta
p.702 Incontinenti pigmenti
Myopic degeneration
staphyloma
Scleromalacia perforans

Angioid streaks:
E.D.
Pseud. elasticum
sickle cell
Paget's disease

hyper vitaminosis A → pseudotumor
papilledema

Gitter cells ...

causes of macular hole

1. u cystoid
2. trauma
3. pre retinal macular fibrosis
4. vitreous traction
5. myopia
6. solar (eclipse)
7. senile macular hole

Cause of u cystoid

1. CRV occl.
   Br. A. Occl.
2. Diabetes
3. Aphakia
4. Epinephrine
5. I.O. Inflammation
   R.P.
6. pars planitis
7. hypertension